The
Natural
Physician's
Healing
Therapies

UPDATED EDITION

MARK STENGLER, NMD
THE NATURAL PHYSICIAN™

Bottom Line Books
www.BottomLineSecrets.com

THE NATURAL PHYSICIAN'S HEALING THERAPIES, UPDATED
Mark Stengler, NMD

Bottom Line Books® Edition 2011
Published by arrangement with Prentice Hall Press, a member of Penguin Group (USA) Inc.

ISBN 0-88723-625-1

10 9 8 7 6 5 4 3 2 1

Bottom Line Books® is a registered trademark of Boardroom® Inc.
281 Tresser Blvd., Stamford, CT 06901
www.BottomLineSecrets.com

The Natural Physician™ is a trademark of Mark Stengler, NMD.

Bottom Line Books® is an imprint of Boardroom® Inc., publisher of print periodicals,
e-letters and books. We are dedicated to bringing you the best information from the
most knowledgeable sources in the world. Our goal is to help you gain greater wealth,
better health, more wisdom, extra time and increased happiness.

Printed in the United States of America

CONTENTS

FOREWORD
BY JAMES F. BALCH, MD   vii

THE NATURAL HEALTH
REVOLUTION   ix

ACKNOWLEDGMENTS   xi

THE NATURAL
HEALING THERAPIES

Acetyl-L-carnitine   1
Aconitum napellus   3
Acupressure   5
Agaricus blazei blazei   11
Aloe   12
Alpha GPC   16
Alpha Lipoic Acid (ALA)   16
Amino Acids   18
Andrographis   21
Antioxidants   22
Apis   29
Arginine   31
Arnica   33
Arsenicum album   34
Artichoke   37
Ashwagandha   38
Astragalus   41
Bach Flower Remedies   45
B-Complex Vitamins   47
Bee Pollen   54
Bilberry   56
Black Cohosh   60
Boswellia   64
Bromelain   66
Burdock   70
Butcher's Broom   72

Butterbur   73
Calcium   76
Calendula   81
Cantharis   83
Caralluma fimbriata   85
Carbo Vegetabilis   86
Carotenoids   87
Cascara Sagrada   90
Cat's Claw   91
Cayenne   93
Chamomile   96
Chlorella   101
Chromium   103
Cinnamon   106
Coenzyme Q10   109
Colloidal Silver   115
Cordyceps sinensis   116
Coriolus Versicolor   118
Cranberry   120
Dandelion   122
D-glucarate   125
DHEA   127
Echinacea   132
Elderberry   138
Enzymes   140
Essential Oils   147
Evening Primrose Oil   149
Exercise   152
Eyebright   156
Fat Reduction   158
Fermented Wheat Germ Extract   166
Ferrum Phosphoricum   168
Feverfew   170
Fiber   172
Fish Oil   179
Flaxseed   187

Food-Sensitivity Therapy 193
Garlic 199
Gelsemium 203
Gentian Root 205
Ginger Root 208
Ginkgo Biloba 212
Ginseng 219
Glandulars 227
Glucomannan 231
Glucosamine 233
Goldenseal 236
Green Tea 240
Guggul 244
Gymnema Sylvestre 246
Hawthorn 250
Horse Chestnut 253
Huperzine 255
Hyaluronic Acid 256
Hydrotherapy 258
Hypericum 263
Ignatia 265
Ipecacuanha 268
Ipriflavone 270
Iron 275
Juicing 281
Kava 284
Lachesis 288
L-carnitine 292
Ledum 296
Licorice Root 298
Lo Han 302
Lomatium 303
Lycopodium 305
Lysine 306
Maca 309
Magnesium 311
Maitake 315
Melatonin 316
Mental Imagery 320
Milk Thistle 322
MSM 326
Multivitamins 331
N-acetylcysteine 334
Nettle 336

Nux Vomica 340
Onion 343
Oregano 345
Passionflower 347
Peppermint 348
Phosphatidylserine 351
Phytonutrients 354
Pine Bark Extract 357
Pomegranate 362
Potassium 364
Prayer 367
Prebiotics 368
Probiotics 370
Progesterone 374
Propolis 379
Pulsatilla 383
Quercetin 388
Red Yeast Rice 391
Reishi 393
Resperate 394
Resveratrol 396
Rhodiola 397
Rhus Toxicodendron 399
Ribose 400
SAMe 403
Saw Palmetto 408
Schussler Cell Salts 412
Selenium 415
Sepia 418
Silicon 422
Sitz Bath 424
Soy 425
Spirulina 429
Stevia 432
St. John's Wort 433
Sulforaphane 437
Sulphur 439
Symphytum 442
Tea Tree Oil 444
Tocotrienols 447
Tryptophan and 5-HTP 448
Turmeric 450
Uva Ursi 454
Valerian 456

Vanadium 458
Vitamin A 460
Vitamin C 462
Vitamin D 468
Vitamin E 474
Vitamin K 480
Vitex 483
Water 488
Wheatgrass 491

Wormwood 492
Xylitol 494
Zinc 496

REFERENCES 500

QUICK CURE FINDER 501

INDEX 515

FOREWORD

I N THE INTRODUCTION to the book *Prescription for Nutritional Healing*, I described the human body as being composed of "millions of tiny little engines." Some of those engines, I went on to say, work in unison while some work independently. All of them are "on call" 24 hours a day.

What I might have added is this: From time to time, some of those tiny engines may need a bit of "fixing." To fix them correctly, you need the correct tools.

Now the tools have arrived, in this wonderfully detailed book, all described and explained by a naturopathic physician who uses those implements of healing with consummate skill every day. Mark Stengler, ND, has treated thousands of people with the natural healing therapies he describes in this book, and his success as a healing physician has won him the respect of peers as well as patients.

I realize, of course, that some people who look through the sections of this book may wonder what I mean by describing these therapies as "healing tools." After all, many of us, when we think "medicine," think first of drugs, surgical tools, and all the high-tech paraphernalia of the operating room. How often do we consider that acupressure, coenzyme Q10, or ginger root could be healing therapies? Did you ever stop to think that mental imagery, prayer, soy, or water could help you preserve or recover your health? Can these healing therapies really help to repair the myriad tiny engines that power your body?

My reply: absolutely.

In fact, in this book of 162 healing therapies, you'll find some of the oldest tools of healing that are known to humankind, alongside some of the newest that today's physicians are researching and exploring. Water, for example. For immunity, for mindpower, for energy, for alertness, for our daily nourishment, we depend on it. If you lack water, all the pharmaceuticals in the world will not be able to save you from the effects of dehydration. A battalion of surgeons wielding scalpels, lasers, X-rays, and cardiac monitors will not be able to rescue your organs from the effects of water depletion, nor can they restore cells that lose their most essential liquid components. Water is absolutely essential for all the engines of your body to work effectively.

Of course, now that I mention it, that may seem self-evident. But too often, the most obvious, natural, beneficial healing ingredients are neglected in favor of more complicated, and sometimes more harmful, modern implements of medical care. When was the last time a conventional medical doctor asked how many glasses of water you drink every day, or described to you the subtle effects of dehydration, or explained how substances like caffeine and caffeine-containing medicines can deplete your body of liquids?

Water is indeed a healing therapy, and an important one at that.

But if some of the therapies in this book seem obvious, others are challenging our foremost medical researchers and biochemists to understand more precisely and definitely how the tiny engines in your body actually work. Take coenzyme Q10—more commonly called CoQ10—as an example. Here's a chemical substance smaller than the eye can see, almost obscured by myriad other components that power our cells and organs, recently revealed to be one of the most important power sources within and around the human heart. As Mark Stengler says so vividly, "When a heart doesn't have enough CoQ10 for proper electronical conduction, it suffers as it starves—and the whole circulatory system pays the price."

As with all the other healing therapies described in this book, Dr. Mark goes on to describe exactly what we know to date about CoQ10, how much you can take, when, for what conditions, and all the ways this essential tool of body maintenance can assist every part of your circulatory system. It's truly another healing therapy. Though not so readily available as water, it's certainly just as important.

In addition to presenting us with an impressive array of healing therapies, this book performs another valuable service that speaks to the very essence of healing. It asks us to look outside the framework of conventional medicine for the assistance we need to maintain and improve our health. Too often, in the current healthcare environment, we begin to believe that physicians and surgeons can repair—or even replace—the body parts that go wrong, get infected, act up, or refuse to work.

To take this attitude is to deny the body's most basic need, which is for attention and maintenance. Fat reduction is just one of the healing therapies in this book that contributes to the maintenance process—so, too, are exercise, fiber, juicing, phytonutrients, and all the vitamins, from A to K. If you follow the guidelines that Mark Stengler provides, you are doing more than fixing or repairing the parts that don't work. You're actually ensuring that you get the longest life and best use from the only body you'll ever have.

Even to a longtime proponent of natural medicine and nutritional healing, as I am, this book offers interesting surprises and remarkable fascinations. It draws on the healing traditions of numerous civilizations from around the world, and also reports practical applications of the healing process that come directly from the journals of a practicing natural physician. Mark Stengler is to be applauded not only for his healing work but also for his persistent exploration of the real frontiers of natural medicine. With this book, we get a share of the knowledge offered by a truly dedicated healer who harmonizes the best of the art and science of healing.

James F. Balch, MD
Coauthor of *Prescription for Nutritional Healing*

THE NATURAL HEALTH REVOLUTION

THE ORIGINAL EDITION of *The Natural Physician's Healing Therapies* was published in 2001. Since then I have had hundreds of people tell me personally how they have benefited from the book. The book has been a great success with more than 350,000 copies sold. A lot has happened in the world of natural healing since then. Thousands of studies demonstrating the efficacy of numerous natural therapies have been released. In addition, I have found great success with several natural remedies in my clinical practice that were not available during the original edition of this book. I am excited to introduce more than 50 new natural healing remedies and therapies in this revised and expanded edition. As well previous therapies from the original edition have been revised and updated to reflect current research and understanding. This revised edition is a completely new book that will help readers achieve a new level of health.

Holistic or natural medicine continues to make inroads to mainstream medicine. Why? First, there are many safe and effective natural remedies and therapies. Millions of Americans have experienced the benefits of holistic medicine and the number of visits to holistic practitioners outnumbers that of conventional medical doctors. Also consumers are becoming more wary of the potential adverse effects of pharmaceutical agents. Third, the amount of scientific evidence for natural remedies is more than ample to convince the skeptical person of potential benefits. Also our healthcare system is bankrupt. Studies show that preventative and safer natural remedies would save many billions of dollars each year in healthcare costs. Lastly, conventional medical schools are starting to offer courses in holistic medicine due to consumer demand. Additionally, the healing professions of naturopathic medicine, chiropractic, Chinese medicine, and other natural healing professions continue to grow.

It is my opinion, and gaining acceptance among other doctors, that preventative and holistic medicine is essential for improving healthcare in America. For example, 51% of Americans suffer from chronic disease. Also, a recent study found Americans have a shorter life expectancy than people in 41 other countries. Two decades ago, we were 11th. While US taxpayers spend more on healthcare than any other country, we continue to fall behind other countries in life expectancy. Though a long life is great, it is important that it be accompanied by a good quality of life. The natural remedies in this book work extremely well to improve one's quality of life.

I believe there are six principles of holistic health. The natural remedies in this book are compatible with all six principles. They are:

1. Do No Harm
2. Tap into the Healing Power of Nature

3. Find the Cause
4. Treat the Whole Person
5. Preventative Medicine Is Your Best Medicine
6. Your Doctor Is Your Teacher

I want you, the reader, to know that the natural remedies and therapies in this book are proven! They are proven in studies as well as in my clinical practice. I trust you will find this book to be a valuable resource.

God bless,

Mark Stengler ND, CHT, MRS
Licensed Naturopathic Medical Doctor
Homeopathic Doctor
La Jolla, California
www.drstengler.com
www.lajollawholehealth.com

ACKNOWLEDGMENTS

To my mother, Mary Stengler, who has always supported me in all areas of my life. To Marty Edelston and the staff at Boardroom Inc., who have been so supportive in the publishing of our successful newsletter "Bottom Line Natural Healing with Dr. Mark Stengler." Thanks to Maria Gagliano, John Duff, and Jeff Herman, for their efforts in the publishing of this book. To the most influential Person in history, the Lord Jesus Christ, who by His grace saved me. "Let us run with endurance the race that is set before us, looking unto Jesus, the author and finisher of our faith, who for the joy that was set before Him endured the cross, despising the shame, and has sat down at the right hand of the throne of God" (Hebrews 12:1–2).

A

Acetyl-L-carnitine

"Ginkgo and the other memory supplements haven't done much for me. Is there anything else I can use for my memory?" asked Betty, a 70-year-old.

Sure there is. Acetyl-L-carnitine (ALC) is well studied and safe, and I have found it helps many people with memory. Within two months Betty was relieved to find that her day-to-day memory was improving.

ALC occurs naturally in the body in the brain, liver, and kidneys. It is formed from other carnitine compounds that are made available from red meat and dairy products. It can be converted into L-carnitine (an amino acid–like substance that has other benefits in nutritional medicine) and vice versa. It can also be made in the body from the amino acids methionine and lysine.

This magnificent nutrient aids the brain in restoring memory and benefits the brain in many ways. It improves energy metabolism in the brain cells and also improves the transmission of nerve impulses. It is one of the few substances that improves communication between the two hemispheres of the brain. It also acts as a potent antioxidant for brain cells, helping to slow the aging process. One of the unique features of ALC is that it is structurally similar to a substance called acetylcholine, a vital neurotransmitter that's needed for many different brain functions, including memory. Interestingly, many Alzheimer's drugs are designed to increase acetylcholine in the brain.

ALC has many other medicinal benefits, including treatment of diabetic neuropathy, male infertility, and some other conditions discussed in this chapter.

DOSAGE

For age-related memory decline as well as Alzheimer's disease: 1,500 to 3,000 mg daily in divided doses

For male infertility: 4,000 mg daily in divided doses or 1,000 mg combined with 2,000 mg L-carnitine

For testosterone deficiency in men: 2,000 mg plus 2,000 mg propionyl-L-carnitine daily

For diabetic neuropathy: 1,000 mg three times daily

For depression in the elderly: 1,500 to 3,000 mg daily

For Peyronie's disease: 1,000 mg twice daily

WHAT ARE THE SIDE EFFECTS?

ALC is well tolerated. Side effects are uncommon but may include digestive upset, skin rash, and agitation.

ACETYL-L-CARNITINE
RECOMMENDATIONS FROM THE NATURAL PHYSICIAN FOR . . .

AGE-RELATED MEMORY IMPAIRMENT

Acetyl-L-carnitine (ALC) has been shown to improve measures of cognitive function and memory in elderly people with age-related mental impairment. It can also delay age-related cognitive decline. For example, a study using 1,500 mg per day for 90 days demonstrated significantly improved memory, mood, and responses to stress in ALC users. A different study found 1,500 mg daily of ALC significantly improved memory. I have also found ALC to be helpful for supporting better memory in younger adults and teenagers.

ALZHEIMER'S DISEASE

Although not a cure, ALC can slow the rate of progression in some people with Alzheimer's disease. Improvements in behavior and memory have been demonstrated. Most studies have shown some degree of benefit.

AMENORRHEA

ALC may have effects on brain chemicals and hormones that control female reproductive hormones. In a preliminary trial, 2 g of ALC daily were given to amenorrheic women who had either low or normal blood levels of female hormones. Hormone levels improved in the women with low initial levels, and half of all the women resumed menstruating within three to six months after beginning supplementation.

DEPRESSION

Research suggests that ALC may benefit seniors suffering from depression. This may be due to increased levels of the brain neurotransmitter acetylcholine.

DIABETIC NEUROPATHY

I have seen several patients with diabetic neuropathy achieve significant improvement from supplementing with ALC. Studies demonstrate that this nutrient increases and regenerates nerve fibers and improves vibration sensation.

Most people notice improvement in two months but up to six months of supplementation may be necessary.

MALE INFERTILITY

Conventional medicine offers little treatment for infertile men with sperm problems. ALC offers benefit, as do other nutrients such as vitamins C, E, and B12; coenzyme Q10, and others.

A study published in *Fertility and Sterility* looked at 60 male infertility patients, ages 20 to 40 years. Participants took 2,000 mg L-carnitine along with 1,000 mg ALC or placebo. Those taking the two supplements for six months had increased sperm motility.

PEYRONIE'S DISEASE

Peyronie's disease is characterized by a bent penis during erection. It is caused by layers of scar tissue under the skin of the penis.

One study compared the benefits of ALC against tamoxifen for 48 men with Peyronie's disease. Researchers found that ALC was significantly more effective and safer than tamoxifen in the therapy for acute and early chronic Peyronie's disease.

❧ TESTOSTERONE DEFICIENCY IN SENIOR MEN

A study published in *Urology* included 120 men, ages 60 to 74. The men were randomized into three groups: one taking testosterone replacement, another taking 2,000 mg ALC combined with 2,000 mg propionyl-L-carnitine daily, and the last taking placebo. Men supplementing ALC with propionyl-L-carnitine were found to have similar results to men taking testosterone but without prostate enlargement. The men noticed improved sexual function, mood, and energy.

Aconitum napellus

"Doctor, is there something natural I can take when I break out into a panic attack?"

Kristina was a new patient, but I was already familiar with her history of chronic anxiety and panic attacks. She was familiar with many of the prescription drugs that she had discussed with other doctors—but she was seeking some form of relief that wouldn't involve the use of pharmaceuticals. I would need to know more about the nature of her anxiety before I made a recommendation.

"Tell me more about what happens to you," I prompted.

"Well, sometimes when I am out in public or before meeting with someone, I get all clammy. My heart starts to race, my body freezes up, and then a wave of fear comes over me—like I'm going to die!"

The natural medicine that instantly came to mind was homeopathic aconite, also known as *Aconitum napellus*. This remedy covers symptoms such as the kind of anxiety that's accompanied by a tremendous fear of death, which is one of the characteristics of a panic disorder. In fact, aconite is one of the main remedies for phobic states as well as anxiety disorders.

I advised Kristina on how and when she could take aconite. Subsequently, she carried it with her wherever she went. As instructed, when she felt a panic attack coming on—which could happen as frequently as every couple of days—she would take a dose of the remedy.

A few weeks later, at a follow-up visit, Kristina reported that the aconite had helped her calm down. A number of times, it helped prevent a full-blown panic attack with that dreaded fear-of-death feeling.

I had explained to Kristina that aconite was not a cure for her condition, but, as she discovered, it did provide some relief. It also fulfilled her own wish for an effective alternative to the pharmaceutical antianxiety medications that had left her with many side effects—including grogginess and what she described as "feeling like a zombie."

There were a number of underlying psychological and biochemical reasons for Kristina's anxiety disorder. The homeopathic remedy would not make those factors go away. What it did, however, is give her relief from the most acute symptoms.

It would be enough if that were the only benefit of aconite. But many homeopathic practitioners have reported other benefits as well. With patients who have suffered from a very violent or traumatic event, such as an earthquake or car accident, practitioners have found that aconite helps relieve some of the symptoms of shock.

HOMEOPATHIC REMEDY VERSUS HERB

The homeopathic remedy called aconite is different from the herb with the same name. Herbal aconite is sometimes used in Chinese medicine in very small amounts. But a homeopathic remedy contains aconite in an almost infinitesimally dilute form—such tiny amounts, in fact, that many scientists have been baffled by the healing effects of homeopathy.

In the remedy Kristina received, the amount of aconite was analagous to one drop in a swimming pool filled with water. For such a small concentration to have such a powerful healing effect sounds bizarre—but again and again, homeopathy has produced results that seem to defy explanation.

In brief, the practice of homeopathy is based on the science of "like cures like." For example, a high concentration of aconite would produce results that were just the opposite of what we wanted. One of my colleagues, for instance, took too much of the herb aconite and was immediately attacked with a number of symptoms that scared the heck out of him—including increased heart rate, elevated blood pressure, sweating, and a feeling of anxiety and of impending doom. We know for a fact that the herb aconite, taken in large doses, is potentially lethal. But in very small concentrations (homeopathic form), it produces symptoms that are precisely the *opposite* of those that my colleague experienced.

That's where "like cures like" comes in— the phrase most commonly used to describe homeopathy. If we know what symptoms are produced by the crude herb, we have guidelines for using the nontoxic homeopathic preparation to *cure* those symptoms. That is to say, a substance that causes symptoms in a healthy person can be used to cure or improve those same symptoms in someone who is ill.

BEATING THE FLU BUG

Aconite is one of the most common remedies for an acute, infectious disease like the flu—and I've experienced the results firsthand. I vividly recall one rainy winter's day in Portland, Oregon, when I felt the symptoms coming on—first the chills, then weakness in my legs, arms, and finally my whole body. Before long, the fever began.

But there was a weird aspect to this start of the flu. I began to have the sensation that something was *seriously* wrong with my body—and that something terrible was going to happen to me. In other words, the physical sensations were accompanied by mental anxiety along with the onset of a sense of fear.

This was strange. As a trained physician, I was not usually aware of any feelings of fear, even when I became ill. Perhaps this is because I'm generally in good health and I trusted in my own vitality. This time, however . . .

So I wondered what was going on—and mentally ran through the usual checklist. Was my blood-sugar low? I had recently eaten, so that didn't seem likely.

Was I stressed-out and just experiencing a stress reaction that I'd never had before? That, too, seemed improbable since I wasn't in a particularly stressful situation at that time.

It soon dawned on me that the fear was actually one symptom of the onset of the flu. For this particular combination of the symptoms, the most effective cure was likely to be homeopathic aconite.

I knew that if aconite is taken in the first hour of a flu, cold, or other infectious disease, it often stops the illness in its tracks. The first dose had an immediate effect. In less than five minutes, I noticed that I had already started to feel calmer.

I took another dose 30 minutes later. The fever broke. Muscle strength began to return. It was actually a strange experience—to feel the sensations of muscle weakness and achiness begin to dissipate within a matter of minutes.

By the end of the day, I was able to continue my regular routine as if nothing had happened. Thanks to the power of homeopathy—and the remedy aconite—I had beaten the flu bug!

CHILDREN'S REMEDY

Every home should have a homeopathic remedy kit that includes aconite. It's one of the most common remedies to use for many minor childhood afflictions, including ear infections, sore throat, croup, flu, and fever. For example, a homeopathic doctor is sure to recommend aconite for high fever if the fever comes on suddenly; if the child is crying, restless, and anxious; and if one cheek is pale and the other red.

There are two key characteristics of a condition that requires aconite. First, the symptoms usually come on very quickly. If it's a fever, for instance, the onset can occur in just a matter of minutes, and the temperature spikes quickly. The second characteristic is that the illness often comes after an exposure to the wind, especially the cold, dry wind. For instance, if a child gets an ear infection after being outdoors on a windy, cold day, I would recommend a dose or two of aconite within the first 30 to 60 minutes after the symptoms begin. There's a good chance the treatment will abort the whole infection.

I've seen a child who has been screaming in pain from an ear infection become calmer—to the point of falling asleep—within 10 minutes of being given homeopathic aconite. Best of all, the symptoms do not return. It's times like these when you say, "Thank goodness for homeopathy."

DOSAGE

Dissolve two pellets of the 30C potency (strength) in your mouth every 15 minutes for the relief of shock, anxiety, panic attacks, or an acute infection like the flu or ear infection. If there is no relief of symptoms within one hour, discontinue use and use a different treatment.

Since aconite can contribute significantly to the relief of anxiety, it is one of the main remedies for women during labor who feel absolutely certain they are about to die.

NOTE: Dosage is the same for all age groups.

WHAT ARE THE SIDE EFFECTS?

As with any homeopathic medicine, side effects are rarely an issue. By taking aconite too frequently, however, you might bring on symptoms of anxiety. Take enough of the remedy to bring symptoms under control, then reduce the dosage or stop taking it.

Acupressure

Dan, a 41-year-old executive, kept rubbing his neck as he described to me the torment that it was putting him through.

"At work, my neck gets so stiff that I get tension headaches all the time. I see a massage therapist once a week, and that helps. I even have one of those special chairs that help my posture. But if there's anything else you can recommend, I'll do it!"

"You can try acupressure," I suggested. "Let me show you some acupressure points you can press on during the day. This will help to reduce the tension in your muscles and promote relaxation."

To start, I demonstrated by pressing on two points on the back of the neck, known as Gallbladder 20. I showed him how to massage those points with his fingertips. Then I introduced him to "Tai Yang," the points near his temple where gentle pressure would relax the muscles almost instantly.

After that we moved on to Yuyao, a spot located in the middle of the eyebrows.

Then I showed him the spot on his hand where pressure would bring relief. "Push on this mound of flesh that pops up between your thumb and index finger, then squeeze the fingertips together. Tender isn't it?

"In traditional Chinese medicine—as practiced by an acupuncturist—this point is known as Large Intestine 4," I explained. "It helps to relieve pain and discomfort of the face and head."

For the next two weeks, Dan worked on the acupressure points I showed him. Periodically during the day, he would stop work for a couple of minutes and apply pressure to these specific acupressure points. He noticed quite a reduction in his neck discomfort. He never experienced any headaches either.

KEEPING UP THE PRESSURE

Many people are aware of acupuncture as a treatment to relieve pain. However, acupressure was used long before acupuncture in China, Japan, and India. Actually, it could be said that most every culture used acupressure to some degree. Simply, it was pushing on "tender" spots to relieve local pain and discomfort. Sometimes, it's what we do naturally—pressing on a sore, aching muscle, for instance. But practitioners in acupressure and acupuncture have identified less obvious, specific points of the body that can contribute to pain relief or healing.

Chinese medicine has relied on acupressure for more than 4,000 years. Today, it remains a major treatment at Chinese hospitals. Its popularity has been growing steadily throughout the world.

CHANNELS OF ENERGY

The traditional Chinese system of medicine focuses on the concept that the life-giving energy called Qi (pronounced *chee*) circulates throughout the body in 12 main channels. Each channel represents a certain organ system—such as kidney, lung, and large intestine. The points that connect to that system are located bilaterally—that is, on both sides of the body. These channels are all interconnected, so they link up to one another.

Along each of the channels, known as meridians, are specific acupressure points that can relieve local pain and inflammation, and also affect pain or tension in other areas of the body. Many of the points can be used to influence the function of internal organs. It is believed that when there is a blockage of Qi circulation in the channels, then disease or illness arises.

To prevent a disease from occurring, or to treat a disease, one must keep the Qi moving. One way to do this is to stimulate the acupressure points where a blockage is occurring. Usually these points are tender to the touch, indicating a blockage. Whether you relieve sore muscles or an internal problem such as digestive upset depends on which points you press. Mental and emotional imbalances can also be helped with acupressure.

CHEMICAL REACTION?

It is not known exactly how acupressure relieves pain or improves the functioning of internal organs. One theory is that the brain releases certain chemicals that inhibit pain and stimulate the immune system. It is also thought that acupressure relaxes trigger points so muscle tension calms down.

Acupressure may improve blood and lymphatic circulation, as well as improve electrical flow along nerves and between cells. Much research is ongoing in this area, including studies funded by the prestigious National Institutes of Health. Acupressure does work and is a major reason why traditional Chinese medicine is one of the fastest growing medical fields.

While someone trained in acupressure can obtain the best results, there are many easy-to-locate points that you can apply pressure to yourself to alleviate discomfort or improve certain conditions. These points are shown in the illustration on pages 8 and 9.

ADMINISTERING AN ACUPRESSURE TREATMENT

Here are four easy steps to follow for self-treatment:

1. Make sure you are relaxed. The room should be free of noise. If possible, you should wear light clothing.
2. Locate the desired point to which you are going to apply pressure. Press on the point using your thumb or fingers. The pressure should be direct, yet not cause great discomfort. Some points may be very tender, indicating a blockage.

   Start with very light pressure, see how you feel, and adjust the pressure accordingly. Press the acupressure point and hold for 10 to 15 seconds.

This can be repeated 5 to 10 times to see if it helps relieve the symptoms.

Chronic conditions will need more treatments to see if the acupressure is working. Some people prefer rubbing or massaging the acupressure points; this is fine to do as well. As the same channel runs on both sides of the body, try to stimulate the points on both sides simultaneously. For example, massaging Gallbladder 20 on both sides of the back of the head helps to relax tense neck muscles. Or, Stomach 36, located four finger widths below the kneecap and one finger width toward the outside of the leg (outside the shin bone on the muscle), can be stimulated simultaneously to improve digestive function.

3. Make sure to breathe while you stimulate the acupressure point. Slow, deep, relaxed breaths are best.
4. Relax in a quiet atmosphere after a treatment and drink a glass of water to help detoxify your body.

WHAT ARE THE SIDE EFFECTS?

Acupressure is a very safe treatment. Temporary soreness of the acupressure point is common and normal. Acupressure should not be applied to open wounds or areas of extreme swelling or inflammation, such as varicose veins.

There are certain points that should not be stimulated on a pregnant woman because of the risk of miscarriage. It is important that pregnant women avoid the use of Gallbladder 21, Large Intestine 4, and Liver 3. Pregnant women should consult with a practitioner of acupressure before self-treating.

ACUPRESSURE POINT LOCATION CHART
(FRONT)

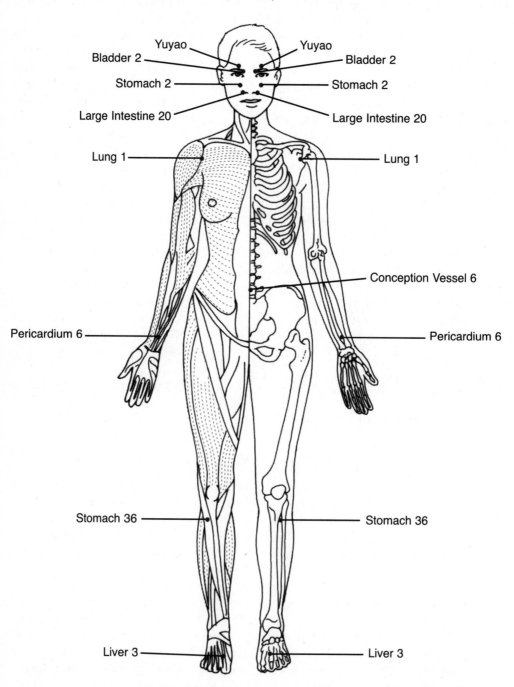

Yuyao

Bladder 2

Stomach 2

Large Intestine 20

Lung 1

Pericardium 6

Stomach 36

Liver 3

Yuyao

Bladder 2

Stomach 2

Large Intestine 20

Lung 1

Conception Vessel 6

Pericardium 6

Stomach 36

Liver 3

(BACK)

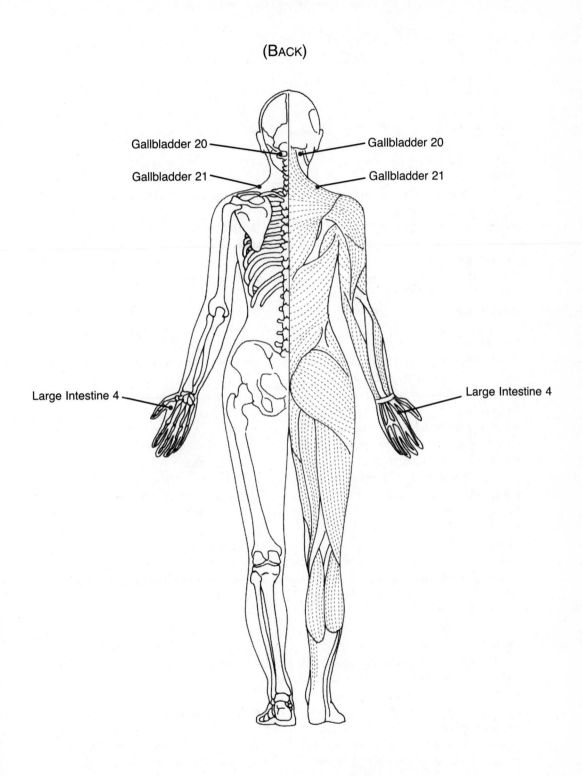

Gallbladder 20

Gallbladder 21

Gallbladder 20

Gallbladder 21

Large Intestine 4

Large Intestine 4

ACUPRESSURE

RECOMMENDATIONS FROM THE NATURAL PHYSICIAN FOR . . .

✤ ALLERGIES

Large Intestine 4, located between the webbing of the thumb and index finger, relieves nasal symptoms and head congestion.

Large Intestine 20, located on the lower, outer corner of each nostril, reduces sneezing and nasal symptoms.

✤ ANXIETY

Pericardium 6, located 2½ finger widths below the wrist crease in the middle of the forearm (palm side), helps relieve anxiety.

✤ COLD AND FLU

Large Intestine 4, located between the webbing of the thumb and index finger, relieves head congestion and sinus discomfort. Gently push on this spot. You want to work this acupressure point on both hands, so after you've treated your left hand, be sure to do the same to the right.

Large Intestine 20, located on the lower, outer corner of each nostril, reduces sneezing and nasal symptoms.

✤ CONSTIPATION

Large Intestine 4, located between the webbing of the thumb and index finger, relieves constipation. Gently push on this spot on both hands.

✤ COUGH

Lung 1, located in the front of the shoulder area, in the space below where the collarbone and shoulder meet, reduces cough.

✤ EYESTRAIN

Stomach 2, located ½-inch below the center of the lower eye ridge (you can feel an indentation), relieves burning, aching, and dry eyes.

Bladder 2, located on the inner edge of the eyebrows beside the bridge of the nose (you can feel an indentation), relieves red and painful eyes.

✤ HEADACHE

The following are all helpful. Choose the point or points that provide the most effective relief for you.

- Gallbladder 20, located below the base of the skull, in the space between the two vertical neck muscles.
- Large Intestine 4, located between the webbing of the thumb and index finger. Gently push on this spot on both hands.
- Liver 3, located on top of the foot in the hollow between the big toe and second toe.
- Yuyao, indentation in the middle of the eyebrow (directly straight up from pupil).

✤ INDIGESTION

Stomach 36, located four finger widths below the kneecap and one finger width toward the outside of the leg (outside of shin bone on the muscle), improves digestive function.

Conception Vessel 6, located two finger widths below the navel, relieves abdominal pain, gas, and other digestive problems.

✤ MUSCLE PAIN

Find the points that are most tender in the sore muscle and gently press on them and release, or massage these points.

◆ NAUSEA

Apply pressure on Pericardium 6, which is located 2½ finger widths below the wrist crease in the middle of the inside of your forearm. This point works so well for nausea that special wrist bands can be bought that stimulate this point. They are used for any kind of nausea, including morning sickness and motion sickness.

Conception Vessel 6, located two finger widths below the navel, relieves nausea and abdominal symptoms. It is also effective for motion sickness.

◆ NECK PAIN

Gallbladder 21, located on the highest point of the shoulder (trapezius muscle), relieves stiff neck and shoulder tension. Feel for a tender spot.

Gallbladder 20, located below the base of the skull, in the space between the two vertical neck muscles, relieves stiff neck and neck pain.

Large Intestine 4, located between the webbing of the thumb and index finger, reduces neck and head discomfort. Gently push on this spot on both hands.

◆ SINUSITIS

The following two points relieve sinus pain and promote drainage:

- Large Intestine 20, located on the lower, outer corner of each nostril
- Large Intestine 4, located between the webbing of the thumb and index finger

Agaricus blazei

An increasing number of doctors and consumers are becoming aware of the medicinal mushroom *Agaricus blazei*. It also has the common names Himematsutake, Agarikusutake, Kawarihiratake, Cogumelo do Sol, and sun mushroom. Preliminary studies have shown promise for its benefiting immune enhancement in people with cancer and hepatitis, lowering glucose levels for those with diabetes, and reducing cholesterol. This mushroom has an extensive history of use as a folk remedy in Brazil and is commonly used in Asian countries, such as Japan, Korea, and Taiwan, for medicinal effects and is cultivated by Brazil, China, and Japan. It is consumed as a food and as a tea.

This mushroom species contains a unique beta glucan complex—one of the highest levels of this out of all the medicinal mushrooms—which appears to activate many components of the immune system. It also has been shown to have antioxidant properties. Animal studies have demonstrated antitumor effects. Although more research is needed on this medicinal mushroom the preliminary studies look encouraging.

DOSAGE

I recommend 1,000 to 3,000 mg daily of a hot water–extracted product.

WHAT ARE THE SIDE EFFECTS?

Agaricus blazei appears to be quite safe. It should be used with caution in those with diabetes as it may lower glucose levels. Also, it should be avoided by those taking immune-suppressing transplant medications.

AGARICUS BLAZEI
RECOMMENDATIONS FROM THE NATURAL PHYSICIAN FOR . . .

✦ CANCER

It has been reported that up to 500,000 people in Japan use hot-water extracts of *Agaricus blazei* for the prevention and treatment of cancer. In a study of 100 women with cervical, ovarian, and endometrial cancers randomized to receive oral Agaricus extract or placebo along with their other treatments, researchers found improved natural killer cell activity (immune cells that kill cancer cells). Also, chemotherapy-associated side effects such as appetite, hair loss, emotional stability, and general weakness were all improved.

✦ CHOLESTEROL

A study of 90 women ingesting an Agaricus extract for eight weeks resulted in an 11% reduction in cholesterol as well as weight loss.

✦ DIABETES

Agaricus has potential for the complementary treatment of type 2 diabetes. A study of 72 people with type 2 diabetes and supplementation of Agaricus extract for 12 weeks resulted in reduced insulin resistance. It also increased the hormone adinopectin, which helps to regulate glucose.

✦ HEPATITIS C

Many of the medicinal mushrooms benefit liver function. Agaricus extract was shown in one study of people with chronic hepatitis C to reduce the liver enzyme GTP in 80% of participants after eight weeks.

✦ HIGH BLOOD PRESSURE

Agaricus has been shown in studies to decrease systolic and diastolic blood pressure. More research is needed to confirm this effect but it could be an added benefit for those using Agaricus for other medical issues.

Aloe

There are more than 300 different types of aloe plants in the world, but aloe vera (also called aloe barbadensis) is the one that people are usually talking about when they mention "aloe." Aloe vera is one of the most popular all-around herbs, because it does so much for the skin: It soothes and smoothes the skin, and reduces healing time if you have any kind of sunburn.

If you have applied aloe vera gel soon after getting a sunburn, you were likely very impressed by how effectively it healed the burn and prevented blisters. In fact, it's so kind to the skin that it's included in many cosmetic products.

But aloe also has medicinal properties when you take it internally. You can take the juice to heal digestive ailments such as ulcers and inflammatory bowel disease (IBD). In addition, it's been known to help heal arthritis, diabetes, and constipation.

The medicinal aloe that's used as a skin gel comes from a different part of the plant from the aloe that's taken internally. The gel comes from the center part of the leaves. That part of the plant is also the source of aloe vera concentrate, a type of aloe vera gel with the water removed. The concentrate, like the gel, is used topically.

To get the aloe vera juice that is usually taken internally, manufacturers remove the latex (which has a bitter taste) and dilute the gel with water. But there's also a product called aloe vera latex, aloe bitter latex, or drug aloe. This is derived from the rind—the lining just underneath the leaf surface—and it's bitter tasting. Bitter latex acts as a powerful laxative.

THE ROLES OF ALOE

Aloe grows in most of the warm, sunny climates of the world. As far back as 550 BC, Egyptians were already using aloe to treat certain skin conditions, according to written sources.

Elsewhere in the world, similar discoveries were made. The Zulu of southern Africa use it to heal wounds, as do the Chinese. In Ayurvedic medicine the bitter latex, taken internally, is one of the medicines used to expel worms.

The plant is also well known for its properties as a laxative. European colonists to Africa, praising the laxative properties, brought some samples back to Europe, where its popularity soon spread. It was also brought to North America from Europe. In fact, if you asked a 19th-century pharmacist anywhere in the western world to recommend some kind of laxative, he would almost certainly have named aloe.

The plant contains many different compounds that account for its diverse medicinal properties. A group of compounds known as anthraquinones, found in the rind part of the leaf, make up the bitter latex and account for its powerful laxative effects.

Another active ingredient is the polysaccharide (long sugar chain) known as acemannan. This compound has been shown to stimulate the immune system. It has strong antiviral effects and is being further investigated in the hope that it will be effective with HIV and cancer.

Aloe also contains prostaglandins and fatty acids (including gamma linolenic acid). These compounds are thought to give aloe some of its wound-healing and anti-inflammatory powers.

Also, many different vitamins are found in aloe including vitamins C, E, B1, B2, B6, folic acid, choline, and beta carotene. Aloe is also a source of many minerals including zinc, which is well known for its wound-healing properties as well. Aloe also contains 20 different amino acids that are known to help with tissue repair.

Scientists still don't know exactly how aloe heals the skin so effectively, though parts of the puzzle are beginning to fit together. It has been shown to stimulate the cells that grow collagen, the protein substance that binds skin together. The polysaccharides are thought to have an anti-inflammatory effect on the skin. The gel that reduces pain contains salicylic acid, the same component that's active in aspirin, so that might account for some of its pain-quelling property. That substance also inhibits many different bacteria and fungus from growing on the skin.

DOSAGE

✒ Gel

The gel can be applied liberally to the skin. You can cut open an aloe leaf and squeeze the gel onto your skin. Any health-food store, pharmacy, and most grocery stores carry aloe gel products. Look for one that contains a high concentration of aloe gel (80% or higher).

🐦 *Juice*

There is not much literature on the proper dosage of juice, which is taken internally. I recommend that people start at 1 teaspoon daily and work up to 6 teaspoons a day. It is recommended to not consume more than 1 quart daily. People with HIV/AIDS use approximately 800 to 1,600 mg per day of acemannan, the active antiviral agent in aloe.

WHAT ARE THE SIDE EFFECTS?

On rare occasions, people have reported allergic skin reactions to aloe vera gel, though I've never seen this side effect. If you do notice your skin reddening or getting itchy, just stop using the gel. For some people it can worsen dry skin.

Using cape aloes (the laxative form) frequently can lead to a condition known as "lazy colon," whereby the lower part of your intestinal tract more or less goes on strike and relies on the laxative effect of the aloe. Side effects with the juice form are rare.

Pregnant women and children under the age of 13 should not use the bitter aloe latex at all. Also, don't ever use this aloe compound if you have intestinal obstruction.

ALOE

RECOMMENDATIONS FROM THE NATURAL PHYSICIAN FOR . . .

🐦 ASTHMA

Aloe vera extract can help treat asthma, but needs to be taken for six months or more before you can tell whether it's effective. My information about this is all secondhand, however. I have never used aloe vera to treat patients with this condition, and I have not met anyone with asthma who has tried the extract as a cure.

🐦 BURNS AND WOUND HEALING

On most of the occasions when I'm recommending aloe vera gel, it's for burns. Either kitchen burns or sunburn are equally well treated with this topical remedy, so it makes sense to have some gel in your kitchen near the stove and also in your beach bag for the shore. It seems to make a dramatic difference in tissue healing.

🐦 CANKER SORES

One study found a special form of acemannan gel—derived from aloe vera—to be more effective than a conventional medication (Orabase) in speeding the healing of canker sores. In a study of 31 children with canker sores, researchers got good results with nearly four out of five. Improvements usually began on the second day of treatment. (While I have not yet recommended aloe for this purpose, the studies are convincing, and I intend to try it myself the next time I get a canker sore.)

🐦 COLD SORES

Aloe cream was shown in one study to increase the healing rate compared to placebo for those with cold sores. Apply aloe gel or cream three times daily to cold sores.

🐦 DIABETES

Researchers in Thailand investigated the effects of aloe on 77 people who had just been diagnosed with diabetes mellitus (type 2). People in the study received either 1 tablespoon of aloe vera juice or 1 tablespoon of an inactive substance that looked and tasted just like the medicine. After taking their doses twice daily for 42 days, people taking the aloe vera juice had significantly lower blood-sugar levels than those who got the "fake" medicine (placebo). In addition, the treated patients had lower triglyceride levels, which meant their blood was in better condition and they were less likely to have strokes or heart attacks. My feeling is that more studies need to be done, but I would certainly consider that this study opens the door to future possibilities.

HIGH CHOLESTEROL

Consuming 10 to 20 mL daily of aloe juice for 12 weeks can reduce total cholesterol by 15%, LDL by 18%, and triglycerides by approximately 30%.

PSORIASIS

This condition can be challenging to treat with either conventional or natural methods. One study showed that a 0.5% aloe vera cream used for four weeks was significantly effective in relieving psoriasis lesions. The aloe cream helped cure four out of five people who used it, whereas the improvement rate was only about 6% among those who used the inactive placebo.

Psoriasis lesions tend to be very dry and flaky. I assume aloe's emollient and anti-inflammatory effects were the reason why it was so helpful in this study. In my experience, not all psoriasis patients find aloe helpful—but a surprising number do.

ULCERS AND INFLAMMATORY BOWEL DISEASE

Aloe juice has become popular as an ulcer treatment in the past few years. One of aloe's constituents, known as emodin, may actually destroy the bacteria *H. pylori*, which is implicated in causing stomach ulcers.

Anecdotally, many people have told me that it helped relieve their long-standing ulcer symptoms. Also, aloe juice is gaining popularity for inflammatory conditions of the digestive tract such as Crohn's disease and ulcerative colitis. One study found that people with mild to moderate ulcerative colitis had significantly reduced symptoms consuming 25 to 50 mL of aloe vera juice twice daily.

VIRAL INFECTIONS AND AIDS

The antiviral component, acemannan, also has a virus-fighting effect against measles, influenza, and herpes simplex viruses. The injection of acemannan was shown in one study to be very effective against feline leukemia virus: 71% of the cats were alive after 12 weeks in what is usually a fatal disease.

Acemannan is showing some promise when used in combination with AZT in the treatment of AIDS. The combination may allow a person with AIDS to use lower dosages of AZT, which would reduce the risk of toxicity and side effects. Studies using acemannan by itself for the treatment of AIDS have been inconclusive.

Alpha GPC

Alpha GPC (which stands for alpha-glyceryl phosphoryl choline) is a fascinating nutrient derived from soy. This nutrient increases the body's levels of the brain-boosting substance phosphatidyl-choline and the neurotransmitter acetylcho-line. It is also a component of cell membranes that may improve nerve cell function. You will find it promoted in holistic medicine for memory enhancement. Studies have shown benefit for those with Alzheimer's disease, dementia, and for stroke recovery.

DOSAGE

I recommend 1,200 mg daily in divided doses.

WHAT ARE THE SIDE EFFECTS?

Alpha GPC is well tolerated. Some users experience digestive upset or headache.

ALPHA GPC
RECOMMENDATIONS FROM THE NATURAL PHYSICIAN FOR . . .

🐾 ALZHEIMER'S DISEASE

Alzheimer's drugs are relied upon to delay the progression or improve the symptoms of this unfortunate disease. However, supplements such as alpha GPC should also be considered.

A multicenter, double-blind, randomized, placebo-controlled trial involved people affected by mild to moderate dementia of the Alzheimer type and treated with alpha GPC (400 mg three times daily) or placebo for 180 days. The study included 261 patients with an age range of 60 to 80 years. Researchers concluded that this substance significantly improved cognitive function after 90 and 180 days of treatment.

🐾 STROKE

An Italian study demonstrated that alpha GPC was helpful for those who had suffered a stroke or transient ischemic attack. The participants were given alpha GPC by injection for the first 28 days, followed by 400 mg of the oral form three times daily for five months. Memory and behavioral function were improved.

Alpha Lipoic Acid (ALA)

"My diabetes doctor gave me a diagnosis of neuropathy—the numbness and pain in my legs are driving me crazy!" exclaimed Paul, a new patient of mine with type 2 diabetes.

"I have a nutrient that works very well for this, Paul, and it's very safe. It is called alpha lipoic acid," I responded. A few months later Paul reported his surprise from a significant reduction in his neuropathy.

The supplement alpha lipoic acid (ALA) (also known as thioctic acid) has become a mainstay in the nutritional treatment of diabetes. This vitamin-like compound is a potent antioxidant that protects cells from damage. It is unique in that it is both water- and fat-soluble, meaning that it has a full spectrum of benefit in all types of tissue in the body. It neutralizes free radicals outside and within cells. This also gives it the unique ability to regenerate the body's use of antioxidants, such as vitamin C, vitamin E, and glutathione. Once inside the cell, ALA is reduced to dihydrolipoic acid (DHLA), which has also been shown to improve insulin sensitivity in people with type 2 diabetes so that their glucose levels can be controlled better.

The human body can synthesize the small amounts of ALA found in foods such as organ meats, red meat, spinach, rice bran, Brussels sprouts, broccoli, tomatoes, and peas. Absorption from ALA supplements is between 30% and 40%.

DOSAGE

For healthy people, 100 to 300 mg is a good general dosage. Those with pre-diabetes or chronic disease should take a minimum of 300 mg. Those with diabetes should take 600 to 900 mg daily in divided doses on an empty stomach (one hour or more before eating or two hours after a meal). For treatment of diabetic neuropathy, take 900 to 1,200 mg daily.

WHAT ARE THE SIDE EFFECTS?

Side effects are not common. Rare side effects include skin rash, digestive upset such as nausea, vomiting, and diarrhea. ALA can reduce blood glucose levels, so people taking diabetes medications should be monitored to see if their medication dosage should be lowered. Safety has not been studied in pregnant and nursing mothers, and therefore they should avoid ALA. One should also supplement biotin and vitamin B1 (thiamin) while taking ALA. This can be in the form of a multivitamin or B-complex.

ALPHA LIPOIC ACID
RECOMMENDATIONS FROM THE NATURAL PHYSICIAN FOR . . .

🔖 CARDIAC AUTONOMIC NEUROPATHY

Up to 25% of people with diabetes develop cardiac autonomic neuropathy, where the heart rate can vary and increase the risk of death. A controlled trial found 800 mg of ALA daily for four months significantly improved two of four measures of heart rate variability compared to placebo.

🔖 CARDIOVASCULAR DISEASE

A study of 28 men and women with peripheral artery disease (characterized by reduced blood flow to the limbs) were able to walk longer with less pain after supplementing with 600 mg ALA daily.

🔖 DEMENTIA

A small, non-blinded trial including nine people with Alzheimer's disease and related dementias who were also taking acetylcholine-boosting medication reported that ALA at a dose of 600 mg daily appeared to stabilize cognitive function over a one-year period.

🔖 DIABETES

ALA can have mild benefits on glucose metabolism for those with type 2 diabetes. A study of 72 people with type 2 diabetes found that 600 mg ALA daily resulted in

(continued)

25% improved insulin sensitivity after four weeks. The researchers also tested 1,200 mg and 1,800 mg ALA daily, and found no increased benefit. However, long-term glucose lowering as measured by hemoglobin A1C levels found no benefit from ALA supplementation. Studies with intravenous ALA have found some benefit for glucose regulation. For those with type 2 diabetes it appears ALA has more benefit for the prevention and treatment of peripheral neuropathy (see below).

🐌 GLAUCOMA

This is a condition where pressure builds up inside the eyeball. A study using 150 mg ALA for one month found improvement in visual function for those with open-angle glaucoma.

🐌 PERIPHERAL NEUROPATHY

The most dramatic effect of ALA is its benefit in treating peripheral neuropathy. This condition is very common in those with diabetes—up to 70% will develop neuropathy. It is characterized by numbness, tingling, or pain in the toes, feet, legs, hands, arms, and fingers. It

generally starts in the feet. Studies using 600 to 1,800 mg ALA have found benefit for those with diabetic neuropathy. The best results have been found with intravenous ALA.

I have also seen ALA help patients with peripheral neuropathy unrelated to diabetes. I have found doses of 900 to 1,200 mg ALA effective for the treatment of diabetic neuropathy. As the studies have shown, wait six to eight weeks before assessing efficacy.

🐌 SKIN AGING

One study in the *British Journal of Dermatology* reported that ALA skin cream (5%) reduced skin roughness in damaged skin. The women in this study were an average age of 54.4 years.

🐌 SMELL

One clinical trial found that 600 mg of ALA significantly improved smell for people who had no sense of smell or reduced ability to smell after an upper-respiratory tract infection. Participants took the ALA for an average of 4.5 months.

Amino Acids

Amino acids are the building blocks of protein and are essential for life. Almost every structure in the body requires amino acids—including enzymes, hormones, muscle, skin, nails, and connective tissue.

When you eat food containing protein, your body acquires a resupply when amino acids are broken down by the digestive system and then absorbed into the bloodstream. Your body will use the amino acids wherever they are most needed.

If you have a deficiency of one or more

amino acids due to your diet, digestive problems, or a genetic predisposition, then you may benefit from taking amino acid supplements. Also, certain illnesses have been shown to improve dramatically with specific amino acid therapy.

There are a number of classic examples of amino acids that help fight disease. Lysine inhibits the herpes virus, while arginine can help to heal burns. Tryptophan reduces depression and anxiety; histidine alleviates allergies; and taurine is effective for helping to prevent heart failure. While these are perhaps the best-known medical uses of amino acids, there are hundreds of other conditions for which the supplements can be helpful.

Amino acids are integral to the whole chain-of-execution process that begins with the "commands" that are given out by DNA, the critical genetic material within your cells. Through activation of amino acids, your body manufactures, or replaces, tissues and organs. So your health is determined, at least in part, by how efficiently amino acids are utilized in the body. Disease can arise when there is a deficiency of amino acids or when they are connected improperly (such as in genetic defects).

There are approximately 20 amino acids that compose more than 50,000 different protein structures in the body. Enzymes, vitamins, and minerals are required for the metabolic pathways that convert amino acids into specific body structures, which include not only whole organs like your stomach, heart, or nerves but also the delicate, transient items like hormones and enzymes. The demand for certain amino acids increases when we are under stress, exposed to environmental toxins, afflicted with disease, and at other times.

THE BIG NINE

There are nine essential amino acids. These must be ingested, as your body cannot manufacture them. The essential amino acids are phenylalanine, tryptophan, methionine, lysine, leucine, isoleucine, valine, histidine, and threonine.

If your gut bacteria, or flora, are healthy, they help synthesize these essential amino acids—and you need them! To put it bluntly, we'd die without these essential amino acids. If these essential amino acids are available, your body can manufacture nonessential amino acids, as long as certain vitamins (such as B6), minerals (e.g., magnesium), and enzymes are available for these metabolic reactions to occur. Examples of nonessential amino acids include tyrosine, taurine, cysteine, arginine, ornithine, glutamic acid, glutamine, proline, and glycine.

FOOD SOURCES

Amino acids are found in protein-containing foods such as meat, eggs, milk, and fish (animal products), and nuts, seeds, soy, corn, and other grains (plant sources). Animal proteins are called "complete" because they contain all the essential amino acids. But even vegetarians can get all the essential amino acids by carefully combining selected plant foods during a 24- to 48-hour period. Spirulina contains all the essential amino acids. Soy comes close to being a complete plant protein. Strict vegetarians can combine whole grains and legumes to achieve all the essential amino acids; for example, by eating peanut butter on whole grain bread or having brown rice with beans.

AMINO ACID THERAPY

The use of amino acid therapy is an emerging field in nutritional medicine. Amino acids are available as supplements. The most common are called free-form amino acids. "Free form" refers to the fact that the amino acids have been "freed" from their protein chain from foods like soy or molasses.

Different amino acids have a variety of different effects. Some amino acids act directly as neurotransmitters. For example, GABA has an inhibitory or calming effect on the body. Other amino acids are precursors that the body converts into neurotransmitters. For example, tryptophan is converted into the serotonin, a neurotransmitter that prevents depression.

Both adults and seniors often benefit from amino acids. Two studies with seniors showed impressive benefits after taking multiple amino acid supplements. These supplements provided 8 to 11 g daily of a blend of amino acids. In one of the studies, reported in the *American Journal of Cardiology*, daily amino acid supplements led to significant increases in muscle after six months—and even more muscle after 16 months. Results in the other study were similar. Multi amino acid supplements, available at most health-food stores, generally provide between eight and eleven different amino acids.

The form known as branched chain amino acids is a group of three essential amino acids known as L-leucine, L-isoleucine, and L-valine. The branched chain amino acids are important for muscle growth and wound healing. They are different in that they are metabolized in the muscle instead of the liver.

DOSAGE

Amino acids can be purchased individually or as blended formulas. These are generally taken for nonspecific reasons—such as to recover from strenuous exercise or for general immune support. Single amino acids are used for therapeutic reasons. For instance, lysine is used specifically for the treatment of herpes.

Amino acids come in different forms. The form best utilized in the body is the L form, as opposed to the D or DL form. The exception to this is DL-methionine or DL-phenylalanine. (The FDA prohibits the sale of D or DL except for the two exceptions noted.)

Amino acids are available in powder, capsule, or liquid format. The typical dose is 500 mg one to three times daily or as recommended by your healthcare practitioner. In some cases, much higher dosages are

required for therapeutic results. (An example is the amino acid arginine, which is used in as high a dosage as 8,000 mg daily for the treatment of heart failure.)

It usually takes at least a few weeks for results to be noticed, but in some cases, improvement can be felt within several minutes. For example, I have had patients tell me their energy or mood improves within 30 minutes of taking amino acids on an empty stomach. As with any supplement, generally, the longer you have had the condition for which you are using the amino acid (or combination of amino acids), the longer it will take to feel some improvement.

Amino acids are best taken on an empty stomach to maximize their absorption. When taken with food, the amino acids compete with each other for absorption.

I usually advise people to work with a nutritional doctor before they begin amino acid therapy. Lab testing of blood (plasma) or urine can help identify deficiencies or imbalances of the amino acids and then specific therapies can be implemented.

WHAT ARE THE SIDE EFFECTS?

Digestive upset (diarrhea, constipation, or flatulence) are the most common side effects but are not experienced by most users.

If you have phenylketonuria (a genetic condition), you should not take phenylalanine (DLPA). Do not take phenylalanine, tyrosine, or tryptophan if you are taking a class of antidepressants known as MAO inhibitors or high blood pressure medications. Persons with liver or kidney disease should not take amino acids unless instructed to do so by their doctor. If you're caring for someone who has a mental illness—or if you have a history of mental illness—be sure to seek the guidance of a doctor before you use amino acid therapy. Avoid the use of arginine if you have herpes.

Pregnant women should not take amino

acids unless instructed to do so by their doctor.

CONDITIONS FOR WHICH AMINO ACIDS MAY BE HELPFUL

Here are some commonly used amino acids and the conditions for which they are used.

Amino Acid	Usage
Arginine	high cholesterol, congestive heart failure, angina, impotence, wound healing, low sperm count
Beta alanine	endurance, muscle mass
GABA	anxiety, depression, seizures, hypertension, hyperactivity
Glutamine	wound healing, inflammatory bowel disease, leaky gut syndrome
L-ornithine	endurance, muscle mass
Lysine	herpes, osteoporosis (For more recommendations, see Lysine, page 306)
Phenylalanine	pain, weight loss
Tryptophan	depression, anxiety, insomnia, migraine headaches, premenstrual syndrome (PMS)
Tyrosine	depression, hypothyroidism

Andrographis

Andrographis paniculata, commonly referred to as andrographis, has gained popularity among nutrition-oriented doctors and the public for the prevention and treatment of the common cold and flu. Interestingly, it is also referred to as Indian echinacea, although the two are not related botanically. It has been used extensively in Asia and India to treat infectious disease.

Components of andrographis have been shown in studies to have antioxidant, antiviral, antibacterial, anti-inflammatory, blood-pressure-lowering, anticancer, ulcer-healing, and pain-relieving properties.

Many studies have been done on the combination of andrographis and Siberian ginseng (*Eleutherococcus*). This combination is known as Kan Jang.

DOSAGE

For the common cold, take 100 mg twice daily of a standardized extract. It is also available commercially in combination with Siberian ginseng (*Eleutherococcus*) for treating the common cold at a combined dose of 400 mg Kan Jang three times daily.

WHAT ARE THE SIDE EFFECTS?

Digestive upset can occur that may be alleviated by taking andrographis with meals or at a lower dose. In one trial people with HIV taking a very high standardized dose reported headache, fatigue, a bitter/metallic taste, and elevated liver enzyme levels. These symptoms are not commonly seen in people without HIV infection. Those taking blood-thinning medications should use caution because andrographis may have blood-thinning properties. Andrographis should not be used by pregnant women or nursing mothers.

ANDROGRAPHIS

RECOMMENDATIONS FROM THE NATURAL PHYSICIAN FOR . . .

🐚 COMMON COLD

Andrographis, especially when combined with Siberian ginseng (*Eleutherococcus*) has been shown to significantly improve symptoms of the common cold when taken within 72 hours of the beginning of cold symptoms. This combination, known as Kan Jang, has also been shown to be effective for upper respiratory infections, including sinusitis.

Use of andrographis can reduce one's chances of developing a cold by approximately 50% after two months of continuous treatment.

In addition, andrographis combined with Siberian ginseng (*Eleutherococcus*) was shown to be effective in alleviating cold symptoms in children.

🐚 FLU

One study of 540 people compared Kan Jang (andrographis plus Siberian ginseng) to commonly used antiviral medications, such as amantadine. Seventy-one people were given 88.8 mg andrographis plus 10 mg Siberian ginseng three times daily, while 469 patients received the conventional antiviral medication for 3 to 5 days. Of those in the Kan Jang group, 30.1% progressed to a complicated flu compared to 67.8% in the control group. The Kan Jang group also experienced a shorter duration of symptoms of approximately six to seven days as compared to the control group's 9 to 10 days. In a second phase of the study, the Kan Jang group's days of sick leave were fewer (7.2 days) compared to the control group (9.8 days). Also, 31.4% of the Kan Jang group developed post-flu complications as compared to 71% in the control group.

🐚 PHARYNGOTONSILLITIS

Andrographis was shown in one study to be similar in effectiveness to acetaminophen in the treatment of fever and sore throat for those with pharyngotonsillitis (infection of throat and tonsils).

Antioxidants

The term "antioxidant" has become a buzzword in the media. Anyone who listens to the radio, watches TV, or reads a magazine or newspaper has heard the term.

But what are antioxidants and what do they do? When I hear people talking about antioxidants, they usually say something like "antioxidants prevent or slow down the aging process" or "they improve immune function." These people are on the right track.

To understand what antioxidants are, let's first discuss the term "free radical." A free radical is an unstable molecule that is missing an electron (charged particle). It is very reactive and potentially damaging to the tissues and organs of the body.

A free radical seeks out another molecule to pair up with to gain another electron. It will steal an electron from another molecule, which in the process creates another free radical.

Free radicals are a natural byproduct of energy production, what biochemists call oxidation. Hence, the term antioxidant means "against oxidation."

LIFE WITH RADICALS

It is impossible to avoid free radicals. When cells "burn" oxygen as fuel to produce energy, free radicals are one of the byproducts of this life-sustaining metabolic process. Research has shown that free radicals are implicated in most diseases, including arthritis, cancer, cataracts, fatigue, heart disease, Parkinson's disease, and even the aging process. Free radicals do have beneficial effects in the body, too, such as killing viruses. However, the levels become too high for the body to neutralize and cell damage can occur.

Our bodies produce certain antioxidants to fight against this continuous onslaught. Other antioxidants are found naturally in foods, including vitamins, minerals, and phytonutrients. Therefore, we can consume valuable antioxidants found in foods that help to quench free radicals. Also, we can avoid foods that produce free radicals, such as fast foods, which are loaded with unhealthy fats such as hydrogenated oils.

In general, it's a great idea to avoid hydrogenated oils (found in margarine, vegetable cooking oils, packaged foods) and saturated fats (found in red meat and dairy products) that lead to the production of free radicals.

In addition to getting a diet that favors antioxidants, we can take antioxidant supplements to ensure adequate levels.

Why all the fuss about using antioxidant supplements? Well, antioxidants are mainly found in plants. How many people are eating seven or more servings of fruits and vegetables a day? The government promotes five servings a day, but seven to ten is what one should consume for optimal health and to prevent diseases like cancer. According to studies, not many people come close to having three servings on a regular basis.

POLLUTION PROBLEMS

There are sound reasons why antioxidant supplements have been in the news so much. As pollution has increased, so has the burden of body stress created by free radicals. Industrial pollution, which contaminates our water, air, and food, has contributed to increased exposure to free radicals and to an increased need for antioxidants.

Radiation from the sun also produces free radicals. Too much exposure to solar rays leads to a much higher free radical load than our body's antioxidant systems can handle. As a result, conditions such as skin cancer, wrinkles, and cataracts develop. As the ozone layer becomes more depleted, the intensity of solar radiation and free radical damage increases.

Unhealthy lifestyle habits such as smoking and drinking alcohol also contribute to free radical damage. Of course, these are controllable factors.

Even high-performance athletes are prone to excessive free radical damage from intensive training. Marathon runners and triathletes are prime examples. It is well known that after exhaustive training and competitive events, many of these athletes become sick with infections or chronic fatigue. High levels of free radicals are to blame for many of these illnesses. Antioxidant supplements can go a long way to protect these athletes.

Certain diseases, such as diabetes, lead to an increased production of free radicals.

Another problem area is digestive health. The result of poor digestion and malabsorption of food is the development of metabolic toxins, and thus free radicals.

Pharmaceutical medications can and often do increase free radical formation, causing damage to the liver and kidneys. I recommend that people who take medications should increase their intake of antioxidants to prevent such side effects.

Paradoxically, free radicals also have a good side. Immune cells use free radicals to destroy bacteria, viruses, and other invading microbes. As a matter of fact, our immune system uses free radicals to kill cancer cells.

Free radicals are also used as messengers in the body. They help to regulate blood pressure and serve other important functions. So the real key is to have a balance between the amount of free radicals and an ample amount of antioxidants to control them.

SHIELDING THE GENETIC CODE

One of the most important functions of antioxidants is to protect the genetic code of our cells, known as DNA. This is important because DNA controls all the cellular activities that go on in the body. One of the more fundamental roles of DNA includes cell division.

According to one leading theory, cancer begins when there's oxidative damage of DNA, which then leads to the uncontrolled division of cells—in other words, tumor formation. This theory would help explain, for instance, why smokers are much more prone to lung cancer than nonsmokers. If we inhale cigarette smoke—or any kind of smoke, for that matter—it damages the DNA in the lungs.

But even without such a clear violation of our defenses, scientists estimate that each human cell's DNA receives thousands of "oxidative hits" a day. So antioxidants are critical to our survival, and they need all the help they can get from the enzymes

in cells that help protect cell DNA from oxidation.

ANTI-ANTIOXIDANT ANALYSIS FLAWED

Researchers from Denmark analyzed data from 68 previous studies, involving more than 200,000 participants, to examine the effects of several common antioxidant supplements on mortality. The findings were published in the *Journal of the American Medical Association* in February 2007. Their conclusion: "Treatment with beta carotene, vitamin A, and vitamin E may increase mortality." This study is a prime example of how data can be cherry-picked to skew results. For instance, of the more than 800 antioxidant studies available for assessment, fewer than six dozen were chosen for review. The average duration of the participants' antioxidant use was only 2.7 years—hardly long enough to ascertain an effect on mortality. Many of the studies analyzed were grossly misrepresentative of the typical supplement regimen. For example, one study included patients who took a single dose of 200,000 IU of vitamin A—a huge and potentially toxic dose, as compared to the recommended daily allowance (RDA) of 3,500 IU to 5,000 IU for adults, and a daily optimal intake of 10,000 IU to 50,000 IU.

Also, many of the studies analyzed had used synthetic forms of vitamin E and beta carotene—though it has been well established that these synthetic supplements do not duplicate the effects of their natural counterparts. I doubt you could even find synthetic vitamin E in a health-food store. It's no surprise that these are the same authors who published a 2004 study attacking antioxidants, without any balanced reporting on the numerous positive studies. Balz Frei, PhD, professor of biochemistry and biophysics at Oregon State University and director of the prestigious Linus Pauling Institute, says, "This is a flawed analysis of flawed data. . . . Instead of causing harm, the totality of the evidence indicates that antioxidants from foods or supplements have many health benefits, including reduced risk for cardiovascular disease, some types of cancer, eye disease, and neurodegenerative disease. In addition, they are a key to an enhanced immune system and resistance to infection." I heartily agree.

DOSAGE

Without a doubt the best way to get antioxidants is from the diet. Phytonutrients and naturally occurring vitamins and minerals in foods are our best supply of antioxidants. Supplemental antioxidants can be beneficial as well. The recommended dosage for antioxidants varies depending on the health of a person. For example, the dosage of the antioxidant for vitamins E and C would be much higher for a person with diabetes than a person who does not have diabetes. I have listed the general daily dosage of the antioxidants in Table 1. These are dosages for a person who wants to take antioxidants for optimal health and for disease prevention.

It is most important to get a full spectrum of antioxidants on a regular basis rather than just to take a few of the antioxidants at higher dosages. Remember, they all work together as a team. I find too many people focusing on one or a few of the antioxidants because of some advertisement they read from a supplement company. Getting the most out of antioxidants can be done through a balanced diet, a full-spectrum multivitamin, or a full-spectrum antioxidant complex supplement. The exception to this rule is when someone has a specific condition, and needs much higher dosages of a single antioxidant.

WHAT ARE THE SIDE EFFECTS?

Side effects are not a problem with normal dosages. High dosages of fat-soluble vitamins like vitamin A can cause side effects, especially if one has liver or kidney disease.

SPECIFIC RECOMMENDATIONS FOR SPECIFIC PEOPLE

In addition to a full-spectrum multivitamin, I recommend the following antioxidants so that the daily total (taking into account what is in the multivitamin) equals the recommended dosage.

Arthritis Patients

Oxidative damage leads to the destruction of joint tissue such as cartilage. These antioxidants have been shown to prevent or slow down this degeneration:

Lipoic acid—100 mg

Vitamin C—1,000 to 3,000 mg

Vitamin E—400 to 800 IU

Selenium—200 mcg

Grape seed extract or Pycnogenol—100 to 200 mg

Athletes

These supplements are recommended to help athletes recover more quickly from training. Studies have shown that vitamins C and E help to reduce muscle soreness after physical activity.

Vitamin C—1,000 mg

Vitamin E—400 to 800 IU

Coenzyme Q10—50 to 100 mg

L-carnitine—500 to 2000 mg

Lipoic acid—100 mg

🐦 Cancer Patients

I recommend the following for those who have a strong genetic susceptibility to cancer or for those who want a more aggressive prevention protocol:

Lipoic acid—100 mg

Mixed vitamin E—400 to 800 IU

Tocotrienols—100 mg

Coenzyme Q10—300 mg

Turmeric extract—900 to 1,800 mg of curcumin

Mixed carotenoid complex—25,000 IU

Chemotherapy and Antioxidants

Many oncologists fear that supplementing with antioxidants (nutrients that neutralize negatively charged molecules called free radicals) may diminish chemotherapy's effectiveness. Recently, researchers from three cancer institutes reviewed 19 studies involving 1,554 subjects who regularly took one or more antioxidant supplements (such as glutathione, melatonin, N-acetylcysteine, ellagic acid, and/or vitamins A, C, and E). Results: In 17 trials, patients taking antioxidants had either significantly or slightly better survival rates and/or tumor response, compared to control groups. Negative side effects from chemotherapy were reported in 17 studies—and in 15 of those, antioxidant users experienced similar or reduced levels of side effects. Check with your oncologist or nutrition-oriented doctor for the latest information on antioxidants with certain types of chemotherapy treatments.

🐦 Detoxification Patients

People in detoxification programs benefit from antioxidants. The process of detoxification itself creates free radicals that need to be detoxified with antioxidants.

Vitamin C—500 to 1,000 mg

Vitamin E—400 IU

Lipoic acid—100 mg

Milk thistle (85% silymarin)—450 mg

Mixed carotenoid complex—25,000 IU

Selenium—200 mcg

Green tea—2 to 5 cups daily

NAC—1,200 mg daily

🐦 Diabetes

People with diabetes have many extra nutritional needs. The following antioxidants are very important:

Vitamin E—800 IU

Lipoic acid—100 to 600 mg

Vitamin C—1,000 to 3,000 mg

Coenzyme Q10—100 to 300 mg

🐦 High Cholesterol and Heart Disease

High cholesterol levels by themselves are not the problem when it comes to heart disease. It is when cholesterol, especially LDL cholesterol, becomes oxidized that an inflammatory response by the immune system leads to plaque buildup in the arteries. These antioxidants are important to prevent this oxidation of cholesterol:

Vitamin E (mixed)—400 to 800 IU

Tocotrienols—100 to 400 mg

Vitamin C—500 to 1,000 mg

Coenzyme Q10—100 mg

Grape seed extract or Pycnogenol—50 to 100 mg

Green tea—1 to 3 cups daily

Smokers

Smoking is a sure way to deplete the body's antioxidants. Supplementing antioxidants can help reduce, but not eliminate, some of the damaging effects. When smokers take antioxidants, the first thing they usually notice is an increase in energy. This is probably because the antioxidants are helping the body detoxify these poisonous chemicals, which frees up energy production of the cells.

Vitamin C—1,000 to 2,000 mg

Lipoic acid—100 mg

Coenzyme Q10—100 mg

Vitamin A—1,500 to 5,000 IU

Selenium—200 mcg

Mixed tocotrienols—100 mg

Mixed carotenoid complex—25,000 IU

Green tea—1 to 3 cups daily

RECOMMENDED FOODS

Many fruits and vegetables are high in antioxidants, and the more you can get in your diet, the better. Here are some of the stars.

- Grapes, strawberries, cherries, and blueberries all contain phytonutrients known as flavonoids that have potent antioxidant activity.
- Red wine and red grape juice have also been shown to have the flavonoids that are protective against heart disease.
- Citrus fruit—including oranges, lemons, and limes—all contain flavonoids.
- Carrots contain the carotenoids that help prevent cancer. These carotenoids are also found in orange and yellow types of squash.
- Cruciferous vegetables, including broccoli, cauliflower, cabbage, Brussels sprouts, and kale, contain various antioxidants. (They also have cancer-preventing phytonutrients such as indoles and sulforaphane.)
- Garlic and onions have antioxidants that help prevent cancer and heart disease.
- Tomatoes are rich in the antioxidant lycopene that helps to prevent prostate cancer.
- Tea contains polyphenols, potent antioxidants that protect humans against cancer and heart disease. Both green tea and black tea have polyphenols (green tea has the higher concentration).

TABLE 1
Sources of Antioxidants

There are many vitamins, minerals, and phytonutrients that are known for their antioxidant activity. The list below will help you find some of the more popular antioxidants and some of the conditions they can help prevent or control. (For more about some of these antioxidants, see other sections.)

SUBSTANCE	INDICATED USE	DOSAGE
Nutritional Supplements		
Vitamin A	Cancer, immune deficiency, respiratory tract infections, vision	1,500 to 5,000 IU
Vitamin C	Arthritis, cancer, heart disease, skin conditions, common cold, heart disease, diabetes, hypertension, liver disease	500 to 3,000 mg
Vitamin E	Arthritis, cancer, heart disease, Alzheimer's disease, smokers	400 to 800 IU
Selenium	Cancer, heart disease, viral infections, HIV	200 to 400 mcg
Carotenoids	Cancer, vision, skin health	Mixed carotenoid complex 25,000 IU
Lipoic Acid	Arthritis, cataracts, stroke, heart disease, liver disease, diabetes, AIDS, Alzheimer's disease, Parkinson's disease, radiation exposure	50 to 300 mg
Grape Seed Extract	Varicose veins, heart disease	50 to 150 mg (Pycnogenol)
Coenzyme Q10	Heart disease, chronic fatigue, hypertension, cancer, gum disease	50 to 300 mg
Lutein	Vision problems (cataracts, macular degeneration)	6 mg daily
Lycopene	Prostate cancer	30 mg daily
Herbal Supplements		
Ginkgo	Alzheimer's disease, age-related memory loss, circulatory problems, asthma	120 to 240 mg of a 24% standardized extract
Milk Thistle	Cancer, liver disease	450 mg of an 85% silymarin standardized extract
Turmeric	Cancer, liver disease	900 to 1,800 mg of curcumin

Apis

"Veronica has just been diagnosed with rheumatoid arthritis in her hands. The pain and stiffness keep her from writing at times," said Veronica's mother who had brought her to my office.

"What does the pain feel like?" I asked Veronica, who was only 10 years old.

"It feels like it's burning and sometimes stinging," she replied.

I put Veronica on a special diet for six weeks. Unfortunately, it did not seem to help as I had expected. I prescribed the homeopathic remedy apis when she came for her next visit. This remedy is indicated in cases of arthritis where there is burning and stinging pain.

Two weeks later, Veronica's mother called me to report that "Veronica's pain is gone."

"That's excellent," I replied. "Veronica needs to keep taking the apis; we need more time to make sure it has a lasting effect."

I kept Veronica on homeopathic treatment for another three months. The last time I talked to Veronica's mother was four years after we started treatment. Veronica's arthritis had not returned.

THE BUZZ ABOUT APIS

Apis is a remedy that is derived from the honeybee—the stinger as well as the whole bee. Think of the symptoms that a bee sting causes such as stinging, burning, swelling, and itching. These are all the symptoms for which apis is beneficial. So a homeopathic doctor may recommend it for bee stings, allergic reactions including hives, arthritis, urinary tract infections, kidney disease, herpes, sore throat, and ovarian pain.

Apis is indicated when symptoms include a lack of thirst, a negative response to heat, and a positive response to cold applications.

APIS

RECOMMENDATIONS FROM THE NATURAL PHYSICIAN FOR . . .

ALLERGIC REACTIONS

Allergic reactions that cause hives or burning and stinging pains that move around the body can be improved quickly with apis. Apis also improves other symptoms of allergic reaction such as swelling of the throat and eyes. These could be allergic reactions to food or to drugs.

(**NOTE:** Seek emergency medical treatment for allergic reactions, especially if you have swelling of the tongue, throat, or face, and/or trouble breathing.)

ARTHRITIS

If you have swollen joints that burn or sting—and if your joints feel better after applying cold compresses—then the condition can probably be alleviated with apis.

BEE STINGS

Apis quickly relieves the pain of a bee sting. This is proof of the homeopathic principle that "like cures like." Take it as soon as possible after getting stung to prevent swelling and other symptoms

(continued)

from getting severe. It is a remedy that should be in your home first-aid kit.

❧ HERPES

Apis is a common remedy for herpes infections. Herpes of the mouth—cold sores that sting and burn and that have a vesicle formation—improves quickly with apis. This also applies to the acute treatment of genital herpes.

❧ INJECTION PAIN

This remedy helps reduce stinging pain from the injection of a needle, such as may be experienced after receiving a vaccine.

❧ KIDNEY DISEASE

Apis is used in acute kidney disease such as glomerulonephritis or nephritic syndrome where there is protein loss in the urine and edema of the body.

❧ MENINGITIS

Symptoms include a stiff neck, high fever, and dilated pupils. Homeopathic apis is most effective in patients whose symptoms are made worse when heat is applied. This remedy can be used in conjunction with conventional treatment.

❧ OVARIAN PAIN

Apis is specific for right-sided ovarian cysts where there is burning and stinging pain. It not only reduces the pain, but also stimulates dissolving of the cysts.

❧ SHINGLES

Apis is one of the primary homeopathic medicines for shingles, especially when there is stinging or burning. Apis helps to relieve the pain and heal the shingles.

❧ SORE THROAT

Apis is very effective for relieving a sore and swollen throat, especially when the sore throat has specific characteristics. Those characteristics include a burning pain (that feels better when you have a cold drink) and a bright red, swollen uvula (the flap of tissue in the middle of the mouth).

❧ TOXEMIA IN PREGNANCY

Apis is a good remedy for toxemia in pregnancy where there is protein in the urine, high blood pressure, and lots of body swelling.

❧ URINARY TRACT INFECTIONS

Urinary tract infections can be helped by apis. This is particularly true for bladder infections that cause scalding pain during urination. If you have a right-sided kidney infection, it's another indication that this remedy will probably work well.

DOSAGE

For acute conditions such as a bee sting or allergic reaction, I recommend taking the homeopathic formulation with a 30C potency every 15 minutes for two doses. Then wait and see if the remedy is helping.

The other option is to take one dose of a higher potency such as a 200C.

For skin rashes, sore throats, and other conditions that are not so acute, I recommend taking a 6C, 12C, or 30C potency twice daily for three to five days, or as needed for continued improvement.

WHAT ARE THE SIDE EFFECTS?

Side effects are not an issue with apis. It either helps or there is no effect at all. It is also safe to use for children.

Arginine

Most well known for its ability to dilate blood vessels, arginine (also referred to as L-arginine) improves circulation and blood pressure. However, this amino acid has many benefits for a wide variety of conditions beyond the cardiovascular system.

Food sources include meat, poultry, fish, dairy products, nuts, seeds, soy foods, legumes, and chocolate. The body can also synthesize arginine from the amino acids L-ornithine and L-citrulline.

Arginine plays a key role in the production of nitric oxide, which causes the dilation and improved blood flow of arteries, including the all-important coronary arteries. Other cardiovascular benefits include reduced blood thickness, reduced free radical damage to lipids, and reduced activity of angiotensin converting enzyme (resulting in lower blood pressure).

People with diabetes are more likely to have suboptimal levels of arginine and should consider supplementation.

DOSAGE

A typical dosage is 5 to 20 g daily, depending on what condition is being treated. Better results may be achieved by simultaneously taking supplemental Pycnogenol at a dose of 120 mg daily. Also, time-release arginine can give more therapeutic effects due to the short half-life (activity in the body) of L-arginine.

WHAT ARE THE SIDE EFFECTS?

Digestive upset occurs with some users. In a study at Johns Hopkins University Medical Center, L-arginine supplements (up to 3,000 mg three times daily) were given to 55 participants, while 59 people got a placebo. The study was cut short because, after six months, there had been six deaths among participants taking L-arginine—and no deaths in the placebo group. In response, researchers recommended that this supplement not be used following a heart attack. It must be noted that the six deaths may have been due to chance. Two participants died from a heart attack or its complications, two succumbed to blood infections unrelated to L-arginine, and two died from unknown causes. In any case, I agree that people who have had a heart attack should not take L-arginine, at least until further studies are done. But for people with no history of heart attack, I believe 3,000 mg L-arginine, taken two to three times daily, is safe and effective in treating hypertension and congestive heart failure, as well as improving blood flow in people with diabetes.

ARGININE

RECOMMENDATIONS FROM THE NATURAL PHYSICIAN FOR . . .

🖜 AIDS-RELATED WEIGHT LOSS

An eight-week double-blind study found that oral supplementation of L-arginine, in combination with hydroxymethylbutyrate and glutamine, increased lean body mass and positively affected immunity.

🖜 ANGINA

There have been several studies demonstrating that oral ingestion of L-arginine decreases angina symptoms (chest pain and pressure) and improves exercise tolerance and quality of life.

🖜 CONGESTIVE HEART FAILURE

L-arginine in conjunction with conventional treatment improves lab measurements such as better kidney filtration and water elimination in people with congestive heart failure. Speak with your cardiologist about adding this amino acid to your treatment program.

🖜 DIABETIC FOOT ULCERS

Interesting preliminary research demonstrates that applying L-arginine (5 g daily) topically to the feet improves circulation in those with diabetes.

🖜 ERECTILE DYSFUNCTION (ED)

A prospective, randomized, double-blind, placebo-controlled study looked at the effect of 5 g a day of oral L-arginine for six weeks on 50 men with ED. Thirty-one percent of men taking L-arginine as compared with 2 of 17 controls reported a significant subjective improvement in sexual function. It should be noted that all nine patients treated with L-arginine and who had improvement had had an initially low urinary nitric oxide level, and this level had doubled at the end of the study.

Taking the supplement Pycnogenol at a dose of 40 mg three times daily may improve the effectiveness of lower dose (1.7 g daily) of L-arginine.

🖜 HIGH BLOOD PRESSURE

L-arginine can reduce blood pressure in healthy individuals and those with type 2 diabetes. I have found that time-release L-arginine works best for this purpose.

🖜 INTERSTITIAL CYSTITIS

L-arginine is one of the few natural treatments studied for helping this painful condition of the bladder and pelvic floor. It has been shown to reduce pain associated with interstitial cystitis. It should be noted that three months of use may be required before significant improvement occurs.

🖜 PERIPHERAL ARTERIAL DISEASE

L-arginine can improve symptoms of intermittent claudication, a condition characterized by cramping and pain of the lower legs due to inadequate circulation.

Arnica

If I had to choose only one homeopathic medicine for doctors to use in their practice, it would be arnica (*Arnica montana*).

Even the staunchest skeptic is likely to be swayed by observing what this homeopathic remedy can do. I doubt that any other medicine exists that can so demonstrably and effectively relieve the effects of physical trauma. I have prescribed arnica for many relatives as well as patients—and almost without exception, they have described the results as "miraculous!"

Not long ago, my sister phoned and, with a great deal of concern in her voice, asked whether I could do anything for my four-year-old nephew. Over the sound of his wailing, she told me how he'd been running through the house, tripped, and banged his head, very hard, on a table. He already had a big goose egg over one eye.

Usually, when people call for advice, I like to ask questions and take time to think about what I am going to recommend—but in this case, it was such a common childhood accident, I only needed to know whether he was fully conscious. Just the background wailing answered that question.

I told my sister to give him a dose of arnica from her homeopathic first-aid kit and to call me back in 15 minutes.

My sister called back and her first words were "It's incredible!"

The wailing had stopped.

"I can't believe it," my sister continued. "I gave him the arnica and within a minute or two I could actually see the bruise decreasing in size. Is that possible?"

"Yes," I replied. "I've seen the same thing myself."

Many times, in fact.

NATURE'S ANSWER TO TRAUMA

Always helpful when someone is recovering from a physical trauma—such as a fall, blow to the body, sprain, or surgery—arnica is most useful whenever there's any kind of bruising. It not only helps prevent the bruise from developing, it also eases the ache or soreness.

CONCUSSION

It's a shame that every emergency room does not use homeopathic arnica. This is especially true in cases of concussions. Although there are many medicines that can relieve pain, I can't think of any that help speed the recovery from a concussion—a condition where the brain is actually bruised. Arnica plays a crucial role with an injury of this kind. It's helpful when there's any kind of head trauma or concussion, whether the result of a car accident, collision, or fall.

Arnica does not only relieve pain, however; it can also help a person refocus when he or she is acting or feeling disoriented. Arnica helps to reduce the swelling of the brain that occurs with a serious head trauma, which is precisely why I strongly recommend it for every first-aid kit. Keep some on hand in your home, office, and car for emergency situations. It can come in handy.

MUSCLE RECUPERATION

Arnica can come to the rescue when your muscles feel sore from overexertion. I vividly remember the aftermath of one workout when—after a long hiatus—I'd gone to the gym and did a number of weight-lifting exercises for my chest and arms.

The next day, I could barely lift my briefcase without groaning. My muscles felt like they'd been hammered with a baseball bat.

Physician, heal thyself! After a couple doses of arnica, the soreness greatly improved, and by the afternoon of the same day, I scarcely felt a trace of the pain that I had experienced earlier. It was a lesson, of course, that I needed to get back in shape more gradually. But even the most consistent athlete is likely to experience occasional strains, sprains, and traumatic body blows. Whatever the sport or cause of the discomfort, arnica can come to the rescue. In fact, I know of many a world-class athlete who keeps a supply of arnica ready to use at a moment's notice.

POST-OPERATIVE SURGERY

According to a study in the *Archives of Facial Plastic Surgery*, homeopathic arnica significantly reduced the area of bruising after plastic surgery.

DOSAGE

A potency of 30C is common, but you can take whatever potency you have on hand. Dissolve two pellets of arnica in your mouth every 15 minutes for the relief of physical trauma. Two to three doses should be sufficient.

(**NOTE:** Dosage is the same for all age groups.)

WHAT ARE THE SIDE EFFECTS?

While there are few side effects, it is best not to use arnica on a regular basis as your response to the remedy may diminish. For instance, I wouldn't advise using it after every workout if you regularly exercise. Instead, take it for more serious injuries or traumatic accidents when it is greatly needed.

Arnica does not interfere with painkillers or other pharmaceutical medicines that may be prescribed for an injury.

WARNING: Do not mistake the herbal form of arnica for homeopathic arnica. The herbal form of arnica (available in creams and tincture) is applied topically to unbroken skin to relieve muscle soreness. The herbal form should not be taken internally.

Arsenicum album

Homeopathy is one of the most fascinating and effective healing therapies. Although it is one of the more difficult therapies to learn, it is one of the most rewarding. Interestingly, tens of thousands of medical doctors (and hundreds of thousands of other practitioners) around the world use homeopathic medicine on a routine basis in their practice.

Millions of people benefit from homeopathy. In Germany, approximately 40% of all medical doctors prescribe homeopathic remedies or refer to practitioners who do. According to Dana Ullman, coauthor of *Everybody's Guide to Homeopathic Medicines*, more than 70,000 registered homeopaths practice in India.

Another country with a strong homeopathic following is Britain, which is home to the Royal London Homeopathic Hospital. Also, the Royal Family has been under homeopathic care since 1930. In France, more than 6,000 physicians practice homeopathy and more than 18,000 pharmacies sell homeopathic remedies.

Homeopathy is one of the fastest growing retail lines in the North American health-food industry. Hollywood celebrities such as Lindsey Wagner and Jane Seymour openly endorse homeopathy and relate the benefits they have received from homeopathic treatment.

There are still many doctors, however, who are resistant to homeopathy in North America. Their minds could be changed by seeing the beneficial effect of a remedy like Arsenicum.

Even though the root word suggests "arsenic," this homeopathic medicine has none of the harmful effects that are commonly associated with the poison called arsenic. Homeopathic physicians in Europe and the United States have been prescribing Arsenicum to patients for more than two centuries without a single case of poisoning.

DRAMATIC PHYSICAL RELIEF

My patient's wife called me one night at around midnight. Her husband was suffering from food poisoning. He was lying on the floor near the bathroom, in agony, having bouts of vomiting and diarrhea. Understandably, he wanted to be close to the toilet.

When I hear of these two symptoms occurring together—vomiting and diarrhea—I prescribe Arsenicum as the homeopathic remedy. Things settled down after my patient took a dose of Arsenicum. His diarrhea improved, as well as the vomiting, and he was able to get some much needed sleep that night.

I recommend Arsenicum when physical symptoms include chills, with worsening of symptoms between 12 a.m. and 2 a.m., burning pains relieved by heat, and thirst for frequent sips of water.

I frequently prescribe Arsenicum for anxiety, asthma, diarrhea, food poisoning, and allergies, although it can be used for many other conditions.

DRAMATIC PSYCHOLOGICAL RELIEF

Arsenicum is not only helpful for physical symptoms, but for psychological states as well.

Jolene was a patient who responded well to Arsenicum. She suffered from a lot of anxiety and worry, had a hard time relaxing, and was constantly on the move. She worried about many things, but particularly her own health. No doctor was able to find anything wrong with her, but for years she went from doctor to doctor to get reassurance that nothing was medically wrong. Jolene would wash her hands several times a day, especially after shaking hands with someone because she had a fear of germs from touching things or people. Her health concerns and general anxiety caused insomnia.

After talking with Jolene, I prescribed Arsenicum. She was very concerned about taking the remedy, for fear of side effects, so I had her take her first dose in my office. This seemed to alleviate some of her concern.

As time passed, Jolene's insomnia gradually improved. Four months later, she reported that she felt calmer in general and had less anxiety. While her anxiety and fears are still a problem, Jolene is able to function more effectively, and, even more important, she has better peace of mind.

Arsenicum is a great remedy for those who are fastidious and feel the need to be in control of things at all times.

DOSAGE

Dissolve two pellets of the 30C potency (strength) in your mouth every 15 to 30 minutes for the relief of acute symptoms, such as diarrhea or anxiety. If there is no improvement of symptoms within one or two hours, discontinue and use a different treatment. For chronic conditions, treatment should be prescribed and monitored by a homeopathic practitioner.

(**NOTE:** The same dosage is effective for people of all ages.)

WHAT ARE THE SIDE EFFECTS?

As with any homeopathic medicine, side effects are not much of an issue. If you take Arsenicum too frequently though, it could aggravate the symptoms you are treating, or bring on other symptoms common to the remedy—such as anxiety or insomnia.

Try Arsenicum for a few days. If your symptoms improve, take it for another week and then stop. If your symptoms return, take it as needed to relieve the symptoms. If your symptoms get worse, or if you are not sure if it is the right remedy, stop using it and see a homeopathic practitioner.

ARSENICUM ALBUM
RECOMMENDATIONS FROM THE NATURAL PHYSICIAN FOR . . .

❧ ALLERGIES

Arsenicum is one of the best hay fever remedies. It is especially indicated for symptoms of burning, watery eyes, and clear nasal discharge or dripping that leaves the upper lip red and excoriated. It is also a good remedy for people with multiple chemical sensitivities.

❧ ANXIETY

Many patients with anxiety have benefited from treatment with Arsenicum. People whose general fears and phobias interfere with their lives may require this remedy. These people are often perfectionists who need to have things exactly to their liking. A key symptom is waking up with anxiety or panic attacks between 12 a.m. and 2 a.m. These people also tend to be restless and have a hard time relaxing because of their anxiety and fears.

❧ ARSENIC TOXICITY

A study done with mice poisoned with arsenic trioxide found that homeopathic Arsenicum had a protective effect on liver enzymes and other markers of metabolism. I have used Arsenicum to help patients detoxify from toxic metal poisoning such as arsenic, mercury, and lead.

❧ ASTHMA

Arsenicum is the most common remedy to treat and prevent worsening of asthmatic attacks. I recommend taking it when the very first symptoms of asthma appear. If it does not help immediately (within a few minutes), then a pharmaceutical bronchodilator should be used. It can also be taken in conjunction with a bronchodilator for quicker relief of symptoms.

WARNING: Do not discontinue the use of your bronchodilator without your doctor's guidance.

❧ CANCER

Arsenicum is one of the chief remedies used by homeopaths for the complementary treatment of cancer. Many homeopathic doctors have observed cases where burning pains that can accompany certain cancers are alleviated with Arsenicum, even when painkilling medications were of no benefit.

❧ DIARRHEA

Arsenicum is used for acute cases of diarrhea, especially when the stools are watery and burning. It is also a great remedy for cases of chronic diarrhea as found in colitis. The diarrhea is often worse from anxiety, cold drinks, and eating fruit. If Arsenicum is the right remedy, relief is noticed after taking only a dose or two.

Acute diarrhea is the leading cause of childhood mortality worldwide. This occurs mainly in third-world countries where poor sanitation, malnutrition, and poor medical care are commonplace.

Oral rehydration treatment can prevent death from dehydration, but does not reduce the duration of individual episodes. A randomized double-blind clinical trial comparing homeopathic medicine with placebo in the treatment of acute childhood diarrhea was conducted in Leon, Nicaragua, in July 1991. Eighty-one children six months to five years of age were included in the study. An individualized homeopathic medicine (some received Arsenicum) was prescribed for each child and daily follow-up was performed for five days. Standard treatment with oral rehydration treatment was also given. The children receiving homeopathic treatment had a statistically significant decrease in duration of diarrhea.

Homeopathic remedies cost only a fraction of what drugs cost. They have no toxicity and are effective against bacteria, viruses, and parasites that cause diarrhea. Antibiotics, on the other hand, treat only bacterial-caused diarrhea.

❧ FLU

People get different symptoms, even with the same strain of flu virus. The symptoms depend in part on how your body reacts to the infection. Arsenicum is helpful for the flu bug that hits and gives you a double whammy of diarrhea and vomiting at the same time. Chills and restlessness are also characteristic of the flu that requires this remedy.

❧ ULCER

Ulcers and gastritis (inflammation of the stomach) can be helped by Arsenicum, especially when the stomach pains are made better by drinking milk. This is the second most common remedy for ulcers after nux vomica.

Artichoke

Artichoke has a long history of use as a medicinal plant by the ancient Egyptians, Greeks, Romans, and 16th-century royalty. Today most globe artichokes grown in the United States are produced in California; worldwide, Italy and Spain produce the most. The outer leaves and "heart"—the bottom of the choke—are eaten. For medicinal supplements the leaves, stem, and root are mainly used.

Artichoke has a long folk history of treating liver and gallbladder disease. Indeed modern studies have shown that constituents in the leaves, such as caffeoylquinic acids, stimulate the flow of bile from the liver. This aids in the release of toxins from the liver as well as bile to the gallbladder. Additional benefits of bile flow include better fat digestion and reduced cholesterol levels.

DOSAGE

Most studies have used 320 to 640 mg artichoke leaf extract three times daily, although higher doses have been used for treatment of high cholesterol (up to 1,920 mg daily).

WHAT ARE THE SIDE EFFECTS?

Side effects are not common with artichoke supplements. Those sensitive to daisies should use these supplements with caution as globe artichoke is a member of the same family (*Compositae* or *Asteraceae*). Also, those with gallstone obstruction should not use supplemental artichoke extract, although those with small gallstones may find benefit from improving bile saturation. Use under the supervision of a doctor. Pregnant women and nursing mothers should not use the supplement form.

ARTICHOKE

RECOMMENDATIONS FROM THE NATURAL PHYSICIAN FOR . . .

🐚 ARTERY HEALTH

Taking 20 mL daily of artichoke juice was shown to improve endothelial function. The endothelium is the inner lining of blood vessel walls. A healthy endothelial lining is critical for the prevention of atherosclerosis and artery rupture.

🐚 HIGH CHOLESTEROL

One double-blind, randomized, placebo-controlled, multicenter clinical trial in Germany involved 143 adults with total cholesterol levels greater than 280 mg/dL. Participants were given 1,800 mg artichoke extract or a placebo daily for six weeks. Total cholesterol was decreased 18.5% in the extract group compared to 8.6% for placebo. More important, LDL cholesterol was reduced 22.9% compared to 6.3% for placebo. Artichoke extract has also been shown to lower trigylcerides. Not all studies have found a cholesterol-lowering effect with artichoke extract.

Test tube studies have shown that flavonoids rich in antioxidants (like those in artichokes) prevent the oxidation or damage of LDL cholesterol. This is thought to be an important process in the development of atherosclerosis.

🐚 INDIGESTION

Bile flow helps with the digestion of fats, proper motility of the digestive tract, and healthful elimination. One trial involving 553 people suffering from a variety of digestive ailments, including indigestion, found that 320 to 640 mg of a standardized artichoke extract taken three times per day reduced a variety of symptoms in more than 70% of participants.

Ashwagandha

In the ancient tradition of Ayurvedic medicine—as practiced in India for thousands of years—the herb ashwagandha (*Withania somnifera*) has been used to treat conditions such as fatigue, chronic disease, impotence, and waning memory. Now, in 21st-century United States, this well-respected herb has a new and even brighter reputation as a much-needed stress reliever.

Sometimes referred to as "Indian ginseng," "winter cherry," or "withania," ashwagandha herb has many similarities to Chinese ginseng. In Ayurvedic medicine, it may be used to treat a number of other diseases besides those already mentioned—including asthma, bronchitis, psoriasis, arthritis, and infertility. Ayurvedic doctors prescribe it in very specific ways that are suited to certain constitutional types. It's often given with the so-called warming herbs, such as ginger, to increase its tonic effect.

Ashwagandha root differs from Chinese ginseng in having a mild sedative action. This makes it well suited for the type A person—that is, someone who's always "on the go" at such a high rate that he or she may be headed for burnout.

MULTITONIC

Research shows that this herb is an excellent adaptogen that helps the body cope with physical and mental stress. Studies show that ashwagandha can help people who have exhaustion from chronic stress, weakened immunity (for instance, if they have cancer), and as a tonic for chronic diseases, especially inflammatory disorders.

This herb also has overall benefits for many body systems. Ashwagandha is unique in acting as a tonic to the nervous system, but also has sedative and antiepileptic effects. It mobilizes different components of the immune system to fight invading microbes and has a modulating or balancing effect if you have inflammation.

A number of animal and laboratory studies have shown this herb has antitumor activity. Ashwagandha has also been shown to have antioxidant activity, so it's helpful in protecting brain cells (which could explain why it helps to prevent memory loss). It also stimulates red blood cell production. Ashwagandha is also said to be a rich source of iron, so it's a potential choice for the treatment of iron-deficiency anemia.

Animal studies have shown that it increases thyroid hormone levels.

More than 35 chemical constituents have been identified, extracted, and isolated in this plant. These include some groups of chemicals such as alkaloids, steroidal lactones, saponins, and withanolides.

Ashwagandha has been used in only a few human studies—far outweighed by the number of animal or test-tube studies that have been done. However, it has remained popular and highly valued through thousands of years of use in Ayurvedic medicine.

DOSAGE

The standard adult dosage is 1,000 to 3,000 mg daily of the root. Or 250 to 500 mg of an 8% withanolide standardized extract.

WHAT ARE THE SIDE EFFECTS?

Since it is nonstimulating, ashwagandha has rare side effects. High doses may cause digestive upset.

ASHWAGANDHA

RECOMMENDATIONS FROM THE NATURAL PHYSICIAN FOR . . .

🌿 AGING

For one full year, 3,000 mg of purified ashwagandha powder or placebo was given to 101 normal healthy male volunteers, all between the ages of 50 and 59. The herb had some physical effects that slowed the effects of aging for all the men in the study. All men showed significantly increased hemoglobin and red blood cell count. Improvements in nail calcium and cholesterol were also noted. In addition, nearly 72% of the men reported improvement in sexual performance.

🌿 ANEMIA AND SLOW GROWTH

Ashwagandha has been shown in two human studies and several animal studies to increase hemoglobin, red blood cell count, and serum iron levels. In a scientific trial that continued for 60 days, 58 healthy children between the ages of 8 and 12 were given milk that was treated with fortified ashwagandha (2,000 mg a day). The herb improved the health factors that contribute to growth—leading to a significant increase in hemoglobin and albumin. Researchers concluded that ashwagandha can be a growth promoter in children—and they also noted that these children were less likely to have anemia.

🌿 ARTHRITIS

Ashwagandha is used in Ayurvedic herbal formulas for the treatment of arthritis and conditions involving inflammation. In a double-blind, placebo-controlled study, 42 people with osteoarthritis were given a formula containing ashwagandha (along with the herbs boswellia, turmeric, and zinc) for three months. Their health was compared with a control group that received a placebo.

The herbal formula significantly reduced the severity of pain and the degree of disability. There were no significant changes in the control of inflammation, however. A more recent double-blind, placebo-controlled study involving those taking ashwagandha extract found a 36.6% reduction of C-reactive protein compared to placebo. C-reactive protein is a marker of systemic inflammation. Also there was a 70.6% reduction in muscle pain.

🌿 FATIGUE

Ashwagandha has been historically used for the treatment of chronic fatigue, especially a patient who shows signs of nervous exhaustion. A double-blind, placebo-controlled human clinical trial was conducted that demonstrated ashwagandha's ability to boost energy and improve overall health. Those taking a standardized form of ashwagandha experienced a 79% increase in energy compared to a group taking placebo.

🌿 INSOMNIA

Ashwagandha extract was shown in one study to improve sleeplessness by 68%. This is thought to be due to the balancing effect on stress hormones such as cortisol and DHEA.

🌿 MEMORY PROBLEMS

Some holistic practitioners recommend ashwagandha for its benefit to the brain.

It helps improve the ability to reason and solve problems as well as improve memory. Practitioners of Ayurvedic medicine who are familiar with these outcomes often recommend it for patients who are starting to experience memory loss. Studies on rats have shown that it improves cognitive function.

❧ STRESS

Ashwagandha appears to help the body cope with the effects of stress more effectively. I am sure that ashwagandha will become as popular as the ginsengs in helping to deal with this all-too-common problem. A double-blind, placebo-controlled human clinical trial where people had been subjected to high levels of chronic stress prior to initiation of the study found that ashwagandha extract had remarkable antistress effects. Researchers found those taking ashwagandha had a 69.9% reduction in an overall measure of stress-related symptoms while those on placebo had no significant change. Significant improvements of stress-related symptoms included irritability, anxiety, insomnia, inability to concentrate, fatigue, sweating, headaches, and muscle pain, as well as heart palpitations. In addition, ashwagandha was shown to significantly lower the stress hormone cortisol while elevating the adrenal hormone DHEA, an effect that is healthy in combating long-term stress.

Astragalus

Jerry had been undergoing chemotherapy for cancer, and he fully understood the ramifications of continued treatment. In addition to side effects such as nausea, chemotherapy contributes to a breakdown of the immune system.

Without question, Jerry was going to continue chemotherapy treatments to control and, hopefully, eradicate the cancer. But at the same time, he wondered what he could do to help protect his immune system while the treatments continued.

I had been down this road many times before, so I was prepared for the question of what Jerry should take to help tolerate the ravages of chemotherapy. As I explained to him, it's especially important to make sure the concentrations of good immune cells, known as white blood cells, don't fall too low. If those immune cells are deficient, serious secondary infections can set in.

"My recommendation is astragalus root," I told him.

This Chinese herb (*Astragalus membranaceus*) is one of the best long-term immune tonics. It is commonly used in China, Japan, and—now—some North American hospitals to protect people against the side effects of chemotherapy treatments.

Acting on my suggestion, Jerry immediately began taking the recommended dose. He reported that his cancer doctors were surprised at how well he tolerated his chemotherapy treatments over the next few months.

After the round of treatments, when his cancer appeared to be in remission, Jerry approached me once again.

"Should I stop taking it?"

My answer was immediate. "No way!"

In fact, I recommended some other detoxifying and immune-building supplements to reinforce and enhance the benefits of the astragalus root. "You need to continue to build your immune system," I reminded him. We mapped out a supplement regimen that would continue for more than a year—both to buttress his immune system and help prevent a recurrence of cancer.

CHINESE TREASURE

Having been trained in Oriental medicine, I have a tremendous respect for the healing powers of Chinese herbs. Among the most treasured of these herbs is astragalus, also known as Huang Qi.

Roughly translated, Huang Qi means yellow energy. The suffusion of energy is suggested by the yellow color of the root, which grows wild in northern China, Taiwan, Mongolia, Japan, and Korea. (In recent years, astragalus has also been grown commercially in North America.) As with many Asian herbs, astragalus has been used for its medicinal properties for more than 1,000 years.

In traditional Chinese medicine, herbalists and Asian doctors prescribe astragalus to help prevent colds and upper respiratory tract infections. It's effective with people who are susceptible to asthma. It's also known as a remedy for poor appetite, weak digestion, and diabetes.

Practitioners of traditional Chinese medicine sometimes recommend astragalus for organ prolapse—that is, conditions like prolapsed uterus or hemorrhoids. In addition, it acts as a natural diuretic, helping to excrete excess fluids and relieve conditions such as edema. Astragalus is also known to heal ulcerations of the skin and help with the underlying cause of weak muscles (due to poor digestion).

As with most Chinese herbs, astragalus is generally used in a formula that's made up of a blend of herbs, and it's a perfectly good addition to soup or rice. In fact, in China, it's not uncommon to use astragalus root as a standard ingredient in cooking.

ACTIVE CONSTITUENTS

There is not a whole lot known about the exact constituents of astragalus that boost the immune system. Large, sugarlike molecules known as polysaccharides probably help to stimulate the "good" immune cells. Astragalus also contains substances called saponins, which have a similar immunity-enhancing effect.

IMMUNE TONIC

Astragalus is one of the best herbs in the world for enhancing the protective effects of the immune system. How does it actually work? Similar to echinacea, astragalus increases the levels of certain immune cells that fight viruses and other microbial intruders. This includes macrophages, which are analogous to a Pac-man that swims around and eats tasty microbes.

Natural killer cells are also activated. These fearless warriors attack and destroy cancer cells and viruses. This is important considering cancer cells develop in our bodies on a daily basis and are kept in check by our immune system.

Astragalus also stimulates the secretion of a powerful antiviral chemical known as interferon, which prevents viruses from replicating. One eye-opening study looked at 28 people over a two-month period and their levels of interferon. Compared with controls, those receiving astragalus had a significant increase in the production of interferon. In addition, the interferon levels remained elevated for two months after astragalus supplementation ended.

What I find interesting is that, for many years now, medical researchers have been trying to use synthetic versions of interferon for immune system enhancement. People with diseases like cancer and hepatitis C are commonly given interferon, but many are forced to discontinue using it because it produces so many side effects. I would suggest that it's time for researchers to focus on finding the active constituents in herbs like astragalus that stimulate the production of the body's own natural interferon, instead of trying to artificially duplicate it. More conventional studies using the whole herb would be even better.

In addition, it's been shown that astragalus has a supportive effect on bone marrow, the core of the bones where white blood cells mature. Animal studies have shown that astragalus increases the army of white blood cells that are needed to fight invading microbes.

Finally, astragalus boosts the levels of antibodies in the body. Antibodies bind foreign invaders and signal the immune system to destroy the most common intruders—bacteria, viruses, fungi, and other microbes.

DOSAGE

Typical adult dosage for the tincture form is 20 to 30 drops three times daily. If you're taking it in capsule form, the recommended dose is 1,000 mg three times daily.

In traditional Chinese medicine, between 8 to 15 g of the root are decocted—that is, boiled in water to extract the crucial ingredients that support and enhance the immune system.

WHAT ARE THE SIDE EFFECTS?

Very high dosages may cause indigestion. In traditional Chinese medicine, astragalus is not prescribed by itself or in high dosages in formulas when a patient has certain kinds of fevers. It should also be used with caution in those with autoimmune disease. Otherwise, it is considered a safe herb to use at all times.

ASTRAGALUS
RECOMMENDATIONS FROM THE NATURAL PHYSICIAN FOR . . .

◄ CANCER

Astragalus is often a key herb in both Chinese and Western herbal formulas for immune support for people with cancer because it enhances the activity of immune cells such as macrophages and natural killer cells that are known to destroy cancer cells.

In one interesting study at the University of Texas Medical Center in Houston, researchers found that astragalus enhanced or restored the function of white blood cells that were taken from people with cancer. In fact, some of the damaged cells were so much improved that they became more active than normal cells taken from people who were cancer free.

As I've mentioned, though, astragalus is rarely administered as a solo cure—and this presents a challenge when we try to figure out what the herb does by itself.

(continued)

Historically, the herb is just one of a blend of Chinese herbs that, together, stimulate immunity. In my own experience, these traditional blends are the most effective. Nonetheless, I have seen patients improve when they only took astragalus, and some studies do find that it's effective by itself.

More commonly, astragalus is used the way Jerry used it—to reduce the side effects of chemotherapy drugs. In Chinese and Japanese oncology hospitals, doctors often rely upon astragalus to reduce the potentially damaging effects of chemotherapy by helping bone marrow produce more white blood cells. Preliminary studies demonstrate that astragalus taken in conjunction with glossy privet (*Ligustrum lucidum*) may increase survival rates in patients being treated conventionally for breast cancer.

Also, astragalus appears to have a protective effect on the liver. In one study, astragalus helped protect the liver against the toxin carbon tetrachloride.

✎ COMMON COLD AND UPPER RESPIRATORY TRACT INFECTIONS

Astragalus is an excellent herb if you're prone to frequent colds and upper respiratory tract infections like bronchitis. One Chinese study looked at 1,000 people with lowered immunity and found they experienced fewer colds, with less-severe symptoms, when they took astragalus either in the form of a nasal spray or a tablet. Reviewing studies like this makes me realize that an herb like astragalus can save a person a lot of time from missed work and family time. It has also been shown to be effective in the treatment of chronic bronchitis.

✎ DIGESTION

Astragalus is known to be a digestive tonic in Chinese medicine. While I have never seen it used by itself for the treatment of digestive disorders, it is an integral component of traditional Chinese digestive formulas.

B

Bach Flower Remedies

"I get very uptight and restless when I fly," said Tina. "Can you recommend something to calm me down? I'm taking a four-hour flight tomorrow, and I don't want to take sleep medication."

"I can recommend the Bach Flower Rescue Remedy," I said. "I'm confident that it will calm you down and help you relax on the plane."

This homeopathic combination of different flower and plant extracts is well known in the natural health field for its ability to calm people (and even pets) during emotional situations.

A few weeks later, Tina reported that regular doses of the Rescue Remedy kept her calm during the flight.

I have found the Rescue Remedy also works well to prevent jet lag. I add 10 drops to a bottle of water and sip it during the flight. Many friends and patients have reported that it works well for them, too.

GIFTS FROM THE GARDEN

In the early 1900s, Dr. Edward Bach developed what he called "the Bach Flower Remedies" from flower and plant extracts. His focus was to find a gentle system of medicine that released emotional blockages and restored emotional and physical health to the patient.

Dr. Bach developed 38 different remedies, each addressing a different emotional state. These gentle extracts have been remarkably effective in promoting emotional healing.

If you are having problems with emotional issues that do not seem to be getting resolved, Bach flower remedies are worth trying. Many patients tell me they have a synergistic effect with their counseling. Others tell me the remedies have helped them break through emotional issues that counseling could not help. I do not recommend Bach flower remedies as a substitute for counseling—but, in my experience, they work well when they're used as supplemental therapy to effective counseling.

These remedies can also help relieve physical ailments. For example, people suffering from stress-induced digestive problems notice a lessening of their symptoms when using the Bach flower stress-related remedies.

DOSAGE

Bach flower remedies come in liquid solutions. The typical dosage is 5 to 15 drops as needed for relief of emotional stress. For long-term use, the remedies are usually taken two to three times daily. For best effect, I recommend you wait at least 10 minutes after eating before taking the remedies.

Many practitioners combine different Bach flower remedies to address multiple issues that patients may be facing. For example, a widow may be given sweet chestnut for feelings of despair combined with the flower remedy heather, which is used for feelings of loneliness.

WHAT ARE THE SIDE EFFECTS?

As with other homeopathic preparations, side effects are not really an issue. The most important aspect of the remedies is to pick the one remedy (or the group of remedies) that best addresses the underlying emotional imbalance.

SELECTING BACH FLOWER REMEDIES

Pick the Bach flower remedy from Table 2 that best matches your emotional symptoms. If more than one of the remedies matches your symptoms, then combine 5 drops of each remedy in a glass of water. The longer you've had an emotional imbalance, the longer you'll need to take the Bach flower remedies. Health-food stores and some pharmacies carry Bach flower remedies.

TABLE 2
Bach Flower Remedies

FLOWER REMEDY	EMOTIONAL THEME
Agrimony	Suppressed grief
Aspen	Fear and anxiety
Beech	Critical and intolerant
Centaury	Weak-willed and seeks praise of others
Cerato	Lack of confidence
Cherry Plum	Fear of losing control
Chestnut Bud	Repeating old patterns
Chicory	Controlling others
Clematis	Lack of motivation and concentration
Crab Apple	Poor self-image
Elm	Feeling of inadequacy, overwhelmed
Gentian	Self-doubt and discouragement
Gorse	Hopelessness
Heather	Loneliness
Holly	Negative feelings
Honeysuckle	Dwelling in the past
Hornbeam	Fatigue of mind and body
Impatiens	Impatience
Larch	Lack of self-confidence
Mimulus	Fear
Mustard	Unexplainable sadness that comes and goes

FLOWER REMEDY	EMOTIONAL THEME
Oak	Struggling against the odds and not giving up
Olive	Mental and physical exhaustion
Pine	Unsatisfaction
Red Chestnut	Overly fearful for others
Rock Rose	States of terror, such as nightmares
Rock Water	People too strict with themselves
Scleranthus	Indecisive
Star of Bethlehem	Emotional trauma
Sweet Chestnut	Despair
Vervain	Argumentative
Vine	Strong-willed to the point of dictatorial
Walnut	Emotional adjustments
Water Violet	Independent
White Chestnut	Persistent worry
Wild Oat	Unfulfilled ambitions
Wild Rose	Indifferent
Willow	Bitterness

B-Complex Vitamins

B-complex vitamins include B1 (thiamin), B2 (riboflavin), B3 (niacin), B5 (pantothenic acid), B6 (pyridoxine), B12 (cobalamin), folic acid, and biotin.

I often refer to these B vitamins as the stress or energy vitamins. However, they do far more than just combat stress and improve energy levels. B vitamins are also effective in preventing certain types of birth defects, cancer, and heart disease, among other conditions.

A patient of mine brought her 75-year-old mother, Dolly, to see me.

"My mother's memory is deteriorating," Theresa told me. "Her doctor said she has age-related memory impairment. It's really bad now. She can't remember where she leaves things and has trouble remembering people's names."

"Did he suggest any course of treatment?" I asked.

"He said there wasn't much he could offer. It's just normal aging."

When I ordered a test to check Dolly's B12 and folic acid levels, I discovered that her B12 level was very low. I had Dolly use a supplement of sublingual B12 (2 mg daily) that also included folic acid. I also recommended an herbal formula that stimulated stomach acid and improved digestive function, as I knew Dolly was probably not getting adequate vitamin absorption from her foods.

Two months later, Dolly returned to my office with her daughter.

"I noticed a great improvement in my mother's memory!" Theresa exclaimed excitedly.

I had Dolly continue the B12 folic acid

supplement for another six months, and then was able to reduce the dosage in half as a maintenance dosage.

RATING: B MINUS

Many people in our society are deficient in one or more of the B vitamins. There are a variety of reasons for this. In a general sense, many of us do not get enough of the B vitamins because we eat refined grains. We lose a high degree of B vitamins when the outer shell of grain kernels is milled.

Another reason is that many of us have a lifestyle that promotes the excretion of B vitamins; for example, we drink coffee and alcohol. In addition, certain medications (birth-control pills, seizure and acid suppressing medications, and steroid medications, to name a few) can also lead to specific B-vitamin deficiencies. Mental stress and physical activity also lead to a greater need for the Bs.

B vitamins are best taken together, hence the term "B-complex." Taking one of the B vitamins by itself for long periods of time may lead to an imbalance in other B vitamins.

There are certain conditions, though, for which high single doses of one or more of the B vitamins are required for therapeutic effects. For example, high dosages of B6 are needed to relieve the symptoms of carpal tunnel syndrome or morning sickness.

Another common example is niacin, which is used in very high dosages for the treatment of high cholesterol levels. Like vitamin C, the B vitamins are all water-soluble. This means they do not need to be taken with meals to be absorbed (unlike fat-soluble vitamins such as A, D, K, and E, which require fat and bile to be absorbed). Also, water-soluble vitamins are more sensitive to the environment as they are more easily lost during cooking and storage.

AGE PROOF

On a microscopic level, aging occurs in large part due to the deterioration of our genes and their ability to provide accurate instructions to cells. This is like having genetic instructions increasingly filled with typos. A solid nutritional foundation protects our genes and slows down this deterioration.

For example, studies show that low levels of B vitamins like folic acid and B12 actually increase gene damage, and that damage is reduced when people consume more of these vitamins. Likewise, Bruce Ames, PhD, of the Children's Hospital Oakland Research Institute in Oakland, California, found that low intake of folic acid and magnesium interfere with normal gene-repair mechanisms resulting in more mutations. More mutations translate to faster aging and a greater risk of disease. Ames has amassed a wealth of scientific data showing that 50 inherited diseases can be improved by taking B vitamins and other supplements.

DOSAGE

B-complex vitamins come in two standard dosages—50 mg and 100 mg. I recommend 50 mg as the daily dosage for most patients because the majority of people I see are already taking a multivitamin, which has B vitamins in it. Therapeutic dosages of individual B vitamins are given in specific profiles for each that follow.

B12 and folic acid are also commonly available in sublingual (under the tongue) form, which gets absorbed directly into the bloodstream from the mouth. This is good for people who have absorption problems. Also, B vitamins are available in liquid form and by injection.

WHAT ARE THE SIDE EFFECTS?

There are few potential side effects from B vitamins, but some people do get nausea and skin flushing, which is associated with vitamin B3 (niacin).

I have had a few patients who cannot tolerate any amounts of supplemental B vitamins. In these cases, an underlying metabolism problem in the liver is often the root cause. This may be helped with a detoxification program and by using lower doses and gradually increasing the dose. Specific B vitamin recommendations follow.

THE B-COMPLEX ROSTER

～ Vitamin B1 (Thiamin)

Alcoholics are at the biggest risk of having a B1 deficiency. Alcohol use, over time, reduces the absorption of B1 through the intestines—and B1 is needed for alcohol metabolism. A deficiency of B1 due to alcoholism can lead to permanent memory impairment, problems with eye movement, and a condition known as Wenicke's encephalopathy, where psychosis or brain damage can occur.

People with epilepsy who use the seizure medication Dilantin are prone to B1 deficiency, as are people with diabetes, Crohn's disease and other digestive conditions involving malabsorption, and several neurological diseases. In addition, antibiotics are known to deplete thiamin.

A high dietary intake of B1 seems to play a role in preventing cataracts. Additionally, patients with diabetic kidney disease (nepropathy) were found to have better kidney function from B1 supplementation.

People with congestive heart failure on loop diuretics such as furosemide (Lasix) are susceptible to B1 deficiency, which may worsen heart function. Also people with chronic fatigue syndrome are more likely to have B1 deficiency.

Good sources of thiamin are whole wheat products, soy, brown rice, peanuts, sunflower seeds, and milk. Therapeutic dosages range from 50 to 8,000 mg daily.

～ Vitamin B2 (Riboflavin)

Vitamin B2 has become popular for the prevention of migraine headaches. One of the theories about migraine headaches is that they are caused by insufficient energy production within brain cells. Riboflavin is an integral factor in cell energy production. Preliminary studies have shown the benefits of riboflavin. One study compared the effects of riboflavin (400 mg) and a placebo in 55 patients with migraine headaches. Riboflavin was found to reduce the frequency and duration of the headaches. Other supplements shown to reduce frequency of migraines include magnesium and coenzyme Q10.

B2 may be important for cataract prevention. A study using the combination of B2 at a dose of 3 mg plus 40 mg of niacin daily demonstrated a lower risk of developing nuclear cataracts compared to placebo.

Several antibiotics and drugs that treat migraines, such as imipramine, can lead to a B2 deficiency.

Symptoms of a riboflavin deficiency can include cracks in the corners of the mouth, inflammation of the tongue (glossitis), visual problems, and seborrheic dermatitis.

Good sources of riboflavin are organ meats, eggs, whole grains, green leafy vegetables, and almonds. A therapeutic dosage is up to 400 mg for the prevention of migraine headaches.

～ Vitamin B3 (Niacin)

Niacin plays a role in many different functions in the body. It remains one of the cheapest and most effective cholesterol-lowering substances that we know about. It lowers all those blood markers that should be low, such as total cholesterol, LDL (the so-called bad cholesterol), lipoprotein A, triglycerides (fats in the blood), and fibrinogen. At the same time, niacin also increases HDL (the so-called good cholesterol), which transports cholesterol away from the blood vessels to the liver.

One of the side effects of this vitamin, as I've mentioned, is what's called the "niacin flush." I had a patient who came to me for natural treatment to reduce his high cholesterol markers. His blood test showed elevations of most of the cholesterol markers, and his protective HDL was too low. He was started at a beginning dose of 1,500 mg of niacin that was to be increased over time. He had a reaction to the niacin. He became hot and clammy, his skin turned red, and he experienced nausea. He said he felt as if he was having hot flashes.

I prescribed, instead, a nonflushing form of niacin called inositol hexaniacinate (although not as well studied as regular niacin, European physicians have used this form of niacin for decades). He started with a dosage of 2,500 mg daily and never had any reactions. Over the next six months, his cholesterol returned to the normal range. Conventional medicine acknowledges that niacin is a potent lipid treatment. Niacin appears to reduce the production of proteins that transport cholesterol and triglycerides in the blood. No drug has the versatile effects of niacin, which includes its ability to:

LDL cholesterol reduced by 5% to 25%

HDL cholesterol increased by 15% to 35%

Triglycerides decreased by 20% to 50%

There is research showing that people who consume higher amounts of niacin (17–45 mg/day) from food and multivita-

mins have a lower risk of developing Alzheimer's disease compared to people who consume less niacin (14 mg/day).

High dietary intakes of niacin also help prevent cataracts. Good sources of niacin are organ meats, peanuts, poultry, milk, eggs, legumes, and whole-grain products. A therapeutic dosage is from 500 to 3,000 mg.

I advise against using time-released niacin, which can be toxic to the liver. Side effects of niacin may include stomach upset, gas, bloating, vomiting, diarrhea, or nausea (these side effects may be reduced by taking nicotinic acid with food); warmth and flushing of the neck, ears, and face along with itching, tingling, and headache.

High doses of niacin should be avoided by pregnant or nursing mothers.

High doses of niacin rarely elevate blood homocysteine levels, a known risk factor for heart disease. Have your levels monitored by your doctor when taking niacin.

Niacin may slow blood clotting and may need to be discontinued before surgery. Discuss this with your doctor.

A derivative of niacin known as niacinamide has many therapeutic effects. They include the treatment of osteoarthritis (3 g daily) and acne (applied topically in cream form), reducing the risk of type 1 diabetes in high-risk children, and improving insulin secretion in those with type 2 diabetes.

❧ B5 (Pantothenic Acid)

I call B5 the adrenal vitamin. The adrenal glands need pantothenic acid to produce stress hormones. Therefore, when people are under chronic stress, whether it be physical or mental, B5 supports the adrenal glands in producing adequate levels of stress hormones such as cortisol. This enables the body to handle stress successfully.

Other conditions are alleviated with vitamin B5. People with fatigue notice a difference when they take pantothenic acid. Vitamin B5 is also commonly prescribed for allergies. A number of my patients reported that B5 was of great benefit in reducing their allergy symptoms.

A different form of pantothenic acid called pantethine has proven to be effective in lowering total cholesterol, LDL, and triglyceride levels while increasing the good HDL. This supplement can also benefit people with diabetes who have elevated triglyceride levels.

Good sources of vitamin B5 are chicken, fish, eggs, organ meats, whole grains, avocados, and cauliflower. A therapeutic dosage is from 500 to 1,500 mg daily of pantothenic acid, or 900 mg of pantethine. (**NOTE:** Many nutritional adrenal support formulas contain pantothenic acid in combination with other adrenal support supplements such as vitamin C, ginseng, and adrenal glandular.)

❧ Vitamin B6 (Pyridoxine)

Vitamin B6 has a multitude of uses. It is intricately involved in amino acid metabolism. A deficiency in B6 can lead to weakness, confusion, depression, and skin conditions like eczema. Drugs that can cause a B6 deficiency include birth-control pills and antibiotics and theophylline (an asthma medication). Smoking contributes to B6 deficiency as well. B6 has been shown to be effective for alleviating PMS.

Vitamin B6 is also important in reducing the risk of cardiovascular disease. Along with B12, trimethylglycine, and folic acid, B6 helps to lower a toxic component of protein metabolism called homocysteine. This metabolite is a causative factor in approximately 10% of heart attacks.

Another condition that B6 can alleviate is carpal tunnel syndrome. This painful condition involves compression of the main

nerve in the wrist from swelling and inflammation as a result of repetitive work (such as typing or carpentry). Carpal tunnel syndrome can also flare up in pregnancy due to fluid retention.

There are many other conditions that are alleviated with B6—including depression, asthma, water retention, diabetes, epilepsy, and morning sickness (for which I have also used injectable B6 with success). I have also treated patients who were suffering from kidney stones. Vitamin B6, along with magnesium, helps to prevent the buildup of the most common type of kidney stones—those composed of calcium oxalate.

B6 at a dose of 50 to 200 mg reduces homocysteine, a protein metabolite that when elevated increases cardiovascular risk.

Good sources of vitamin B6 are meats, poultry, fish, eggs, walnuts, peanuts, bananas, and whole-grain foods. A therapeutic dosage is 50 to 200 mg. (**NOTE:** Too much B6 supplementation can lead to nerve toxicity. Symptoms may include tingling and changes in coordination. This may happen with dosages above 200 mg. Most reported cases occur in people who have taken dosages of above 500 mg for a prolonged period of time.)

❧ Folic Acid

Folic acid is important for the brain. It can be helpful for those who suffer from depression and poor memory, especially the elderly.

One of the most important functions of folic acid is to prevent neural tube defects in newborns (the incomplete development of the spinal cord and/or the brain) as well as cleft palate. The majority of these defects can be prevented with daily folic-acid supplementation of 400 to 800 mcg. Taking the folic acid before conception gives the best results. It can reduce the risk of a neural tube defect by 60% if taken one month prior to conception and during the first trimester. A deficiency of folic acid can also contribute to depression.

As I mentioned earlier, folic acid is important for preventing the buildup of homocysteine, thus reducing the risk of heart disease in genetically susceptible individuals. In addition, maintaining lower homocysteine levels also helps in preventing osteoporosis.

As with B12, folic acid is required for cell division.

Folic acid deficiency competes with iron for the most common vitamin deficiency in the world. A deficiency of folic acid can lead to anemia, gingivitis, depression, memory problems, and many other symptoms. Drugs that can lead to a deficiency of folic acid include barbiturates, corticosteroids, estrogen, chemotherapy medications such as methotrexate, birth-control pills, antacid medications, and many others. Commonly used nonsteroidal anti-inflammatory drugs (NSAIDs), such as aspirin or ibuprofen, taken in large doses may cause folic acid deficiency. Also, inherited problems with folic acid metabolism are common and can be overcome with supplementation. Depending on the population, 50% of individuals may have inherited one copy (C/T), and 5% to 25% of individuals may have inherited two copies.

Studies show that dietary intake of folic acid as well as supplementation reduces the risk of colorectal cancer, particularly for women with strong family history of colorectal cancer. Doses of greater than 249 mcg for men and 400 mcg for women are most protective. The consumption of dietary folic acid reduces the risk of breast cancer in women. In addition, dietary intake

of folic acid has a protective effect against pancreatic cancer. Also people taking antidepressant medications may get better results by taking folic acid supplementation. The topical application of folic acid can help reduce gingivitis in pregnant women. A study in the Netherlands found that supplementing 800 mcg of folic acid daily slowed the rate of age-related hearing loss. Supplementation has also been shown to reduce the symptoms of vitiligo. Last, nutrition-oriented doctors use folic acid along with B12 for the treatment of precancerous changes of the cervix.

Folic acid is found in high concentrations in green leafy vegetables such as spinach, chard, and kale. Other sources are asparagus, organ meats, orange juice, and whole-grain foods. A therapeutic dosage is 400 to 2,000 mcg.

🐦 B12

Vitamin B12 works in tandem with folic acid for many biochemical processes such as cell division and formation of the myelin sheath (the covering of nerve cells).

Many vitamin users refer to B12 as the energy vitamin. I have seen many patients with fatigue experience tremendous boosts of energy after receiving B12 injections. Other conditions that are alleviated by taking supplemental B12 include asthma, depression, multiple sclerosis, shingles, and chronic fatigue.

B12 is one of the critical nutrients to lower homocysteine, a substance that increases the risk of heart disease.

Drugs known to deplete B12 stores in the body include birth-control pills, stomach acid blockers, antibiotics, and some seizure medications.

A deficiency of B12 will result in anemia. In addition, the nervous system is quite dependent on adequate levels of B12. Memory loss is a symptom, especially in the elderly. As a matter of fact, physicians have reported cases of suspected dementia that actually turned out to be B12 deficiencies, which were improved with B12 supplements. British researchers assessed mental function of 1,562 men and women, ages 65 and older, three times over a 10-year period. Participants who had greater imbalances in these two blood markers showed faster cognitive decline. Their conclusion was that B12 supplementation could slow cognitive decline by one-third.

We know that brain degeneration is associated with Alzheimer's disease and is used as a marker for the disease's progression. Researchers from England, Norway, and Australia examined 107 men and women ages 61 to 87 without cognitive impairment at the beginning of a five-year study. Blood tests to assess vitamin B12 status and magnetic resonance imaging (MRI) scans of the brain were conducted annually. Researchers found those with the highest vitamin B12 levels were six times less likely to lose brain volume than those with the lowest levels.

Other signs of B12 deficiency include a beefy, red tongue and diarrhea. Blood and urine tests can be done to evaluate the levels of B12 in the body.

Vegetarians may require B12 supplementation as animal foods contain the highest quantities. They can take whole-food supplements such as spirulina and chlorella, which contain B12, or a B-complex supplement can be taken on a regular basis. Approximately 20% of seniors in the United States have a vitamin B12 deficiency. The ability to absorb this nutrient can diminish as people age. This certainly can predispose them to mood, fatigue, memory, and other problems. The solution is to take supplemental B12. The most effective method is either a B12 injection once monthly or the regular consumption of sublingual B12, which is absorbed in the veins underneath the tongue.

One study found an effective treatment for people with chronic fatigue is twice weekly injections of B12 at a dose of 5 mg. I have verified B12 injections do help patients with chronic fatigue even when their blood B12 levels are normal.

Other food sources of vitamin B12 are liver, eggs, fish, cheese, milk, meat, dark green leafy vegetables, asparagus, organ meats, orange juice, and whole-grain foods. A therapeutic dosage is 400 to 2,000 mcg.

❧ Biotin

Biotin is a B vitamin known for its benefit to nails and hair. It is manufactured by *Bifidobacterium bifidus*, a group of friendly bacteria that reside in the intestines. Therefore, a suspected biotin deficiency in an infant or adult should also be treated with probiotic supplements containing these helpful and necessary bacteria. As the bifidus bacteria in the intestines manufacture biotin, it is logical that antibiotics can deplete body stores of biotin.

Biotin is also helpful for cradle cap, also known as seborrheic dermatitis. Yellow scales that may be greasy or dry form on the scalp of an infant or adult. Many cases of infant cradle cap have been reported to respond to biotin supplementation. Of course, you must check with your pediatrician before giving any supplement to your baby.

Studies have shown that biotin supplementation can be helpful for improving blood-sugar control in both type 1 and type 2 diabetes. It has also been shown to help peripheral neuropathy for those with diabetes. Also biotin can help improve the thickness of the nails in those with preexisting brittle nails. Nutrition-oriented doctors like me use biotin for hair loss or thinning hair. It can also be used topically in commonly available shampoos.

Good sources of biotin are brewer's yeast, liver and other organ meats, milk, cheese, soybeans, eggs, cauliflower, mushrooms, and whole-wheat products. A therapeutic dosage to strengthen nails and hair in adults is 1,000 to 3,000 mcg daily. For cradle cap, a breast-feeding mother can take 6,000 mcg daily or the infant can be given 200 to 300 mcg daily.

Bee Pollen

I can usually figure out a way to help my patients when they complain of allergy problems. There are many good remedies for hay fever symptoms—the sinus pressure, headache, fatigue, runny nose, sneezing, and itchy nose that seriously impinge on your quality of life. But one spring, when I had exactly those symptoms myself, I found it impossible to come up with natural treatments that were any help at all. I was just plain miserable—and, I'll admit, more than a little humbled by the fact that I couldn't heal myself.

Of all the remedies that I'd considered for myself, however, there was still one that I hadn't tried. Some colleagues, and even a number of patients, had told me that bee pollen products had helped them to relieve or cure their allergies.

Up to that point, I'd had no reason to use or recommend bee pollen. On the other hand, I'd never been so taxed for ideas. I wasn't having any success at all with the homeopathic and nutritional supplements that normally worked so well. So why shouldn't I test bee pollen on myself?

I began to take bee pollen capsules. The product I used was harvested from a bee farm in Peace River, Alberta.

Typically, people are advised to take 2 to 4 capsules daily of bee pollen for a therapeutic effect. Being an aggressive supplement taker, I started at 8 capsules daily. On the first day of use, I did not notice any change in symptoms, but by the sixth day, most of my hay fever symptoms had disappeared.

Ecstatic with the results, I was still fearful that my symptoms would come back, so I stayed on a regimen of 8 capsules per day, which is about double the dose that's usually recommended. (Bee pollen is nontoxic, so I knew I was perfectly safe taking the higher dosage.) When I remained allergy-free, I decided to try a reduced dose, and within three weeks I was down to 4 capsules per day. Still, no symptoms—so in another week, I reduced my dosage to 2 capsules daily.

I stayed on the 2-capsules-a-day schedule for another two months, then stopped taking the bee pollen. I knew there was a risk of the symptoms returning because I'm in an area (San Diego) where there are different types of pollens all year round. But the hay fever was gone for good.

THE BUZZ ABOUT POLLEN

Produced by flowering plants, pollen clings to bees as they go about their business of gathering nectar. It's sometimes referred to as "nature's superfood" because it includes a wide spectrum of nutrients, from vitamins A and C to the B-complex vitamins and amino acids. Among the other nutrients are carotenoids, calcium, magnesium, copper, iron, potassium, and flavonoids such as rutin and quercetin—all of which are believed to give bee pollen a large part of its antiallergy effect. In addition, it contains those hard-to-get trace minerals such as silicon, molybdenum, boron, and sulfur. It also contains life-sustaining enzymes and plant hormone structures known as sterols, which are thought to have hormone-balancing effects.

Bee pollen is used to treat or prevent many different conditions, from arthritis and allergies to depression and fatigue. Many people who are active in sports rely on bee pollen to increase their energy and endurance. It is said to have benefits for the reproductive system as well.

DOSAGE

The typical adult dosage for chronic health conditions is 2 capsules daily (equivalent to 500 to 1,000 mg). For the relief of acute symptoms, higher dosages of 4 to 8 capsules or more may be used, as long as there are none of the side effects mentioned below.

WHAT ARE THE SIDE EFFECTS?

The most talked-about concern is that people who are allergic to bee stings should not use bee pollen. Experts state that bee pollen allergies are quite rare—but they do occur, and in some cases can be quite severe. If you've ever had an allergic reaction to bee stings, avoid bee pollen completely.

A small percentage of users may also experience digestive upset.

Even if you've never had an allergic reaction to bee stings, I'd advise that you test a very small amount of bee pollen— just to make sure—before you take a whole capsule. Open one capsule and place a small amount of the powder on your tongue. If you have any allergic symptoms at all—such as wheezing or a rash—don't take any more.

Some bee pollen products are tainted with contaminants from air pollution (pesticides, herbicides) and environmental chemicals (heavy metals). Therefore, I advise that you only use a product from a company that uses a quality bee pollen source and tests their product to make absolutely sure it is not contaminated.

BEE POLLEN
RECOMMENDATIONS FROM THE NATURAL PHYSICIAN FOR . . .

❧ ALLERGIES

It is thought that the pollens in bee pollen have a desensitizing effect on the immune system. In other words, you may be allergic to certain pollens that are in very small concentrations in the pollen that bees have collected. When you take bee pollen, your immune system starts to become desensitized to the point where you can tolerate more of these pollens, with less allergic reaction. Essentially the bee pollen has a homeopathic effect.

❧ ARTHRITIS

After one lecture, I met a 64-year-old man who appeared healthy and full of vitality. Ten years before, he said, he had visited a naturopathic doctor for treatment of rheumatoid arthritis. By the time he went to see that doctor, his arthritis was so bad that he couldn't even walk. He was in a wheelchair.

As he told his story, his wife stood beside him nodding her head in agreement.

(continued)

"When did you get better?" I asked, since his condition had obviously improved.

He told me his doctor had given him a bottle of bee pollen and specified a daily dose. The man was told to return to the clinic in two weeks.

In those two weeks, he recalled, his symptoms improved so much that he was able to walk into the doctor's office on his own.

Needless to say, I had just met a great believer in bee pollen. Since then I have paid more attention to this remedy and have met a number of people who have had success with it. While the effects are not so dramatic for everyone with arthritis, bee pollen is used by natural health-care practitioners around the world to help alleviate arthritis symptoms.

ENERGY BOOST

Bee pollen is a popular supplement among many athletes, who report that it helps them train hard and recover quickly. Many athletes report that it helps increase stamina.

IMMUNE SUPPORT

Bee pollen is reported to help strengthen the immune system. People susceptible to recurring colds and respiratory tract infections may be helped.

Since bee pollen is so high in nutrients, you might want to take it if you're detoxifying. When you detoxify, you reduce the intake of foods that normally keep your immune system in good working order.

Bilberry

"The eye doctor says my eyes are going bad. I guess it's just part of aging," said 72-year-old Maureen.

"Oh, a lot of things get blamed on aging," I said. "Tell me more about your eyes."

"Well, I can't read as well as I used to," Maureen continued. "But what really bothers me is that my doctor said I am developing bad cataracts. He said if they get worse over the next year or two I will need cataract surgery, and I don't want surgery of any kind!"

"Let me take a look," I said.

While examining Maureen's eyes through my ophthalmoscope, I could see clouding in the lenses of each. But I didn't think surgery was called for—and told her that.

"Compared to a lot of people your age, your eyes look pretty good. If we get you on a good, comprehensive protocol now we should be able to halt any further progression of the cataracts."

"What is it that can help me?" asked Maureen.

"Lots of good things," I said. "You need to increase the fruits and vegetables in your diet, and take some antioxidant supplements. One of the main supplements you need to take on a regular basis is bilberry."

Fortunately, it was easy to convince Maureen to try this herb. She had already heard about it from a friend, and was wondering about its effectiveness. What I told her confirmed her assumption that it would be helpful.

Ten months later, Maureen had her eyes examined by an ophthalmologist. She was told that her cataracts had not worsened at all, and, if anything, had slightly improved. There was no doubt in my mind that bilberry extract was benefiting Maureen.

TRIED AND TRUE BLUE

Bilberry (*Vaccinium myrtillus*, European blueberry) is one of the more popular herbs in Europe and North America. Millions of Europeans are fond of bilberry jam, and many eat the berries. Thousands rely on it for its medicinal benefit for the eyes and as a tonic to the circulatory system.

Bilberry fruit has been used medicinally since the Middle Ages; historically, for the treatment of scurvy. (Bilberry is high in vitamin C and flavonoids.) Bilberry leaves and the fruit are also known to have an astringent effect. This is why it was and still is used today for diarrhea and urinary tract infections. It is also used medicinally for diabetes, varicose veins, and other circulation-related conditions.

The German Commission E, the government-backed medical board in Germany that helps regulate herbal medicine, lists bilberry as a treatment for acute diarrhea, and mild inflammation of the mucous membranes of the mouth and throat. Modern interest in bilberry was sparked during World War II when British Royal Air Force pilots reported that consuming bilberry jam improved their nighttime vision and accuracy on bombing missions. Almost 20 years later, scientists began studies on bilberry and its benefit for the eyes.

A POTENT SPECIAL PIGMENT

Researchers have concluded that potent antioxidants called anthocyanosides are responsible for many of the healing properties of bilberry. This antioxidant effect reduces cellular damage and breakdown. As a result, anthocyanosides improve circulation through the smallest areas of circulation—through the capillaries.

Bilberry actually strengthens the capillary walls, thus preventing easy bruising, bleeding, varicose veins, and poor circulation. In addition, improved circulation allows valuable nutrients to flow efficiently to specialized structures such as the retina of the eye. This is why visual problems such as cataracts, macular degeneration, and poor night vision can be prevented and treated with bilberry.

The special pigment in bilberry also has a natural anti-inflammatory effect, making it potentially useful for conditions such as rheumatoid arthritis.

DOSAGE

For most adults, I recommend a standardized extract containing 25% anthocyanosides, at 160 mg twice daily. For adults with more severe problems, the dosage may be increased to 160 mg three times daily. For example, for a case of inflamed varicose veins (phlebitis), a dosage of 480 mg daily should be taken for a week or longer until the inflammation calms down, and then 320 mg can be taken as a maintenance dosage. Most of my patients notice improvement with 320 mg and take bilberry on a long-term basis.

Bilberry is most commonly taken in capsule form. It is also available as a tincture and in tablet form as well. As I mentioned, people in Europe use bilberry as a fruit the way we use its cousin, the blueberry, but it takes a lot of fruit to equal one capsule: You'd have to eat three bowls of bilberry fruit to equal what is found in 320 mg of a standardized extract!

My guess is that blueberries have very similar properties to bilberry. Studies have shown that blueberries are also high in antioxidants.

Incidentally, these same types of antioxidants are found in red grapes, which have been shown to reduce the risk of heart disease.

(Both red wine and red grape juice, containing these antioxidants, are often recommended.)

WHAT ARE THE SIDE EFFECTS?

There is no known toxicity with bilberry. It does have a blood-thinning effect, however.

Therefore, if you are on blood-thinning medication, let your doctor know that you are taking bilberry. This may require your doctor to prescribe a lower dosage of the pharmaceutical blood thinner you are taking.

BILBERRY

RECOMMENDATIONS FROM THE NATURAL PHYSICIAN FOR . . .

❧ CATARACTS

Cataract surgery is very common in the United States. Oxidative damage from sunlight exposure is the leading cause of cataracts. Bilberry and its antioxidant properties are well recommended for those with cataracts.

Of course, it makes more sense to take it on a preventative basis or in the early stages of cataract development rather than waiting until the onset of cataracts. I also recommend antioxidants, such as vitamins A, C, E, selenium, carotenoids, zinc, and a few others, to be taken for the treatment of cataracts, along with bilberry, for a more aggressive treatment.

The power of bilberry and vitamin E in preventing the progression of cataracts was shown in a randomized, double-blind, placebo-controlled study. This high-quality study found that the combination of bilberry (360 mg) and vitamin E (100 mg) daily for four months prevented the progression of cataracts in 97% of 50 people with mild senile cataracts. As an added bonus, no side effects were reported. This study is encouraging as it demonstrates that a lot of people with early-stage cataracts could avoid surgery with safe supplements such as bilberry and vitamin E.

❧ DIARRHEA

European doctors recommend bilberry for the treatment of acute diarrhea, although I have never used it for this. It is said to have an astringent effect on the mucous membranes, thus relieving diarrhea. The German Commission E recommends it for "nonspecific, acute diarrhea."

❧ EYESTRAIN

Many of my patients report eyestrain and headaches from working on their computers all day long. Most people notice their eyes feel much better after they take bilberry. Patients tell me their vision improves, their eyes get less tired and bloodshot, and they are less prone to headaches. Bilberry is quite helpful for anyone who has to spend long hours in front of a computer screen. (But for anyone who has to sit in front of a computer many hours a day, I also recommend the new flat computer screens—which emit less radiation—and advise taking regular breaks.)

❧ GLAUCOMA

Glaucoma is a disease that causes pressure to build up in the tissues of the eye. This is the result of fluid not being able to drain properly out of the eye chambers.

Glaucoma is a serious condition and is the second leading cause of blindness after macular degeneration. Bilberry may have a protective effect against glaucoma by improving the strength of the eye tissues. Although I have not seen any studies supporting this, many holistic physicians recommend bilberry for this condition.

HEMORRHOIDS

Bilberry strengthens the capillary walls, thus preventing the buildup of fluid in the blood vessels and surrounding tissues. In addition, it promotes circulation through the blood vessels. These actions make bilberry effective for the prevention and treatment of hemorrhoids.

I was impressed by a study that examined 51 pregnant women who took bilberry extract. Bilberry significantly improved the pain, burning, and itching associated with their hemorrhoids. After reading this study, I now consider bilberry for the prevention and treatment of hemorrhoids and varicose veins in pregnant patients.

MACULAR DEGENERATION

The macula is the portion of the retina in the back of the eye responsible for fine vision. Degeneration of the macula leads to a slow or sudden loss of central vision. Macular degeneration is the leading cause of blindness in people 55 years and older.

There are two types of macular degeneration—dry and wet. There is hemorrhaging of blood vessels in the wet type. Bilberry treatment is most indicated for the dry type, which is more common. Free radical damage from smoking and sunlight appears to be the underlying cause of macular degeneration. Risk factors also include hypertension and atherosclerosis. Bilberry's antioxidant effect may offer protection against macular degeneration.

A protocol of antioxidants (such as lutein, zinc, carotenoids, vitamins C and A, and grape seed), along with bilberry and ginkgo extract is what I routinely recommend to people with this condition.

NIGHT VISION

Research has shown that bilberry improves energy production in the eye, critical to good night vision. Bilberry extract demonstrated significant improvements in pilots' speed-adaptation ability to light changes. While one study has challenged this assumption, we know that bilberry has been helpful for people in the past. Since it's nontoxic, there's no reason why you shouldn't try it for a while to find out whether it improves your night vision.

RETINOPATHY

Bilberry fruit has shown to be of benefit for those with disease of the retina, as is commonly found in those with diabetes or high blood pressure.

VARICOSE VEINS

Many of my female patients over the age of 40 want natural treatments for varicose veins. Bilberry improves circulation, so it's certainly one of the better herbs to use. In the same study where researchers studied the ability of bilberry supplements to reduce hemorrhoid symptoms in pregnant women, doctors saw that it improved varicose veins as well.

My patients who use bilberry for varicose veins report that it noticeably improves the appearance of their veins and prevents them from getting worse. Bilberry works nicely in combination with the herb horse chestnut and grape seed (or Pycnogenol) extract for varicose veins.

Black Cohosh

"I have a hot flash every hour of the day; it's driving me crazy! The doctors I have seen all recommend hormones. I assume there is something else you can recommend?"

Kristy, a 50-year-old patient of mine, was going through the transition of menopause and wanted nothing to do with the standard prescription of synthetic hormones.

I asked whether she had heard of the herb black cohosh.

"Well, yes," said Kristy, "but does it actually work? Remember, I am having hot flashes all day long, I need something strong!"

"I don't think you will be disappointed."

I talked to Kristy two weeks later, and she said her hot flashes had decreased to a frequency of about three a day. Then I followed up again, about six weeks after she began treatment. Kristy reported she no longer had any hot flashes at all. As an added bonus, she also had less depression and insomnia—two problems that had started when she began menopause.

These are the kinds of results I have come to expect from black cohosh. As you will read, this menopause-specific herb is effective in other areas as well.

A Closer Look

Black cohosh (*Cimifuga racemosa*) is also known as "black snakeroot" because of its black roots—the part of the plant that's used for medicinal purposes. This member of the buttercup family grows wild in the eastern forests of the United States. Other similar species grow in China, Japan, Korea, and Siberia. Commercial black cohosh farms in Europe now supply much of the raw materials for the North American herbal industry.

Native American Indians—particularly the Iroquois and Cherokees—used black cohosh for many different reasons including menstrual cramps, childbirth, arthritis and sore muscles, coughs and upper respiratory tract complaints, and snakebites. It was also used by "eclectic medical doctors," as practitioners of herbal medicine were called in the 1800s and early 1900s. Naturopathic doctors also used it later on in the early 1900s for headaches, heart conditions, and as a digestive tonic. Black cohosh is also known as "bugbane," since the strong smell of the flowers works as a natural insect repellent.

Black cohosh was imported to Germany in the early 1900s. Since the 1940s, German research has heavily influenced the various uses and scientific validation of black cohosh. Today, black cohosh is the most popular herbal treatment for the symptomatic relief of menopausal symptoms. It can be found everywhere—in health-food stores, pharmacies, grocery stores, and even on the Internet.

Active Ingredients

Most of the studies done on black cohosh have used an extract containing 2.5% triterpene glycosides that include the markers actein and cimicifugoside. Researchers disagree on exactly how black cohosh relieves menopausal symptoms. There is some literature that supports the idea that taking black cohosh lowers the hormone LH (lutenizing hormone).

During menopause, estrogen and progesterone levels drop, while the pituitary gland increases levels of the hormone LH. The rise in LH is believed to be one of the causes of menopausal symptoms. The inhibition of LH release by the pituitary gland is a leading factor in the relief of menopausal symptoms.

Some researchers feel that estrogen-balancing chemicals in black cohosh—known as "phytoestrogens"—may act to relieve menopausal symptoms as well, but recent research has not shown this to be the case.

DOSAGE

Black cohosh supplements are available in capsule, tablet, and tincture form. The tea form is also available, though it's not commonly used.

As a standard dosage, I recommend a black cohosh extract standardized to 2.5% triterpene glycosides. The typical dosage used in studies for the relief of menopausal symptoms was 80 mg of the tablet or 80 drops of tincture. Most women notice improvement within four weeks of starting supplementation. Other women can notice improvement with as little as 20 to 40 mg of a black cohosh extract.

For severe menopausal symptoms or for women who do not see improvement at 80 mg, I recommend using 160 mg daily. In time, usually after six months or longer, the daily dosage may be reduced to 80 mg. A similar dosage can be used for other conditions such as fibromyalgia or arthritis.

LENGTH OF USE

The duration of menopausal symptoms varies from woman to woman. I have had women tell me they have been having hot flashes and other menopausal symptoms for more than five years.

How long can you take black cohosh? Many books quote the German Commission E, which states that black cohosh should not be used for more than six months. The commission's recommendation appears to be based on the fact that no studies have yet shown whether side effects occur with long-term use. However, it is important to note that there is no information showing that long-term use is detrimental.

Historically, black cohosh has been used for long periods of time without problems. I have to disagree with the commission on this one. I and other experts in the field of herbal medicine find no problem with prescribing black cohosh on a long-term basis. It is no doubt safer than long-term hormone replacement therapy.

WHAT ARE THE SIDE EFFECTS?

Though side effects are uncommon, a small percentage of users get digestive upset. This may be corrected by taking black cohosh with food.

Clinical studies involving more than 1,700 patients over a three- to six-month period showed excellent tolerance of black cohosh. Using higher dosages than I recommend may result in headaches and dizziness. Black cohosh should not be used during pregnancy or while breast-feeding.

The media got all worked up from a negative black cohosh report from the Australian Therapeutic Goods Administration (ATGA), a regulatory body in that country. It announced that it had become concerned about a possible relationship between black cohosh and liver disease. The mainstream American media got ahold of this story and, in some cases, has chosen to portray black cohosh as dangerous. But is there any merit to this warning by the ATGA? Let's take a look at how Australian regulators reached their conclusion about black cohosh. They cited 47 reports of liver toxicity among black cohosh users that were collected worldwide. In Australia, four patients were hospitalized, and two of these required liver transplants. But the ATGA did not disclose what criteria it used to interpret the data. For example, the ATGA didn't say what brands or dosages of black cohosh products were involved in the cases or whether the products were analyzed to confirm their content. Some of the products involved in the ATGA's report contained a variety of herbs, not just black cohosh. All these factors make it difficult to judge the merit of the ATGA's warning.

What's more, in a contradictory statement, the ATGA wrote, "Considering the widespread use of black cohosh, the incidence of liver reaction appears to be very low." This statement comports with a 2004 finding by the US National Institutes of Health that there was no evidence that black cohosh causes liver toxicity.

CANCER SAFETY ISSUES

Studies have shown that black cohosh is safe to use by women with a history of breast or uterine cancer. For example, one study showed that black cohosh does not have the same effects that estrogen does—that is, the breast cancer cells whose growth is dependent on estrogen were not stimulated by black cohosh. As a matter of fact, just the opposite; black cohosh inhibited the cancer cells from proliferating. For example, a 2007 study published in *Maturitas*, a European health journal, found that black cohosh extract not only had no hormonal effect but also decreased estrogen formation in normal breast tissue. In addition, a very interesting National Institutes of Health–sponsored study concerning black cohosh and cancer, published in the *International Journal of Cancer* in 2007, compared the supplement use of 949 women with breast cancer to 1,524 control subjects. They discovered that women who took black cohosh had a 61% lower risk of breast cancer!

This study underscores the point I emphasize about the hormonal effects of black cohosh. It alters the levels of hormones already present in the body, as well as hormone cell receptors, instead of supplying actual hormones as in hormone replacement therapy.

BLACK COHOSH

RECOMMENDATIONS FROM THE NATURAL PHYSICIAN FOR . . .

❧ ANXIETY AND DEPRESSION

Black cohosh is effective for anxiety and depression that is associated with menopause. In the study I cited earlier, 85% of the 629 menopausal women who were given black cohosh extract had improvement in their anxiety and irritability, and almost 83% had improvement in their depression, with 46% no longer having any symptoms of depression.

Another study showed that black cohosh relieved anxiety and depression more effectively in menopausal women than the antianxiety drug diazepam. That is remarkable considering that diazepam is a powerful sedative drug. But the connection makes sense, because hormone imbalance leads to chemical imbalance in the brain's neurotransmitters (messengers). By balancing the ratios of the hormones estrogen and progesterone with black cohosh, you can indirectly balance the brain's chemicals and relieve symptoms such as anxiety and depression.

ARTHRITIS AND FIBROMYALGIA

Black cohosh has a natural anti-inflammatory effect. This makes it helpful in reducing pain, stiffness, and soreness associated with all types of arthritis. Arthritis pains are also a common symptom associated with menopause. Hormonal changes can result in circulation and immune system imbalances that may lead to joint inflammation.

It is also one of the better herbs to use in cases of fibromyalgia. In this condition, muscle pain is more of a problem, as opposed to joint pain. Black cohosh has a muscle-relaxing effect and reduces some of the soreness from which people with fibromyalgia invariably suffer. Women ages 25 to 45 are most commonly afflicted with fibromyalgia.

I have found a strong connection between hormone imbalance and fibromyalgia. I believe black cohosh's hormone-balancing qualities are one of the main reasons it helps improve fibromyalgia.

MENOPAUSAL SYMPTOMS

Black cohosh is one of the best natural therapies a woman can use to relieve menopausal symptoms. All the clinical studies on black cohosh that I have seen relate to its benefit for menopausal women. The vast majority of the studies have been done in Germany and the results are impressive to say the least. At least eight studies have shown that it can relieve menopausal symptoms, including hot flashes.

In a study of 629 menopausal women who used black cohosh extract for six to eight weeks, 80% noticed improvements within the first four weeks of use. These are very impressive results, considering that hormone replacement can take four to eight weeks to begin to relieve menopausal symptoms. Symptoms that were noticeably improved included nervousness and irritability, hot flashes, headache, insomnia, vertigo, heart palpitations, ringing in the ears, and insomnia.

Another interesting double-blind study followed 80 menopausal women for 12 weeks. Women were given black cohosh, synthetic estrogen, or a placebo. Women who were given the black cohosh had the best results in relieving menopausal symptoms including reduced anxiety and decreased hot flashes. This study is quite powerful as it proves the effectiveness of black cohosh over estrogen replacement.

Women who still have their ovaries may be able to switch from estrogen replacement therapy to black cohosh extract. I have done this with several women by slowly reducing their hormone replacement while starting them on black cohosh extract or a menopausal formula containing black cohosh. Researchers have studied women who were making the transition from hormones to black cohosh. For example, one study involved 50 women who were taking hormone replacement to relieve menopausal symptoms. Out of the 50 women, 28 were able to make the switch to black cohosh without being given additional hormones.

My patients tell me they feel better both physically and mentally when they switch from synthetic hormones to natural therapies like black cohosh extract. Psychologically, they feel safer getting

(continued)

off hormones that have a reputation for causing cancer and other diseases.

Keep in mind that black cohosh has not been shown to reduce the risk of osteoporosis or heart disease. These factors need to be addressed on an individual basis. It is also helpful for menstrual cramps and may be included in PMS formulas.

⁓ MENSTRUAL CRAMPS AND PMS
Black cohosh helps to reduce menstrual cramps by relaxing the smooth muscles of the uterus. While it does not have as strong an antispasmodic effect as the herb cramp bark, it can help relieve the cramping associated with PMS and dysmenorrhea (painful menses).

Boswellia

In the news some time ago was a well-known basketball player who had been diagnosed with a rare kidney disease. He was forced to stop playing, at least temporarily, while he waited to find whether he was a candidate for a kidney transplant. With the tragic news of this player's health problems, the spotlight turned on the long-term use (some would say abuse) of anti-inflammatory medications. These medications are given, as a matter of course, to many professional athletes. But other people take them, too, and in so doing they may run the risk of kidney, liver, and gastrointestinal problems.

For anyone who has been taking anti-inflammatory pharmaceuticals, herbs such as boswellia (*Boswellia serrata*) offer an effective and much safer natural alternative.

My own knowledge of traditional herbal remedies, such as this one, comes from the experience of healing remedies that date back many generations. Boswellia is one of these valuable herbs that originates in Ayurvedic medicine. It is often used to treat inflammatory conditions like rheumatoid arthritis, osteoarthritis, and cervical spondylitis. It also has been used in traditional Ayurvedic medicine for diarrhea, chronic lung disorders, menstrual disorders, and skin problems.

Though the use of boswellia was initiated in India, today it is commonly prescribed in the West, particularly Europe and now North America.

Boswellia serrata—a branching tree found in India, Northern Africa, and the Middle East—is a close relative of frankincense (*Boswellia carteri*), which contains similar compounds. When the bark of the Boswellia tree is stripped away, the trunk yields a milky gum resin. Constituents found in this resin include oils and triterpenic acids.

The boswellic acids are among those triterpenic acids, and most of the anti-inflammatory properties are thought to come from the boswellic acids. When you're looking for boswellia on the shelf, you want an herbal product that is "standardized to boswellic acids."

It is believed that the boswellic acids interfere with leukotriene synthesis. That could explain why it brings some relief. Leukotrienes are hormonelike compounds that cause pain and inflammation.

DOSAGE

I recommend 1,200 to 1,500 mg of a standardized extract containing 60% to 65% boswellic acids taken two to three times daily.

WHAT ARE THE SIDE EFFECTS?

Boswellia appears to be very safe. Animal studies have shown no toxicity problems. It is known to occasionally cause mild diges- tive upset. Safety for pregnant and nursing women has not been established, so until testing is done, I'd advise pregnant women to avoid taking it.

BOSWELLIA
RECOMMENDATIONS FROM THE NATURAL PHYSICIAN FOR . . .

ᵔᵔ ARTHRITIS

Boswellia has been traditionally used for both rheumatoid arthritis and osteoarthritis. But there are many other kinds of arthritis as well, and boswellia is now quite popular in the natural healthcare field as a natural anti-inflammatory for all the different types.

One researcher who reviewed 11 German clinical studies found that boswellia had been beneficial for 260 people who did not respond well to conventional treatments. Researchers found that standardized boswellia extract significantly reduced swelling and pain and usually reduced morning stiffness for people with rheumatoid arthritis.

Even more impressive was that some people were able to reduce their intake of NSAIDs (nonsteroidal anti-inflammatories). The dosage used in most studies was 1,200 to 1,500 mg of extract in capsules that were taken two to three times daily—so people were getting a total of 3,600 to 4,500 mg of extract each day.

Researchers in India found that this herb performed as well as the anti-inflammatory drug Valdecoxib. The study involved 66 participants (ages 40 to 70) with osteoarthritis of the knees who took either BSE (333 mg three times daily) or Valdecoxib (10 mg once daily) for six months. Those taking BSE showed significant reduction in pain and stiffness after two months—and benefits lasted for one additional month after the herbal extract was discontinued. Participants who took Valdecoxib noted improvement after one month, but benefits lasted only as long as the drug was taken. The authors of this study stated, "In terms of safety, efficacy and duration of action . . . BSE was superior to Valdecoxib."

A randomized, double-blind, placebo-controlled crossover study found boswellia extract to be very effective and safe for osteoarthritis of the knees.

It is important to note that NSAIDs, the pharmaceutical medicines most often taken for arthritis, help to relieve pain and inflammation, but may actually accelerate cartilage degeneration. Boswellia does not cause this cartilage degradation. It actually reduces the breakdown of cartilage building blocks known as glycosaminoglycans.

More research needs to be done before we'll know whether boswellia slows down or halts the underlying disease process that's associated with arthritis. But we do know that boswellia works very well when combined with glucosamine sulfate and MSM for the treatment of osteoarthritis.

(continued)

🐾 ASTHMA

Preliminary studies have shown that boswellia extract can help reduce the frequency of asthma attacks and improve breathing for those with asthma.

🐾 CROHN'S DISEASE

Boswellia has been shown to be helpful for Crohn's disease due to its anti-inflammatory effects on the digestive tract.

🐾 INJURIES

Boswellia, along with other natural products with natural anti-inflammatory properties (such as bromelain, MSM, and vitamin E), should be considered for the prevention and treatment of athletic injuries and other kinds of muscle and joint problems.

🐾 RHEUMATOID ARTHRITIS

Studies are conflicting for the benefit of boswellia and this condition, yet I find it helpful along with other natural nutrients such as MSM, fish oil, devil's claw, and turmeric.

🐾 ULCERATIVE COLITIS

Boswellia is useful in alleviating the inflammation associated with inflammatory bowel disease (IBD). In a six-week study involving 42 people who had ulcerative colitis symptoms, researchers found that boswellia extract was just as effective as the high-powered pharmaceutical drug sulfasalazine in producing remission.

Bromelain

"Mark, you should see the bruise I have on my shoulder. It's massive!"

For my friend Les, such bruises came with the territory. He was in the midst of hockey playoffs. Bruises like this had happened before and they would surely happen again—as long as he stuck with the sport.

"Do you still have any bromelain left?" I asked, reminding him of the remedy I'd given him just a week before.

"Oh yeah, I still have some left."

I have noticed that many people completely forget that they have supplements on hand that may be precisely what they need.

"How about taking two tablets every couple of hours?" I suggested.

It was no more than two days later that Les returned to tell me that the bruising—along with the shoulder pain—had improved remarkably.

I wasn't surprised. It was the kind of results I'd come to expect from bromelain.

PLUNDERING THE PINEAPPLE

Bromelain is actually a group of protein enzymes derived from the pineapple plant, whose healing powers were described in the medical literature as far back as 1876. Though the active enzymes are found in the fruit as well as the stem, commercial products are made exclusively from the stem.

Bromelain is used for many purposes— as a digestive aid, natural blood thinner, anti-inflammatory, mucus-thinning agent, immune system enhancer, and for skin healing. It also helps improve the absorption of certain supplements (such as glucosamine) and drug medications such as antibiotics.

One of bromelain's unique actions is to reduce inflammation in people who have conditions such as arthritis or heart disease. It can also help control the inflammatory process after an injury. It breaks down blood clots at the site of an injury, so swelling is reduced and, at the same time, there's increased circulation to the site of injury or inflammation. Bromelain also helps control some of the body's naturally produced chemicals that tend to increase an inflammatory reaction after an injury.

DOSAGE

The dosage of bromelain is designated in two different ways with regard to supplements. One is milk-clotting units (MCU) and the other is gelatin-dissolving units (GDU). Look for products that are standardized to 2,000 MCU per 1,000 mg, or 1,200 GDU per 1,000 mg. Most people require a dosage of 500 mg three times daily between meals.

WHAT ARE THE SIDE EFFECTS?

Side effects are rare with bromelain. However, allergic reactions can occur in sensitive individuals. Increased heart rate and palpitations have been observed in some people at dosages near 2,000 mg. Those on blood-thinning medications should check with their doctor before using bromelain.

MAXING YOUR ANTIBIOTICS

Bromelain is used in many countries to increase the absorption and utilization of antibiotics.

In one study, 53 hospitalized patients were given bromelain in various combinations with appropriate antibiotic medications. Their conditions included a wide range of health problems, such as pneumonia, bronchitis, skin staphylococcus infection, thrombophlebitis, cellulitis, pyelonephritis (kidney infection), and abscesses of the rectum. Twenty-three of the patients had been on antibiotic therapy without success. Bromelain was administered four times a day along with antibiotics or by itself.

To compare, a control group of 56 patients was treated with antibiotics alone.

Of the 23 patients who had been unsuccessfully treated with antibiotics, 22 responded favorably to the combined treatment. The rate of improvement was across-the-board, for every type of disease, when patients were given the combination of bromelain and antibiotics.

For doctors involved in the study, it was an eye-opener. Many had not realized that bromelain was able to potentiate the effects of antibiotics in this way.

I hope we'll see larger-scale studies in the near future. Such promising results suggest that people may be able to take lower doses of antibiotics if they simultaneously take bromelain. (Many doctors are eager to reduce the rampant overuse of antibiotics, which is leading to ominous new strains of resistant bacteria.)

Those with weak or compromised immune systems could be the greatest beneficiaries of combination treatments with bromelain and antibiotics. Infants, seniors, and AIDS patients are particularly good candidates for the combined therapies.

BROMELAIN

RECOMMENDATIONS FROM THE NATURAL PHYSICIAN FOR . . .

ARTHRITIS

Bromelain is a popular component of natural arthritis formulas. It is helpful for both osteoarthritis and rheumatoid arthritis.

One study found that the supplementation of bromelain enabled people with rheumatoid arthritis to reduce their corticosteroid medications. In addition, patients noticed significant improvements in joint mobility and also noticed less swelling. This study is encouraging because many people suffer side effects from corticosteroid therapy—and the less medicine they have to use, the better. If bromelain supplementation can reduce the amount of steroids needed, the risk of serious side effects decreases as well. In addition, bromelain has been shown to help reduce mild knee pain in healthy adults.

My experience is that most people with arthritis can maintain a good quality of life if they take the opportunity to try bromelain and other natural treatments.

BURNS

A specially prepared bromelain cream has been shown to eliminate burn debris and speed up the healing of burned skin.

CANCER

Various studies have looked at a link between bromelain treatments and cancer deterrence or recovery. In one study, 12 patients with ovarian and breast tumors were given 600 mg of bromelain daily for at least six months. (Some treatments continued for several years.) Resolution of cancerous masses and a decrease in metastasis was reported.

Bromelain in doses more than 1,000 mg daily have been given in combination with chemotherapy drugs such as 5-FU and vincristine, with some reports of tumor regression.

Although I do not rate bromelain as one of the more potent anticancer herbs, it is worthy of more study. For those who are using chemotherapy to fight cancer, the addition of bromelain offers the promise of making the therapy more effective.

CARDIOVASCULAR DISEASE

Holistic practitioners have expressed a great deal of interest in using bromelain for treatment and prevention of cardiovascular disease. We know that bromelain helps break down fibrinous plaques in the arteries, allowing for more efficient circulation. In theory, at least, this is a sure way to help prevent strokes.

When we take routine tests to determine whether people are at risk of cardiovascular disease, fibrin is one of the markers that we're beginning to look at routinely. (In other words, a lot of fibrin in the blood is one indicator that stroke could be somewhere on the horizon.) The fact that bromelain can help "break down" this fibrin is significant. In one study, bromelain administered at a dosage of 400 to 1,000 mg per day to 14 patients with angina (chest pain) resulted in the disappearance of symptoms in all patients within 4 to 90 days.

Bromelain also has the potential to

break down plaque, the fatty deposits that impair blood flow through the arteries. The enzyme has been shown to dissolve arteriosclerotic plaque in rabbit heart arteries. While more studies need to be done, I've talked to many practitioners who notice that their heart patients do better on bromelain.

DIGESTIVE PROBLEMS

Bromelain has long been used as a digestive aid in the breakdown of protein, and there are now many "digestive-enzyme formulas" that routinely include bromelain as one of the key ingredients. Either bromelain alone or the enzyme formulas can be helpful for people who have digestive conditions such as colitis or irritable bowel syndrome (IBS). In addition, we know that incomplete protein breakdown is implicated in immune reactions that lead to inflammatory conditions such as arthritis.

INJURIES

Bromelain's most well-known use is in the treatment of injuries, and it definitely helps to reduce pain and swelling if you have bruises. In one early clinical trial, doctors gave bromelain to 74 boxers who regularly suffered bruising on the face, lips, ears, chest, and arms. When bromelain was given four times a day, all signs of bruising disappeared by the fourth day among 58 of the boxers.

A control group, comprised of 72 boxers, were given a placebo—a look-alike capsule made up of inert substances. In that group, 62 of the boxers needed 7 to 14 days before the bruises cleared up. (Only 10 were free from signs of bruising after four days.)

RESPIRATORY MUCUS

Bromelain thins mucus. If you have bronchitis and another kind of respiratory-tract condition, you'll probably discover that dosing with bromelain will help you expel the mucus more easily. For similar reasons, taking bromelain has been shown to improve cases of sinusitis.

SURGERY RECOVERY

Bromelain is a valuable supplement in helping people recover more quickly from surgery.

In one study, patients who were given bromelain supplements 2 to 4 days before surgery were able to recover from pain and inflammation more quickly than those who didn't take the enzyme. The bromelain-takers took an average of 1.5 days to be pain free, compared with an average of 3.5 days for those who went without it. Without bromelain, it took an average of 6.9 days for inflammation to go down, but only about 2 days for those who had bromelain supplements.

In my opinion, supplements such as bromelain should be routinely given to those recovering from surgery. Just think of all the days of suffering patients could avoid!

THROMBOPHLEBITIS

In studies, bromelain has been proven very effective in the treatment of vein clots, as thrombophlebitis is commonly called.

VARICOSE VEINS

Bromelain has value in the treatment of varicose veins. I do not rate it as effective as horse chestnut and some of the other herbs, but it certainly helps.

Burdock

"This cleansing formula contains burdock root. I have never heard of it before. What does it do, Dr. Stengler?" asked Wendy, a patient of mine.

"Burdock is a great herb to help a person detoxify," I replied. "In your case, I think it will help with your chronic eczema. If we get your digestion working better and liver filtering toxins more efficiently, then your skin should also improve. Burdock works to do all these things."

Burdock (*Arctium lappa*) is an amazing herb to use for detoxification. It supports the liver, our primary organ of detoxification. It also supports kidney detoxification and destroys impurities of the blood such as harmful bacteria and yeast. An underrated aspect of detoxification is lymphatic drainage, which burdock also enhances. Burdock seeds act as a natural diuretic to flush out water-soluble toxins.

BURDOCK BASICS

Burdock exemplifies an important class of herbal medicines called "alteratives." An alterative herb improves general health by balancing and tonifying body functions. Alteratives improve nutritional status through improved digestion and elimination. They are sometimes referred to as "blood purifiers" as they help cleanse the liver and blood. They often are rich in minerals, phytonutrients, and other nutrients that stimulate metabolism and healing.

They are also referred to as "tonics," as they tonify and optimize different organ systems of the body. They also help indirectly with energy production by improving the body's overall level of health. Alteratives generally have low potential for toxicity and can be used on a long-term basis.

Burdock is native to Asia and Europe, and is grown in North America. North American herbalists and naturopathic doctors mainly use the roots for their medicinal properties, but the leaves and fruits are also used. A related species, common burdock (*Arctium minus*), can also be effective.

Burdock root contains many different constituents including inulin, phytosterols, polyacetylenes, arctic acid, volatile acids, tannins, vitamin A, iron, calcium, sodium, and other minerals. It is said to be "cooling" in terms of its effect on body temperature.

Burdock is an excellent herb for skin disorders such as acne, eczema, psoriasis, and rashes. Its hormone-balancing qualities are useful for the treatment of PMS and relieving menopausal symptoms. It is also used for diabetes, arthritis, and gout. This herb will improve digestion and help detoxify the lymphatic system. In addition, burdock will tonify the urinary system and help treat fevers and sore throats.

It has often been included in herbal cancer formulas as well.

DOSAGE

I recommend that adults take 20 to 30 drops (0.5 mg) or 300 to 500 mg of the capsule form two to three times daily with meals.

WHAT ARE THE SIDE EFFECTS?

Burdock is very safe; however, there are a few caveats. Those who have chronic diarrhea should start with a low dosage at first, as burdock stimulates the digestive organs. In some people, prolonged use of burdock seed can cause urinary tract irritation. Burdock should not be taken during pregnancy.

BURDOCK

RECOMMENDATIONS FROM THE NATURAL PHYSICIAN FOR . . .

❧ ACNE AND SKIN CONDITIONS

Burdock is my favorite herb for the treatment of acne—with vitex and milk thistle not too far behind. I have seen dramatic effects from the use of burdock in the past to improve low- to moderate-grade acne. I find it consistently helps my patients.

It works well because it treats all the root problems of acne: hormonal imbalance, poor digestion, inefficient liver activity, intestinal and skin bacteria and yeast overgrowth, and general toxicity.

Improvements are usually noticed within four to six weeks of consistent use, although teenagers may need to take it longer before they see results.

It is also a favorite for the treatment of eczema.

Along with sarsaparilla, burdock is one of the best herbs for psoriasis. For an aggressive treatment of psoriasis, I'd recommend taking both burdock and sarsaparilla together.

❧ CANCER

Burdock is often a component of Western herbal formulas targeted toward cancer. While cancer can be a complex disease, many researchers detect a connection between cancer and "toxicity" in the body.

Burdock improves detoxification and supports the immune system. In addition, its hormone-balancing properties may be beneficial for hormone-dependent cancers. (Research on natural therapies and cancer is limited.)

❧ CONSTIPATION

Bowel movements are easier when the liver and gallbladder secrete more bile. This is why it is a good idea to take burdock with meals to help improve digestion and elimination.

❧ DIABETES

Animal studies have shown that burdock improves glucose tolerance. This is attributed to the inulin—the substance that makes up between 20% and 40% of the root.

❧ FEVER AND INFECTION

Burdock is "cooling." The seeds are known to be especially effective in helping to reduce fever. It is also used for sore throats and mouth sores.

❧ INDIGESTION

As a bitter herb, burdock stimulates most of the digestive organs to work more effectively. Over time, this herb can help strengthen weak digestive organs and improve digestion.

❧ PMS AND MENOPAUSE

The liver works to metabolize all the hormones in the body. The better the liver is working, the better the overall hormone balance. PMS is caused by a hormone imbalance, which burdock helps to correct. Also, as a "cooling" herb, it helps reduce hot flashes.

❧ URINARY TRACT INFECTIONS

Burdock is used to help support kidney function, and for the treatment of chronic urinary tract infections.

Butcher's Broom

"These dang hemorrhoids are killing me. I can't sit or lie down. And there is no way I am getting the rubber band treatment or surgery like my friends have had!"

Jim, a 65-year-old retired farmer, was living with the classic problem of a modern-day average person—the excruciating and embarrassing pain of hemorrhoids. In his case, we were able to relieve his rectal symptoms without drugs or surgery. One of the main components of his treatment was a capsule extract of butcher's broom.

Untold numbers of people have hemorrhoids—and a quick tour of pharmacy shelves will quickly reveal how many products are available. But whether you take those products or have conventional treatments, the "cure" usually isn't lasting. Fortunately, nature has provided remedies that shrink hemorrhoid tissue and without side effects.

One such herb is butcher's broom (*Rusculus aculeatus*). Coming from an evergreen bush that's a member of the lily family—native to the Mediterranean and northwest Europe—the herbal preparation is actually made from the rhizome that grows along the ground.

A Good Venotonic

Butcher's broom has a long and noble history as the chosen preparation for hemorrhoids and varicose veins. Long ago, its bundled branches were made into brooms that were used by butchers—hence the name. But these days the herbal preparation comes in various bottled and packaged forms that suggest neither butcher shop nor busy sweeper.

The active constituents in butcher's broom are believed to be ruscogenins. They work to treat hemorrhoids by constricting blood vessels and reduce inflammation in the hemorrhoidal tissue.

Butcher's broom is a classic example of what is called a venotonic, which simply means that it improves the tone of the venous wall. If you have hemorrhoids, the veins have become weakened because of swelling and abrasion. So a venotonic is exactly what you need for treatment.

Dosage

I recommend a standardized extract that gives you a total dosage of 100 mg of ruscogenins daily. Creams that contain butcher's broom extract are widely available in Europe, but you can find ointments at some stores in the United States.

What Are the Side Effects?

There are no known side effects for butcher's broom.

BUTCHER'S BROOM
RECOMMENDATIONS FROM THE NATURAL PHYSICIAN FOR . . .

HEMORRHOIDS

Butcher's broom can be used for treatment of an acute hemorrhoid condition or on a long-term basis to keep hemorrhoid tissue from becoming engorged and inflamed.

In studies, researchers have usually given butcher's broom combined with flavonoids and vitamin C—which is the formula I recommend for maximum healing benefits.

VARICOSE VEINS

Butcher's broom is a venotonic, so it can also be used for varicose veins.

A study was done of 40 people with chronic venous insufficiency. They had various symptoms—such as varicose veins in the legs, edema (swelling caused by buildup of fluids), itching, and leg cramps—that indicated poor venous blood flow. Those taking the butcher's broom extract in combination with a flavonoid improved significantly without side effects.

Butterbur

"Doctor, I have tried all sorts of different natural remedies for my migraine headaches. I use pharmaceuticals when they get bad, but I would prefer a more natural approach." Those were the words of Laurie, a 45-year-old with a 10-year history of migraine headaches. As I spoke to her further, I found out she also experienced severe hay fever three months out of each year. During this time, the frequency of her migraines increased. I told her that improving her diet and digestion, and identifying other triggers of her migraines, would treat the root causes of her headaches. However, since she was so prone to migraines, I prescribed the plant extract of butterbur (*Petasites hybridus*). Laurie was thrilled to eventually achieve a substantial reduction in her headaches and allergies using this natural extract.

Butterbur has a history of more than 900 years for its use as a medicinal remedy. Other common names for this plant include blatterdock, bog rhubarb, and butter-dock. In the past it was used to treat fevers, coughs, asthma, digestive ailments, and skin wounds. Today it is used primarily for the prevention of migraine headaches and treatment of hay fever, bronchitis, and asthma. It is also applied topically for the treatment of wounds.

The parts of butterbur used for medicinal effects are the root, leaf, and rhizome. Butterbur extracts contain several compounds, including volatile oils, tannins, and alkaloids. The most active constituents of butterbur are sesquiterpene compounds, known as petasin and isopetasin. Commonly used commercial products are often standardized to contain certain levels of petasin and isopetasin. Butterbur is thought to help migraines, allergies, and asthma through its anti-inflammatory effects—it inhibits the inflammatory compounds known as leukotrienes and histamine. In addition, it seems to have antispasmodic effects on smooth muscle and blood vessel walls. In addition to reducing histamine, butterbur appears to decrease the responsiveness of mast cells to allergens. It is mast cells that release histamine in response to allergens.

DOSAGE

For migraine prevention in adults, take 50 to 100 mg of an extract standardized to 15% petasin and isopetasin twice daily with meals. Children ages six to nine with migraines should take 25 mg twice daily; children ages ten and older, 50 mg twice daily. For hay fever, take a standardized product containing 8 to 16 mg of petasin per dose three to four times daily.

WHAT ARE THE SIDE EFFECTS?

Butterbur is well tolerated. Occasional side effects may include digestive upset, headache, itchy eyes, and fatigue. You will read in the literature that butterbur contains substances known as pyrrolizidine alkaloids, which can be toxic. However, the standardized extracts recommended in this chapter have these substances removed and are not of concern. One example of a common trade name without these alkaloids is Petadolex, available through various supplement companies. Look for labels that note that the product is free of pyrrolizidine alkaloids.

BUTTERBUR
RECOMMENDATIONS FROM THE NATURAL PHYSICIAN FOR . . .

✦ ALLERGIES (HAY FEVER)
Butterbur is commonly used in Europe for the treatment of hay fever and is gaining popularity in the United States. I find it is helpful for patients with hay fever, especially for those prone to headaches as the result of allergies. A double-blind, randomized study of 330 participants with hay fever (allergic rhinitis) compared butterbur to fexofexanidine (Allegra) and placebo. Both treatments were found to be superior to placebo, and they were found to be comparable to one another in efficacy. Another study found butterbur to be as effective as cetirizine (Zyrtec).

✦ ASTHMA/BRONCHITIS
In folk medicine, the leaves of butterbur were used to treat asthma and coughing associated with mucus. One Polish study demonstrated that butterbur improved lung ventilation in patients with asthma or chronic obstructive bronchitis. I have not had experience yet using this botanical for these conditions.

✦ MIGRAINE HEADACHES
Butterbur extract is safe and effective for the prevention of migraine headaches in adults and children. A three-arm, parallel-group, randomized trial study published in *Neurology* involved 245 people, ages 18 to 65, who had had at least two to six migraine attacks during the preceding three months. Participants who took butterbur standardized to contain 75 mg twice daily for four months had their migraine attack frequency decrease an

average of 48% as compared to 26% for the placebo group. Another study with adults using 50 mg daily found those taking butterbur extract had a responder rate (improvement of migraine frequency greater than or equal to 50%) that was 45% versus 15% in the placebo group.

There is also evidence that butterbur extract can decrease the frequency of migraine headaches in children ages 6 to 17, as published in the medical journal *Headache*. That multicenter, prospective open-label study involved 108 children and adolescents between the ages of 6 and 17. Participants suffered from migraines diagnosed for at least one year. Depending on the child's age 50 to 150 mg of butterbur root extract was given for a period of four months. Treatment progression was recorded in migraine journals especially designed for children and adolescents. Overall 77% of all patients reported a reduction in the frequency of migraine attacks. Overall attack frequency was reduced by 63%, and 91% of patients felt substantially or at least slightly improved after four months of treatment. Undesired effects (reported by 7.4% of patients) included mostly burping. No serious adverse events occurred and no adverse event caused a premature discontinuation of the study.

C

Calcium

All the milk ads say you need calcium from cow's milk for strong bones and healthy teeth. True enough. Calcium is essential for strong bones—as long as you're getting many other minerals as well—and it's certainly beneficial for teeth. But there are more food sources of calcium than milk, and many of them are actually *better* than milk.

But let's look at the mineral itself before we get to sources.

Calcium is required by every cell of your body for a multitude of different actions.

This is the mineral that helps your muscles contract, keeps your nerves lively, facilitates cell division, and helps arrange for the release of neurotransmitters, the chemical signals that scoot between nerve cells. Among its other valuable services, calcium helps your heart beat, your blood clot, and your hormones stay active. It's a factor in enzyme reactions and sperm motility.

So important is calcium that it makes up almost 2% of your body weight, more than any other mineral. No question about it— for good health and vitality, you have to consume and absorb enough calcium on a regular basis.

TABLE 3
Calcium

If you are lactose intolerant or have other kinds of problems with dairy products, here are some alternative food sources that can help you meet your daily requirements of calcium:

FOOD SOURCE	SERVING SIZE	CALCIUM (IN MG)
Wakame (sea vegetable)	½ cup	1,700 mg
Agar (sea vegetable)	¼ cup	1,000 mg
Nori (sea vegetable)	½ cup	600 mg
Kombu (sea vegetable)	¼ cup	500 mg
Sardines with Bones	½ cup	500 mg
Salmon	3 ounces (canned)	150 mg
Tempeh	1 cup	340 mg
Collard Greens	1 cup	355 mg

FOOD SOURCE	SERVING SIZE	CALCIUM (IN MG)
Calcium-Enriched Rice or Soy Milk	1 cup	300 mg
Almonds	1 cup	300 mg
Spinach	1 cup	280 mg
Yogurt	1 cup	270 mg
Sesame Seeds	½ cup	250 mg
Kale	1 cup	200 mg
Broccoli	1 cup	180 mg
Tofu	1 cup	150 mg
Walnuts	¼ cup	70 mg
Black Beans	1 cup	60 mg
Lentils	1 cup	50 mg

SOME NOTABLE DEFICIENCIES

We have an epidemic of calcium deficiency in North America. Only 10% of adults get the recommended amount of calcium each day. Our kids aren't getting enough, either. Approximately 70% of teenage boys and 95% of girls get less than the minimum amounts recommended in standard nutrition guidelines. Of course, this deficiency is particularly alarming among the teenage girl population, since females are particularly susceptible to bone loss, and postmenopausal women are much more likely to have fragile bones if they don't get enough calcium in their earlier years.

As for postmenopausal women, they too seem oblivious to the risks of underconsumption of calcium. Most American women get 600 mg of calcium daily, which is far below the 1,200 mg per day that's recommended by the National Academy of Sciences. Is it any wonder that approximately one out of every three postmenopausal women will develop osteoporosis?

This dreaded condition accounts for more than 1.5 million fractures each year.

Now comes the question that nutritionists and doctors haggle over all the time: Given that we need more calcium, what are the best sources?

Most conventional doctors will immediately say cow's milk. It's true, milk does contain calcium. One 8-ounce serving of skim milk contains 302 mg. So, at least theoretically, a postmenopausal woman could meet her calcium requirement with just four glasses of milk every day.

But that's not quite the whole story.

First of all, some people simply don't tolerate cow's milk very well. If you lack the enzyme lactase—as many of us do—it's difficult to digest milk sugar (lactose), and you're likely to have symptoms of gas, bloating, nausea, abdominal cramps, and diarrhea. According to *The Merck Manual*, 75% of adults have some degree of lactase deficiency. For those of northwest European descent, lactase deficiency is much lower, around 20%, but that's a small proportion of the world's population. At the other extreme, 100% of Chinese have lactase deficiency, so all Chinese are lactose intolerant to some extent. Roughly 75% of African Americans have lactase deficiency, as do a high number of those from Mediterranean descent.

Another problem is that cow's milk and the products derived from cow's milk tend to create excess mucus. I have seen many patients with chronic sinusitis and upper respiratory tract problems (including chronic bronchitis and asthma) who improve as soon as they go on a dairy-free diet. The same is often true of children who have reoccurring ear infections, since those conditions just get worse when the children have too much mucus.

Some researchers suspect a link between cow's milk and hardening of the arteries, while others suspect that consumption of cow's milk may be a factor in autoimmune diseases such as lupus and rheumatoid arthritis. Cow's milk is also known to be a common cause of iron-deficiency anemia because it can create the conditions for internal bleeding. (Anemia is a possibility any time there's excessive blood loss.)

For children who get more than 24 ounces of whole cow's milk daily after the first year of life, there's an additional risk of iron deficiency because milk has little iron, may replace foods with higher iron content, and may cause occult (hidden) gastrointestinal bleeding.

Studies have also shown that cow's milk is a major cause of chronic constipation in children.

ARE YOU LOSING CALCIUM?

While milk isn't quite the calcium hero that it's made out to be, some other common foods are worse villains than we recognize.

There are a number of foods, beverages, and habits that can cause you to lose calcium. It has been proven that soda, sodium, alcohol, and sugar all promote the urinary excretion of calcium. Also, you likely will lose more calcium if you have a diet that's high in animal protein. Smoking causes calcium loss, too. It's also been shown that hormonal imbalances and poor digestive function can contribute to a calcium deficiency.

You should also be aware of the dietary factors that *improve* the absorption of calcium. Vitamin D, vitamin C, and the mineral magnesium are among the nutrients that help your cells absorb and use calcium.

DOSAGE

The National Academy of Sciences recommends the following for daily calcium intakes. These doses apply to males as well as females. In my view, you should be getting at least these amounts—and for most people, more is better. I especially feel that children eight years and younger should be getting closer to 500 mg daily of supplemental calcium.

DIETARY REFERENCE INTAKE

0 to 6 months: 300 mg

6 to 12 months: 500 mg

1 to 10 years: 600 to 800 mg

11 to 18 years: 800 to 1,000 mg

18+ years: 800 to 1,500 mg

Pregnant/lactating mothers: 400+ mg

For a calcium supplement, I recommend calcium citrate or calcium citrate-malate, or microcrystalline hydroxyappatite or a chelated calcium. Studies show that these are the forms best absorbed by the body.

The carbonate form is not so well absorbed and it buffers stomach acid—that is, gets in the way of the stomach acid that's needed for calcium absorption. If calcium carbonate is used, higher amounts are required due to the decreased absorption.

Make sure to use a reputable brand, as some calcium supplements have been found to be contaminated with lead. Avoid dolomite, bone meal, and coral calcium: These calcium supplies are poorly absorbed, and some sources have a history of lead contamination.

I recommend most adults and children take 500 to 1,000 mg daily of a good-quality calcium supplement. You'll probably need at least this much added to whatever calcium is in your diet, because dietary deficiencies are so common. Make sure to take a high-potency multivitamin that contains other vitamins and minerals needed to absorb and utilize calcium effectively.

Also, use calcium supplements that contain magnesium, as this mineral is very important in helping your body absorb and use as much of the calcium as possible. Magnesium should be taken at half or equal to the amount of calcium each day. If you take a magnesium supplement that's separate from the calcium supplement, you'll find it in many acceptable forms— as magnesium citrate, chelate, or glycinate aspartate, fumarate, malate, and succinate. You'll need 500 to 600 mg daily of magnesium as well as vitamin D—1,000 to 2,000 IU daily.

Calcium supplements are best absorbed if you take them with food. Your body releases hydrochloric acid when you eat, which helps with the absorption process.

WHAT ARE THE SIDE EFFECTS?

At one time, doctors thought high calcium intake could raise your risk of kidney stones—but studies have shown this isn't so, especially in the case of calcium citrate. Any dosage below 2,000 mg is safe. People who have been diagnosed with thyroid problems—in particular, hyperparathyroidism—should not supplement calcium unless under a doctor's supervision. You'll also need to follow a doctor's guidance if you have kidney disease.

Calcium does interfere with iron and zinc absorption. If high levels of iron and zinc are required, then take them at different times of the day, away from calcium. For example, if you're taking iron for anemia, take a separate iron supplement, and make sure it's a couple of hours before or after you take your calcium.

CALCIUM

RECOMMENDATIONS FROM THE NATURAL PHYSICIAN FOR . . .

❧ HEARTBURN

Calcium carbonate has been shown to reduce the symptoms of heartburn by neutralizing stomach acid. It works well for this purpose but isn't the best long-term calcium to take for your general health. However, occasional use for heartburn is fine.

❧ CIRCULATORY PROBLEMS AND HEART DISEASE

By taking calcium supplements, you'll excrete more saturated fat, which is a dietary factor that contributes significantly to heart disease. At the same time, you'll *decrease* the absorption of cholesterol, thus lowering blood cholesterol levels. Because calcium has both a fat-removing and cholesterol-lowering effect, it may reduce your risk of stroke and heart attack.

❧ COLON CANCER

Colon cancer ranks number two, after lung cancer, among fatal cancers. Many human and animal studies show that you'll have a decreased risk of colon cancer if you take more calcium in foods and supplements.

❧ DIABETES

Population studies suggest that an increased intake of calcium from diet and supplements, alone or in combination with vitamin D, is associated with a lower risk of developing type 2 diabetes compared to lower calcium intake.

❧ GROWING PAINS

I have found that almost 90% of all cases of growing pains in children are related to a deficiency of calcium, magnesium, vitamin D, or all three. Unfortunately, many family doctors still do not recognize this solution to what can be an excruciating problem for a child.

❧ HIGH BLOOD PRESSURE

Calcium should definitely be one of the supplements prescribed for high blood pressure. Studies show that calcium has a mild blood pressure–lowering effect. It is theorized that calcium helps relax the muscle cells that line your blood vessel walls, thus decreasing pressure inside the arteries. I find it works very well in combination with magnesium, potassium, vitamin C, and coenzyme Q10.

❧ MUSCLE CRAMPS AND SPASMS

Calcium deficiency is often the underlying problem when people have muscle problems. Again, it works well in combination with magnesium and potassium. I've found that chronic muscle spasms often disappear after people take calcium and magnesium supplements for a week or two. Calcium along with magnesium is also effective for pregnant women experiencing muscle cramps.

❧ OSTEOPOROSIS

Calcium is constantly flowing in and out of bones. Bone density decreases when we're not supplying enough absorbable calcium to make up for daily losses.

Studies have shown that calcium supplementation slows down bone loss.

The *New England Journal of Medicine* reported that postmenopausal women who added 1,000 mg of calcium to their normal daily diets experienced a 43% reduction in bone loss when compared with women who weren't getting the supplements.

PMS

Along with magnesium and vitamin B6, calcium supplementation has been shown to help alleviate PMS. It takes one to two cycles of supplementation for significant reductions in PMS symptoms.

PREGNANCY

Calcium appears to reduce the risk of pregnancy-induced high blood pressure. It also lowers the risk of a pregnancy-related condition called preeclampsia—higher blood pressure combined with

increased water retention and more loss of protein in the urine. I recommend calcium to pregnant women to prevent these two conditions and also to prevent the muscle cramps and spasms that frequently occur during pregnancy.

TOOTH LOSS IN THE ELDERLY

Calcium supplementation along with vitamin D has been shown to help prevent tooth loss in the elderly.

WEIGHT LOSS

A randomized, double-blind, placebo-controlled trial was performed with 36,282 postmenopausal women, ages 50 to 79. Those taking 1,000 mg of calcium plus vitamin D were less likely to gain weight compared to those taking a placebo. Other studies have shown that calcium from food or supplements can help with weight reduction and lean body mass.

Calendula

One of the most practical botanicals to have in the home medicine cabinet is *Calendula officinalis*, also known as marigold. I routinely recommend it for cuts, scrapes, eczema, and infections of the skin. One weekend I got a call from a patient who was quite concerned about an infection developing on his lower leg. He had cut his leg in a pool and now a red streak was beginning, a sign of an infection. Since he had type 2 diabetes we both knew he was more susceptible to infections. I recommended the topical application of calendula liquid extract every two waking hours. When I checked in with him the following day he was happy to report the redness had disappeared and over

the following days his leg healed up without a problem. Surprisingly few studies have been done on calendula. Yet I and other holistic practitioners find it consistently to be effective, particularly for skin conditions.

Traditionally the leaves and flowers of the calendula plant have been used for their medicinal qualities. Today most products contain extracts from the flower portion. Calendula has been used for the treatment of all types of skin ailments, including varicose veins, ulcers, bee stings, and various types of skin inflammation. It also been used internally to heal inflammation of the digestive tract lining ranging from the mouth (gingivitis), to ulcers of the stomach or intestines, and hemorrhoids. Additionally, it has been used topically for the treatment of conjunctivitis of the eyes.

Calendula is rich in anti-inflammatory pigments known as flavonoids, which are thought to be responsible for a lot of its wound-healing benefits. It also contains carotenoids, antioxidants important for tissue health, as well as constituents known as triterpene saponins.

DOSAGE

Calendula is commonly available in various topical ointments, including salves, creams, soaps, and gels. This makes it easy to apply for skin conditions and I usually recommend it be applied four times daily for acute skin problems or twice daily for chronic skin issues such as eczema. Also, it is available in tincture or tea form, which can be used for mouth rinses, oral ingestion, or topical administration. One cup of the tea form consumed two to three times daily is a normal oral dosage. Calendula is also available in homeopathic pellet form, which is used for skin conditions, especially skin infections.

WHAT ARE THE SIDE EFFECTS?

Side effects are not common. Rarely there are skin allergies to calendula, but I have not seen this to be a common problem. Caution is noted for those with ragweed allergy.

CALENDULA
RECOMMENDATIONS FROM THE NATURAL PHYSICIAN FOR . . .

➥ BURNS
Minor burns can be helped with calendula topical application. It helps to heal and soothe burns. St. John's wort oil is most effective for burns; the two can be used together.

➥ CELLULITIS
This is a bacterial infection of the skin, often beginning in the lower leg. It can be serious, spreading quickly throughout the body and it requires medically supervised treatment. Calendula can be used topically for this condition even when antibiotics are used internally. I have also used the homeopathic form for the treatment of this condition.

➥ CONJUNCTIVITIS
Also known as pinkeye, this is a viral or bacterial infection of the eyelid and eyeball. Calendula has an antiseptic action and reduces the burning sensation. I find it works best when combined with euphrasia (eyebright) and mixed with saline solution for administration into the eye. Five drops of each herb in an ounce of saline solution applied four times daily works well.

➥ CRACKED NIPPLES
The drying, cracking, bleeding, and irritation of the nipples of breast-feeding mothers can be helped with topical calendula application. The gel form works well for this purpose. I have prescribed it to several women with success without any other treatment.

➥ ECZEMA
Calendula can clear up very mild cases of newly developed eczema, and it helps to control chronic cases in a non-suppressive fashion.

❧ RADIATION DERMATITIS

A study published in the *Journal of Clinical Oncology* involved 254 patients who had been operated on for breast cancer and received postoperative radiation therapy. After each session, participants were randomly given an application on the irradiated fields of either a common topical pain-relieving drug known as trolamine (128 patients) or calendula (126 patients). The occurrence of acute skin inflammation of Grade 2 or higher was significantly lower (41% versus 63%) with the use of calendula than with trolamine. Additionally, patients receiving calendula had less frequent interruption of radiotherapy and significantly reduced radiation-induced pain.

❧ RASHES

One of the first natural treatments that should be tried for any rash is calendula; in most cases it will have benefit. The underlying cause for the rash (contact allergy, food sensitivities, etc.) of course needs to be treated for a complete cure.

❧ ULCERS

Calendula has been traditionally used to treat stomach ulcers and inflammatory bowel diseases such as ulcerative colitis. I have not used it for these conditions, although it appears to be very safe to do so. A preliminary study published in the *International Journal of Tissue Reactions* found calendula ointment to be statistically significant in accelerating wound healing.

❧ VARICOSE VEINS

The topical application of calendula has a minor benefit for reducing the appearance of swollen veins of the lower legs.

Cantharis

One night I got a call from a relative of mine. Her husband, Darrel, had been burned in an accident at work, and he was in serious pain.

Darrel worked at an oil compressor station, and he had received steam burns on his thigh when one of the pipes broke. The pain was excruciating.

This all occurred in the dead of winter, where the temperature was about 4 degrees below Fahrenheit. Though he was in severe pain, Darrel managed to pull off his jeans before he got into his truck and raced to the hospital some 20 miles away. So it happened that around 7:00 on a bitter winter's evening, a man came running into the emergency room of an Alberta hospital, clad only in his underwear.

Darrel was given some cream for second-degree burns, along with a shot of morphine. He took home some pain medication as well as antibiotics to prevent a secondary bacterial infection. His wife had picked him up from the hospital.

When I received the call from Darrel's wife, many hours had passed since his release from the hospital, but the pain-relieving medications weren't helping.

I recommended that he take homeopathic cantharis that was in their homeopathic first-aid kit. Thirty minutes later, I called again to find out how he was faring. He reported a dramatic reduction in pain. A short time after my call, I later learned, he fell asleep and slept soundly for the rest of the night.

The next day, when Darrel saw the doctors at the emergency room, they asked how he'd coped with the pain overnight. He pulled out his bottle of cantharis and said, "I quit using the pain medication because it was not helping. Instead, I have been using this. I really do not feel much pain at all!"

The attending doctors looked at him in disbelief. They had no idea what cantharis was.

A BEETLE BONUS

In my view, many burn victims could be spared a lot of pain and agony if emergency-room doctors knew a lot more about homeopathic remedies such as cantharis.

The cantharis preparation comes from the blister beetle, sometimes called the Spanish fly. The beetle contains a chemical called cantharadin, which can raise blisters and cause severe inflammation on human skin. Based on the homeopathic premise that "like cures like," this is the perfect substance to use in a homeopathic dilution to heal burns. It's very effective with second-degree burns—the kind that raise blisters on the skin. It also helps relieve pain and

promote healing if you have a third-degree burn, the most severe kind.

Homeopaths tell of cases of hospitalized patients with the severest of burns who have gotten relief from cantharis. Other homeopathic remedies to consider include Arsenicum and *Urtica urens*.

Cantharis is also one of the best remedies for urinary tract infections, especially bladder infections.

DOSAGE

Cantharis is generally used for severe acute burns and bladder infections, so I recommend using the highest dose possible. I typically use a 200C potency or higher. Most health-food stores and pharmacies carry the 30C potency as the highest strength. This, too, can work; it just needs to be taken more often, such as two to four times daily. If it helps, but wears off, then contact a homeopathic practitioner for a stronger potency.

WHAT ARE THE SIDE EFFECTS?

I have never seen any side effects with cantharis. If it doesn't help, it does nothing at all, in which case you should simply try a different remedy.

CANTHARIS
RECOMMENDATIONS FROM THE NATURAL PHYSICIAN FOR . . .

BURNS

While cantharis is most helpful for the type of burns that raise blisters, I have also found it helpful for severe sunburns. I found myself recommending it just a few days before my wedding, when one of my best men got a nasty-looking sunburn. (I didn't make him feel any better by commenting that he resembled a baked salmon—but it was true, his whole upper body was bright pink.) So he got a high dose of cantharis (and also aloe vera gel) just to get him to the church on time. Surprisingly, he had no blistering or peeling, and none of the typical sunburn pain!

For burns that cover a large area of the body, one homeopath recommended dissolving two pellets of cantharis in a bottle of purified water. Spray the solution over the burn areas as needed during the day.

🐾 URINARY TRACT INFECTIONS

Cantharis is very effective in the first stages of a urinary tract infection, especially if you've experienced a burning sensation while urinating. One source describes this as "each drop passes as if scalding water."

Cantharis is prescribed if blood accompanies the stream of urine, which often happens with bladder infections, or if there's dribbling as a result of the infection. Cantharis can be combined with antibiotics to speed recovery and reduce urinary pain, especially if the infection has spread to the kidneys.

Caralluma fimbriata

"I just need something to help me with my appetite and I know I could lose weight. I am exercising, eating relatively healthy, but I find myself never satisfied with the amount I am eating . . . and so I eat more!" revealed Brynn, a 40-year-old accountant.

"There are a number of supplements and drugs people can use to reduce their appetite, but many are dangerous to your health," I told her. "There is one I have used with patients successfully, and it is very safe. It is called Caralluma."

Caralluma is a roadside shrub found in many parts of India as well as areas of Africa, the Canary Islands, Arabia, southern Europe, Sri Lanka, and Afghanistan. For centuries it has been consumed like a vegetable—boiled or eaten raw. It was used by tribesmen to suppress hunger and thirst during long journeys. It is listed by the Indian Health Ministry's compilation of medicinal plants as a vegetable and "famine food."

An Indian herbal product manufacturer has conducted some interesting research on this plant and using it in the supplement form. They found that 1,000 mg of an extract is equivalent to 100 g of raw Caralluma consumed as a food for an appetite- and thirst-quenching effect. It is thought that components known as pregnane glycosides are responsible for its appetite- and thirst-suppressive effects on the brain.

DOSAGE

Take 500 mg two times a day, 30 to 45 minutes before meals, usually breakfast and dinner.

WHAT ARE THE SIDE EFFECTS?

Occasionally digestive upset and headache is reported. Digestive symptoms tend to go away after a week of continual supplementation. Caralluma is not recommended for pregnant women or nursing mothers. Children should only use it under a doctor's supervision.

CARALLUMA FIMBRIATA

RECOMMENDATIONS FROM THE NATURAL PHYSICIAN FOR . . .

☙ APPETITE SUPPRESSION AND WEIGHT LOSS

I find about 80% of patients seeking weight loss notice an obvious improvement from Caralluma extract. There have been two studies done with Caralluma examining its effect on appetite suppression and weight loss. The first study, at St. John's National Academy of Health Sciences in Bangalore, India, involved 50 participants who walked for 30 minutes daily and took Caralluma or a placebo. Those taking Caralluma showed only a slightly greater average weight loss after eight weeks (1.94 pounds) than the placebo group (1.12 pounds). However, the average loss in waist circumference was 2.75 inches in the Caralluma group versus only a 1.29-inch loss in the placebo group. Loss of abdominal girth correlates with reduced body fat.

In the second study, at Western Geriatric Research Institute in Los Angeles, overweight patients took the regular dose of Caralluma or a placebo for four weeks. Participants were instructed not to change their daily activity pattern (exercise) or their food intake for four weeks before starting the trial and during the four weeks of the trial. Out of 18 patients who took the Caralluma and completed the trial, 15 lost weight. Eleven patients lost an average of six pounds, with the highest loss nine pounds. The other four participants lost one to two pounds. Of the patients taking a placebo who completed the trial, three gained one pound each, one lost one pound, and the other two dropped out due to minor digestive upset.

Carbo Vegetabilis

Toni had been suffering from digestive problems for several months. She experienced bloating, gas, and—most troubling of all—belching. Amazingly, she would belch all day long, several dozens of times and it was an understandable embarrassment for her. Her family doctor ran tests and never found any abnormalities. His recommendation was to "change your diet," although he did not define how it should be changed. Toni actually had tried various diets, without much benefit for her digestive problems. When asked if I had something that could dramatically help her belching I replied, "I have just the medicine that should do the trick." Sure enough her

belching was considerably improved in only a few weeks of taking homeopathic carbo vegetabilis, or carbo veg, as many homeopathic prescribers call it.

Carbo veg not only helps several digestive symptoms, but also is effective for many lung conditions. This includes asthma, bronchitis, and pneumonia. Those requiring this remedy often have those symptoms accompanied by a "weak feeling." This homeopathic is derived from vegetable charcoal, that is, charcoal from birch or beech.

DOSAGE

The homeopathic 30C potency is commonly available in health-food stores. For the treatment of acute conditions, take two pellets of a 30C potency four times daily for up to three days. For chronic conditions, take the same dose twice daily for two to four weeks and stop using if symptoms return.

WHAT ARE THE SIDE EFFECTS?

I have not seen side effects with this homeopathic remedy. Normally it either works or it doesn't. As with any homeopathic medicine, if it is taken indefinitely, it can cause the same symptoms one is trying to treat.

CARBO VEGETABILIS
RECOMMENDATIONS FROM THE NATURAL PHYSICIAN FOR . . .

ANXIETY/PANIC ATTACKS

Carbo veg can be helpful for acute anxiety and panic attacks, including feelings of anxiety along with shortness of breath and the desire to be fanned or be in the open air.

ASTHMA

Although not a cure for asthma, this remedy can help reduce asthma symptoms such as shortness of breath with a desire for open air. Also, it can help when asthmatics get shortness of breath at night requiring them to sit up.

BRONCHITIS AND PNEUMONIA

As with asthma symptoms, carbo veg can be quite helpful for lung infections where there is shortness of breath and a desire for fresh air or to be fanned. It can be used in combination with antibiotic therapy.

CONGESTIVE HEART FAILURE

Symptom relief of shortness of breath, cold hands and feet, and bloated appearance may be achieved with carbo veg.

DIGESTIVE UPSET

There are many uses for carbo veg in the treatment of digestive ailments. Just as activated charcoal is used medicinally to reduce gas and bind toxins, this homeopathic preparation can help a variety of gastrointestinal complaints. These include belching, acid reflux, bloating, and indigestion.

Carotenoids

"As you can tell, I'm a sun worshipper. So I already know you're going to recommend sunscreen," said Barb, a 35-year-old fitness trainer. She assured me that she already did that—and she was also trying to limit the time she spent in the sun. "But besides that . . . ?"

"Antioxidants are what I recommend," I answered. "A diet rich in fruits and vegetables is your best choice. There are many antioxidants in the multivitamin that you are taking. But I also recommend a mixed carotenoid complex. The carotenoids act as antioxidants to protect the skin and help absorb the sun's ultraviolet rays."

"My multivitamin contains beta carotene. Is that one of the carotenoids?" asked Barb.

"Yes, it is." But I also wanted her to know that she might need more than that. "Most multivitamins do not contain a mixed carotenoid complex," I noted. "There are several carotenoids besides beta carotene. As a matter of fact, it appears that getting a combination of them are more important than taking any single one by itself."

Researchers estimate that more than 700 different carotenoids exist in nature. Fruits and vegetables are rich in carotenoids, especially ones with bright colors such as red, yellow, orange, purple, and dark green.

WHAT ARE CAROTENOIDS?

Carotenoids are actually fat-soluble pigments that are responsible for the brilliant colors in the full spectrum of the fruit and vegetable rainbow. Apart from their colorful contribution, they are also responsible for protecting the plant from oxidants formed during photosynthesis.

Beta carotene is the most well-known carotenoid but not necessarily the most potent. Other important carotenoids that have been the focus of recent research include alpha carotene, cryptoxanthin, lutein, lycopene, and zeaxanthin.

Some of the carotenoids are converted into vitamin A, but many are not. Essentially, nature has intended for us to get a mix of carotenoids.

In general, the brighter the food, the greater the carotenoid concentration. For example, a pale orange carrot contains less beta carotene than a dark orange carrot. General sources include carrots, pumpkins, squash, sweet potatoes, broccoli, peas, collard greens, kale, peppers (all colors), spinach, apricots, cantaloupe, papaya, peaches, tangerines, tomatoes, watermelon, and cherries.

Most supplements use a mixed carotenoid complex from the sea algae *Dunaliella salina* from the waters of Australia.

A FULL SPECTRUM OF HELP

As a whole, the carotenoids are protective against a variety of cancers and cardiovascular disease. They also enhance the immune system and act as antioxidants.

Specific carotenoids are known to benefit specific organs of the body. For example, the carotenoids lutein and zeaxanthin (found in high concentration in spinach and dark green leafy vegetables) appear to be important in protecting against macular degeneration. Lycopene is carotenoid found in high concentration in tomatoes and appears to be protective against prostate cancer.

Carotenoids are important for proper lung function as they suppress free radicals from air pollution. A study of 528 people ages 65 to 85 years old found that persons with high blood levels of beta carotene, lycopene, and alpha carotene had significantly better lung function than those with low levels of these nutrients.

Studies have shown that carotenoids help to prevent the damaging effects of the sun's ultraviolet rays on the skin. A recent study showed that 25 mg of a natural carotenoid complex protected against sunburn after eight weeks of supplementation. (However, the combination of carotenoids and vitamin E worked better to provide protection after four weeks of use.)

DOSAGE

I recommend taking one capsule of a mixed carotenoid complex. A blend can be found in a high-potency multivitamin or separately. A typical soft gel carotenoid complex will contain a mixture similar to the following:

Beta carotene—25,000 IU

Lycopene—5,000 mcg

Alpha carotene—492 mcg

Cryptoxanthin—115 mcg

Zeaxanthin—98 mcg

Lutein—74 mcg

Specific conditions require higher dosages of the individual carotenoids.

It is important to note that zinc, vitamin C, and thyroid hormone are required for the conversion of carotenoids to vitamin A.

Note that carotenoids are helpful in preventing many health problems, especially for the conditions listed below.

WHAT ARE THE SIDE EFFECTS?

The carotenoids are nontoxic. A yellowish discoloration of the skin (carotenemia) can result from taking too high a dosage. The discoloration goes away when the dosage is reduced.

CAROTENOIDS
RECOMMENDATIONS FROM THE NATURAL PHYSICIAN FOR . . .

❧ CANCER

It has been well documented through population studies that carotenoid-rich diets are protective against a variety of cancers. Specifically, the carotenoid lycopene seems to have powerful preventive effect, especially in guarding men against prostate cancer.

Interestingly, lycopene is the most abundant carotenoid in the prostate gland. Researchers feel that lycopene is better absorbed from tomato sauce as opposed to raw tomatoes.

A six-year Harvard study of 48,000 male physicians found that men who consumed tomato-rich foods (tomatoes, tomato sauce, and pizza) at least 10 times a week, had a 35% decreased risk of prostate cancer compared with those men who had less than a serving and a half of those high-lycopene servings every week.

Men have asked me whether it makes sense to use lycopene as a supplement for prostate cancer. One study has been done.

In this study researchers looked at 30 men with localized prostate cancer who were scheduled to undergo surgical removal of the prostate. For three weeks prior to surgery, the participants were randomly assigned 30 mg of lycopene supplement or a placebo—that is, a sugar pill that resembled the real supplement. After the men underwent surgery, follow-up examinations showed that the treated group had smaller tumors than the group of men who received the placebos. Also, the PSA value had declined in those taking lycopene. PSA is a "marker" that is used to help doctors determine the presence of prostate cancer, so a decline in PSA was considered an excellent indicator that the lycopene was having a beneficial effect.

One study showed that high-lutein diets were associated with a 17% decrease in colon cancer risk, and young people with a diet high in lutein had a 34% lower risk of colon cancer.

(continued)

Many studies have shown a protective effect of beta carotene, especially in early-stage cancers of the mouth and esophagus—though studies have shown the protection is not powerful enough to help prevent lung cancer in smokers.

Overall, for cancer prevention it makes sense to eat a diet rich in carotenoids. If supplements are used, then mixed carotenoid supplements make the most sense to me. Higher dosages of lycopene—30 mg daily—are a good idea for men with prostate cancer.

CARDIOVASCULAR DISEASE

Carotenoids also appear to be important for the prevention of cardiovascular disease. This may be due to their protective effect, since they help to prevent the oxidation of cholesterol.

One study showed that eating a diet rich in carotenoids may reduce the risk of angina. Researchers found that people with the highest levels of alpha carotene, beta carotene, and beta cryptoxanthin were on average 50% less likely to develop angina.

MACULAR DEGENERATION

This condition is the leading cause of blindness in the United States. The macula—the part of the retina responsible for visual acuity—deteriorates. Population studies show that the risk of developing age-related macular degeneration is significantly reduced in people whose diet is rich in fruits and vegetables containing beta carotene.

Lutein and zeaxanthin are two carotenoids that appear to be even more important. These carotenoids are found in dark green vegetables such as spinach, kale, and collard greens. They function in the macula to absorb light and protect our eyes against light's damaging effects.

A survey of 876 elderly individuals showed that those whose intake of these two carotenoids was high were 56% less likely to develop age-related macular degeneration.

OSTEOPOROSIS

Low levels of carotenoids may predispose one to osteoporosis. More study is needed to confirm this link.

SUNBURN

Lycopene is a very good carotenoid for preventing sunburn. Eating fruits and vegetables rich in lycopene and supplementation can help reduce how easily your skin gets red from sun exposure. Supplementation has been shown to reduce how easily the skin turns red from ultraviolet radiation, too.

Cascara Sagrada

"This is so unlike me . . . my bowels haven't moved in three days and my stomach is bloating up! In a few days I have to travel to Washington and I am concerned." So said Jack, a 42-year-old writer.

"Okay, let's get you on some cascara for the next day or two to get things moving," I replied, assuring Jack the situation could be quickly resolved.

Virtually every health-food store carries cascara sagrada, also referred to as sacred bark. This herb has a long traditional use for the acute treatment of constipation. It is native to British Columbia (Canada),

Washington, Oregon, and northern California. The aged, dried bark of cascara is rich in hydroxyanthraquinone glycosides called cascarosides. These substances stimulate motility (contraction) of the large intestine so fecal matter is expelled.

DOSAGE

Most people use the capsule form. Normally 500 to 1,000 mg taken twice daily will get the bowels to move in a day or two. In tincture form, ½ to 1 teaspoon can be taken twice daily. If you cannot achieve relief of constipation in four days, or if you develop abdominal pain, see your doctor. Also make sure to drink adequate water—64 to 80 ounces daily when constipated.

WHAT ARE THE SIDE EFFECTS?

This herb should not be used by pregnant or breast-feeding women. For children under the age of 10 it should be used under the guidance of a doctor. It should also be avoided by those with abdominal pain and inflammatory bowel disease such as ulcerative colitis and Crohn's disease. It should not be used long term—such as longer than a week—as it may result in the colon becoming lazy and worsening bowel function. Too frequent bowel movements and loose stool over long periods of time may also cause electrolyte imbalance, such as potassium deficiency.

CASCARA SAGRADA

RECOMMENDATIONS FROM THE NATURAL PHYSICIAN FOR . . .

CONSTIPATION

Acute constipation is the only condition for which I prescribe cascara. I have spoken with many people who use cascara on a long-term basis for constipation. I believe this is a mistake because it is not treating the root of their constipation, and ultimately makes their bowels more sluggish. Instead they should focus on adequate fiber and water intake, exercise, avoiding food sensitivities, developing better stress coping mechanisms, and reestablishing flora balance, all of which improve constipation. However, cascara is a good short-term treatment for acute constipation and is readily available in health-food and drug stores.

Cat's Claw

I occasionally will see a patient who grew up in Peru or has traveled there. I ask these folks about their thoughts on the botanical cat's claw. Their eyes usually light up, and they tell me how popular it is in that country, where it is revered for its medicinal uses, especially among Peruvian Amazonian tribes. Cat's claw, also known as *uña de gato* or by its botanical name *Uncaria tomentosa*, is a superstar among the Peruvian and Brazilian people and has become popular in the United States as well. It grows in the Amazon region of Peru and neighboring countries. Native healers of Peru use cat's claw for treating arthritis, cancer, liver ailments, ulcers and other digestive ailments, and skin conditions. Locals also use it on a preventative basis to prevent disease.

This woody vine can reach 1,000 feet in height. The inner bark of the vine is boiled as a decoction by locals, whereas extracts of the root are used for medicinal purposes in US supplements. In Germany and Austria, cat's claw is used as a standardized extract and regulated as a pharmaceutical medicine. Europeans often use a different species, known as *Uncaria guianensis*, and both species are used in South American botanical medicine. Cat's claw is available by prescription only in Europe and is used by doctors in those countries for immune enhancement for people with cancer. Most of the commercially available cat's claw has been harvested in the wild of Peru and Brazil.

Cat's claw has a history of being used by South American folk healers for the treatment of cancer. In the 1970s, this caught the attention of European researchers, who began to explore its medicinal qualities. There has been little scientific data published, however, in regard to the use of cat's claw for cancer or other diseases. Reviews of clinical studies done on cat's claw suggest it has immune modulating and anti-inflammatory properties. Brazilians believe cat's claw is useful as a treatment for urinary tract cancers.

Several dozen compounds have been isolated in cat's claw. One group known as pentacylic alkaloids has been shown to have immune-stimulating properties. This botanical has also been shown to have antioxidant, anti-inflammatory, antiviral, blood-pressure-lowering, and immune-modulating effects. Animal studies have demonstrated that cat's claw enhances phagocytosis, the increase in activity of white blood cells that fight infectious microbes. Overall, more studies are required to further explore the benefits of cat's claw. Studies in human beings have shown posi-

tive results for those with rheumatoid arthritis and osteoarthritis, which are included later in this chapter. Clinically, doctors like me find this botanical to benefit patients in need of immune system modulation and as an anti-inflammatory agent.

DOSAGE

The dosages vary for cat's claw depending on whether the product is standardized or not. Check the label for directions. Generally a dosage of 1 to 2 mL of the tincture form is taken twice daily or standardized capsules are taken as directed on the label.

WHAT ARE THE SIDE EFFECTS?

Cat's claw is considered to be nontoxic. However, there is not a lot of literature in regard to side effects. It is therefore not recommended for pregnant or nursing mothers. Use for autoimmune conditions is controversial, although it was shown in one study to benefit rheumatoid arthritis. For these conditions it is best used under the guidance of a doctor.

CAT'S CLAW
RECOMMENDATIONS FROM THE NATURAL PHYSICIAN FOR . . .

❧ CANCER

Holistic practitioners may prescribe cat's claw for the complementary treatment of cancer. It is used for its immune-modulating properties. There is limited data on this use, but I see no problem when it is used under the guidance of a doctor.

❧ LYME DISEASE

Cat's claw is used as a complementary treatment for the treatment of Lyme disease, caused by a spirochete bacteria called *Borrelia burgdorferi*. Practitioners report beneficial results, although I am unaware of any formal studies.

❧ OSTEOARTHRITIS

Forty-five patients with osteoarthritis of the knee were involved in a study on cat's claw extract (*Uncaria guianensis* species). Thirty were treated with cat's claw extract and fifteen with placebo for four weeks. Blood markers were assessed at the beginning and end of the four-week trial. Pain, medical, and subject assessment scores and adverse effects were collected for weeks 1, 2, and 4. Knee pain associated with activity was significantly reduced and benefit was noted within the first week of treatment for the cat's claw group. Knee pain at rest and knee swelling were not significantly improved. Researchers found no harmful effects on blood or liver function or other significant side effects compared to placebo.

❧ RHEUMATOID ARTHRITIS

Forty patients with rheumatoid arthritis were enrolled in a randomized 52-week, two-phase study and were receiving the medications sulfasalazine or hydroxychloroquine in addition to cat's claw or a placebo. Researchers found benefit from cat's claw supplementation. After 24 weeks of treatment with the cat's claw extract (*Uncaria tomentosa* species), results showed a greater reduction of the number of painful joints compared to placebo. Only minor side effects were noted.

Cayenne

Spicy food lovers crave it, people with pain need it, and those with heart disease swear by it.

Cayenne or red pepper is actually the berry of the *Capsicum annuum longum* plant. Cayenne literally means "to bite" and the hot sensation one senses from eating cayenne makes it a popular spicing agent in foods. Cayenne is used medicinally for improving circulation and improving digestion. Topically it has become popular for reducing pain and itching.

The typical color for cayenne is red. However, there are other capsicum varieties that vary in color from yellow to purple to orange. They all tend to be spicy except for paprika, which is a different variety of *Capsicum annuum* and has a milder, sweeter taste. The degree of pungency, which is calculated in heat units, of dried capsicum and/or the oleoresin extractive is what determines the value and usage.

Cayenne peppers have been consumed by the people of South America and the East Indies for thousands of years. Interestingly, the term "chili" is the Aztec name for cayenne pepper. In the 15th century, Dr. Diego Alvarez Chanca, who accompanied famed explorer Christopher Columbus, brought cayenne seeds from the Caribbean Islands back to Italy from the New World. Cayenne then spread to Africa, India, and throughout northern Europe and temperate zones around the world.

Cayenne has been used in traditional and folk treatments for a variety of conditions including asthma, fevers, poor circulation, respiratory tract infections and sore throats, digestive problems, and cancers. Topically it has been used to treat toothaches and muscle pain. In China and Japan, it has been used topically to treat frostbite and muscle inflammation. Herbalists use it in formulas to improve absorption and circulation of other herbs and supplements in the body.

A well-researched active component in cayenne is capsaicin. This substance is responsible for the intense heat produced by the fruit. It works to relieve pain when applied topically or taken internally. It depletes substance P ("P" stands for "pain") from nerve fibers, which ultimately blocks the pain sensation. Creams and gels containing capsaicin are FDA approved for arthritis and pain such as diabetic neuropathy.

Research has also shown that cayenne has antioxidant properties, reduces cholesterol, and has a blood-thinning effect by reducing platelet aggregation.

Cayenne is such a potent spice that it may seem contradictory to use it for pain relief. But many holistic practitioners as well as conventional medical doctors recommend the topical use of cayenne to relieve joint and muscle pain. Because the capsaicin blocks the neurotransmitter substance P, the nerves to the skin and spinal cord do not receive any "pain signals." This is also the chemical that gives cayenne its hot taste.

When cayenne is first applied, you may feel a burning, stinging sensation as substance P actually increases for a short time. But as you use cayenne for a longer time, the sensations diminish as substance P activity decreases.

Some people, including me, have stomach irritation when we eat cayenne or take a cayenne supplement. But I've found that this reaction isn't universal—it all depends on the person. Whatever your reaction, however, there's no evidence that chili peppers damage the intestinal tract. On the contrary, one study has shown that capsaicin actually inhibits the growth of the bacteria *H. pylori*, which is implicated in many cases of stomach ulcers.

Cayenne has also been praised as a natural ingredient that improves circulation. Many herbalists and supplement companies claim that cayenne helps to "clean out" the arteries and reverse the effects of atherosclerosis. More studies must be done before we can be sure of these effects, but I do believe cayenne benefits the heart and cardiovascular system based on the feedback I get from patients. It's also known to be a great source of antioxidants such as vitamins A and C, and phytochemicals that protect against cellular damage. Some laboratory studies have also shown that cayenne reduces cholesterol levels and acts as a natural blood thinner.

Cayenne is used by many herbalists and naturopathic doctors in formulas for sore throats, upper respiratory tract infections, and sinusitis. It helps to reduce congestion and inflammation of these areas.

DOSAGE

For internal use, take 5 to 10 drops in water, or 400 to 500 mg in capsule form up to three times daily. For topical application, use a cream standardized to 0.025% to 0.075% capsaicin. Apply to the affected area of pain up to four times daily.

WHAT ARE THE SIDE EFFECTS?

Some people do experience digestive upset from taking cayenne internally. The cream form, which is applied to the skin only, has been shown to be very safe in clinical studies—though some people may initially experience a burning sensation that goes away after three or four days. **CAUTION:** The cream should not be applied on open skin or near the eyes.

Cayenne probably has blood-thinning properties, so you should let your physician know you're taking the drops or capsules if you happen to be on blood-thinning medications.

CAYENNE

RECOMMENDATIONS FROM THE NATURAL PHYSICIAN FOR . . .

ARTHRITIS

Studies have shown capsaicin cream effective for osteoarthritis. Keep in mind, however, that this approach alleviates the pain, not the underlying cartilage deterioration. Supplements such as glucosamine sulfate, SAMe, and antioxidants (selenium, vitamin C, alpha lipoic acid) help to regenerate cartilage tissue and should also be used simultaneously.

Rheumatoid arthritis can also be helped with capsaicin cream.

DIABETIC NEUROPATHY

Diabetic neuropathy is the nerve damage related to a diabetic condition, and it's characterized by pain and abnormal sensations in the legs and feet. In studies, researchers have found that capsaicin is effective in relieving this kind of pain. When researchers tried the cream with 49 patients who had moderate to severe diabetic neuropathy, it was found that 90% of the people who took capsaicin had pain reduction by the eighth week of use. Remember, capsaicin is the active ingredient in cayenne.

Other studies have confirmed this benefit as well—so cayenne is a simple, nontoxic way to relieve nerve pain if you have severe diabetic neuropathy. To make the treatment even better, I recommend adding alpha lipoic acid, vitamin B12, and ginkgo biloba, which work internally to reverse this painful condition.

HEART DISEASE

Cayenne has been shown to reduce the risk of heart disease by reducing cholesterol and triglyceride levels. Despite the lack of studies about this effect, hundreds of people have testified to the tremendous benefits they have experienced from supplementing with cayenne.

As a natural blood thinner, cayenne helps promote optimal circulation through the arteries of the body and heart. It is theorized that cayenne improves

(continued)

circulation through the coronary arteries. It is a great herb to include in herbal cardiovascular formulas.

◈ PSORIASIS

This painful and itchy skin condition is one of the most stubborn conditions to treat because flare-ups can occur almost any time. The best long-term treatments involve herbs, supplements, and therapies that will help balance the internal environment. However, topical treatments with capsaicin have also proven effective.

For difficult cases, capsaicin is a treatment to consider.

◈ SHINGLES

The pain from shingles can be excruciating. I've had patients who couldn't even lie on their side on the examining table because the pain was so bad. Yet these "worst cases" are, fortunately, the very ones who are likely to benefit the most from treatment with cayenne.

When tested in controlled studies, capsaicin has relieved shingles pain in about 50% of users. I usually like to combine this treatment with other therapies, including vitamin B12 injections, acupuncture, and homeopathic remedies. Capsaicin cream can be used to help relieve pain while these other natural therapies are working internally for a long-term cure.

◈ SURGERY RECOVERY

Surgery can be traumatizing enough, but when you have additional nerve pain after surgery, life can be pretty miserable. Fortunately, capsaicin cream has proven helpful for people who have had nerve trauma and lasting pain after surgery.

Several studies support this recommendation. In a study of 23 patients who had mastectomies for breast cancer, researchers found that a cream with 0.075% capsaicin significantly reduced pain levels. These types of pain studies are encouraging because, so often, physicians don't know how to treat postsurgical nerve pain except with more surgery or with pharmaceutical pain medications, many of which have side effects. (Other natural treatments that work well include acupuncture and homeopathic remedies such as hypericum.)

Chamomile

You'll routinely be offered chamomile tea in many restaurants and homes in Germany. It's an herb with a pleasant taste—so tasty, in fact, that even hard-core coffee-lovers can be found drinking it from time to time. If you ever need a tonic, too, to help anyone in the family overcome stomach upset, chamomile (*Recutita matricaria*) is the one to choose.

Much of chamomile's medicinal effects are targeted toward the digestive tract and nervous system. It's a synergistic combination, since the state of your nervous system is quite likely to dictate the health of your digestive system. In a world where high stress predominates, chamomile offers welcomed relief to "jangled nerves."

Chamomile has a rich history of use around the world. Ancient Egyptians, Greeks, and Indian healers relied on chamomile for its healing properties. It's a leading treatment for digestive conditions in many parts of Africa. It's officially considered a drug rather than an herb in many parts of the world—notably in Belgium, France, and the United Kingdom.

It comes in many forms. You'll easily find chamomile tea in the supermarket. The tinctures and capsules are in many health-food stores and pharmacies. Chamomile is even used as an ingredient in shampoos. (It brings out blond highlights, as well as acting as a cleanser.) Widely used as a homeopathic remedy, it's also a popular essential oil that's much valued for its aroma.

A CHOICE OF TEAS

Two species of chamomile are used medicinally. German chamomile, also known as *Matricaria chamomilla* or *Matricaria recutita*, is the species of chamomile that has been most frequently used in research. This is the variety I recommend for patients. There's also a Roman chamomile, but I prefer the German. According to my sources in the health-food industry, German chamomile is not contaminated by pesticides and other chemicals that are frequently found in Roman chamomile products.

Researchers have identified two major classes of active constituents in chamomile. Essential oils in the herb appear to have potent anti-inflammatory and antispasmodic effects. This accounts for the many beneficial ways it soothes the gastrointestinal tract by relieving spasms, preventing gas, and even helping to ward off ulcers.

Chamomile also enhances antiviral and antibacterial activity, promoting the proliferation of substances that help fight off infection.

Because of its anti-inflammatory properties, chamomile is also used topically for the treatment of skin disorders such as eczema. Even pets can benefit from this herb. I recall the time when my wife's cat had a very painful-looking patch of ulcerated skin on its belly—an area where a patch of hair was missing. The vet wanted to prescribe antibiotics and a topical cortisone cream. Instead, we used a treatment of fresh cool chamomile tea applied topically to the wound a few times each day. Within a week this raw-looking flesh wound had healed up nicely.

Another group of important compounds in chamomile is the flavonoids. Flavonoids promote an antianxiety effect. Scientists have shown that they do this by binding to special receptor sites in the brain, helping to induce a state of relaxation. Flavonoids also add to the anti-inflammatory effects of chamomile.

DOSAGE

～ *Tea*

Chamomile works best, I've found, when you brew fresh tea. When the chamomile flowers are freshly steeped in boiling water, the essential oils form a high concentration. Also, just taking the time to make a fresh cup of chamomile tea is therapeutic. It's a way of saying, with your actions, "My health is important so I will take the time to make a health-promoting cup of tea."

I recommend steeping ½ to 1 teaspoon of dried chamomile flowers in a cup of freshly boiled water. Just one fresh cup helps to relieve digestive cramps and flatulence—and reduces anxiety, too—and you can have several cups during the course of the day.

Traditionally, mothers gave their infants a teaspoonful of freshly made chamomile tea to help relieve colic. I recommend it—but make sure the teaspoonful of tea is room temperature or cooler before giving it to a baby.

❧ Tincture

I recommend 10 to 30 drops (0.5 mL) of the tincture form. For best results, add this tincture to ½ cup warm water. The tincture and the warm liquid combine to help relieve spasms in the digestive tract.

Infants also respond well to this mixture, but you only need to mix a few drops of chamomile tincture in the warm water.

❧ Capsule

You can get chamomile capsules, but often the capsulized herb is combined with other herbs to create a formula. I recommend that adults take 250 to 500 mg in the capsule form three to four times daily.

❧ Creams

Chamomile is used in creams and salves for various skin conditions such as rashes. Apply as directed on the container.

WHAT ARE THE SIDE EFFECTS?

A number of herbalists have suggested that people should avoid use of chamomile if you're allergic to plants in the ragweed family, but I haven't seen any clinical evidence to support this view.

The warning signs would be reactions like an outbreak of hives, difficult breathing, or digestive upset. Of course, you should stop taking chamomile if you have any of these reactions. But millions of people use chamomile each year, and I haven't seen any reports of these adverse reactions.

CHAMOMILE

RECOMMENDATIONS FROM THE NATURAL PHYSICIAN FOR . . .

❧ COLIC

Chamomile can be a godsend for parents whose child is suffering from colic. While experts do not agree on the cause of colic, it is clear that many cases are related to abdominal pain from the buildup of intestinal gas. Chamomile with its antispasmodic action can relieve colic in short order.

To prevent a flare-up of colic, administer ½ to 1 full teaspoon of cooled-down chamomile tea every 10 minutes or so until the infant stops fussing or crying. Quite often, parents will comment that after taking the chamomile the infant will pass gas, then settle down.

An even better way to use chamomile for colic is by giving the child the homeopathic form. Mix a pellet in water, and when it's completely dissolved, give the child ½ teaspoon.

Herbal combinations can be very effective, too. In one study, 69 infants who were prone to colic were given a variety of different teas. Of those who got an herbal tea consisting of chamomile, vervain, licorice, fennel, and lemon balm for seven days, 57% had fewer colic symptoms.

Whether you're giving the child herbal or homeopathic forms of chamomile, be sure to treat the underlying cause as well. If the infant is still breast-feeding, the mother should avoid eating chocolate, peanuts, cow's milk, and spicy foods. Some children have an adverse reaction to cow's milk-based formulas and even soy formulas.

EARACHE

While the herbal form of chamomile can be used to treat mild cases of childhood earaches, I consider the homeopathic form to be almost a wonder remedy. If the child is very irritable and holds one ear in pain, I would give the homeopathic cure. Chamomilla, the homeopathic form, is particularly recommended if one cheek is red while the other is pale, and the earache is so acute that nothing will settle down the child.

I remember one child who was brought into my clinic screaming and kicking from the intense ear pain. Examining the child's ear, I could see that she had a middle ear infection. The parents were at their wit's end—but they didn't want to treat their daughter with antibiotics.

Five minutes after I gave the girl one dose of chamomilla, she was asleep in the mother's arms. When I saw the child the next day, the parents told me the child had slept through the night and was back to her regular self. I have seen dozens of cases like this, and so have other colleagues who practice homeopathy.

FLATULENCE

To help relieve flatulence, many people combine this herb with other digestive tonics such as fennel, peppermint, and ginger.

INSOMNIA

Chamomile is one of the herbs to consider using before you go to bed if you occasionally have a problem with insomnia. I find this herb also works well in a combination formula with herbs such as valerian, oatstraw, skullcap, and passionflower.

IRRITABLE BOWEL SYNDROME (IBS)

IBS is a condition characterized by abdominal pain, flatulence, constipation, and/or diarrhea. In many cases, this all-too-common condition is correlated with high stress levels. Many stress-reduction techniques are helpful—including exercise, prayer, and counseling. But along with those strategies, I recommend chamomile to help relax the nervous system.

When you're more relaxed, digestive organs work more efficiently. In addition, the antispasmodic effect of chamomile provides pain relief for anyone with IBS.

I recall working with Michael, a 34-year-old mechanic, who had a fairly typical case of IBS. His worst symptom was the buildup of gas, which often caused great abdominal pain. In addition to testing Michael for food sensitivities, I recommended he drink a cup of chamomile tea with each meal.

Michael reported a dramatic improvement within two weeks. His condition greatly improved over time—only flaring up when he ate too much fast food. Even when he had a flare-up, however, the chamomile helped alleviate most of the discomfort.

MENSTRUAL CRAMPS

Chamomile can be used to relieve the pain of menstrual cramps, particularly when combined with herbs such as cramp bark.

If you are experiencing menstrual cramps, I recommend placing a hot water bottle over the lower abdomen and taking chamomile every 15 minutes.

(continued)

In its homeopathic form, chamomilla is also quite effective for menstrual cramps. My wife, Angela—who is also a natural doctor—once suffered from cramps so badly that she had to lie down. I came to see her between patients one day and found her lying on a table in one of the exam rooms. She said she felt like she was going to die.

I immediately gave her a dose of chamomilla, and within 10 minutes the pains greatly subsided. An hour later, she was back seeing patients with me.

Angela later told me that after taking the remedy, she passed a huge clot, which was likely causing most of her discomfort.

❧ SKIN

The use of chamomile in natural skin products continues to become more popular. Its anti-inflammatory effect makes it valuable for rashes of all types. European practitioners recommend that it be added to baths for skin ailments.

One study found chamomile to be effective in speeding up the healing of skin abrasions after tattoos were surgically removed with abrasive materials.

❧ STRESS

The nerve-relaxing properties of chamomile make it a popular herb for anxiety. Although not so strong as the nerve-soothing herbs kava root or valerian, it does work well for mild cases of anxiety. It's often included in herbal formulas, particularly for people whose muscles get very tight and tense from stress.

❧ TEETHING

Homeopathic chamomilla is the number one remedy for children who have discomfort and pain from teething. Not only does it provide relief from the pain, chamomilla also helps alleviate the diarrhea that can accompany teething. (Homeopathic doctors look for a green stool color to determine whether chamomilla is the remedy of choice.)

You can give a child chamomilla in the usual homeopathic form or in the form of teething tablets. Herbal teas or tinctures also help, but I've found they don't work so well as the homeopathic form.

❧ ULCERS

Chamomile has a rich herbal history of use in the treatment of ulcers. One of its key components, azulene, is believed to promote healing in the mucus layer of the stomach. Animal studies have demonstrated the antiulcer effects of chamomile.

One old-time naturopathic doctor taught me a treatment that I have frequently given to my patients. First, I have the patient drink ½ cup of chamomile tea, then lie down on her back. Fifteen minutes later, the patient drinks another ½ cup and lies on her left side. After 15 minutes and another ½ cup of chamomile tea, the patient shifts to her stomach. A final dose, and she lies on her right side for the last 15 minutes.

As the doctor had indicated, having someone shift positions in this way allows the chamomile to settle in different areas of the stomach, and 15 minutes is enough time to let the healing properties go to work on the contacted tissue.

The highly regarded German medical doctor and herbalist Rudolph Weiss states in his book *Herbal Medicine* that "chamomile does not merely give symptomatic relief in these cases [of ulcers], but directly effects a cure. . . ." But he also notes that large doses of chamomile tea or tincture need to be given for prolonged periods of time for complete healing to occur.

I would recommend at least two months of continuous use.

Chlorella

One of the most popular super foods in the health-food industry is chlorella. I remember using this product more than 20 years ago to support detoxification and energy levels. Chlorella is green algae that grows in freshwater. It is a single-celled plant. Out of the many thousands of different species of algae, approximately 15 are edible. There are different species used medicinally. The name chlorella is derived from the Greek, *chloros* meaning "green" and *ella* meaning "small."

Chlorella is a whole food supplement available in different forms. The two most common are tablet and liquid. It is also commonly found in blends of "green" formulas in capsules, powders, granules, and liquids. Reputable products use a commercial process in their preparation that breaks down the cell wall to make chlorella digestible.

Chlorella contains a powerhouse of nutrients and is a significant source of chlorophyll, protein (some products contain ½ to ¾ g of protein per 3 g chlorella), carbohydrates, lipids, fiber, nucleic acids, vitamins, and minerals. More specifically it is composed of several key amino acids, as well as vitamin C, beta carotene, chlorophyll, lutein, thiamin (B1), riboflavin (B2), pyridoxine (B6), niacin, pantothenic acid, folic acid, biotin, choline, vitamin K, lipoic acid, inositol, phosphorus, calcium, zinc, iodine, magnesium, iron, copper, protein, dietary fiber, omega fatty acids, and vitamin B12.

Test tube and animal studies suggest chlorella has antitumor, antibacterial, antifungal, and antiviral activities.

DOSAGE

Follow directions on the label since the concentration of each product is different. Studies have used up 10 g of the tablet form.

WHAT ARE THE SIDE EFFECTS?

I have not found side effects to be very common with chlorella. Digestive upset can occur but normally this will dissipate with a reduced dosage and time. A small percent of people may experience some initial fatigue, presumably due to detoxification occurring from the chlorella. Stools may be green from the chlorophyll content of chlorella.

CHLORELLA
RECOMMENDATIONS FROM THE NATURAL PHYSICIAN FOR . . .

✎ BREAST-FEEDING

Dioxins are chemical toxins formed from chlorine-containing materials in waste (such as polyvinylchloride [PVC] plastics) burned in medical and municipal incinerators or from the burning of fuels such as wood, coal, or oil. They are associated with a variety of health problems, including cancer, developmental and learning problems in children, and hormone imbalance. They can be passed from the breast milk of a mother to the child. Most dioxins that get into the human body are ingested from food. A Japanese study gave healthy pregnant women 6 g chlorella for six months and then investigated the effects on dioxin and IgA (a beneficial immune system antibody) concentrations in breast milk. Researchers found chlorella supplementation resulted in reduced dioxin levels and increased levels of IgA.

✎ COMPLEMENTARY CANCER TREATMENT

Chlorella is a gentle nutritional support to support those undergoing conventional cancer treatments. With its concentrated chlorophyll and nutrient content I believe it supports more effective detoxification for the cellular waste products generated by these treatments. One study found that taking chlorella tablets (up to 20 g daily plus 150 mL liquid extract daily) may help people with brain tumors (glioma) better tolerate chemotherapy and radiation.

✎ FATIGUE

Chlorella is a good supplement to use for overall nutrition and detoxification for those with fatigue. It complements other nutrients recommended in this book for the nutritional treatment of these symptoms. Some patients with fatigue cannot tolerate energy-enhancing supplements. Chlorella, being more of a food-based supplement, is generally tolerated quite well by those with sensitivities.

✎ FIBROMYALGIA

This is a chronic, painful condition of the muscles and tendons that involves several "tender points." A double-blind, placebo-controlled, crossover study published in *Phytotherapy Research* found that chlorella was effective in relieving the symptoms of fibromyalgia. Participants supplemented with 10 g chlorella tablets and 100 mL of liquid chlorella, or a placebo along with 100 mL of liquid chlorella. Another trial found benefit as well.

✎ GENE EXPRESSION AND HEALTH PROTECTION

A relatively new field known as nutrigenomics involves the use of food products and nutrients to favorably affect gene expression. The effect of chlorella was studied on 17 people with risk factors for lifestyle-related diseases and 17 healthy participants over a 16-week period, including a four-week post-observation period. Blood tests and gene expression profiles were completed before and after chlorella intake. Researchers confirmed that in both groups chlorella intake resulted in noticeable reductions in body fat percentage, serum total cholesterol, and fasting blood glucose levels. Also, gene expression analysis found effects of chlorella, including insulin-signaling pathways involved in lowering glucose levels.

HIGH BLOOD PRESSURE

One study found that chlorella supplementation had benefit in stabilizing blood pressure for people with mild to moderate hypertension. Although chlorella is not a primary supplement I use to treat high blood pressure it can be an adjunctive treatment. It would also be a good choice for those who have high blood pressure as the result of toxic metal accumulation such as mercury or cadmium.

TOXIC METALS

Small human and animal studies have demonstrated that chlorella assists the body in detoxification of toxic metals such as mercury and cadmium.

ULCERATIVE COLITIS

This is an inflammatory condition that involves ulceration of the gut mucosa of the colon and rectum. One pilot study lasting two months looked at chlorella supplementation with 10 g tablets and 100 mL of the liquid form for people with ulcerative colitis. For those who completed the study a sigmoidoscopic examination found significantly less inflammation. The decrease in stool frequency was also significant. Patients filled out a questionnaire that revealed much higher quality of life during the study.

VEGETARIANISM

Vegetarians often supplement chlorella to increase their vitamin B12 levels. One study in the *Journal of Nutrition* found that nori (a type of seaweed) and chlorella increased blood levels of this vitamin. However, some experts question whether this form of vitamin B12 is an active form usable in the body. More research is required to confirm whether chlorella supplements can be relied upon as a primary vitamin B12 source.

Chromium

"Mark, I have been following the exercise program you recommended and have been doing pretty well on my diet. But there is one little problem—well, it's actually a big problem. I can't stop eating those sweets. I crave them all day long!"

Susan, a 33-year-old mother of three, had made it her goal to lose 20 pounds of "leftover pregnancy weight." But this craving for sweets—certainly a common problem—was making it impossible.

"Let's have you take some chromium to

help with your blood-sugar regulation," I suggested. "Maybe you crave sweets because your body wants to compensate for low blood-sugar levels."

Any kind of sweets—whether chocolate, candy, or soda—gives you an instant "blood-sugar fix." Unfortunately, those foods also cause blood-sugar irregularity and cause insulin levels to rise, leading to fat storage. (Insulin is the hormone produced by your body that helps open the gates of your cells to blood-sugar and, therefore, fat storage.)

When Susan heard that chromium would help reduce sweet cravings, her response was predictable: "Great, I would like to get started on it right away!"

She reported four weeks later that her sweet cravings were much improved. Chromium was "doing the trick," to use her phrase.

TRACE-MINERAL POWER

Chromium is a trace mineral, meaning that our bodies only require very small "trace" amounts. While we need many milligrams of some vitamins and minerals, a trace mineral like chromium is fine if it comes in microgram dosages—that is, one-thousandth of the other requirements.

Chromium facilitates the uptake of glucose (blood-sugar) into the cells so that it can be "burned" for energy. Admittedly, the hormone insulin is the substance that's mainly responsible for transporting glucose into the cells—but chromium teams up nicely with the hormone to carry out the delivery function.

Without insulin, serious disease such as type 1 diabetes can occur. Commonly called juvenile-onset diabetes, this type occurs when the pancreas does not secrete enough insulin. People with type 1 diabetes need regular injections of insulin so that their cells can get a sorely needed, steady supply of glucose.

Type 2 diabetes (adult onset or noninsulin dependent) usually occurs later in life and has a different type of pathology. This is not a disease where there is a lack of insulin; rather, it occurs when the cells are insensitive to insulin. If the insulin doesn't unlock the door of the cell, glucose can't get in. It's like a taxicab pulling up to the door—but the passengers can't get out and go in the building.

Chromium—and another trace mineral called vanadium—both have the keys to help get the doors unlocked. By enhancing the action of insulin, the trace minerals help glucose penetrate the cells.

But apart from playing a role as a "glucose tolerance factor"—as it's sometimes called—chromium is good for a variety of other applications. We are learning more about a condition called "Syndrome X," which occurs when people have an inherited problem—they can't metabolize carbohydrates (including sugar) very effectively. If someone has high blood-sugar levels because of Syndrome X, that person is going to have increased levels of the hormone insulin—and if you have elevated insulin levels, you're prone to many health problems including obesity, high blood pressure, fatigue, and heart disease, to name a few. Minerals like chromium are a godsend for people with Syndrome X, as it optimizes the cells' ability to metabolize carbohydrates.

Chromium is found in whole grains. Deficiencies are quite common, because most of the grains found in processed or packaged food are highly refined and just don't have enough chromium content. Meat and brewer's yeast are also rich sources of chromium.

DOSAGE

If you have no blood-sugar or weight problems and want to take an extra chromium supplement just to see how you feel, I recommend 200 mcg daily. Many multivitamins now contain this amount. But if you're supplementing with chromium specifically for weight, you should generally take 400 to 600 mcg daily.

If you have diabetes or blood-sugar problems (for example, hypoglycemia), the recommended dose is between 400 and 1,000 mcg daily. But anyone taking these dosages should have their blood-sugar and medications monitored by a doctor.

Chromium picolinate is the type that has been most widely researched in reliable studies. It works hand-in-hand with the trace mineral vanadium to help regulate blood-sugar.

WHAT ARE THE SIDE EFFECTS?

Dosages at 1,000 mcg and lower appear to be very safe and nontoxic. If you're taking drugs for diabetes, however, the addition of chromium can affect your need for pharmaceutical medication. Often, diabetic pharmaceutical medications (insulin or type 2 diabetic drugs) need to be reduced or the blood-sugar levels can get too low. That's why it's essential for anyone with diabetes to discuss their plans with a doctor before starting a supplement program with chromium.

CHROMIUM

RECOMMENDATIONS FROM THE NATURAL PHYSICIAN FOR . . .

❧ CHOLESTEROL AND TRIGLYCERIDES

Chromium has been shown to lower total cholesterol and triglycerides by about 10% in people with type 2 diabetes and also those who do not have diabetes. Both of these effects help to lower your risk of heart disease. It also increases the good cholesterol HDL. While the improvements are not dramatic, it makes sense to include chromium for improved heart health.

❧ DEPRESSION

Studies show chromium supplementation can be of benefit for those with mild depression (dysthymia) and those with atypical depression.

❧ DIABETES AND HYPOGLYCEMIA

Anyone with diabetes or hypoglycemia should definitely be supplementing with chromium. The fact that chromium makes the cells more sensitive to insulin has been borne out by studies done with people who had type 2 diabetes. Often, those who have type 2 diabetes have a chromium deficiency, which appears to make them more susceptible to the condition.

In one study, for instance, researchers examined 29 overweight individuals who also had a family history of diabetes. Using the usual methods of controlled experiment, some of the patients received 1,000 mcg (1 mg) of chromium daily, while others received a placebo. After four months, the patients were tested again, and researchers found that the chromium-takers had a 40% reduction in insulin resistance. The same improvement was maintained at the end of eight months. This study suggests the need for people who have a strong family history of diabetes to begin chromium supplementation on a preventative basis, especially if they are overweight.

A study published in *Diabetes Care* involved 37 people with type 2 diabetes. People were randomized to receive a diabetic drug plus placebo or a diabetic drug plus 1,000 mcg of chromium for six months. Those receiving the medication plus chromium had significantly improved insulin sensitivity and glucose control. Those receiving the medication

(continued)

plus placebo had a significant increase in body weight, percent body fat, and total abdominal fat. Another study looked at the effect of chromium on elderly people with diabetes, average age 73 years. The participants supplemented 200 mcg twice daily for three weeks. The other group was a control group. Significant differences in the fasting blood level of glucose compared to the baseline (190 mg/dL versus 150 mg/dL) were found at the end of the study.

On the heels of research like this, the arguments for taking chromium are compelling. The trace mineral is nontoxic—so why not try this natural therapy (along with lifestyle changes), if it can help prevent this disease?

When I started my practice more than 16 years ago, I saw a patient who was showing the early warning signs of diabetic retinopathy, an eye disease—potentially leading to blindness—that's directly related to high blood-sugar levels. From the patient's description, I realized that his diet varied enormously from day to day—yet it seemed like he would benefit from chromium supplementation, so I started him on 400 mcg a day. Six months later he told me that the medical doctor whom he'd been seeing could no longer find any evidence of retinopathy. The physician simply recommended that

my patient continue to do whatever he had been doing. Such a reversal of the condition was rare, his doctor noted.

I find that hypoglycemia also responds well to chromium supplementation. One small study of eight females with hypoglycemia found that their condition was alleviated when they took 200 mcg for three months.

🍃 POLYCYSTIC OVARIAN SYNDROME

Chromium supplementation at a dose of 500 mcg twice daily has been shown to help with glucose balance in women with polycystic ovarian syndrome. Insulin resistance is a root problem with this condition and chromium can help.

🍃 WEIGHT LOSS

Human studies have shown that chromium supplementation at doses of 200 to 400 mcg can help people lose weight and increase lean muscle mass. Larger studies need to be done—but, in the meantime, I've seen this type of regimen help about 50% of the patients I've treated with similar amounts of supplementation. Remember that it may take a couple of months before the beneficial effects start to show.

The supplements work best when the doses are combined with a steady, good diet and regular exercise.

Cinnamon

Medicinal spices have become a media item of interest in recent years. Cinnamon has long been revered as a medicinal spice since biblical times. Ancient Egyptians used it as a medicinal herb, beverage flavoring, and embalming agent. Not only does cinnamon add a pleasurable taste to foods but it also has several health benefits. Cinnamon comes from the inner bark of small evergreen trees native to tropical southern India and Sri Lanka. After the inner brown bark is peeled off the tree, it curls up into tubes.

It is used as a spice and as a flavoring agent in personal products such as cosmetics or pharmaceuticals. It has been an important component of traditional herbal therapy in China and India for centuries. It is commonly used in Chinese and Ayurvedic medicine for treating digestive conditions, infections, arthritis, menstrual problems, and for enhancing circulation. Cinnamon has become popular in supplement form in Germany and North America as well, especially for reducing glucose levels. As a food, it is available as cinnamon sticks or ground-up powder.

It is important to realize that there are more than 200 varieties of cinnamon. The most popular are Ceylon cinnamon (*Cinnmamomum zeylandicum* and *Cinnamomum verym*) and Chinese cinnamon (*Cinnamomum aromatic*). Often *Cinnmamomum zeylandicum* is referred to as "true cinnamon." This type of cinnamon is produced in Sri Lanka, India, Brazil, Madagascar, and the Caribbean. The Chinese variety is known as "cassia." It is produced mainly in China, Indonesia, and Vietnam. The cassia form is more popular in North America, likely due to its cheaper price. Some cinnamon powders contain a blend of different cinnamon species.

The most well-studied supplemental form of cinnamon is a proprietary water-soluble extract of *Cinnamomum burmannii*. It is standardized to substances known as type-A polymers.

Cinnamon contains various types of therapeutic ingredients. These include volatile oils such as cinnamaldehyde, eugenol, and trans-cinnamic acid. The volatile oils have been shown to have antifungal, antiviral, bactericidal effects, and antioxidant properties. Cinnamon also contains phenolic compounds and tannins such as catechins.

DOSAGE

Four cinnamon powder studies have used 1 to 6 g daily to reduce cholesterol and glucose levels. In supplement form, the most well studied is a water-soluble extract known as cinnulin PF, available from various manufacturers. The dose is 250 mg twice daily before meals.

For the tincture, the dose is 3 to 6 mL three times daily. For infusion or decoction, it's 0.5 to 1.5 g in 150 mL water three times daily.

WHAT ARE THE SIDE EFFECTS?

Cinnamon is well tolerated. Those taking diabetes medications may require a lower dosage since cinnamon may reduce their glucose levels. Extremely high amounts may have blood-thinning effects, although it's unlikely one would consume amounts high enough to be a problem. Studies with pregnant women and nursing mothers are lacking so supplementation with cinnamon by these groups should be avoided.

CINNAMON

RECOMMENDATIONS FROM THE NATURAL PHYSICIAN FOR . . .

🐾 CHOLESTEROL

A study of 60 people with type 2 diabetes involved people divided randomly into six groups. Three groups consumed 1 to 6 g cinnamon daily in capsule form while the other three groups received a placebo. Researchers found that after 40 days, among those receiving 1 to 6 g, the mean reduction of fasting triglyceride levels was 23% to 30%, LDL cholesterol 7% to 27%, and total cholesterol 12% to 26%. In contrast, there were no significant changes in the placebo groups. However not all studies have found this same benefit.

🐾 CIRCULATION

Cinnamon is used in Asian and Western herbal formulas to promote circulation. Indeed I have found that patients notice a warming sensation, especially in the hands and feet.

🐾 COLDS AND FEVERS

Cinnamon twig is used in Asian formulas for the treatment of the common cold and other upper respiratory tract infections, as well as fever.

🐾 DIABETES

A 2003 study in *Diabetes Care* found 1 to 6 g cinnamon powder daily reduced fasting glucose levels by 18% to 29%. Yet other studies did not find any significant changes in terms of a blood-sugar-lowering effect. A small 2009 study in the *American Journal of Clinical Nutrition* found that 3 g cinnamon reduced insulin levels after ingesting rice pudding without

significantly lowering blood glucose levels. It is possible that over longer periods of time participants' glucose levels would have been lowered. More research is needed to confirm the glucose-lowering effects of cinnamon powder.

A special type of cinnamon extract known as Cinnulin PF has been shown to significantly decrease fasting blood-sugar compared to placebo. It also showed statistically lower body fat, enhanced lean body mass, lower systolic blood pressure, and improvements in various antioxidant measures.

🐾 DIGESTION

The German Commission E Monographs, which summarize therapeutic uses of herbal medicines, approved the internal use of cinnamon for loss of appetite, mild spastic condition of the gastrointestinal tract, bloating, and flatulence. Also, cinnamon has been shown to promote intestinal motility and help break down fats. You will find cinnamon a common component of Asian and Western digestive tonic formulas.

🐾 MENSTRUAL CRAMPS AND HEAVY BLEEDING

Cinnamon bark is commonly used in female-related herbal formulas, particularly Chinese formulas to reduce menstrual cramps and heavy periods.

Coenzyme Q10

Several pictures come to mind when someone mentions the supplement coenzyme Q10 (also referred to as CoQ10). One is that of the heart. I see this big, red pumping muscle contracting and relaxing. Inside the heart cells are tiny explosions where energy is being created. Within these cells I see the spark plug. The spark plug is CoQ10.

Without coenzyme Q10, heart cells could not produce energy, known as ATP. Though the heart is the most famous center of operations for CoQ10, it's found in other body cells as well—and in all of them, it's important for energy production.

But the heart suffers most when there's a lack of CoQ10. It beats slowly. Its contractions are wimpy. Its rhythm goes awry. When a heart doesn't have enough CoQ10 for proper electrical conduction, it suffers as it starves—and, of course, the whole circulatory system pays the price.

Fortunately, when new CoQ10 comes on the scene, recovery can be noticeable and rapid. As CoQ10 saturates the heart cells, life returns; the heart resumes its strong, regular series of rhythmical contractions; tissues fill with more oxygen as blood flow improves; and energy abounds.

BETTER VESSELS

Not only does CoQ10 improve heart cells, it also renovates the highways and byways of all our blood vessel walls. Subjected to constant pounding from the surge of blood flowing through them, our arteries and veins can get damaged over time as the pressure builds. As those blood vessels absorb some of the coenzyme Q10 that's circulating through the body, the walls relax and blood pressure drops. Blood flow hits an optimum level—not too fast and not too slow, but just right to deliver oxygen and nutrients to the tissues.

The blood vessel walls are safer when blood pressure is lower—hence, the premium that we place on "normal blood pressure." As pressure rises, so does the risk of heart attack or stroke.

FUEL FOR THE ATHLETIC SET

Though exercise is certainly healthful, committed athletes get so much of it that their bodies produce what are known as metabolic byproducts, including free radicals. These are runaway substances that, left unchecked, can cause rapid cell aging.

By taking low levels of antioxidants such as CoQ10, the body counteracts some of the effects of these free radicals. Athletes can become more resistant to fatigue and immune-system breakdown. Therefore, anyone who is involved in rigorous physical activity would do well to supplement at least a minimal amount of CoQ10.

A UBIQUITOUS SUBSTANCE

With so many benefits for the body, in so many places, it's appropriate that CoQ10 should also be known by the medical term ubiquinone. A ubiquitous substance, found in all the cells of the body, coenzyme Q10 was originally discovered in 1957 by scientists from the Merck pharmaceutical company. They used the number 10 in reference to its biochemical structure (10 isoprenoid units on its side chain), but apart from assigning the name that stuck, they didn't do much to explore its properties.

The Japanese began testing CoQ10 on

humans in 1963, and by 1976 it was "placed on the formulary" (that is, accepted as a medicine) for Japanese hospitals. In 1978, Peter Mitchell was awarded the Nobel Prize in Chemistry for his studies of energy production in the human body, which led to hypotheses on how CoQ10 works and how it relates to heart disease.

From that time on, hundreds of studies on CoQ10 have been done in Japan, the United States, and other countries. (So much of the research has been done by Dr. Karl Folkers of the University of Texas that he is often referred to as the "father of coenzyme Q10.") By the mid 1990s coenzyme Q10 was widely accepted in the health-food industry as a popular supplement to help improve heart health. Unfortunately, even today, there are many cardiologists who do not recommend CoQ10.

CoQ10 is found in high amounts in meat and fish. Nuts are also a source as are some vegetables like broccoli and spinach. The body manufactures CoQ10 from the amino acid tyrosine. This synthesis requires the action of vitamins C, B2, B6, B12, folic acid, niacin, and pantothenic acid. Another important function of CoQ10 is that it works to recycle vitamin E.

DOSAGE

If your health is good but you just want to take coenzyme Q10 for prevention, I'd recommend 50 to 100 mg daily. It does make sense to supplement with CoQ10, whatever the state of your health, as cardiovascular disease can sneak up on just about anyone (it's the leading cause of death in the United States) and CoQ10 is one of the best antioxidants for the entire cardiovascular network.

If you have cardiovascular disease or any other serious illness (such as cancer), you should take between 300 and 450 mg daily.

CoQ10 is available in different forms. You can get soft gel capsules, sublingual tablets, and powder-filled capsules. Coenzyme Q10 creams are now available as well, to help prevent aging of the skin.

CoQ10 is best taken with meals.

WHAT ARE THE SIDE EFFECTS?

Coenzyme Q10 is very safe, but we don't know about its effects on pregnant or lactating women, or higher dosages on young children. Until it has been tested, I would not recommend it to these groups unless a patient has an urgent medical problem, such as a heart condition, that warrants its use (and then, only with the supervision of a doctor).

CoQ10 may interfere with the action of the blood-thinning drug Coumadin. If you're taking that pharmaceutical, let your doctor know that you plan on supplementing with CoQ10 so that your blood-clotting ability can be closely monitored. Personally, I have never seen a bad interaction between Coumadin and CoQ10, but some problems have been reported in the medical literature. Additionally, I have noted some patients experience insomnia when CoQ10 is taken in the evening, presumably due to its energy-enhancing effects.

COENZYME Q10

RECOMMENDATIONS FROM THE NATURAL PHYSICIAN FOR . . .

ᴥ ANGINA

If you have this symptom of heart disease, it actually feels like your heart is being squeezed, or you experience the sensation of a great pressure in the chest. Angina is almost always caused by a lack of oxygen to the heart muscle. Because the arteries are partially blocked by plaque—a buildup related to high cholesterol—your heart isn't getting enough blood flow to provide oxygen to the heart muscle. Spasm of the coronary arteries can also lead to angina.

Several studies have shown CoQ10 to be effective for this condition. Pharmaceutical medications are useful for treating acute episodes of angina, but CoQ10 is the supplement of choice for prevention of future attacks. I have had outstanding results in patients who have had a history of angina. Sometimes I recommend CoQ10 by itself while, for other patients, I favor combining it with magnesium, hawthorn berry extract, and cactus extract (*Cereus grandiflorus*).

ᴥ ARRHYTHMIA

People who have this condition say they have the sensation that their heart is missing a beat. Coenzyme Q10 has a stabilizing effect on the electrical conductivity of the heart, so it helps to prevent arrhythmia. Studies have shown it to be effective in nearly one-quarter of cases where people are having a particular kind of arrhythmia related to premature ventricular contractions.

Magnesium, L-carnitine, and potassium supplements are also indicated for arrhythmias.

ᴥ ATHEROSCLEROSIS

When cholesterol and other fatty substances go through an oxidation process in the arteries, they begin to damage blood vessel walls. As a result, plaque builds up as your immune system reacts to what's going on inside the blood vessel. If this process continues undeterred, it can lead to the blocked condition commonly called "hardening of the arteries" or atherosclerosis. But that process can be slowed or stopped if you make dietary changes and use coenzyme Q10 to inhibit the oxidation of cholesterol and other fatty substances in the body.

ᴥ CANCER

Researchers have discovered that anything we do to bolster the immune system can also help fight cancer, and we know that CoQ10 is required as a nutrient for a healthy immune system. Many holistic doctors recommend CoQ10 in high dosages (300 mg or higher) along with other therapies in the treatment of cancer. Five cases of metastatic breast cancer have been documented in which there was complete reversal of metastasis with high doses of CoQ10 (390 mg). Obviously, there need to be more studies done on CoQ10 and cancer. It does make sense, though, to at least use it as a complementary therapy when treating cancer.

(continued)

❧ CARDIOMYOPATHY

This is a disease of the heart that results in a reduced heart contraction force. Cardiomyopathy may be caused by a variety of factors, including viral infections, nutritional deficiencies, and autoimmune reactions. The progression of this disease can lead to congestive heart failure, where the heart refuses to pump. (If the heart isn't jump-started again, congestive heart failure can be fatal.)

One study looked at 34 people with severe cardiomyopathy who were given 100 mg of CoQ10 daily. Eighty-two percent of the people showed improvement—as measured by heart tests—after the therapy. Their two-year survival rate was 62%, compared with a second group of people who only had conventional therapy. (Of the latter group, the two-year survival rate was only 25%.)

❧ CHRONIC FATIGUE SYNDROME

A small study at the University of Iowa found CoQ10 supplementation was effective for 69% of users with unexplained chronic fatigue syndrome. Those with fatigue usually note some benefit from CoQ10 supplementation.

❧ CONGESTIVE HEART FAILURE

If you have this condition, the heart simply "gives out" as a pump, and your system is deprived of blood. Shortness of breath, fatigue, and water retention in the lungs and lower legs are common symptoms of this disease. Coenzyme Q-10 is a must for all patients with congestive heart failure. When combined with conventional CHF drugs, studies show it improves quality of life, decreases hospitalization rates, and decreases symptoms of heart failure including shortness of breath, peripheral edema, enlarged liver, and insomnia. Also, a clinical study involving men and women with low serum CoQ10 levels and decreased ejection fraction (how much the heart pumps out) was studied in relation to CoQ10 supplementation. After three months, the subjects experienced a 24% to 50% increase in their left ventricular output. I recommend 300 to 600 mg daily of coenzyme Q10 supplementation for those with CHF under a doctor's guidance.

❧ DIABETES

People with diabetes have been found to have low levels of CoQ10. Theoretically, they have a higher need for this natural substance because the disease increases the need for antioxidants. I recommend that people with diabetes should take CoQ10 as part of an antioxidant regimen.

❧ DRUG DAMAGE

Several drugs deplete the body of CoQ10. Adriamycin, a chemotherapy drug used for various types of cancer, can cause irreversible heart damage and possible heart failure. Coenzyme Q10 works as an antioxidant to protect the heart from the damaging effects of this chemotherapy agent. One study of children with cancer who were being treated with Adriamycin showed that CoQ10 had a protective effect when they were given 200 mg daily.

Beta blockers are a class of drugs that also deplete CoQ10. These medications are commonly used for conditions like high blood pressure and arrhythmia.

Interestingly, beta blockers can lead to congestive heart failure in people, though it isn't known whether the heart failure is a side effect of the beta blocker or is caused by depletion of CoQ10. While more research needs to be done in this area, it seems prudent to take CoQ10 as a preventative supplement if you're taking a beta blocker.

Millions of North Americans take cholesterol-lowering drugs, and many of these drugs have well-reported side effects. CoQ10 is a very important supplement if you're taking a class of cholesterol-lowering drugs known as HMG CoA reductase inhibitors such as Atorvastin, Mevacor, Pravachol, and Zocor. These drugs work by inhibiting the enzyme HMG CoA reductase that is required by the liver to manufacture cholesterol. This same enzyme is also involved in the synthesis of CoQ10. If you are taking a lot of this class of medicine, it can lead to tissue depletion. One study found that people taking atorvastin (Lipitor) had blood CoQ10 levels reduced by 50% after 30 days.

For anyone taking these kinds of drugs, I recommend an additional dose of 100 to 200 mg of CoQ10. (I also recommend other liver-protective substances such as alpha lipoic acid and milk thistle.)

Some psychoactive drugs, including tricyclic antidepressants and phenothiazines, also deplete CoQ10 levels. Some heart conditions such as arrhythmias, congestive heart failure, and heart attacks have been associated with the use of these medications. Taking CoQ10 will help you protect yourself against the cardiac toxicity of these drugs.

🐚 HAIR LOSS INDUCED BY WARFARIN (COUMADIN)

There is preliminary research that CoQ10 supplementation may help prevent hair loss caused by the drug warfarin (Coumadin).

🐚 HEART ATTACK

Taking 120 mg of CoQ10 daily decreased the risk of cardiac events in people with a recent heart attack who were at risk for blood clots. When CoQ10 supplementation was given within 72 hours of a heart attack and given for one year, it significantly lowered the risk of cardiac events including nonfatal and fatal heart attacks. If you or a loved one have had a recent heart attack, speak to your doctor about immediately supplementing CoQ10.

🐚 HIGH BLOOD PRESSURE

Coenzyme Q10 can be very helpful for blood pressure. In a study published in *Pharmacotherapy*, more than 50% of patients with high blood pressure were able to stop taking between one and three blood pressure medicines just four months after starting CoQ10 supplements!

Taking 120 mg daily of CoQ10 for 12 weeks significantly lowered systolic blood pressure by about 26% in some people with isolated systolic hypertension. CoQ10 can help lower blood pressure for those with type 2 diabetes and those on existing medications.

🐚 MALE INFERTILITY

Coenzyme Q10 has been shown to improve the fertility potential of sperm. This may occur because CoQ10 is an

(continued)

energizing substance that could literally help the sperm to swim more rapidly or more strongly. It is also likely that CoQ10 protects the sperm from the damaging effects of free radicals.

CoQ10 is well worth trying for low sperm counts or poor motility. When I recommend it, I often suggest other supplements as well, including the amino acid arginine, and vitamins B12, C, E, zinc, and L-carnitine.

MIGRAINE HEADACHE

CoQ10 is an excellent supplement to prevent migraine headaches. A Thomas Jefferson University study followed 31 migraine patients who were given 150 mg of CoQ10 daily. After three months of treatment, participants reported that the average number of attacks per month fell from 4.85 to 2.81, and that the number of days the migraines lasted also was significantly reduced. A different double-blind, placebo-controlled study by the same institution gave 42 participants a placebo or CoQ10 at 100 mg three times a day for three months. Migraine frequency diminished by half in 47% of the patients taking CoQ10, compared with 14% of placebo users. CoQ10 users also reported less nausea.

MITRAL VALVE PROLAPSE

Mitral valve prolapse means that one of the heart valves is not closing properly as your heart contracts and expands. CoQ10 helps this condition. In a study published in the journal *Molecular Aspects of Medicine*, heart function was restored to normal in 87% of mitral valve prolapse patients receiving 2 mg of coenzyme Q10 per kg of body weight per day for eight weeks. (Coenzyme Q10 may normalize heart function in mitral valve prolapse patients.)

MUSCULAR DYSTROPHY

This refers to a group of genetic diseases characterized by progressive muscle weakness. Most of us have become familiar with this disease through the annual Jerry Lewis telethons. Dr. Folkers has shown in two small studies that CoQ10 improved physical performance in people with this disease. He recommends people with muscular dystrophy supplement with CoQ10 indefinitely, as it has been proven safe and it improves quality of life. CoQ10 is well worth trying, and I would recommend L-carnitine as well.

PARKINSON'S DISEASE

A study at the University of California–San Diego found CoQ10 supplementation of up to 1,200 mg daily provided less disability developed in subjects assigned to coenzyme Q10 than in those assigned to placebo.

PERIODONTAL DISEASE

Several studies have shown that CoQ10 improves the health of the gums—a significant finding, since more than 30 million Americans suffer from gum disease. In theory, CoQ10 improves oxygenation of the gum tissues and also has a supportive effect on the immune system. So it not only helps the gums heal, it also helps to suppress the bacteria that lead to gum inflammation and erosion.

CoQ10 is definitely worth trying if you have chronic bleeding gums due to gingivitis. I recommend taking the supplement for several months before your dentist makes an assessment of progress.

CoQ10 is now available in special tooth-pastes for people with gum disease.

⁓ PHYSICAL PERFORMANCE

CoQ10 can help athletes. A randomized, double-blinded, placebo-controlled, three-crossover study involving 17 healthy volunteers looked at the effect of the level of fatigue and supplementation of 300 mg per day of CoQ10. Researchers found CoQ10 resulted in reduced fatigue and improved physical performance.

⁓ SKIN HEALTH

I have noticed that skin creams containing CoQ10 have come onto the market. Although I was skeptical at first, there is research showing that creams containing antioxidants such as CoQ10 and vitamin C do, indeed, help to protect the skin. It could be that these products help the rehydration of the skin, giving it a more youthful appearance.

CoQ10 also helps protect the skin against the ultraviolet radiation from the sun.

Colloidal Silver

"My bronchitis seems to have gotten worse over the past few days. I am feverish and have all this green gunk coming up. All the natural things I have tried on my own haven't helped. And you know I have bad reactions to most antibiotics. What do you recommend?" asked Steve, a 49-year-old lawyer.

"I am going to give you colloidal silver; it's the closest thing we have in natural medicine to an antibiotic, except it doesn't have the same toxicity potential," I replied.

An insider secret among holistic doctors and practitioners is the potent germ-killing ability of colloidal silver. The term *colloidal* refers to particles (in this case, of silver) suspended in solution. Colloidal silver can be used to treat virtually all types of infection, including bacteria, viruses, fungi, and parasites. It directly kills microbes while simultaneously stimulating good white blood cell activity and the production of hydrogen peroxide, a substance that also destroys infectious agents.

Antibiotic resistance is a major problem today because bacteria adapt and are unaffected by many existing drugs. Antibiotics normally

kill bacteria by one of three mechanisms: destroying their outer cell membranes, disrupting internal activity in the cells, or interfering with cell division of bacteria through actions on their DNA. Colloidal silver appears to affect all three mechanisms, and when you combine that with its immune enhancement and generation of hydrogen peroxide, you can see why it is such a potent natural germ-killing substance. Many colloidal silver products have such a small particle size that they readily enter the cells of bacteria and inflict damage to the microbes without causing toxicity in the host body. It appears that particle size and charge are the most important qualities of a good colloidal silver product.

Using silver as a medicine is nothing new. As a matter of fact, from 1900 until the 1940s silver was used by mainstream medicine to treat infections. The advent of antibiotics and the non-patentability of colloidal silver led to its loss of favor among conventional doctors. Going back further into history, it has been recorded that Russian armies used silver to clean drinking water during World War I and World War II and silver was used by ancient Greek and Roman physicians to treat infections.

DOSAGE

A product containing 10 parts per million for acute infection can be taken at a dose of 1 teaspoon every one to two waking hours for five days. The dose for children is generally half the adult dosage. Do not take colloidal silver on a long-term basis (longer than seven days) without the guidance of a doctor knowledgeable in its administration.

WHAT ARE THE SIDE EFFECTS?

I have never seen any side effects with the supplemental use of colloidal silver. The average consumption of silver from water and food is approximately 350 mcg. One teaspoon of a 10 parts-per-million solution of colloidal silver is equivalent to 50 mcg

silver. More research needs to be done on the long-term intake of colloidal silver and potential side effects. I use it with patients for the internal and external treatment of acute infections. There has been a lot of press in recent years about a condition known as argyria. This occurs when too much or too high a concentration of silver is ingested and the body is unable to excrete it from the tissues where it deposits, including the skin. As a result there can be a permanent discoloration of the skin and fingernails, which it turns gray or bluish gray, or even darker on exposure to strong sun exposure. Quality colloidal silver products that use 10 parts-per-million or higher strengths used for short periods of time do not seem to pose any risk for this condition.

COLLOIDAL SILVER

RECOMMENDATIONS FROM THE NATURAL PHYSICIAN FOR . . .

🦊 INFECTIONS

As described in the introduction colloidal silver can be used for the short-term treatment of acute infections. I commonly use it to treat respiratory tract infections. It can be taken internally and applied topically for skin infections, as well. Since it has antifungal and antiparasitic effects, it can also be taken internally for infections of the digestive tract. Some holistic doctors use lower doses for the long-term treatment of conditions such as Lyme disease.

Cordyceps sinensis

One supplement I have used with hundreds of patients over the years to combat fatigue and revitalize libido is Cordyceps. The American public first got wind of this supplement in 1993 when a group of Chinese runners broke nine world records in the World Outdoor Track and Field Championships in Germany. It was claimed

by the Chinese coach that supplements of Cordyceps had greatly benefited his team. Athletes around the world quickly began using Cordyceps to boost energy and stamina and this popularity crossed into the public arena.

Classified as a medicinal mushroom, Cordyceps is a fungus that in the wild grows on and acquires nutrients from several species of caterpillars, hence its common name of caterpillar fungus. It also has the nick-names winter worm and summer grass. It is found in nature at high altitudes such as the mountaintops of China, Nepal, and Tibet, although it is commercially produced with modern commercial fermentation tech-niques in China and the United States.

Most studies done on Cordyceps have been done on an isolated wild strain known as Cs-4. In traditional Chinese medicine, Cordyceps is considered to benefit the lung and kidney channels. Elderly people in China use it as a tonic for rejuvenation and stamina.

DOSAGE

Take 800 to 1,600 mg daily of a standard-ized extract from *Cordyceps sinensis* strain Cs-4.

WHAT ARE THE SIDE EFFECTS?

Cordyceps should be avoided by people with organ transplants using immunosup-pressive agents and with caution for those taking blood-thinning medications (it has a mild blood-thinning effect).

CORDYCEPS SINENSIS
RECOMMENDATIONS FROM THE NATURAL PHYSICIAN FOR . . .

~ FATIGUE
I have found Cordyceps is quite helpful for people with fatigue problems, includ-ing those with chronic fatigue syndrome. Cordyceps was shown to benefit seniors with fatigue, cold intolerance, dizziness, and memory, among other symptoms. Animal studies suggest Cordyceps improves the production of ATP (cellular energy). Also Cordyceps appears to improve adrenal gland function.

~ HEART HEALTH
Human and animal studies have demon-strated that Cordyceps can reduce cho-lesterol and triglyceride levels while increasing levels of HDL cholesterol. It may also benefit those with congestive heart failure by improving coronary artery circulation.

~ HEPATITIS B
One study found Cordyceps extract improved liver function for those with chronic hepatitis B.

~ KIDNEY TOXICITY AND FAILURE
Cyclosporine is a drug used to suppress the immune system for those undergoing organ transplant. This medication has the potential side effect of kidney damage. Cordyceps at a dose of 3,000 mg was shown in one study to decrease kidney toxicity in kidney transplant recipients taking cyclosporine. One study also found Cordyceps had a protective effect against kidney toxicity from aminoglycoside anti-biotics.

~ LUNG CONDITIONS
Cordyceps can have benefit for asthma, chronic bronchitis, and other respiratory diseases. I have commonly used it with benefit as part of a holistic protocol for those with chronic bronchitis and chronic obstructive pulmonary disease with benefit.

(continued)

🐌 SEX DRIVE

Cordyceps has been used historically in traditional Chinese medicine to enhance sex drive and has been shown to do so in Chinese studies. This is a non-hormonal way to help those with low libido.

Coriolus Versicolor

"I had colon surgery several months ago to remove a cancerous tumor. Since then I have greatly improved my diet. Is there a particular supplement you would recommend to help my immune system and possibly prevent a recurrence?" asked Don, a real estate broker.

"One of the best supplements you could and should be taking is coriolus, also known as turkey tail. It not only boosts immune function but has been shown to have benefit on your condition," I replied. As I reviewed the literature on coriolus with Don he quickly let me know that he was eager to get started on it right away.

Coriolus is a very well-studied medicinal mushroom. It has been the subject of more than 400 published studies and is routinely used, especially in Japan and China, for its immune-enhancing properties. In recent years holistic doctors and consumers in the West have become acquainted with its immune-stimulating benefit.

Coriolus has an interesting history. More than four decades ago, a chemical engineer for a Japanese pharmaceutical company observed his neighbor with late-stage stomach cancer treating himself with coriolus because it was a traditional remedy for cancer. The engineer convinced his company to study the mushroom and over time developed an extract from it known as polysaccharide-K (PSK). The K stands for the first letter of Kureha Chemical, the company that developed PSK and later the anti-cancer drug known as Krestin. Krestin went on to become a top-selling cancer drug in Japan. Chinese researchers later developed their own extract known as polysaccharide-peptide (PSP).

Coriolus grows throughout the world, including the United States. In the West, coriolus is referred to as "turkey tail" due to its fan-shaped, multicolored cap. Coriolus is also known as *Trametes versicolor*. In Japan, coriolus has been a folk remedy for cancer, and in traditional Chinese medicine it is used to treat lung infections and hepatitis as well.

Special long-chain sugars known as polysaccharides, also known as beta glucans, are found in coriolus. These unique beta glucans are absorbed into the bloodstream and stimulate the immune system's response. In addition, they appear to be toxic to cancer cells.

DOSAGE

Take 1,500 to 2,000 mg of an extract twice daily.

WHAT ARE THE SIDE EFFECTS?

This mushroom extract is quite safe. It should be avoided in people with organ transplants using immunosuppressive agents.

CORIOLUS VERSICOLOR

RECOMMENDATIONS FROM THE NATURAL PHYSICIAN FOR . . .

❧ CHEMOTHERAPY AND RADIATION COMPLEMENTARY THERAPY

One of the things I appreciate about coriolus is that it has human studies demonstrating that it reduces the side effects of chemotherapy and radiation in a safe and effective manner. For example, a study published in the *Lancet* examined the effect of coriolus polysaccharides (PSK) in addition to standard chemotherapy with patients who had undergone curative stomach removal. A total of 262 patients were randomly assigned standard treatment alone or with PSK, with minimum follow-up time of five years. The survival rate of the group using the combination of PSK and chemotherapy was 73% after five years. The group receiving chemotherapy alone had a survival rate of 60%. Researchers concluded that PSK had "a restorative effect in patients who had been immunosuppressed by both recent surgery and subsequent chemotherapy."

Another study, at the University of Shanghai, examined if coriolus polysaccharides (PSP) had any benefit for treating the side effects of chemotherapy or radiation. The study involved 650 people with cancer undergoing chemotherapy and radiation who were given either PSP or a placebo. Participants' side effects were monitored, and researchers determined that those receiving PSP had markedly fewer side effects than those receiving placebo.

❧ COMPLEMENTARY CANCER TREATMENT

Unlike many supplements, coriolus has data derived from human subjects in the complementary treatment of various cancers. It is most commonly prescribed for those undergoing treatment for esophageal, lung, stomach, and colon cancer. For example, a 10-year study of 185 people with non-small-cell lung cancer receiving radiation found PSK to be effective in protecting and promoting immune function. The study found that "as a result of administering PSK as adjutant treatment to patients with epidermoid carcinoma of the lung showing satisfactory tumor shrinkage after radiotherapy, the five-year survival rate of the patients with stages I or II disease, as well as stage III was 39% and 22%, respectively, compared with the non-administered group's 16% and 5%. These differences are statistically significant." In addition, patients ages 70 years or more who received the combination of PSK and radiation had a significantly higher survival rate than those who only received radiation.

In a different 10-year, randomized, double-blind trial, researchers studied the effects of coriolus (PSK) with 56 patients and also studied another 55 patients who received a placebo, all after surgical operations on their colorectal cancers. The rate of patients in remission (or disease-free) was significantly higher (more than doubled) in the PSK group than in the placebo group.

Cranberry

The medical community scoffed for decades at the notion that cranberry juice could clear up urinary tract infections. It was widely regarded as nothing more than a folk remedy.

Yet there's a rich history behind this tart berry (*Vaccinium macrocarpon*), and many people have reported medicinal benefits. Although I like to see scientific studies, the many stories of its healing power added up to strong empirical evidence. Now the research has caught up with the folk history. A number of studies in the last decade have shown that cranberry is quite effective for the prevention and relief of urinary tract infections.

Cranberry has long been used for medicinal purposes by Europeans as well as Native American Indians. It won acceptance as a cure for urinary tract infections—but beyond that, it was used to deal with gallbladder attacks, liver and stomach problems, and for the prevention of scurvy. (Both vitamin C and flavonoids, which are contained in cranberry, help to prevent scurvy.)

Today, cranberry juice and supplements are used by millions around the world—and the medical community has become more accepting. In the past few years, many more conventional physicians have been recommending cranberry for their patients.

The fruit called cranberry comes from the vine of a plant that belongs to the same genus (*Vaccinium*) as bilberry and blueberry. It grows in North America in marshlike conditions, such as the famous "cranberry bogs" of Cape Cod, Massachusetts, and southern New Jersey.

I mainly recommend cranberry for the prevention and treatment of urinary tract and prostate infections. Research has shown that cranberry inhibits growth of the bacteria *E. coli*, which is the culprit most commonly associated with urinary tract infections. As a food source, cranberry provides ample vitamin C and flavonoids for people who need higher amounts for conditions such as varicose veins and cataracts.

DOSAGE

❧ *Juice*

It is important to drink the unsweetened form of cranberry juice. "Regular" cranberry juice—the kind that appears on most supermarket shelves—is sweetened with sugar that suppresses the immune system and feeds harmful bacteria.

For anyone dealing with urinary tract infections, I recommend 8 ounces of unsweetened cranberry juice four to five times daily. If the tart taste is too much for you, dilute the juice with water. For long-term use and prevention of urinary tract infections, I recommend having one or two 8-ounce glasses of unsweetened cranberry juice daily.

❧ *Capsules and Tablets*

If you take cranberry in capsule form, the dosage varies depending on the potency of the product. In the past, the capsules had such a low concentration of cranberry that you'd have to take eight capsules or more to get the same therapeutic effect as four 8-ounce glasses of the juice. Currently, the standardized capsules and tablets have higher concentrations. You can take three to four capsules or tablets daily to achieve therapeutic benefit.

WHAT ARE THE SIDE EFFECTS?

There are no reported side effects. However, I would recommend anyone with diabetes to check with his or her doctor first before using cranberry juice on a long-term basis. The naturally occurring fruit sugars could cause blood-sugar problems. But if you have diabetes, you might be able to avoid spiking blood-sugar levels by taking cranberry juice with your meals.

CRANBERRY

RECOMMENDATIONS FROM THE NATURAL PHYSICIAN FOR . . .

PROSTATE INFECTIONS

Known as prostatitis, prostate infections are more common in men who have an enlarged prostate gland—a condition that occurs in about half of all men over the age of 50. E. coli is the most common bacteria associated with prostate infections.

An enlarged prostate pinches on the urethra (urinary tube), causing a slowdown or backup of urine flow. As a result, bacteria and other microbes are more likely to grow in the urethra, leading to infection. Cranberry can help prevent this problem.

URINARY TRACT INFECTIONS

It was generally believed up until the last decade that cranberry juice prevents urinary tract infections by lowering the pH of urine. A lower pH makes for an inhospitable environment for bacteria like E. coli.

But studies done in the 1990s demonstrated that phytochemicals in cranberry—known as proanthocyandins—prevent bacteria from attaching to the bladder wall and urinary tract. Researchers also discovered that the sugar molecule fructose helped prevent a certain strain of E. coli from adhering to the urinary tract cells. Finally, a 1998 study in the New England Journal of Medicine demonstrated that cranberry prevents the fimbriae (analogous to arms and hands of bacteria) from attaching to the urinary tract walls. In research, cranberry's cousin blueberry was found to have a similar action.

I recommend cranberry juice or cranberry extract in supplemental form be used by people who have been taking prescription antibiotics for a urinary tract infection—especially if they have any kind of kidney infection. This simultaneous use optimizes the chances of a quick recovery.

A 1994 study in the Journal of the American Medical Association found that regular consumption of cranberry juice significantly reduced the frequency of bacteria and pus in the urine of elderly women. In this six-month study, the 153 women drank less than one pint of cranberry juice every day—with the usual "control group" drinking a placebo drink that had a similar flavor to cranberry. Improvements were noticed in the cranberry drinkers within four to eight weeks.

Consuming 500 mg of cranberry extract in capsule form was shown to be nearly as effective as the antibiotic trimethoprim in the prevention of urinary tract infections for women with a history of UTIs. The advantage of cranberry extract over antibiotics is that it does not destroy the good flora in the body, which can lead to fungal overgrowth and digestive problems.

D

Dandelion

One person's weed is another's healing herb. The same dandelion (*Taraxacum officinalis*) that so many homeowners set out to pull, eradicate, or destroy has a rich history of medicinal use in Europe, China, Japan, and Russia. Even in the United States, this herb has been used for detoxification for more than a century.

Dandelion root is revered for its ability to tonify the liver. The leaves have a natural diuretic effect—that is, they'll help remove excess water from the body. In addition, the whole plant is a nutritious and healing food. You can use the leaves in salads or in teas. The roots can be roasted and used as a coffee substitute, while the flowers have gone into a variety of alcoholic beverages, including dandelion wine and the after-dinner liqueur schnapps.

WEEDING OUT THE GOOD STUFF

Dandelion is a rich source of minerals such as magnesium, potassium, manganese, copper, phosphorous, sodium, iron, and silicon. The leaves are also rich in vitamin A. According to Dr. Bernard Jensen, author of *Foods That Heal*, "Dandelion greens have more vitamin A than almost any other vegetable."

Other nutrients found in dandelion include the B-complex vitamins as well as vitamin C, vitamin D, vitamin K, and calcium. Choline, a relative of the B-vitamin family is also found in relatively high amounts in dandelion. This nutrient is important for preventing and treating a fatty liver, and it also serves as an aid in bile production.

The chemical constituents of dandelion lend additional healing properties. One of the more important chemicals, taraxacin, which has a bitter taste, is thought to stimulate the digestive organs. It plays a role in prompting the liver and gallbladder to release bile. Improved bile flow is important because it helps the liver detoxify (that is, get rid of toxic chemicals) more effectively.

Dandelion also contains two hormone-balancing constituents: taraxerol and taraxasterol. It's one of the premier herbs recommended for hormone-related conditions like PMS.

Pectin is also found in dandelion. This is a type of fiber that helps to relieve constipation and reduce cholesterol levels. It also binds with toxins, which helps get rid of them. (The toxic substances that bind with pectin pass more readily through your digestive system.) Finally, dandelion contains a type of resin that helps in eliminating lung congestion, so it's a helpful remedy for coughs.

Dandelion ranks alongside milk thistle as the most frequently recommended herbs to help patients who need liver detoxification. Doctors who use natural healing methods are often concerned with the overall condition of the liver because it performs so many functions. Among other things, it detoxifies the chemicals and pollutants that get into our body, produces bile to help digest fats, stores and helps to regulate blood-sugar, and metabolizes hormones. As one expert noted, the liver performs more than 5,000 different enzymatic reactions every second. It's no wonder so many conditions can be helped by improving liver health. Just by treating the liver, we can sometimes resolve numerous conditions, ranging from physical problems such as indigestion and hepatitis to the emotional imbalances that contribute to irritability and depression.

Dosage

Dandelion root is most often taken in the capsule form. A typical adult dose is a 250- to 500-mg capsule taken three times a day with meals. Since the dosage may vary depending on the strength of the extract, I recommend that you follow the directions on the label.

If you're taking the tincture form, 20 to 30 drops with each meal is an average dose.

You can have dandelion leaf tea any time you need the benefits of its diuretic effect, as it will help you get rid of excess water and reduce bloating. Use 1 heaping table-spoon of dandelion leaves per cup of water. If you pick local dandelion to make a tea or add the leaves to your salad, be sure you're getting the plant from an area that has not been sprayed with herbicides.

Dandelion leaf is also available in both capsule and tincture form.

What Are the Side Effects?

While the dandelion plant is not toxic, some people get loose stools because it increases bile flow in the body. Therefore, it's not advisable to take capsules, tincture, or tea if you have diarrhea.

Some people are allergic to dandelion. Don't take it if you get an inflammation—contact dermatitis—when the leaves touch your skin. Dandelion should not be used if you have bile duct obstruction, acute gall-bladder inflammation (cholecystitis), or intestinal blockage. Also don't take dandelion to relieve gallstones unless you have been given a dosage that's prescribed by a knowledgeable herbal practitioner.

The German Commission E states that dandelion is a safe herb for women to use during pregnancy or while breast-feeding.

DANDELION
Recommendations from the Natural Physician for . . .

⚘ CONSTIPATION, FLATULENCE, AND INDIGESTION
Poor bile flow can lead to chronic constipation. If you have enough fiber in your diet and consume plenty of water but still have constipation problems, then it is a sign that the liver needs some work. Your bowels move more easily with some dandelion to increase the bile flow. Unlike pharmaceutical laxatives—which should only be used for a short time—you can take dandelion root in any of its forms for a few months and then gradually discontinue it. Once the liver and gallbladder are "tuned up," the bowels should move on their own without continual use of the herbal remedy.

(continued)

Indigestion or flatulence might be caused by insufficient stomach acid or bile production. If you're having these problems, dandelion is helpful because it stimulates natural actions and secretions of the digestive organs. Taken with meals, over time, it helps "retrain" the digestive organs so they'll function more effectively.

Dandelion is especially helpful if you have any problems digesting fats. When that's the case, it's usually because bile flow is insufficient.

☙ DIABETES

Dandelion root can be helpful for the long-term treatment of diabetes. It contains inulin, which is known to help balance blood-sugar levels. When you improve liver health by taking an herb like dandelion, you're assisting one of the organs that's most essential for blood-sugar regulation.

☙ EDEMA

I have had several elderly patients come to see me for the treatment of edema in their lower legs and ankles. That's the swelling or bloating that's caused by fluids in the extremities. Dandelion leaf extract works very nicely without side effects to substantially reduce this swelling.

I have determined in some cases that water retention is due to a weak heart. If the heart doesn't contract forcefully, water can back up in the tissues, which is a common symptom of congestive heart failure. Conventional medical tests such as an EKG (electrocardiogram) and ultrasound can reveal whether you have symptoms of congestive heart failure. To treat the heart weakness along with the edema, I not only recommend dandelion but also add herbs like hawthorn berry and nutrients like CoQ10 and L-carnitine.

I commonly recommend dandelion leaf for edema that occurs with pregnancy, when many women experience swelling of the hands and ankles. Dandelion leaf extract will usually help reduce some of the bloating. One of the benefits of dandelion leaf as a diuretic is that it does not cause the loss of potassium. (Potassium loss is a common side effect of some pharmaceutical medications that are prescribed for relief of edema.)

☙ GOUT

Dandelion has traditionally been used for the treatment of gout because it helps lower the levels of uric acid—and excess uric acid is often responsible for this problem. From my own observations, dandelion doesn't have dramatic effects in the short term, but it can be helpful on a long-term basis. (Cherries and celery seed extract are also excellent for relieving gout.)

☙ HEPATITIS

A valuable herb when it comes to liver problems, dandelion has been shown to improve liver function and alleviate the symptoms of liver toxicity. So it's well-suited as a treatment for hepatitis. If you are taking medication for hepatitis, you should continue to follow your doctor's advice, but dandelion can help improve bile flow so that there is no backup of bile in the ducts. Most herbal liver formulas contain dandelion root as one of the main herbs.

❧ HIGH BLOOD PRESSURE

I almost always recommend dandelion leaf in the treatment of high blood pressure. It acts as a natural diuretic so that blood volume is reduced, which has the effect of relieving high blood pressure.

Prescription blood-pressure medications, which are mostly diuretics, work on the same premise. But I prefer dandelion leaves over medication because of the way some pharmaceuticals cause potassium depletion.

An ideal herbal formula for high blood pressure includes dandelion leaf, hawthorn berry, viscum, and valerian. I've found that this combination is successful in a high percentage of cases, and many patients are able to reduce their pharmaceutical medications. At the same time, I always emphasize the importance of keeping your doctor informed if you have high blood pressure— and you should never discontinue a blood-pressure medication without the approval of your doctor.

❧ LOSS OF APPETITE

Dandelion root, like many other bitter herbs, can help restore your appetite. Just a daily cup of dandelion tea may be enough to improve appetite if you haven't been feeling hungry.

❧ PMS, MENOPAUSE, AND HORMONE BALANCING

Dandelion root is excellent for conditions related to hormone balance. The liver has to metabolize hormones, so you may develop a hormone imbalance if this organ is not working effectively.

In Chinese and naturopathic herbal medicine and in many other natural healing systems, optimizing liver health is considered very important if you want to treat conditions such as PMS, irregular menstrual cycles, or the symptoms associated with menopause.

In addition to helping out the liver, dandelion has two chemical constituents—taraxerol and taraxasterol—that help balance hormones as well.

❧ WEIGHT LOSS

If you take dandelion leaf tea or extract, you'll encourage the excretion of water, which leads to weight loss. It's not an easy weight-loss route, however, because it just reduces fluids without affecting the underlying causes of being overweight.

D-glucarate

I had a conversation with Dr. Thom Slaga, a well-known researcher at the prestigious American Cancer Research Center in Denver, Colorado. We were discussing his ongoing studies of a naturally occurring nutrient called glucaric acid.

Dr. Slaga piqued my interest with his explanation. Glucaric acid, he said, is a potent phytonutrient (plant nutrient) that helps the body detoxify toxic substances. This amazing phytonutrient, he went on to say, seemed to prevent certain types of cancers in animals. It was soon to become available as a supplement, in a form known as calcium D-glucarate, often referred to as D-glucarate.

I was struck at once by the possibility that D-glucarate might offer tremendous benefits for my patients. If this supplement stood up to scientific scrutiny, it was just what I was looking for. I had been intrigued about the new frontier in natural medicine—the role of phytonutrients and whole-food extracts—and here was a supplement that represented the latest discovery in that frontier.

TOMORROW'S BREAKTHROUGH TODAY

I would expect that we will all be hearing a lot more about this breakthrough supplement in the coming years. As a medical advisor for the health-food industry, I am sometimes privy to leading-edge research years before it becomes public knowledge. Often, new supplements are slow to be accepted. But I expect calcium D-glucarate will prove to be one of the most important nutritional supplements on the market.

The phytonutrient occurs naturally in fruits and vegetables such as apples, broccoli, alfalfa, cherries, and grapefruit. In this naturally occurring form, it's known as glucaric acid. When it's made into a supplement, calcium is added to help improve absorption.

Most people don't eat enough fruits and vegetables to get therapeutic amounts of phytonutrients like glucaric acid. That's where the supplement comes in handy. We would have to eat 7 to 10 servings of fruits and vegetables a day for cancer prevention, according to current recommendations. Living in a world where fast food is the norm, most people struggle to get two servings a day. By taking glucaric acid in supplemental form—as D-glucarate—we can take a step toward cancer prevention by making up some of that daily deficit.

LIVER SUPPORT

D-glucarate helps the liver metabolize or "burn up" some dangerous toxins, prevent-

ing these chemicals from causing harm. The toxins include carcinogens—that is, cancer-causing agents—as well as certain hormones. In the liver, D-glucarate helps the toxins turn into a water-soluble form, after which they can be excreted in urine.

When toxins enter the body, they go through two main detoxification phases in the liver. Phase one breaks down the compound and turns it into what's called an intermediate form, which is less toxic. Then the less-toxic form enters phase two, where it becomes water-soluble. If either one of these phases doesn't work correctly, the toxic substances continue to circulate in the body, causing damage. Eventually, these toxins get stored in tissues such as the brain, bone, or fat—or they build up inside other organs.

D-glucarate is important in the process because it helps carry out phase-two detoxification efficiently. But it does more than remove cancer-causing chemicals. In addition, D-glucarate helps metabolize hormones and many other potentially harmful substances.

HORMONE BALANCER

While healthy levels of hormones help the body function properly, excessive amounts of certain hormones can cause serious problems. Studies have shown that unhealthy levels of hormones like estrogen, progesterone, testosterone, and other hormones can cause cancer. For example, excess levels of estrogen and some estrogen-related compounds have been associated with breast, uterine, ovarian, and prostate cancers. Calcium D-glucarate has been shown to inhibit the incidence of breast tumors in animals. In one study, supplementing 2% of the animals' diets with D-glucarate produced dramatic results, among them:

- A 50% inhibition of beta glucoronidase. This is an enzyme that, by reversing the beneficial breakdown of hormones, allows risky amounts of hormones to build up in the body.
- A 23% reduction in the levels of estradiol. Estradiol is one of the estrogens known to promote breast and uterine cancers, so the reduction of estradiol is the equivalent of a reduced risk of cancer. (It also reduces the levels of toxic estrogen metabolites.)
- A fourfold reduction in the numbers of tumors.

❧ Getting Balance Back

It's quite common for people to suffer from hormone imbalances, so all of us can benefit from eating foods that contain D-glucarate as well as taking the supplemental form. I particularly recommend supplements for women who have a family history of breast cancer. Women who have had breast cancer, or are currently being treated, can also use this supplement, because it may help correct the underlying hormonal imbalance that is likely one of the root causes of the cancer. I also recommend it for women who are using birth control pills. I commonly use it in combination with the phytonutrient indole 3 carbinol.

Women and men on hormone-replacement programs would do well to take D-glucarate on a preventative basis to prevent the toxic buildup of these hormones. Men with an enlarged prostate or those trying to prevent or treat prostate cancer should be on this supplement. We now know that testosterone and estrogen imbalances are implicated in this hormone-sensitive gland.

In addition to its cancer-preventive properties, D-glucarate is generally effective in detoxification—that is, removing many different harmful compounds from the body. It makes a lot of sense for those on any type of detoxification program to get this nutrient into their body at therapeutic levels.

Dosage

Toxicity studies have shown D-glucarate to be very safe. I generally recommend patients take 400 mg daily as a preventative dosage and up to 2,000 mg if they're on a detoxification program. Studies as high as 10,000 mg a day have been done with calcium D-glucarate with no side effects reported.

I usually recommend the capsule, which is most readily available and is convenient to use. But you can also get D-glucarate in tablets and in powdered drinks.

The supplement does not require a prescription. You can purchase it at health-food stores, pharmacies, and some grocery stores.

DHEA

My suspicions were confirmed by the test.

Bob, a 51-year-old businessman, had come to me complaining of a profound feeling of burnout. As a result, I'd sent out for a saliva DHEA hormone test. It showed that his DHEA levels were very low for his age.

"You have the DHEA levels of a 70-year-old," I told him. "That helps to explain why you feel burned out. It also helps to explain why your libido is so low."

"What can we do to get it back to normal?" Bob asked.

"Anything you can do to cut down on stress will help," I answered. "The way you perceive stress is important, too."

We discussed some of the approaches he could take to help alter his approach to stressful situations and control his response.

Then we moved on to the subject of nutrition and herbal supplements.

"I want you to start taking 50 milligrams of DHEA daily," I said. "Your levels are so low that you need the supplementation."

Bob felt a surge in his energy levels over the next two months. Also, he reported that his wife was pleasantly surprised to find his sex drive had been renewed.

He was also surprised that a single supplement could make such a difference. Though he had been to several physicians before seeing me, he said that I was the first to request the DHEA hormone test that showed what the problem was.

FROM THE ADRENALS

Dehydroepiandrosterone (DHEA) is a steroid hormone that is mainly secreted by the adrenal glands, which are located on top of both kidneys. It was first identified in 1934 and since then more than 5,000 research studies have been completed on it.

In the past decade, some enthusiastic researchers have referred to it as a "fountain of youth" and an "antiaging" hormone. That's based upon the way DHEA levels decline as we age. They tend to peak in people when they reach the age of 30. After that, there's a general decline until, by age 70, DHEA levels are about 20% of those of a young adult. Since it seems to be associated with youthful energy, appearance, and immunity, DHEA has many applications.

DHEA is the most abundant steroid hormone in the body. It serves as a precursor to other hormones such as testosterone, androstenedione, and estrogen. It also has many direct effects on the body. For example, population studies show that higher DHEA levels are associated with the prevention of heart disease and cancer. It has a profound benefit to the immune system and is thought to be an important factor in autoimmune conditions.

DHEA is found in very high concentrations in the brain and is thought to play an important role in memory and cognitive function. Depression may be related to low levels of DHEA. Doctors are increasingly recommending hormones like DHEA for the treatment of chronic inflammatory conditions such as arthritis. Hormone specialists also recommend it as part of a comprehensive treatment for osteoporosis. It may also benefit women suffering from menopausal hot flashes.

DHEA supplementation appears to protect against bone loss (osteopenia). It also improves cognitive function in people who are taking prednisone, the hormone that's most often prescribed by medical doctors to help prevent bone loss.

DOSAGE

The dosage for DHEA should be determined by a doctor well-versed in natural hormone replacement.

The starting dose I recommend is based on the levels determined by the saliva or blood test. For many of my patients who have low levels of DHEA, I recommend a starting dose of 5 to 50 mg of DHEA daily. I then monitor their levels and observe their subjective symptoms to find the right dosage for them.

People with conditions such as lupus may require 200 mg or more daily. I do not recommend that people routinely take a DHEA supplement without knowing what their levels are. DHEA is often used in conjunction with its precursor, a hormone known as pregnenelone.

DHEA is available over the counter in capsule form. It is also commonly used by doctors in the sublingual, microionized capsule, and transdermal forms.

WHAT ARE THE SIDE EFFECTS?

Even though DHEA is available over the counter, this hormone—as with any hormone—should be used with caution. One of the first side effects that typically occurs is an acne breakout, especially on the back.

Too high a dosage of DHEA can cause masculine effects in women, such as facial hair growth. This is reversible when the dose is lowered.

The long-term effects of DHEA supplementation are unknown at this time. It is unclear whether it will cause problems for people who have hormone-dependent cancers such as breast and prostate cancers. Until we know the possible side effects for people with those conditions, I would not advise taking DHEA.

Women who are pregnant or breast-feeding should not take DHEA unless instructed to do so by a physician under special circumstances.

DHEA

RECOMMENDATIONS FROM THE NATURAL PHYSICIAN FOR . . .

ALLERGIES

Some people with chronic allergies, especially multiple chemical sensitivity, notice reversal of their condition after taking a DHEA supplement.

CHRONIC FATIGUE SYNDROME

I have had some patients with chronic fatigue syndrome respond quite dramatically to DHEA supplementation. In all cases the patients had tested low in DHEA before therapy was started. DHEA is an effective supplement for those with adrenal fatigue, where the adrenal glands produce suboptimal levels of DHEA to help one be more resistant to stress and fatigue. It has also been shown to be helpful for those with Addison's disease, where there is failure of the adrenal glands to produce stress hormones such as DHEA and cortisol.

CIRCULATORY HEALTH AND HEART DISEASE

DHEA may have a protective effect against heart disease. The Massachusetts Male Aging Study looked at the relationship between heart disease and levels of DHEA. The study included men between the ages of 40 and 70. There was an inverse relationship found between the levels of DHEA and heart disease.

DEMENTIA

Stress hormones such as cortisol and DHEA appear to play a role in dementia and diseases such as Alzheimer's. More research needs to be done in this area but DHEA appears to have a beneficial effect on aging brain function.

DIABETES

DHEA may be a key supplement for those with diabetes. Benefits have been shown in animal studies. Many holistic doctors report benefits with patients who have diabetes. It helps to prevent infections, build immunity, and improve wound healing.

(continued)

HIV

A longitudinal study showed a relationship between low serum DHEA levels in HIV-infected men and a more rapid progression to AIDS. Since there is currently no cure for HIV, we must use all possible means to help people with this condition, including hormones such as DHEA.

IMPOTENCE

I have found DHEA to be helpful for some men with impotence, which may be because DHEA is converted to testosterone. Researchers from the University of Vienna who tracked the results of DHEA replacement therapy in a group of 40 men found that the hormone was helpful for impotence (erectile dysfunction). The men—who were all between the ages of 41 and 69—were given DHEA supplements or inactive placebos over a 24-week period.

All of the men in the study had been experiencing early loss of erection, which made them unable to complete intercourse. The study showed that the men who took DHEA—as opposed to the placebo—had improved sexual response in a number of areas. They reported improved erectile function, orgasmic function, sexual desire, intercourse satisfaction, and overall satisfaction.

INFLAMMATORY BOWEL DISEASE (IBD)

Researchers evaluated DHEA and cortisol levels in patients with ulcerative colitis and Crohn's disease. DHEA was found to be much lower in IBD patients than in a group of healthy people.

Although treatment with a cortico-steroid such as prednisone can inhibit adrenal hormone production, these DHEA deficiencies were found even in patients who had not been subjected to previous treatment with corticosteroids. Researchers also found that as DHEA levels rose and cortisol levels dropped, the patients who were being monitored showed fewer signs of inflammation.

LUPUS

I have found DHEA supplementation to be helpful for some female patients who have lupus. Many other doctors of natural medicine report similar experiences. I find it to be a good alternative to prednisone therapy, especially when combined with other naturopathic therapies such as homeopathy and nutrition.

In one study, some women with systemic lupus erythematosus were given 200 mg of DHEA daily, and others were given a placebo. Those given DHEA had better improvement as rated by the patients and physicians, while there were more flare-ups of the disease in the group that was given the placebo. Those taking DHEA were also able to reduce their dosage of prednisone while those taking the placebo had to slightly increase their dosage.

MENOPAUSE

DHEA decreases (as do estrogen, progesterone, and testosterone) in women going through menopause. DHEA can be helpful in increasing libido, reducing hot flashes, and protecting against bone loss. In rare cases it may help relieve vaginal dryness and thinning of vaginal tissue.

❧ OSTEOPOROSIS

DHEA should be considered as part of an aggressive treatment protocol for those who have osteoporosis, as it appears to prevent bone loss.

❧ PREDNISONE TAPERING

DHEA is an excellent hormone to use to help people lower their dosage or discontinue using the drug prednisone. Long-term prednisone use can damage the immune system, liver, and kidneys, and cause osteoporosis. Making the transition from prednisone to DHEA must be done under the guidance of a knowledgeable physician.

❧ SCHIZOPHRENIA

DHEA has been shown to improve symptoms associated with schizophrenia. Use only under the guidance of a doctor.

❧ SKIN

The oral supplementation of DHEA has been shown to improve skin thickness, sebum production, and skin hydration and to decrease facial skin pigmentation in elderly men and women.

❧ STRESS

In a study published in *Biological Psychiatry*, researchers at Yale University and the Veterans Administration National Center for Post-Traumatic Stress Disorder reported that having a higher level of DHEA is associated with an improved ability to cope with extreme stress.

❧ WEIGHT

A study published in the *Journal of the American Medical Association* found DHEA supplementation with 50 mg resulted in significant reductions in abdominal fat in seniors. DHEA was also shown to improve insulin resistance.

Echinacea

It's not unusual to get calls at my office from patients wondering what to do about the cold or flu that just hit them. My first thought is: What natural supplements can they get quickly, right off the shelf?

Well, just about anyone can find echinacea (pronounced *eck-in-ay-sha*) at a nearby store. It's one of the five top-selling herbs in North America. In fact, it's a worldwide bestseller, as herbalists and doctors in Europe have been prescribing echinacea for decades. Carrying the popular name of purple coneflower (so-called because of its beautiful, purple, daisy-like petals), echinacea is renowned as an herb that enhances the immune system. It's commonly used to treat a number of conditions from flu and the common cold to a range of other infectious diseases.

THE SNAKEBITE CONNECTION

Native Americans of the Plains are believed to be the first to use echinacea. As today, it was a remedy for colds, coughs, and sore throats, but also toothaches, battle wounds, and even rattlesnake bites.

During the latter part of the 1800s, Plains settlers adopted the purple coneflower as a common remedy; and by the 1920s, echinacea was being sold as a commercial product and prescribed by the many physicians who were comfortable with herbal medicines.

Dr. H.C.F. Meyer of Pawnee, Nebraska,

was a keen commercial promoter. Adding his own recommendations to what he had learned from Native Americans, Dr. Meyer sold echinacea as a "cure-all" for various ailments. His reputation was considerably enhanced by the claim that he had successfully treated 613 cases of rattlesnake poisoning. One doctor gave the following candid account of Dr. Meyer's personal echinacea experiment:

"With the courage of his convictions upon him, he injected the venom of the crotalus (rattlesnake) into the first finger of his left hand; the swelling was rapid and in six hours up to the elbow. At this time he took a dose of the remedy, bathed the part thoroughly, and laid down to pleasant dreams. On awakening in four hours, the pain and swelling were gone."

INFECTION FIGHTER TO THE RESCUE

I can't say I have had any patients come to me for the natural treatment of rattlesnake bites. (If I did, I would quickly hurry them off to a hospital emergency room for a dose of up-to-date antivenom.) But it's interesting to note that echinacea does have the special property of preventing the spread of infectious substances to tissues.

Echinacea as a healing remedy was introduced to Europe during the 1930s. Since then the preponderance of scientific research on echinacea has been done in Western Europe, especially Germany, where the government plays an active role in funding natural medicine research. But Canadian and American researchers have recently made similar strides in echinacea research, with clinical studies and biochemical analysis of the healing herb.

More than 400 studies to date have looked at the pharmacology and clinical uses of echinacea. Not all studies have shown efficacy of the herb, but most of the research indicates that echinacea helps reinforce the immune system.

Echinacea is consistently one of the best-selling herbs in North America and Europe. More than 10 million units are sold annually in Germany alone.

Though there are nine species of echinacea, *Echinacea purpurea* and *Echinacea angustifolia* are the two most often used commercially. Most clinical studies are done with these species, especially *purpurea*.

TONGUE-TINGLING CHEMICALS

Scientists have not reached a consensus about the active ingredients in echinacea. Though researchers acknowledge the herb has many immune-boosting properties as well as anti-inflammatory and antimicrobial effects, they're not sure what chemicals or combination of chemicals are responsible.

It's known, however, that echinacea contains caffeic acid derivatives such as cichoric acid and polysaccharides. The plant also has compounds known as alkylamides that are thought to be important. (Alkylamides are the substances that make your tongue tingle and go numb if you take a hefty dose of straight echinacea.)

Some of these compounds are water-soluble and some are alcohol-soluble. When tinctures, pills, or tablets are being created from echinacea, the manufacturer must go through an elaborate process to extract the compounds. Recent research done at the University of British Columbia in conjunction with the University of Alberta has shown that the ratio of the actives in echinacea is important for optimal immune response. So in other words, not only is it important to have active constituents in echinacea products, but to also have them in a specific ratio or blend.

A BOON IN PREGNANCY

Pregnant women have to be careful about anything they eat, which includes supplements, so I'm often asked whether echinacea is safe to use during pregnancy. My answer is yes. Echinacea has a long history of use by herbalists and naturopathic doctors for the treatment of acute infections during pregnancy. If a pregnant woman has a cold, flu, or urinary tract infection, I would not hesitate to recommend echinacea. Side effects or problems with the pregnancy or health of the baby have not been reported. In fact, my wife used echinacea during her entire first pregnancy with no adverse effects.

A study by the Hospital for Sick Children in Toronto, in conjunction with the Canadian Naturopathic College, has confirmed the safety of echinacea use during pregnancy. A group of 206 women who used echinacea during pregnancy for upper respiratory tract infections were analyzed along with a control group of 198 pregnant women who had upper respiratory tract infections but never used echinacea. The researchers found no association with the use of echinacea and birth defects. There were also no differences in the rate of live births or spontaneous abortions between the two groups.

AROUSING IMMUNE CELLS

Echinacea doesn't work like the pharmaceutical antibiotics that "kill" microbes like bacteria. Instead, echinacea arouses the immune cells that patrol and defend the body against these invaders. It increases the number and activity of disease-fighting white blood cells, and it activates antiviral chemicals such as interferon. Echinacea can even activate the immune cells that fight tumors. In addition, research has shown that the chemicals in echinacea have the power to inhibit an enzyme released by bacteria, called hyaluronidase. Bacteria normally produce this enzyme to penetrate into human tissue. Echinacea prevents this from happening.

Researchers in a German study found clear evidence that echinacea helps to promote good immune cells, called phagocytes. One group of people were given 30 drops of echinacea three times daily for five days, while people in the control group were given a placebo. The level of phagocytes was measured at the beginning and throughout the study. At day three, the phagocyte activity of those taking echinacea increased by 40%. By the fifth day, phagocyte activity had increased 120%. When people stopped taking echinacea, immune-cell activity dropped off sharply. After three days, there was no difference in immune-cell activity between the group taking echinacea and the control group.

Leading researchers now feel that echinacea may actually be more of an immune-modulating herb, meaning it has a balancing effect on the immune system. As research continues, this may mean that echinacea may be more valuable than just boosting immune function.

VIRUS SLAYERS

While there are a host of modern antibiotics for killing bacteria, modern medicine has a limited arsenal of weapons to defeat viral infections. This presents a problem for the many doctors who rely on conventional pharmaceuticals in their medical practice. More than 65 million people in the United States each year "catch" the common cold, while another 108 million get the flu—and these are just two of the infectious diseases caused by viruses. Others include genital herpes, which affects an estimated 45 million people, as well as hepatitis C, which afflicts 170 million people in the world. Even a simple viral infection like a viral sore throat poses a challenge for any doctor who relies exclusively on antibiotics and other conventional prescription medications.

Echinacea, like some other immune-enhancing herbs, has a direct antiviral effect. Even better, it seems to summon all the resources of the immune system to help destroy viral invaders.

It also works well in combination with other antiviral plants and herbs. I like to prescribe echinacea in a formula called the "virus cocktail," which is comprised of echinacea, lomatium, astragalus, reishi, and licorice root. The synergistic blend of these herbs tends to be more effective than any one herb by itself.

BENEFITS FOR ATHLETES

Sports medicine specialists studied the effect of echinacea on men who participated in triathlons—those grueling events that involve long-distance swimming, running, and cycling. It is well known that triathletes are at an increased risk for infection because they train so exhaustively for each event. Among the participants of the study, some took a placebo, others were given a mineral supplement (43 mg of magnesium), while a third group took 8 mL of *Echinacea purpurea* daily. All three groups of athletes took the supplements for 28 days before a triathlon.

During training, one-quarter to one-third of the athletes taking a placebo or mineral supplement ended up getting colds. (Those taking magnesium missed 13 days of training, while those in the placebo group missed a total of 24 days.) None of those who were taking echinacea showed any cold symptoms, and none missed any training days.

BACTERIA AND FUNGUS

Since echinacea enhances the action of your immune cells, it is also effective against bacterial, fungal, and yeast infections. This is especially helpful if you're fighting a bacterial infection, because many bacteria are now resistant to antibiotics (because they're overprescribed by doctors for things like viral infections). If needed, there is no problem using echinacea in combination with antibiotics. As a matter of fact, I find when people are on antibiotics for a bacterial infection and use echinacea simultaneously, they recover more quickly.

At least one study—which included 4,190 patients—confirmed this observation. Researchers divided the patients into two groups and gave about half of them an antibacterial formula that included echinacea (along with two other herbs—thuja and baptisia). Along with that formula, the patients received antibiotics that were chosen by the doctors. For comparison, the rest of the patients received only antibiotics, with no herbal formula.

The results showed the effectiveness of taking herbal antibacterial agents along with antibiotics. In the group that got an echinacea-based formula plus an antibiotic, people were cured significantly faster and there was a lower incidence of recurring infection than in the group of people who just got an antibiotic. Also, the symptoms of "sore throat" and "difficulty in swallowing" were improved much more efficiently in the first group than in the second group.

DOSAGE

Echinacea is generally available as a tincture, capsule, tablet, or cream in the United States. It's also possible to take it in the form of an injection, though this method is mainly used in Germany.

Glycerine (alcohol-free) tinctures are available. These are good for kids, who especially enjoy the berry-flavored varieties.

Echinacea is one product that I find works very well as a standardized extract.

Tincture

I recommend 20 to 60 drops of the tincture every two to three hours for acute infections or twice daily for long-term use.

Capsule

I recommend 500 to 1,000 mg every two to

three hours for acute infections or twice daily for long-term use.

NOTE: High-potency, quality echinacea products are standardized to contain active ingredients such as alkylamides, cichoric acid, and polysaccharides.

Some controversy surrounds the length of time one can use echinacea. Many authors state that echinacea should not be used on a long-term basis. However, there are no studies showing that long-term use is harmful or that echinacea loses its effectiveness.

I generally recommend patients use echinacea for acute infections until they are completely over the illness. For those who are very susceptible to infections, especially during the winter, and do not want to change their lifestyle, echinacea can be used on a long-term basis (although it is not so effective as improving diet, reducing stress, and exercising). Long-term use of echinacea throughout the winter season is common in European countries.

WHAT ARE THE SIDE EFFECTS?

There has been no reported toxicity with echinacea, but two patients of mine have had allergic reactions, with some throat swelling after they started taking echinacea. Such a reaction has the potential of being life threatening. In both cases, I recommended that my patients avoid using echinacea and switch to other immune-enhancing herbs instead.

There have been some concerns about echinacea affecting fertility. An animal study that appeared in 1999 suggested that echinacea might adversely affect fertility—but, in my view, the research was seriously flawed. Researchers directly exposed hamster eggs to echinacea extract and concluded that at high concentrations echinacea impaired or prevented the sperms' ability to penetrate the eggs.

The flaw of the study is that echinacea is broken down in the digestive system to various components, each of which is highly diluted. Putting echinacea directly on sperm or hamster eggs does not replicate what happens in real life. Perhaps there will be further studies that give us a better idea of echinacea's effects on fertility, but this one isn't worth taking seriously.

ECHINACEA
RECOMMENDATIONS FROM THE NATURAL PHYSICIAN FOR . . .

🐎 AUTOIMMUNE CONDITIONS

There's some controversy about prescribing echinacea to patients who have autoimmune diseases—that is, conditions that become worse when the immune system is overactive. The German Commission E, the government-backed medical board that helps regulate herbal medicine, recommends that echinacea should not be used in those who have tuberculosis, leukosis, collagenosis, multiple sclerosis, AIDS and HIV, lupus, rheumatoid arthritis, and other autoimmune conditions. The assumption is that echinacea will worsen the hypersensitivity of the immune system, causing a flare-up of problems.

While I often agree with many of the commission's recommendations, many physicians point out that there have not been any studies showing that echinacea is harmful for autoimmune conditions. I have not seen or read any reports where a patient with one of these conditions was made worse from using echinacea, despite the fact that millions of people take it every year.

That said, echinacea would not be my first choice for a condition like multiple sclerosis, rheumatoid arthritis, or other autoimmune diseases. But when my patients with these conditions have an acute infection, such as a cold or urinary tract infection, I do recommend echinacea and other immune-enhancing herbs to fight off the infection. Usually these herbs are helpful; in any case, they don't seem to aggravate the autoimmune disease.

Interestingly, German physicians commonly use echinacea as a topical cream to relieve rheumatoid arthritis symptoms. These same doctors also frequently recommend echinacea be taken internally for its natural anti-inflammatory effects. Furthermore, newer research is showing that many autoimmune conditions are due to the immune system reacting to infectious agents, and cross reacting with the body's own tissue at the same time. In theory, this would make echinacea helpful for these conditions. More studies are needed to tell us exactly what effect— both good or bad—echinacea has for people with inflammatory or autoimmune conditions.

❧ COMMON COLD

I have found that echinacea can help prevent the common cold as well as reduce the symptoms and shorten the duration— but results differ. Some people respond almost miraculously, while others get no benefits at all. Overall, though, echinacea is more effective than over-the-counter medicines, which only help to reduce some of the symptoms of a cold and do nothing to assist the immune system or battle the infection.

One clinical study looked at the effectiveness of *Echinacea purpurea* for 120 patients who had the initial symptoms of the common cold, with "acute, uncomplicated upper airways infection." When these patients took 20 drops of echinacea every two hours for the first day— and thereafter three times daily—they fared much better than another group that took a placebo. At the end of the 10-day study, patients were questioned about the intensity of their illness and the time it took them to improve. The time to improvement was significantly shorter. In the echinacea group, people averaged four days to recover, while those in the placebo group took an average of eight days to recover.

In an analysis of 14 studies, University of Connecticut researchers found that echinacea supplements slashed the odds of catching a cold by an impressive 58%. The herb also reduced the length of a typical seven-day cold by about a day and a half, according to an article published in *Lancet Infectious Diseases*.

❧ FLU

Yes, there are a few antiviral drugs that can help treat the flu. However, the clinical data on these drugs does not impress me very much. The most commonly prescribed drug, amantadine, isn't at all effective in the first two or three days. This is a real drawback because most people experience their worst symptoms during the first 72 hours of a flu attack.

(continued)

Fortunately, my clinical experience has shown that herbs like echinacea can often help with symptoms the first 24 hours. This is supported by research—but the research also suggests that the size of the dose is an important factor. In a study of 180 men and women between the ages of 18 and 60, researchers compared three different groups. The first group took a placebo. The second got 90 drops of *Echinacea purpurea* every day, which is the equivalent of a 450-mg dose, while the third group received double that, or 900 mg daily. Symptoms of all participants were evaluated after three to four days and again after 8 to 10 days. The results showed that 90 drops of tincture had little effect, but the people who took 180 drops were significantly better off, with less-severe symptoms that lasted for a shorter time.

✍ SKIN CONDITIONS

In North America, echinacea has not quite caught on as a topical treatment for skin conditions. But many European makers of skin products are including the herbal ingredient.

A review of 4,958 clinical cases focused on the effectiveness of echinacea ointment. The main researcher in the study concluded that the ointment was highly effective for many skin conditions. These included 1,453 patients with wounds, 900 with varicose ulcers, 629 with eczema, 26 with burns, 222 with herpes simplex, and 212 with inflammatory skin problems. More than 90% positive results occurred when the ointment was used to treat burns, wounds, and herpes.

✍ VAGINITIS

Recurring vaginal yeast infections can be quite troublesome for women. One German study looked at 203 women with this condition. Of the 60 women taking echinacea (while the rest took a placebo or other medicines), only 10 had recurrences of yeast infections.

Elderberry

"This flu is nasty, my muscles ache all over, and I have a terrible cough. Do you think I need antibiotics?" asked Jennifer, a patient of mine. After examining her, I explained that influenza is caused by a virus, which had led to her cough and muscle aches. My primary solution for Jennifer was elderberry syrup. This botanical is an amazing flu fighter and also has the bonus of treating coughs.

Also known as European or black elderberry (*Sambuccus nigra*), North American elderberry, or elder, this plant grows in North America and Europe. The berries and flowers are the medicinal components used in herbal formulations. The dried berries have a long history of being consumed as a food. Native American healers used elderberry for treating coughs, respiratory tract infections, and skin conditions. Elderberry has been popular in European folk medicine for the treatment of various ailments. In 400 BC, Hippocrates referred to the elder tree as his "medicine chest." It continues to be a popular botanical in Austria, which is the world's leading elderberry-producing country.

Elderberry flowers and berries contain flavonoids known as anthocyanins that have potent antioxidant and anti-inflammatory effects. These substances appear to inhibit influenza replication and boost immune system activity.

DOSAGE

For treating the flu and cough, adults should take 15 mL (1 tablespoon) elderberry juice–containing syrup (Sambucol) four times daily and children 15 mL (1 tablespoon) twice daily.

WHAT ARE THE SIDE EFFECTS?

The standardized elderberry syrup used in the studies is very safe and was well tolerated by children and adults in the study when taken for three to five days. I have patients use it short term for the treatment of infections.

ELDERBERRY

RECOMMENDATIONS FROM THE NATURAL PHYSICIAN FOR . . .

ᕦ COUGH

While mainly studied for the treatment of the flu, elderberry syrup can be effective in the treatment of coughs.

ᕦ FLU

Two studies have demonstrated that elderberry syrup is effective in treating influenza. A randomized, double-blind, placebo-controlled Norwegian trial, involving 60 men and women between the ages of 18 and 54, was designed to determine the efficacy of a standardized elderberry syrup for the treatment of influenza. Patients were screened for participation between December and February, when influenza infection is most prevalent. All volunteers selected for the study had a fever and at least one respiratory influenza symptom. Influenza type A virus was isolated from 54 patients and influenza type B from 6 patients. Patients were randomized to receive either a standardized black elderberry syrup preparation or a placebo syrup.

Participants supplemented with 15 mL of elderberry or placebo four times per day, starting within 48 hours of the onset of the influenza-like symptoms and continuing for five days. Symptoms were relieved on average four days earlier and use of rescue medication was significantly less in those receiving standardized elderberry extract as compared with placebo. None of the patients reported any adverse events during the study.

An earlier trial was conducted in Israel with both children and adults. Significant improvement of symptoms, including fever, was noted with 93.3% of the elderberry group within two days, compared to 91.7% of the placebo group not showing improvement until day 6. Complete resolution of symptoms was achieved within two to three days in approximately 90% of the elderberry group. Overall standardized elderberry syrup reduces the duration of symptoms of the flu by about 56%.

Enzymes

"I travel a lot on business," said Jeremy, a 35-year-old in the software business. "I wish I could eat good food all the time—but it's just impossible."

Dependent on restaurant food, often obliged to eat with customers, at the mercy of in-flight meals, Jeremy was having increasing problems with his colitis.

"I know what will help a lot," I replied. "Enzymes!"

When taken with meals, enzymes help with digestion. I recommended that Jeremy always have a bottle with him wherever he traveled, just to prevent flare-ups.

In addition, I recommended a number of other herbs to take in combination with the enzymes. Last of all, "I still want you to follow the diet recommendations we talked about."

From that point on, Jeremy started taking the enzymes with every meal, whether or not he was in-flight, on the road, or eating hotel food. Not only would these enzymes help to repair his digestive tract, they would also help increase the supply of enzymes produced by his own body.

Enzymes are protein molecules found in every cell in humans, animals, and plants. As you read this sentence, millions of enzymatic reactions are occurring, regulating all the chemical reactions that occur in your body.

Enzymes perform many life-sustaining functions. Some, known as digestive enzymes, help break down food so the nutrients can be absorbed from the digestive tract into the bloodstream. Others, called metabolic enzymes, are involved in energy production, detoxification, immunity, and many other important activities.

All the vitamins and minerals found in food, or taken as supplements, require the action of enzymes to make them active. Those nutrients also boost enzyme activity, since these molecules require what are called cofactors—magnesium and other minerals—to help them function. In addition, coenzymes such as B vitamins or coenzyme Q10 are needed to activate the enzyme. Working together, the enzymes, cofactors, and coenzymes sustain the energy creation that sustains every one of our living cells.

There is no doubt that a healthy body requires a rich supply of enzymes. Though many supplement programs focus on our vitamin and mineral requirements, we may see more interest in enzyme therapies in the future. An increasing number of nutrition-oriented doctors are beginning to make enzymes a central focus of healing therapies.

BEST SOURCES

There are several ways our bodies get life-sustaining enzymes. Some are manufactured by our body organs. Our saliva glands, stomach, and liver all produce enzymes—and the pancreas is the major factory.

Raw foods are another important source because plants produce enzymes to sustain their own metabolic activities. Raw fruits and vegetables provide many of the nutrients we need to help replace our enzymes, but they do have to be raw. You don't get the same boost from these foods when they're cooked, because the enzymes in food are destroyed when temperatures hit 140 degrees Fahrenheit.

Besides getting enzymes from raw fruits, vegetables, herbs, and seeds, you can also get a good supply from juices. It's best to drink juice that's as freshly made as possible if you want to get the highest amount of vitamins, minerals, phytonutrients, and enzymes from that source.

Other food sources of enzymes include fermented foods such as yogurt, kefir, sauerkraut, miso, tempeh, and natto (fermented, cooked soybeans). You can also get good, healthy doses from wheatgrass, alfalfa, algae (chlorella, spirulina), and raw honey.

You can also take supplements for a boost. The three main forms of supplements provide plant, microbial, and animal enzymes. Research has shown that the body uses these enzymes for different activities such as digestion and other metabolic functions. Another category of supplements—whole-food supplements—may contain some live enzymes, though not in such high concentrations as enzyme supplements.

THE DEPLETION EFFECTS

Enzyme deficiency may be a major factor in chronic disease. Since our cells can't possibly function without enzymes, it's reasonable to conclude that any deficiency could contribute to health problems. So if you're not getting enough enzymes from your diet—particularly if you don't eat enough raw fruit and vegetables—it's reasonable to make sure you take supplements.

Studies have shown that the average American eats approximately two servings of fruits and vegetables daily. This is a far cry from the government-recommended five to seven servings or the seven to ten servings advocated by most nutritional experts. Even when we do eat these foods, we're usually getting them after they've been cooked, when the enzymes have been destroyed by frying, boiling, steaming, baking, or microwaving.

Enzymes are also destroyed by pesticides, herbicides, food preservatives, additives, colorings, and flavor enhancers. They're also depleted by other substances, such as smoke and other air pollutants, excessive sun (UV rays), and medications. Illness also depletes enzymes; in addition, they can be diminished by the free radicals produced during normal cell activity or by the physical demands of increased activity.

Enzymes are critical to good digestion, so you may need to get additional enzymes to improve digestion. While your body produces many different enzymes to assist in the assimilation of food (see Table 4), you might need to take enzyme supplements to help these internally created enzymes break down food more efficiently. This can be very helpful for people with digestive conditions such as IBS, Crohn's disease, or other inflammatory bowel disorders.

Also, people with food sensitivities and general digestive weakness (gas, bloating, diarrhea) can benefit from enzyme supplementation. Keep in mind that a lot of chronic illnesses are caused at least in part by the malabsorption of food and nutrients, which creates toxic byproducts that get into the bloodstream. Therefore, supplements such as enzymes can indirectly help conditions such as arthritis, cancer, fatigue, and allergies.

TYPES OF SUPPLEMENTAL ENZYMES

As mentioned, there are three main types of enzymes that you can purchase commercially.

❧ Plant Enzymes

The two best examples are bromelain from pineapple and papain from papaya. Both of these supplements can be taken with meals to help with the digestion of protein. If you take either of them—especially bromelain—on an empty stomach, they help to prevent inflammation. These enzymes assist with the breakdown of protein, but not other foodstuffs such as carbohydrates and fats.

Microbial Enzymes (Fungal Enzymes)

This group of enzymes has a much broader scope of use—especially for digestion—than the plant enzymes. All the microbial enzymes are derived from the fermentation of fungus. Though some people in the health industry commonly refer to microbial-derived fungal enzymes as plant enzymes, they actually come exclusively from fungi rather than other types of plants. The fungi are fermented in a specific way to produce a full spectrum of enzymes.

The two most common types of fungi are *Aspergillus oryzae* and *Aspergillus niger*, which are grown on a base of wheat or rice bran that's been enhanced with other substances that encourage good enzyme growth. Extracted from the fungi, the enzymes then go through a purification and separation process. They're dried, concentrated, and analyzed by a quality-control technician.

European doctors give microbial-derived enzymes by injection, using the intravenous form in the treatment of disease. I often recommend the supplement form of microbial-derived enzymes because of their potency, purity, and stability. I've found that full-spectrum fungal enzyme formulations are extremely helpful to people who need to improve their digestion. They can also help with tissue repair from injuries.

Animal Enzymes

These are derived from animal organs. Typically, pancreatic enzymes are derived from pig or sheep pancreas, while bile enzymes and salts are derived from ox gallbladder. Some of these formulations seem to be unstable—which means they quickly break down (and therefore lose their effectiveness) when they're exposed to stomach acid.

To get around this problem, the extracts are made into tablets with a special coating (enteric coating) to avoid being destroyed by stomach acid. Many researchers state that even with the enteric coating, many of the enzymes are still destroyed by stomach acid.

The other concern I have with animal enzymes is the issue of purity. Seeing as the extracts are ground up pancreatic tissue, can the consumer be guaranteed that all contaminants are removed, including things such as viruses? I have not seen this issue fully addressed by manufacturers. However, many people do get therapeutic benefits from pancreatic extracts—and studies show they work.

Given the choice among plant, microbial (fungal), and animal enzymes, however, I generally choose microbial-derived enzymes.

TABLE 4

Where From and What For?

Enzymes are produced in many different parts of the digestive system, and they perform a wide variety of functions in the breakdown of food. Here's an overview of some of the most important and what they do:

ENZYME(S)/SOURCE OF PRODUCTION	LOCATION OF ACTIVITY/ACTION
Amylase (ptyalin)/Saliva glands	Mouth/Breaks down carbohydrates
Gastric lipase/Stomach	Stomach/Breaks down fats
Renin/Stomach	Stomach/Breaks down milk protein
Pepsin/Stomach	Stomach/Breaks down protein
Proteolytic/Pancreas	Small intestine/Breaks down protein
Amylolytic/Pancreas	Small intestine/Breaks down carbohydrates
Lipolytic/Pancreas	Small intestine/Breaks down fats
Peptidases/Small intestine	Small intestine/Breaks down protein
Amylolytic/Small intestine	Small intestine/Breaks down sugars
Lipase/Small intestine	Small intestine/Breaks down fats

A WRAP-UP OF COMMERCIAL ENZYMES

Most of the following enzymes can be purchased individually. More commonly, they're part of multi-enzyme formulas.

- *Alpha galactosidase:* The best known of these alpha glactosidase products has the brand name Beano. The enzyme helps break down the carbohydrates that cause gas formation from eating beans. It is also found in full-spectrum microbial-derived enzymes.
- *Amylase:* Breaks down carbohydrates. *Sources:* Plant, microbial, animal.
- *Bromelain:* Breaks down protein and has natural anti-inflammatory effect. (See Bromelain, page 66.) *Source:* Plant (pineapple stem or fruit).
- *Cellulase:* Breaks down fiber. *Source:* Microbial.
- *Chymotripsin:* Breaks down protein and reduces inflammation. *Source:* Animal.
- *Dipeptidyl Peptidase:* Breaks down protein, especially gluten and casein. *Source:* Microbial.

(continued)

- *Invertase:* Breaks down carbohydrates, especially sugar. *Source:* Microbial.
- *Lactase:* Breaks down milk sugar (lactose). Found in milk products (LactAid) as well. *Source:* Microbial.
- *Lipase:* Breaks down fats. *Sources:* Microbial, animal.
- *Maltase:* Breaks down carbohydrates, specifically maltose. *Source:* Microbial.
- *Nattokinase:* Breaks down fibrin clots and acts as blood thinner. *Source:* Microbial.
- *Pancreatin:* Breaks down proteins, fats, and carbohydrates. *Source:* Animal (derived from cow or hog pancreas).
- *Papain:* Breaks down proteins and has a natural anti-inflammatory action. *Source:* Plant (papaya).
- *Pepsin:* Breaks down protein. *Source:* Animal.
- *Phytase:* Breaks down phytic acid of plants. *Source:* Microbial.
- *Sucrase:* Breaks down the sugars sucrose and maltose. *Source:* Microbial.
- *Trypsin:* Breaks down protein and has natural anti-inflammatory effect. *Source:* Animal.

DOSAGE

Different measurements are used for enzymes. Microbial-derived enzymes have different units of measurement than animal- and plant-derived enzymes.

When enzymes are taken as a digestive aid, the typical dosage is one to two capsules with each meal. Some people may need to take three capsules with each meal for a better digestive effect.

The dosage for plant enzymes is the same, but you don't want to take them with meals if you're using them for their anti-inflammatory effect or to heal wounds. Instead, take them between meals.

Enzymes should be kept away from heat and moisture when they're in storage. They should also not be exposed to light. Make sure the lid to the enzyme supplement container is closed tightly.

Individual enzymes can be taken between meals for specialized therapeutic effects. For example, proteolytic enzymes—such as bromelain or protease—help to reduce inflam-

mation and heal injuries and wounds when used in higher concentrations between meals. Practitioners use lipase enzymes to help metabolize triglycerides. Follow the directions on the container.

I mainly recommend the use of microbial-derived enzymes derived from *Aspergillus oryzae,* as do many health professionals. They are a very concentrated source of enzymes and appear to be more stable than animal enzymes. If you do use animal-derived pancreatic enzymes, then make sure they are enteric coated.

WHAT ARE THE SIDE EFFECTS?

Side effects are not common with enzymes. However, a small percentage of people get gas and bloating when they first start taking them. These initial symptoms are often the result of the digestive system "rebalancing" itself as yeast and undesirable bacteria are killed from the changes in the digestive flora. Less often, it could be a sensitivity reaction, in which case the symptoms will not go away.

Those with active ulcers or a history of ulcers should avoid the use of protein (protease) enzymes as they can further irritate an ulcerated stomach. If you suffer from ulcers and also need digestive support, you can obtain digestive enzyme formulas that are made without protein enzymes.

Persons with blood-clotting disorders, those on blood-thinning medications, and people about to undergo surgery should avoid the use of protein (protease) enzymes or nattokinase as they can thin the blood,

especially when taken between meals. ~ might be able to use digestive enzyme formulas that contain proteolytic enzymes, as long as you take them with your meals—but be sure to consult with your doctor first.

If you're allergic to pork, avoid porcine-derived animal enzymes.

People always ask if they can take microbial (fungal-derived) enzymes if they have *Candida* (yeast overgrowth). I have not seen a problem in these cases. The enzymes come from yeast, but in the end-product of the whole extraction process, no yeast are left in the formulation.

ENZYMES
RECOMMENDATIONS FROM THE NATURAL PHYSICIAN FOR . . .

❧ ARTHRITIS

Poor digestion is one of the major factors associated with the development of arthritis. Enzymes help to reduce the toxic load in the body and improve the absorption of nutrients. This is especially important for people who have rheumatoid arthritis. Proteolytic enzymes like bromelain help to reduce inflammation. (For more information, see Bromelain, page 66.)

❧ AUTOIMMUNE CONDITIONS

If you improve the absorption of foods, it means you're getting more and better nutrition, and that helps anyone who has an autoimmune condition. There's a well-established connection between poor intestinal absorption (leaky gut syndrome) and autoimmune diseases. Inflammatory chemicals are released in the body when the immune system reacts to poorly digested proteins.

❧ CANCER

Proteolytic enzymes are used by holistic cancer specialists to help break down cancer cells. Also, full-spectrum enzymes enhance digestion, which helps to improve the nutritional status of the body and makes for a healthier immune system.

Many cancer clinics in Europe and now the United States use enzyme therapy as a complementary therapy in the treatment of most types of cancers. Dr. Nicholas Gonzales, a medical doctor who practices in New York City, has raised quite a few eyebrows in the medical community with his successful natural treatment of cancer. The results of his clinical trial showed that a treatment protocol consisting of diet, nutritional supplements (which included megadoses of animal-derived pancreatic

(continued)

enzymes), and detoxification was significantly more successful than conventional therapy (chemotherapy) for inoperable pancreatic cancer. For example, his patients had an 81% survival rate after one year as compared with a 25% average survival rate for those undergoing conventional treatment for the same cancer. Currently, a large-scale study of Dr. Gonzales's enzyme treatment of advanced pancreatic cancer is about to get underway and is being funded by the National Institutes of Health's National Center for Complementary and Alternative Medicine, with collaboration from the National Cancer Institute.

CARDIOVASCULAR DISEASE

Nattokinase is an enzyme that is extracted from the traditional Japanese food natto, which is made from fermented soybeans. It enhances the body's natural ability to dissolve fibrin. Nattokinase is a more aggressive approach to cardiovascular disease prevention than other natural therapies—and is generally recommended for those with elevated fibrinogen or a history of heart disease. Researchers in the United States and Japan have found it to be a potent natural agent that can effectively and safely prevent blood clots without any side effects. With careful monitoring, some holistic practitioners are able to help some patients on blood thinners such as warfarin switch to nattokinase. To prevent heart disease, take a supplement providing 2,000 fibrinolytic units (FU) daily (not with meals). For those with atherosclerosis, take a supplement that provides 2,000 to 4,000 FU of nattokinase twice daily under the supervision of a healthcare professional.

Supervision is important with all anti-coagulants since there is the danger that too much can lead to hemorrhage and too little to heart attack or stroke. Nattokinase should not be taken with other blood thinners such as aspirin or warfarin.

COLIC

One technique that can help improve colic is to add full-spectrum microbial-derived enzymes to the baby's formula. Just by adding one enzyme you help to predigest the proteins and other foodstuffs in the formula so that they can be more easily digested. Breast-feeding mothers can take enzymes with meals so that the food they eat is broken down better—but consult with your doctor first. Taking enzymes makes it less likely that food allergens will be passed through breast milk.

DIGESTIVE DISORDERS

This is a huge category of conditions that really includes pretty much every digestive disorder. Simple indigestion, flatulence, and chronic diarrhea can be helped with enzyme supplementation.

Those with Crohn's disease, irritable bowel syndrome, and ulcerative colitis should definitely consider supplementing with enzymes to help get their condition under control. Enzymes are helpful to prevent indigestion when eating a large meal or food that is hard to digest. (My occasional pizza binges are accompanied with enzymes.)

FOOD SENSITIVITIES

Supplements that improve digestion can help improve or eradicate food sensitivities. While avoiding the foods that may be causing a food-sensitivity reaction, you can also help the condition by taking enzymes.

❧ INJURIES

Proteolytic enzymes have long been used for the treatment of injuries, particularly athletic injuries. They help decrease inflammation and swelling, and stimulate immune activity in the repair of the injury. Bromelain is the most well-known proteolytic enzyme for these

kinds of treatments. Microbial-derived protease is also effective.

❧ SKIN RASHES

Chronic skin rashes can be the result of poor intestinal health. The irritation from toxic metabolites of poor digestion can cause inflammation of the skin. Along with dietary improvement, enzymes help to decrease this toxic load and, over time, can improve various skin conditions.

❧ VIRAL INFECTIONS

A number of people have told me that they took proteolytic enzymes (microbial-derived) on an empty stomach to help fight viral infections such as the common cold and flu. Advocates of this type of therapy say that the enzymes help to break down the protein coat (capsid) that surrounds the virus. Though I'm not aware of any studies that validate this use, many popular European pharmaceutical products include a combination of proteolytic enzymes and "cold drugs" together in a formula.

Essential Oils

Modern research has demonstrated the medicinal effects that various aromas can have on the mind and body. Today essential oils are becoming popular again to help calm the nerves, improve concentration, fight infections, and treat many other ailments. Essential oils are highly fragrant, complex, and volatile substances with unique aromas. The olfactory system (sense of smell) transfers nerve messages to the

brain. This can result in beneficial effects on emotions, hunger, pain, and memory.

These aromatic extracts are concentrated from the parts of plants, including leaves, fruits, flowers, roots, spices, needles, twigs, and wood. Physical methods are used to extract the essential oils; usually steam distillation but including other techniques, such as cold pressing.

Essential oils are used in the practice of aromatherapy. This involves using specific aromatic extracts to assist the body in healing or preventing disease. The practice of aromatherapy has been around for thousands of years. It was commonly used by Egyptians to enhance health and in religious ceremonies. The Greeks adopted the use of aromatherapy from the Egyptians and also believed certain scents had therapeutic properties. Hippocrates also used aromatherapy for different specific ailments. Moving along to the 1920s, French chemist René-Maurice Gattefossé then coined the term *aromatherapy*. After an accidental burn of his arm he dipped it into the nearest cold liquid, which was lavender oil. He was surprised how quickly his pain was relieved and that his burn healed without scarring. Gattefossé's work was continued by Jean Valnet who used essential oils to treat gangrene in wounded soldiers during World War II.

There is a difference between essential oils and vegetable oils or fatty acid supplements like flax oil. Essential oils are volatile so they evaporate quickly when exposed to air. Many essential oils are too strong to apply undiluted on the skin or to breathe in. For topical applications, they are diluted in carrier oils like sesame or almond oil. For inhalation, they can be inhaled directly or made into a steam inhalation or diffusor.

DOSAGE

The amount used depends on the carrier technique being used. It is best to follow the guidance of a practitioner trained in aromatherapy. Following are general dosage recommendations. For massage, 10 to 20 drops of an essential oil are added to one ounce of a carrier oil. One can sniff an essential oil directly or put 2 to 3 drops on a tissue to inhale periodically throughout the day. For steam inhalation, 3 to 6 drops of essential oil can be added to a heat-proof bowl filled halfway with hot water. While sitting, place a towel over your head to trap the steam and inhale for a few minutes. For diffusers, follow the directions that come with the machine, which usually involve only a few drops.

WHAT ARE THE SIDE EFFECTS?

Essential oils should always be diluted before being applied to the skin. Also, try a small amount on a limited area of your skin before applying to larger surface areas. Do not apply to broken skin. Some essential oils, like tea tree oil, when diluted can be used as mouthwashes. They are also available at health-food stores as commercial products already in a safe dilution. However, never swallow essential oils. If you are pregnant or nursing, use aromatherapy only under the guidance of your doctor. People with asthma should be cautious inhaling essential oils.

ESSENTIAL OILS
RECOMMENDATIONS FROM THE NATURAL PHYSICIAN FOR . . .

✒ AGITATION
A study of 70 older adults with dementia found that lavender oil was effective in reducing agitation.

✒ DEPRESSION
A four-week, double-blind, randomized trial of adults with mild to moderate depression found that the combination of lavender essential oil and a pharmaceutical antidepressant (imipramine) to be more effective than imipramine alone. Researchers also found the combination to work earlier than the drug treatment alone.

✒ DIGESTIVE UPSET
Peppermint oil has been shown in studies to help postoperative nausea as well as a rare condition called difficult esophageal spasm.

✒ HAIR LOSS
Bald spots, medically termed *Alopecia areata*, were shown in one study to be helped by the topical application of

lavender and other essential oils. The formula included rosemary (3 drops or 114 mg), thyme (2 drops or 88 mg), lavender (2 drops or 108 mg), and cedarwood (2 drops or 94 mg), all mixed with 3 mL jojoba oil and 20 mL grape seed oil. Each night, the mixture was massaged into the scalp for two minutes, with a warm towel placed around the head to increase absorption. The study was a seven-month, randomized, double-blind, controlled trial involving 86 people with *Alopecia areata*. Those receiving a placebo were given carrier oil only. Hair growth was noted in up to 44% of patients receiving the lavender mixture compared to 15% in the placebo group.

🍃 MEMORY

A study in the *International Journal of Neuroscience* assessed cognitive function and mood in 144 volunteers randomly given essentials oils of ylang-ylang, peppermint, or a no-aroma control. Peppermint was found to enhance memory, whereas ylang-ylang impaired it and lengthened processing speed. In terms of subjective mood, peppermint increased alertness and ylang-ylang decreased it, but ylang-ylang significantly increased calmness.

🍃 WELL-BEING

Eighty women not receiving treatment for psychological disorders who were staff or students at the University of Wolverhampton found that adding lavender plus grape seed to their baths improved their overall mood.

Evening Primrose Oil

Few supplements are as confusing to people as the essential fatty acids (EFAs)—probably because "fatty" has such a sinister connotation. But the "essential fatty acids" are not at all synonymous with weight gain or poor health or any of the other things that "fatty" seems to imply. Rather, they're essential to life itself.

The human body doesn't "manufacture" EFAs, so we either have to attain them from our diet or through supplementation. They're what we need to help build the basic structure of our cells and also to help those cells function as they should. They're also the essence of what's good about evening primrose oil (*Oenothera biennis*).

Evening primrose oil—commonly referred to as EPO—is an essential fatty acid supplement comprised of oil that's extracted from the seeds of evening primrose. For a number of years, an increasing number of holistic doctors have been recommending it for treatment of women who have PMS symptoms and cyclical breast pain. It's also recommended for eczema, diabetic neuropathy (the nerve damage experienced by some people who have diabetes), and arthritis pain.

Evening primrose oil is high in the group of essential fatty acids known as omega-6. It's not hard to get omega-6 fatty acids from other food sources, because it's in red meat and most vegetable oils such as safflower and sunflower. But evening primrose oil does have one other very special constituent, which is the main reason why so many people can benefit from it. This constituent is known as gamma linolenic acid (GLA). In fact, evening primrose seeds yield between 7% and 10% GLA. (Other plant sources of GLA include borage and black currant seed.)

GLA is an essential fatty acid that is required for proper brain development and function. Infants receive GLA from breast milk. As GLA is metabolized in the body, it's transformed into other chemical substances (metabolites) that help control inflammation, prevent blood clots, reduce some kinds of muscle cramping, and balance hormones. Some people actually need a direct source of GLA to help prevent nerve damage from diabetes or conditions such as eczema. Therefore, they benefit from a direct source like EPO.

DOSAGE

The amount of evening primrose oil that should be used depends on your weight and, of course, the condition you're treating. The most important aspect of evening primrose is the amount of GLA that is contained in each dose. Evening primrose oil capsules usually come in 500-mg sizes—and from that, you should be getting about 50 mg of GLA.

There's also an oil form, which is usually more cost effective. Adults with specific conditions such as eczema and PMS can benefit from 150 to 400 mg of GLA daily, which means taking between 1,500 and 3,000 mg of evening primrose oil. (For some diseases, such as neuropathy, higher doses are needed.)

The optimum doses for children are between 50 and 200 mg of GLA, or 500 to 2,000 mg of evening primrose oil capsules.

For those taking evening primrose oil on a preventative basis, I recommend 500 to 1,500 mg daily in combination with an omega-3 oil such as flaxseed, hemp, or fish oil. Most people are deficient in omega-3 fatty acids, so it is important to take eve-

ning primrose with omega-3 fatty acid-rich foods or supplements.

As with other fats, evening primrose is best taken with meals. It is wise to make sure you are taking some extra vitamin E each day (400 IU), because it helps maximize the benefits of the fatty acids. In fact, many of the oil blends contain vitamin E, which helps prevent the oils from becoming rancid.

I also recommend taking a multivitamin if you're taking evening primrose oil. You need a variety of different vitamins and minerals for essential fatty acid metabolism. Vitamin C, vitamin B6, magnesium, zinc, and biotin are among the important nutrients needed for optimum metabolism.

WHAT ARE THE SIDE EFFECTS?

A few people experience digestive upset and headaches when they take evening primrose oil, especially if they don't take it with meals. These side effects usually go away when the dosage is reduced. (Before reducing the dosage, however, try taking evening primrose oil with meals.)

My biggest concern with EPO is that it needs to be balanced with dosages of omega-3 fatty acids. Long-term solo use of EPO, without simultaneous doses of omega-3s, may set the stage for disease or worsen existing conditions. I have patients come into my office saying that they have been taking evening primrose oil because they heard or read that it is good for their nails, hair, menopause symptoms, and many other things. In some cases it has worsened their problem because they were not simultaneously taking omega-3s and creating an essential fatty acid imbalance.

Natural physicians are particularly concerned that people may worsen existing diseases like heart disease, arthritis, and cancer with unbalanced EPO supplementation. Using evening primrose oil in the short term (a few months) is unlikely to cause any kind of harm—but, still, I always recommend taking EPO in a blend with omega-3 fatty acids such as fish oil, flax oil, or hemp oil.

EVENING PRIMROSE OIL

RECOMMENDATIONS FROM THE NATURAL PHYSICIAN FOR . . .

ARTHRITIS

For most people who have rheumatoid arthritis, I've seen best results from oil blends that contain omega-3 fatty acids and some GLA. Flaxseed or fish oil supplementation seems to do the most good.

ATTENTION DEFICIT DISORDER (ADD) AND ATTENTION DEFICIT/ HYPERACTIVITY DISORDER (ADHD)

I usually recommend the fatty acid DHA for children who have attention-deficit problems. However, some children need extra amounts of GLA to help this condition—and for them, I'll specify an oil blend containing DHA and GLA. Fortunately, we now have blood tests that can measure the levels and ratios of the essential fatty acids, and based on these, we can develop specific fatty-acid formulas that are best for each individual. Studies have shown the combination of fish oil and evening primrose oil can improve the symptoms of ADHD.

DIABETES

Neuropathy is a common complication that affects 30% of people with diabetes. Often the first signs of this condition are "pins and needles" feelings in the feet and hands. In several studies it has been shown that nutritional therapies are beneficial, especially evening primrose oil. People with diabetes often have problems converting linoleic acid into GLA, and a defi-ciency of GLA leads to circulation problems, so insufficient oxygen reaches the nerves. Evening primrose can be a big help because it's a direct source of GLA.

Researchers in one study looked at the effects of GLA on 84 people who had type 2 (adult-onset) diabetes. All participants had neuropathy symptoms such as tingling, burning, weakness, and impaired reflexes. They were given either 12 capsules of evening primrose oil containing 480 mg of GLA or a placebo capsule with no active ingredients. During the following year, the patients in the study met with their doctors every three months for evaluations. The researchers used 16 different ways to measure neurological damage or improvement. Among the people who took evening primrose oil, there were greater positive changes in all 16 measurements.

Studies like this show the value of evening primrose oil and GLA for people with diabetic neuropathy. My feeling is that even better results would be attained with an oil blend of omega-3 and omega-6 fatty acids. Better yet, you may be able to prevent a condition like diabetic neuropathy by taking these oils well before symptoms of neuropathy ever show up. I recommend combining the essential fatty acids with supplements like ginkgo, bilberry, alpha lipoic acid, vitamins E and

(continued)

B12, and folic acid. This is a very powerful, comprehensive, nutritional approach for diabetic neuropathy.

ECZEMA

Children with eczema tend to have an inherited problem of converting linoleic acid into GLA. Studies have shown that their mothers also have a history of eczema and have low levels of GLA in their breast milk. They also have higher levels of linoleic acid, signifying a conversion problem.

Studies show that internal use of evening primrose oil provides relief from itching but can take up to four months of continuous use to be fully effective. Again, I would recommend it be taken in an oil blend with fish or flax oil.

Adults with eczema can also benefit from evening primrose oil. A study of 52 adults with eczema found that evening primrose oil was very effective in reducing skin redness and damage.

OSTEOPOROSIS

The combination of fish oil, evening primrose oil, and calcium has been shown to improve bone density in seniors.

PMS AND CYCLICAL BREAST TENDERNESS

Evening primrose oil can be helpful as part of a comprehensive nutritional approach for treating PMS. It helps reduce symptoms of irritability and depression, and it can also help prevent fluid retention. Some women find that it takes care of monthly breast tenderness and pain— but it may take four months or more of supplementation before evening primrose oil begins to be really effective.

British doctors use evening primrose oil as a first choice treatment for cyclical breast pain and fibrocystic breast syndrome. For these conditions, I recommend a combination of evening primrose oil, omega-3 fatty acids, vitamin E, and the herb vitex.

Exercise

"I'm a mess," said Cheryl, a 31-year-old mother of three. "I've gained a lot of weight, I'm tired all the time, and I'm depressed."

"You used to be fit and energetic," I said. "What's happened?"

"Since I had the baby, I've just been falling apart," Cheryl replied.

As I was taking a comprehensive history, I began to suspect that a large part of Cheryl's health problems stemmed from a single source.

"You're doing lots of good things," I told her. "Your diet is good; you have a positive attitude toward your family, and you're actively involved in a women's group to help reduce your stress. However, you're not taking time out to exercise."

There were a lot of other things I could have done to help her, such as homeopathic and herbal treatment. But I knew that until we got her moving with some simple exercise, we were not going to get the results that Cheryl needed and deserved.

"Cheryl, what type of exercise did you enjoy doing in the past?" I asked.

"I used to like walking and swimming," she answered.

"Are you willing to start back on one of those two exercise programs?" I asked.

"I'll do the walking," she replied, "but I don't want to go swimming at this point.

I'm embarrassed by the 30 extra pounds I put on over the last five years."

So walking became the mantra. She started doing 10 minutes every other day for the first two weeks. Then she increased the time to 15 minutes, five times a week.

Three months later, Cheryl was doing 30 minutes of brisk walking five times a week. She had lost 10 pounds, was feeling more energetic, and her depression had greatly improved. After just three months, she knew she still had a way to go—but now she had the confidence and motivation to continue. I was certain she could take her health to a higher level.

As an added bonus, she had seen her relationship with her family improve, too. She was less irritable with her kids and husband—partly because she felt better about herself, psychologically, and also because her vitality and energy were on the rise.

THE BENEFITS OF MOVING AND SHAKING

I wrote this section after coming back from a three-mile run. I felt great—and knew why. Every time anyone does exercise like this, there's a surge in endorphins and enkephalins—the body chemicals that make you feel good. I was highly motivated to discuss this major component of health and vitality.

Exercise is essentially some form of movement. This ranges from walking to jogging, from biking to playing tennis, to dancing and tai chi, and all the other forms of movement you can think of.

Many people think of a gym when they hear the word "exercise." For some people this brings up images of large muscular men or women grunting and groaning as they lift weights. They equate "exercise" with painful exertion.

My goal here is to get you motivated to exercise and then to select exercises that excite you. I also want you to realize the benefits of exercise and what it can do for you physically and mentally. In addition, I want to give you a sense of what *kind* of exercise you may want to be doing.

GETTING STARTED

The first step to a successful exercise program is to get motivated. Think of the health improvements you can get by exercising. Also, think how the quality of your life will improve when you lose weight, gain muscle, and have an abundance of energy.

With more exercise, many areas of your life can improve, including relationships and work. Exercise is also an effective way to increase sex drive and libido naturally in men and women.

Next, think about what will happen if you don't exercise. See yourself as out of shape, having less energy, and your body "falling apart." It's not a pleasant sight. Make up your mind right now that you will begin to figure out and implement an exercise program immediately. Feel good about it and get excited.

I think it's a mistake to select an exercise that you don't really like. For example, a friend invites you to go jogging, so you go, but you really have no interest in jogging. You would rather go swimming. If you pick an exercise that you don't have an interest in, you are not likely to stick with it. For an exercise program to be worthwhile, you have to stick with it over the long term. Studies show that if you abruptly stop exercising, within a couple of weeks you lose most of the benefits that you gained.

Besides motivation, compliance is everything when it comes to getting the benefits of exercise and sticking to an exercise program long term. By choosing one or two forms of exercise that you really enjoy, you increase your chances of sticking with it. Exercise should be something to which you look forward. It's something from which you can gain energy.

CHOOSING THE MIX

When choosing your exercise program, focus on aerobic work first. By this I mean walking, jogging, biking, swimming, tennis, dancing—any activity that keeps you constantly moving.

By contrast, there is also anaerobic exercise—such as weightlifting—but it's secondary. For example, weightlifting can improve muscular strength, muscle mass, and bone density. It is also good for the heart and cardiovascular system. However, I recommend beginning with an aerobic exercise program, and then adding an anaerobic exercise like weightlifting.

A combination of cardiovascular training like walking or swimming (or many others) plus some form of resistance training like weights is best. This works all the systems of the body.

Don't feel you have to engage in vigorous physical activity to get the benefits of exercise. A study of more than 72,000 female nurses found that women who walk briskly five or more hours a week cut their risk of heart attack by 50%.

FREQUENCY AND LENGTH OF EXERCISE

The frequency and length of exercise depends on your current level of health. Your doctor and a fitness trainer can best determine this. In general, moderately healthy people should start with 10 to 15 minutes of aerobic exercise three times a week and work up from there.

Over time, the length of the exercise period can be increased to 30 to 45 minutes, and the frequency should be four to six times a week. If you experience muscle soreness, and it does not seem to be going away, then cut down the frequency and length of your exercise. If you're starting a weightlifting program, be sure to work with a personal trainer.

If you want some guidance in starting an exercise program, I recommend *Weight Training for Dummies* by Liz Neporent and Suzanne Schlosberg and *The Aerobics Program for Total Well-Being: Exercise, Diet, and Emotional Balance* by Kenneth H. Cooper.

WHAT ARE THE SIDE EFFECTS?

Initially, muscle soreness will be the most common side effect as your body becomes accustomed to the exercise. This soreness will become less of a problem after the first three weeks. Proper form is required for weightlifting; otherwise, injuries can occur. In addition, proper warm-up and post-exercise stretching are important to prevent soreness and injuries.

EXERCISE

RECOMMENDATIONS FROM THE NATURAL PHYSICIAN FOR . . .

❧ ANXIETY AND DEPRESSION

Exercise reduces the effects of stress on the body and should be an important part of a treatment program for anyone with these conditions. It also stimulates the release of chemicals in the brain that are important for mood.

A study reported in the *Journal of Epidemiology* showed that those who participated in exercise, sports, and physical activity experienced a decrease in depression, anxiety, and malaise.

❧ ARTHRITIS

The right kind of exercise can be helpful for the different forms of arthritis. For example, swimming is a good choice of exercise for someone with rheumatoid arthritis or osteoarthritis as it is gentle on the joints. Exercises performed improperly, such as running on a hard surface or using an improper weightlifting technique, can aggravate arthritis.

❧ DETOXIFICATION

Regular exercise is helpful for anyone in a detoxification program. It promotes increased circulation and lymphatic drainage. It also causes sweating, and thus stimulates detoxification.

❧ DIABETES

Exercise increases insulin activity, reduces total cholesterol and triglycerides, and increases the good HDL cholesterol in those who have diabetes. It stimulates blood flow that is more easily impeded in someone with this condition. However, anyone who has diabetes should be monitored by his or her doctor, and follow an exercise program under medical supervision.

❧ FATIGUE

By expending energy, you can actually increase your energy and vitality level. This is the paradox of exercise, which works well to increase energy levels when done within the parameters of a person's exercise limits. On the other hand, over-exercise can lead to fatigue.

❧ HEART DISEASE

It is a well-known fact that exercise reduces the risk of most cardiovascular diseases. Part of this effect comes from the lowering of cholesterol and triglycerides, and the increase in good HDL cholesterol. It also helps to reduce the effects of stress, another big risk factor for heart disease. Exercise also strengthens the heart muscle. However, anyone who has heart disease should be monitored by his or her doctor, and follow an exercise program under medical supervision.

❧ HOT FLASHES

Regular exercise has been shown to reduce the number of hot flashes that women experience during menopause.

❧ IMMUNITY

Exercise done in moderation strengthens the immune system. For example, breast-cancer risk is reduced in women who exercise. But it's important to note

(continued)

that overtraining, as seen sometimes in marathon runners or triathletes, for example, can lead to suppression of the immune system. Again, balanced exercise is the key.

🦋 OSTEOPOROSIS

It is undisputed that weight-bearing exercise stimulates the growth of bone cells and thus increases bone density. Actually, swimming and some other forms of less weight-bearing exercise have also proven to be effective. This is why exercise is so important to prevent and help treat osteoporosis.

🦋 PMS

Regular exercise is quite helpful for women who consistently suffer from PMS.

🦋 STRESS

Exercise is one of the most effective techniques to alleviate the effects of stress on the body and mind.

Eyebright

"My eyes are irritated, they feel hot and itchy, and see how red they are! These allergies seem to have set right in my eyes," exclaimed Kayla, a college student. My recommendation was to apply eyebright (*Euphrasia officinalis*) herbal drops preserved in saline solution to her eyes. Kayla noticed benefit after her second application.

Eyebright is a traditional herbal treatment for irritation of the eyes. Naturopathic doctors and herbalists commonly recommend it topically and sometimes internally for eye inflammation such as allergies, conjunctivitis, and blepharitis. For close to 15 years I have seen this herb work wonders for acute eye conditions, but the active constituents in eyebright are unknown.

DOSAGE

For eye irritation, I have patients dilute 3 to 5 drops of the tincture form in ½ ounce of saline solution (preferably in a disposable cup) to make an eyewash. The patient washes the eye three times daily. Use a different disposable cup for each eye. For internal use, a typical dosage is 3 mL of the tincture form or 500 mg of the capsule or 1 cup of the tea three times daily. The homeopathic form, known as euphrasia, also works well internally for the treatment of irritated red eyes related to eye strain, conjunctivitis, or allergies. Two pellets of a 30C potency taken four times daily is a typical dose.

WHAT ARE THE SIDE EFFECTS?

While I have not seen a problem with the eyewash I have used with patients there is always the possibility of eye irritation. Topical application to the eyes without proper sterility could lead to infection. The internal use of eyebright is considered safe. Internal use should be avoided by pregnant and nursing women since there are no specific safety studies in this regard.

EYEBRIGHT

RECOMMENDATIONS FROM THE NATURAL PHYSICIAN FOR . . .

ALLERGIES

Redness, itching, and irritation of the eyes related to allergies such as hay fever are a good indication for eyebright. The topical and/or internal use of this herbal remedy is helpful for most people with allergies that affect the eyes. Complementary natural therapies include quercetin, nettles, and vitamin C.

COMPUTER EYE IRRITATION AND FATIGUE

Fatigued and irritated eyes from staring at computer screens can be helped by eyebright. Improvements are usually noted quickly with this approach.

CONJUNCTIVITIS

This is a condition of inflammation or infection of the outermost layer of the eye and eyelids. I have found topical treatment and internal use of homeopathic eyebright to work well for most patients, including cases of pinkeye, a viral infection of the conjunctiva.

EYELID INFLAMMATION

For this condition, known as blepharitis, eyebright can be a very helpful treatment.

Fat Reduction

"I have tried many different diets over the years. With some of them, I improved for a period of time, but the weight keeps coming back. I don't know why my body wants to carry around this extra 30 pounds."

Betty's words were an echo of the words I'd heard many times from many other patients. A 32-year-old homemaker with two children, she was very familiar with a number of books and weight-loss programs—and she had tried more than one. Nothing, so far, had worked for her, but she still believed there was a "simple secret" to losing fat and lowering her weight.

"My secret for helping people lose weight? It's simply to treat the cause of the weight problem."

My answer obviously puzzled her. "And what's the cause of my weight problem?" Betty asked.

"That's what we need to find out today," I answered. "I believe there are seven main causes of weight problems. One is genetics. Some people just are genetically programmed to store more fat. However, they can overcome this with a strong program.

"Two is diet. You need to have a diet or nutritional program that is compatible with your metabolism.

"Three is exercise. It is very important to burn that fat and speed up your metabolism. The trick is finding an exercise program that you enjoy, and getting the maximum benefit without having to kill yourself with endless hours of workouts.

"Four is hormone balance. Most women have hormonal imbalances such as high estrogen and/or low progersterone levels. In addition, blood-sugar balance is connected to the hormone insulin, and is very important. Blood-sugar that goes up and down stimulates the release of insulin, which causes fat storage. If your hormones are out of whack, your metabolism is messed up.

"Five is toxicity. If you are full of toxins, your enzyme systems cannot work properly. As a result, your body stores fat and retains water. Detoxification is often important for people with weight problems.

"Six is nutritional deficiencies. They can interfere with your metabolism.

"Seven is the emotional and spiritual component. Suppressed or unresolved issues in these areas can be a major contributor to weight problems. For example, I talk to patients all the time who overeat or eat junk food because they're filling a void for their loneliness, depression, or some other emotion."

"Sounds pretty comprehensive," said Betty.

"Yes, it is. People with weight problems have a problem in one or more of these areas. From your health history and the metabolic testing, I can pinpoint exactly why you have the problem and then together we can correct it. This will not only help you lose weight in a safe manner, but you'll keep it off for good."

Betty's response was optimistic. But even

when she declared "I feel very hopeful about this," I could sense that her optimism was tinged with reservations. After all, this wasn't the first time she'd tried.

But by the next year, she no longer had hesitations about the program. She lost 25 pounds. Her total cholesterol dropped 20 points, and her blood-sugar levels balanced out. She also knew that it wasn't a passing phase of dieting or weight loss. She had no problem keeping the weight off—and her optimism was sustained by a new sense of vitality and self-esteem.

THE SEVEN CAUSES OF WEIGHT PROBLEMS

Think of being overweight as a symptom of an underlying imbalance. When you identify why you have the weight problem, you can shed those extra pounds more quickly and with less effort.

I've found that it's quite feasible for you, on your own, to go through the seven causes of weight problems. If you do an honest evaluation of the cause or causes, you can make your own analysis of why you are having difficulty losing weight and keeping it off. Whether you're male or female, young or old, your weight problem is certain to relate, in some way, to one or more of these seven causes. But it's up to you to decide which of these are more pertinent than the others.

1. Genetics

You may come from a family that tends to have weight problems. Quite often, when a number of people in the same family are overweight, it's easy to conclude that "it's in the genes."

But is it?

Except in rare cases, the notion that you are genetically "doomed" for fat accumula-

tion just isn't true. What we really are talking about is genetic tendencies or genetic predisposition. Everyone comes into the world with some distinct, genetic predispositions, and it's true that people can have a genetic makeup that makes them more prone to having weight problems. If you already have a predisposition toward being overweight, and you're in a family where people consume a lot of high-calorie foods—well, between genetics and lifestyle, you are, indeed, in a situation that makes weight gain a near certainty. However, you can overcome or reduce your fat-storage tendency by focusing more on the other six causes. It just takes a little more work.

2. Diet

The biggest problem with general weight-loss diets is that they put everyone on the same regimen. Any diet that does this is destined to fail for a certain percentage of people.

Everyone is biochemically unique and responds differently to different foods. Food preferences are as unique as taste in clothes. But you may "wear" one diet a lot better than you do another one. Some people do better on a vegetarian diet, while others do worse. Others do fine on a diet that focuses more on protein foods. Also, I have seen some people do well on a diet that's custom-designed for a specific blood type.

Deciding which diet is for you may be a process of trial and error unless you see a physician. However, I have found some successful diet guidelines that will help you turn on your body's fat burners.

Watch Your Sugar Intake

The average American consumes 125 pounds of sugar a year. It is no wonder this country has a weight problem. Consumption of refined carbohydrates, which are essentially simple sugars, leads to a condition known as insulin resistance.

Your body responds to simple sugars by releasing insulin, which transports blood-sugar (glucose) into the cells. The rapid release of sugar into the bloodstream results in insulin "spikes"—so called because if you charted your blood glucose during the day, you'd see times when insulin spiked upward on the chart. This response helps get glucose into the cells, but when you have those sudden spikes of insulin, it has the effect of causing fat storage.

But there's another response, as well, that occurs over time. If you consume a diet of refined sugars for very long, the cells' response to insulin becomes sluggish, leading to the condition known as insulin resistance. When glucose isn't transported into the cells so efficiently—because of this insulin resistance—the body stores it as fat.

Refined carbohydrates that you should try to avoid or minimize include pastas, white rice, non-whole-wheat grain products such as white bread, and most bakery items. You'll also want to avoid sugars such as white and brown sugar, corn syrup, dextrose, fruit juices, and maple syrup. Of course, candies and chocolate bars fall into the "unwanted" category.

These are probably foods that you eat at nearly every meal, so you may be wondering what's left. As a rule of thumb, I'd advise that you stick to what nature has provided by eating whole foods such as fresh vegetables. Based on the same principle, whole-grain pastas and breads are better to eat because the grain is unrefined, and brown rice is better than white rice. These foods have fiber—among other good nutrients—and the fiber helps slow the release of sugar into the bloodstream.

But there's another fact to remember about refined carbohydrates. They can actually be consumed in moderation if you also eat high-fiber foods like vegetables, whole grains, and legumes. The reason for this is that each food has what is called a glycemic index.

People always ask about fruit juice, which is concentrated sugar. Fruit juice can be consumed in limited amounts as long as you don't drink it on an empty stomach and you have it with foods that will slow the sugar absorption. For example, drinking fruit juice along with fish and salad would have much less effect on fat storage than drinking fruit juice by itself.

The best way to avoid refined sugars is to prepare meals yourself or eat with a discriminating eye when you eat out.

One ray of hope: Natural sweeteners such as lo han, stevia, and xylitol (all described in this book) can safely be used. It's actually sweeter than sugar and does not adversely affect blood-sugar levels, even in people with diabetes. It can be purchased as a liquid or powder at health-food stores and some grocery stores.

Watch Which Fats You Eat

The wrong types of fats worsen insulin resistance and contribute to fat deposits. Avoid saturated fats—those found in red meat and dairy products. They not only worsen your weight problem, but also increase your risk of heart disease and certain cancers.

Avoid fake fats, too. These synthetic fats include trans fatty acids as found in fried foods, margarine, and products containing partially hydrogenated oils (such as cookies and crackers). Instead, focus on healthy omega-3 fats that are highly concentrated in cold-water fish such as salmon, mackerel, and herring. Omega-3s are also found in flaxseeds, flaxseed oil, and walnuts.

Stay away from oils that are rich in omega-6, such as sunflower, corn, soy, and most other cooking oils. Use heart-healthy and fat-friendly extra-virgin olive oil instead.

Balance Your Carbohydrates, Proteins, and Fats

The ratio of carbohydrates, proteins, and fats is important in a successful program of fat reduction. Many weight-loss books advocate certain proportions among these three components of the diet. In general I find that a lot of people lose weight more efficiently on a diet that emphasizes a little more protein and less carbohydrates and fats. A major reason this works is because people consume less refined carbohydrates when they focus on getting more protein. Also, protein does not cause blood-sugar spikes and thus does not generally cause fat deposition.

The trick is to eat high-quality proteins such as fresh fish, nuts, seeds, and relatively high-protein plant foods such as soy and corn. Other good animal sources include organic eggs and poultry.

I find that a good general diet for fat reduction has approximately 40% to 50% carbohydrates, 30% fat (mainly "good fats" such as omega-3s), and 20% to 30% protein. Don't stress yourself by trying to calculate the percentages of calories that fall into each category for each meal. Instead, simply make sure you include a good protein, a complex carbohydrate, and a good fiber source in each meal.

Find what proportions of carbohydrates, proteins, and fats are optimum for you and adjust the percentages accordingly. In general, you will attain a percentage close to what I recommend, and will turn on the fat burners while shutting down the fat storers.

Counting Calories Is a Factor

Calories are a factor in fat reduction. The higher the number of calories from food, the more energy you must expend burning them off. However, the real issue is focusing on quality foods in moderate portions.

If you focus on quality foods and the right ratio of the different types of foods, the calorie count will remain at a level where you can lose weight. However, you should have a good grasp of where your calorie count is on a regular basis.

Eat Smaller Meals

Eating smaller, more regular meals throughout the day helps to quell the appetite and level the blood-sugar. This is a long-term strategy for fat reduction.

Do Not Skip Meals

I would say 30% of all my weight-loss patients tell me on our initial visit they skip breakfast. Never skip a meal. This is a signal to the body to conserve energy and store fat.

If time is an issue, prepare breakfast the night before or make yourself a protein shake by combining 1 scoop of soy or whey protein powder with soy or rice milk and 1 to 2 tablespoons of ground-up flaxseeds. Add some blueberries or another fruit that you like.

This takes a whopping two minutes and supplies you with protein, carbohydrates, good essential fatty acids, and fiber. It will help to level out your blood-sugar and prevent fat storage. It will also increase your energy and mental sharpness as opposed to being tired and mentally dull from skipping breakfast.

Harness the Power of Plant Foods

Don't forget the power of plant foods when you're on a fat-reduction diet. Vegetables and some fruits are excellent sources of fiber, which helps to bind fat from foods and expel it in the stool.

Fiber also helps to slow the release of sugar from foods into the bloodstream. This is especially true of soluble fiber—found in oat bran, dried beans, peas, rice bran, barley, and apple skin.

Plant foods are also excellent sources of phytonutrients that aid the body in many ways, including the process of "burning fat"—that is, fat metabolism.

You can get the full spectrum of amino acids from the combination of various plant foods. They are also very important for detoxification. That's significant because proper detoxification removes toxins that cause fat storage and water retention.

Watch Your Water Intake

Drinking an adequate amount of water is critical for weight loss. Dehydration, even at a marginal level, actually causes the body to store water, and water retention is a large factor in weight gain. In addition, water is essential for detoxification.

You should drink at least six to eight 8-ounce glasses of water daily (48 to 64 ounces). Also, avoid those substances that cause dehydration such as caffeine (coffee), salt, and alcohol.

Identify Your Food Sensitivities

One of the ways I expedite the weight-loss process for my patients is to identify their food sensitivities. Different people are sensitive to different foods. Food sensitivities cause water retention and make metabolism and detoxification more sluggish.

Many of my patients who have had food-sensitivity testing report that they lost extra weight by avoiding the foods to which they are sensitive. (See Food-Sensitivity Therapy, page 193.)

Consistency Is the Key

Harvard School of Public Health and Louisiana State University researchers assigned 811 overweight men and women, ages 30 to 70, to one of four low-calorie diets comprised of different percentages of protein, fat, and carbohydrate combinations. The dieters participated in group and individual counseling sessions. After six months, participants lost an average of 13.2 pounds, about 7% of their starting weight. After two years, each diet group lost, and regained, about the same amount of weight (an average loss of 8.8 pounds), regardless of the carbohydrate, protein, or fat content of their diet. All of the diets reduced cholesterol and blood-pressure levels. I found this study very interesting and want to point out two important facts. The first is that, regardless of the type of calorie-reduced diet a person follows, the key in the long run is consistency. The ability to follow a diet for long periods of time is critical. Second, regular personal or group counseling sessions are very important to staying consistent with a diet. I would also note that in clinical practice I find that different diets (varying protein, carbohydrate, and fat intake) can work more effectively for some individuals. Through metabolic testing and individualized diet plans I can normally achieve an average weight loss greater than what was found in this study.

Yet consistency by the patient is required to maintain the weight loss.

❧ 3. Exercise

Without question, exercise is a cornerstone of any fat-reduction and weight-loss program, but it may be a challenge to find an exercise program you like so that you will stick with it long term. Fat reduction will also be fastest if you do aerobic exercise such as walking, jogging, swimming, biking, or dancing, because you burn fat more efficiently.

Weightlifting isn't such an efficient fat burner, but it does increase your body's metabolism—and a combination of the aerobic activities along with some weightlifting (called "anaerobic") is ideal.

Sports such as racquetball or tennis are excellent, too.

How often should you exercise and for how long? That depends on your current level of health. Your doctor and a fitness trainer can best determine the optimum periods.

In general, moderately healthy people should start with 10 to 15 minutes of aerobic exercise three times weekly and work up from there. Ideally, the time of exercise should be 30 to 45 minutes (or longer) and the frequency should be four to six times a week. If you're just starting a weightlifting program, work with a personal trainer who can help you begin at a reasonable level without risk of injury. You can always build up to heavier weights or more repetitions over time.

❧ 4. Hormone Balance

Hormones are powerful chemicals that control your body's metabolism. One of the most important in the fat-reduction equation is the thyroid gland. It is well known that if thyroid hormone is low, cell metabolism slows down and weight gain is a pretty sure thing.

Many physicians, including me, believe that hypothyroid (low thyroid function) is epidemic in our society, especially among women over the age of 25. Unfortunately, blood tests often do not pick up borderline cases of low thyroid.

The best diagnostic procedure is to have a thyroid panel done by your doctor (including the tests called "free T3" and "TSH"). Saliva thyroid hormone tests have recently become available. Also, take your temperature each morning at the same time for five days straight. Temperature is an indication of thyroid function, and if the temperature reading is consistently below 98.2 degrees Fahrenheit, then you have a sluggish thyroid.

If you do have low thyroid, I recommend you find a holistic doctor for natural thyroid support. I don't favor conventional thyroid hormone replacement (with the medication Synthroid) because it weakens the thyroid. Over time, patients on Synthroid need to take increasingly higher dosages to equal results.

Estrogen and progesterone balance is also very important for weight loss. Many women have too much estrogen relative to progesterone, a condition referred to as "estrogen dominance." I find that synthetic estrogen and progesterone lead to water retention and hinder thyroid function.

Testosterone and growth-hormone deficiency can also lead to fat deposition, especially in men. Women given synthetic hormone replacement for menopause almost always start to gain weight and increase water retention. The birth-control pill has similar effects.

(For more about natural hormone-balancing options, see Black Cohosh, Vitex, and Progesterone.)

The last issue of hormone balance is the concept of insulin resistance, which I described earlier. The consumption of refined carbohydrates leads to insulin spikes that promote fat storage. Over time, the cell insulin receptors become less sensitive to insulin so the body stores the glucose as fat.

Another condition known as "Syndrome X" also comes into play. This refers to a cluster of conditions. Insulin resistance is part of the equation, but added to that are two of the following—high cholesterol, high triglycerides, or high blood pressure, or obesity. (The "apple shape" figure is a general sign of Syndrome X—that is, with excess fat around the belly, hips, and thighs.) Researchers feel that anyone who has Syndrome X is only one step away from developing diabetes.

❧ 5. Toxicity

Toxins—such as pesticides, herbicides, and other chemicals—that get into the body from the environment wreak havoc on your body's enzyme systems. Toxins known as heavy metals, such as mercury and lead, are particularly dangerous and can suppress thyroid function. They also impair the detoxification process and lead to water and fat accumulation.

Toxins that accumulate as the result of poor digestion are also a problem. For a thorough detoxification program, I generally advise people to work with a holistic doctor who can help you identify the toxins that may be stored in your body and then work with you to help eliminate them. But if you follow a good diet, exercise, and take nutritional supplements, you are already enhancing the detoxification process.

❧ 6. Nutritional Deficiencies

Nutritional deficiencies are widespread in a society like ours, because we consume monumental quantities of refined and synthetic foods. Many different vitamins and minerals are involved with fat metabolism in one way or another.

Specifically, I find that chromium, vanadium, and alpha lipoic acid are of particular help in regulating blood-sugar levels, and thus preventing fat storage. Dosages of 400 mcg of chromium picolinate or chelate, 100 mcg of elemental vanadium, and 100 to 200 mg of alpha lipoic acid are useful.

Zinc and magnesium are required for proper insulin function. A dosage of 30 mg daily is good for zinc, and a dosage of 500 mg is good for magnesium.

Beyond that, a high-potency multivitamin is helpful as an insurance policy for nutritional support.

Nutrients that help to speed up metabolism include D-ribose, L-carnitine, resveratrol, and coenzyme Q10.

An essential fatty acid source such as ground-up flaxseeds, or flaxseed or fish oil is recommended to help metabolize fats and for proper insulin function.

Nutritional deficiencies cause cravings for sweets and fatty foods, which translate into fat gain.

❧ 7. Emotional and Spiritual Factors

Many people have weight problems because of past emotional traumas. As a result, they use food to help dampen, reduce, or control emotional pain. I often see this problem in people who have been divorced or been through difficult relationships. People who have suffered physical and sexual abuse often have eating disorders, too—and one manifestation of that could be excessive weight gain because of bingeing or alternate bingeing-and-starving.

Is this an issue for you?

One way to answer that question is to consider whether eating is actually something that compels you. Though you might use food this way—to make yourself feel temporarily "good"—the reality of what it does for you is probably quite different. The excessive food consumption makes you gain weight, which actually decreases your energy levels and vitality. Far from feeling better about yourself, you're more likely to feel reduced self-esteem.

If this is an issue for you, it must become the first thing you address. Work with a counselor or spiritual counselor such as a pastor to overcome the emotional and spiritual traumas that are the underlying cause of your weight problem and unhappiness.

Are you looking for a miraculous weight-loss product you can take without changing your eating habits or doing exercise? I have not yet found such a product—at least, one with no side effects—and I seriously doubt that it exists.

However, you can use certain products that may aid in fat reduction as part of the comprehensive program outlined in this section. These products fall into two broad categories that are worth considering: nutritional supplements and natural stimulants. While I do not recommend the stimulants, I discuss them in this section because they are so popular.

NUTRITIONAL SUPPLEMENTS

Many nutritional supplements on the market are described as weight-loss products, even when there are few good studies to back up their use. There are a number of products that may be promising, but, as I've noted below, some have only been tested in animals.

❧ Caralluma fimbriata
This vegetable extract can help with appetite suppression and fat burning. See page 85.

❧ Conjugated Linoleic Acid (CLA)
Promoted as a weight-loss promoter, antioxidant, cancer fighter, and immune system enhancer, conjugated linoleic acid (CLA) is found in red meat. It helps glucose get into muscle cells more effectively, thus preventing glucose from being converted into fat. It also helps fats enter the cell membranes of muscle and connective tissue, where the fat is burned for fuel. Studies show CLA significantly reduces body fat mass and also lowers appetite. *Dosage:* 1,000 mg three times a day with meals.

❧ D-ribose
This naturally occurring sugar improves cellular metabolism. See page 400.

❧ Glucomannan
This type of fiber reduces appetite and glucose levels. See page 231.

❧ Hydroxycitric Acid (HCA)
This extract is derived from the rind of Garcinia cambogia, a fruit grown in Southeast Asia. Laboratory and animal research has shown it helps with weight loss by reducing the conversion of carbohydrates into stored fat. It has been shown to suppress appetite in animals, and seems to have no side effects. Whether it will prove effective in human studies remains to be seen. *Dosage:* 500 mg three times daily before meals.

❧ L-carnitine
This amino acid–like substance can help in the battle of fat, especially in seniors. See page 292.

❧ Pyruvate
This is an altered form of the sugar molecule. In human and animal studies, pyruvate seems to aid in weight loss when people

combine it with a low-fat diet. That doesn't imply, however, that you can take pyruvate on its own—without other dietary alterations—and expect to reverse weight gain. *Dosage:* 6 to 30 g daily.

🐦 *Resveratrol*

Preliminary research shows resveratrol helps with insulin resistance and cell metabolism. See page 396.

NATURAL STIMULANTS: BE WARY

Many weight-loss stimulants are popular, but I don't recommend them. These "natural stimulants," as their name suggests, actually stimulate the nervous system and help prompt the release of adrenaline. That hormone, produced by the adrenal gland, promotes the burning of fat for fuel.

The drawback of these products is that they may have serious side effects. People may have a variety of reactions to these stimulants, such as anxiety, insomnia, chronic fatigue, heart abnormalities, and elevated blood pressure. If you already have one of these conditions, the addition of natural stimulants can make the symptoms more severe.

I am also concerned about their effect on the thyroid and adrenal glands. I advise people never to take natural stimulants for long periods of time. When the thyroid and adrenal glands are overstimulated, they don't function as well (call it "wearing out")—and when their function is inhibited, other health problems can arise.

🐦 *Caffeine*

Good old caffeine is a stimulant that increases the metabolic rate and may curb appetite. As many people have discovered, too much caffeine may cause anxiety, insomnia, heart palpitations, elevated blood pres-

sure, and trembling. Caffeine also increases urinary frequency and can lead to hyperactivity. Smaller amounts in multicomponent supplements seem to be fine, except for people sensitive to caffeine.

🐦 *Guarana* (Paullina cupana)

Guarana seeds were originally used as a medicine by indigenous peoples of the Amazon forest to treat diarrhea, reduce hunger, and relieve arthritis. It contains guaranine, which is a stimulant that is very similar in its structure and effects to caffeine. People use it as an alternative to ephedra and caffeine supplements. It is thought to have fewer side effects than other natural stimulants.

Fermented Wheat Germ Extract

Wheat germ has long been esteemed as a health food. The "germ" is the most nutritious part of the wheat seed. Today fermented wheat germ extract (FWGE) has been shown in studies to be most helpful to people battling cancer. More than 20 peer-reviewed publications describing cell, animal, and human studies support the use and benefits of FWGE as an adjunct therapy for the disease, meaning one that is used as part of a broader treatment program. As a matter of fact it is one of the most well-studied natural products for complementary cancer therapy.

FWGE appears to have several mechanisms of action, including starving cancer cells of glucose (their fuel source), and thus promoting cancer cell self-destruction by activity and enhancing the activity of some immune cells. Wheat germ contains benzoquinones, chemicals that seem to have anticancer properties, and fermentation increases their concentration.

This substance has also been show in preliminary studies to have benefit for those with autoimmune conditions, including rheumatoid arthritis.

FWGE is very different from the wheat germ granules and wheat germ oil you can buy at health-food stores. It comes in a powder and is sold in many of these stores, as well as by health professionals and online, as a dietary supplement in the United States. I routinely prescribe it to patients who consult with me at my clinic for the complementary treatment of cancer because studies show it improves cancer survival rates.

DOSAGE

In the morning before breakfast take one packet containing 8.5 to 9 g of FWGE daily mixed with eight ounces cold water or any other beverage that contains less than 10 mg vitamin C per eight-ounce serving. Store the packets at room temperature or (best) in the refrigerator.

WHAT ARE THE SIDE EFFECTS?

Side effects have not been shown to be a problem with FWGE. People occasionally have digestive upset that can be helped by dividing the dose in half twice daily. Do not take vitamin C supplements or beverages containing high amounts of vitamin C within two hours of ingesting FWGE. Those who should not consume FWGE include pregnant or nursing mothers, those who have had an organ or tissue transplant, those suffering from bleeding gastrointestinal ulcers, gluten-sensitive enterophaties (celiac sprue), malabsorption syndrome, fructose intolerance, or those who have hypersensitivity to gluten or wheat germ.

FERMENTED WHEAT GERM EXTRACT
RECOMMENDATIONS FROM THE NATURAL PHYSICIAN FOR . . .

❧ CHEMOTHERAPY-INDUCED INFECTIONS

Researchers studied 22 children and teenagers who were diagnosed with and treated for different types of cancer. The 11 children who received FWGE had significantly fewer infections and fevers while receiving chemotherapy.

❧ COLORECTAL CANCER

A study of 170 patients who had received conventional treatments for colorectal cancer found that those who took 9 g of FWGE daily in addition to their treatment for six months had less risk of developing new cancers. The cancer spread for only 8% of the patients receiving FWGE, compared with 23% of those getting only conventional treatment.

❧ ORAL CANCERS

Researchers tracked 22 patients with oral cancer who took FWGE and compared them with 21 patients not receiving the supplement. Those who took FWGE reduced the risk for cancer progression by 85%.

❧ MELANOMA

For one year, FWGE was given to 22 patients with advanced (stage 3) melanomas, and their progress was compared

(continued)

with 24 similar patients not receiving FWGE. Patients taking FWGE were half as likely to die from melanoma during this time.

✎ᵕ OTHER CANCERS

Numerous animal and cell studies suggest benefits from FWGE for leukemia and breast cancer, as well as ovarian, gastric and thyroid cancers. In one study, laboratory rats received both FWGE and vitamin C in the treatment of lung, skin, and colon cancers. The combination prevented the cancer from spreading, but vitamin C alone did not. In another study, FWGE worked better alone than it did with vitamin C to treat kidney cancer.

✎ᵕ RHEUMATOID ARTHRITIS

FWGE has been shown in preliminary studies to benefit people with rheumatoid arthritis (RA). In a yearlong study patients with RA had significant reduction in stiffness after 6- and 12-month follow-ups. Also, dosages of steroid medications could be reduced in half of the participants.

Ferrum Phosphoricum

Ferrum phosphoricum, abbreviated as ferrum phos, is an important homeopathic remedy for treating anemia and fevers. This remedy is a combination of the minerals iron and phosphate.

Iron is an integral component of red blood cells, helping to bind oxygen so that it can be stored in the cells. Iron is in the food we eat, and a certain amount is added when you cook with cast-iron pots and pans.

The homeopathic form of iron—ferrum phos—is what I recommend to improve the cellular uptake of iron. It's just what you'll need, for instance, if you have iron-deficiency anemia.

A number of health and lifestyle factors can contribute to this type of anemia. Some women suffer from iron-deficiency anemia because of heavy blood loss during their menstrual cycle. Bleeding from injuries is another possible cause. You also have to be alert to the possibility of anemia if you're on a strict vegetarian diet and have digestive and absorption problems. Plant foods are low in iron, and the iron in plant foods cannot be absorbed as well as the iron that comes from meat.

Ferrum phos does not actually supply the body with doses of iron; rather, it works to increase the absorption of iron from the foods we eat. More important, it helps to increase the uptake of iron by our red blood cells. Even if you take high doses of iron supplements to offset low-iron blood, the supplements don't help if the iron cannot be incorporated into your red blood cells and, from there, get carried to other iron-starved tissues.

When Rebecca came to me for treatment of iron-deficiency anemia, she already recognized that an irregular and very heavy menstrual cycle might be contributing to her constant feeling of tiredness. I noticed at once that she had large black "shiners" under her eyes, which is a symptom of iron deficiency.

For the previous three months, she had been taking large doses of iron supplements (120 mg daily) as her doctor had recommended—but during that time, her anemia had not improved. Subsequently, the doctor had used injections—and these may have been somewhat more effective, but Rebecca reported the injections were also very painful.

There was more. Because of Rebecca's heavy monthly blood flow, her doctor had prescribed birth-control pills, hoping that the pills would help regulate her menstrual cycles. But Rebecca had experienced severe nausea and headaches and had finally refused to use the pill any more. Furthermore, the benefits were slight. After two months of supplements, injections, and birth-control pills, her blood tests showed only slight improvement.

After talking with Rebecca, I had her stop the injections and began her on a treatment that focused on the use of ferrum phos along with a multivitamin that had a relatively small amount of iron in it. I reasoned that Rebecca's cells were, obviously, not assimilating the iron effectively. Instead of trying to force more iron into her body, I wanted to make changes at the cellular level that would help improve the way her cells utilized and incorporated the iron.

There was another reason to recommend ferrum phos as soon as possible. In women like Rebecca who have iron-deficiency anemia associated with heavy menstrual bleeding, a cycle develops, leading to worsening conditions. The anemia actually promotes even heavier menstrual bleeding. So I knew that until we got the anemia under control, it would be difficult—if not impossible— to get the bleeding under control.

Rebecca took the ferrum phos diligently. Within three weeks her bleeding became lighter and within six weeks her menstrual cycle became regular again. Blood tests showed a 50% improvement in her red blood cell levels and ferritin levels (storage levels of iron). The dark eye shiners disap-

peared and her skin color improved. Rebecca's improvement continued over the next three months until her iron and red blood cells were back to normal.

DOSAGE

For the treatment of iron-deficiency anemia I recommend ferrum phos 3x or 6x to be taken three times daily. For a more aggressive treatment of anemia, you can also take the herb yellow dock, which contains small amounts of iron and enhances the digestive absorption of iron.

For the treatment of acute illnesses, I recommend the 30C potency or higher. Take the ferrum phos as needed until you feel the relief of symptoms. (However, lower potencies of 3x and 6x also work well for some acute illnesses.)

WHAT ARE THE SIDE EFFECTS?

I have never seen any side effects with ferrum phos supplementation. It is a homeopathic remedy, so there's no danger of iron toxicity, even with children.

FERRUM PHOSPHORICUM
RECOMMENDATIONS FROM THE NATURAL PHYSICIAN FOR . . .

✒ ANEMIA

I would not hesitate to give ferrum phos supplementation on a long-term basis for severe anemia. I also recommend it during pregnancy to help women maintain normal iron levels.

✒ BLEEDING

Ferrum phos is a good remedy to any kind of bleeding, especially nosebleeds and minor cuts. You can crush the tablets of ferrum phos and apply the powder directly to scrapes and cuts.

✒ EARACHE

Ferrum phos is one of the more common remedies used for childhood ear infections. Homeopathic physicians are most likely to prescribe it if the child's face is flushed and the child has a fever of 102 degrees Fahrenheit or higher.

I also notice whether the child acts sick. Oddly enough, ferrum phos is most effective as an earache remedy for a child who does not even seem to be sick but continues to play around and act as if nothing were wrong.

I also examine the child to find out whether the right ear tends to be more painful than the left. If so, again, it's an indication that ferrum phos may be the most effective earache remedy.

✒ FEVER

Ferrum phos is also an excellent remedy to help control fevers, especially in younger children. It helps to calm down a fever—unlike fever-reducing pharmaceutical medications that tend to suppress the fever rather than reduce it. Because fever helps to stimulate the immune system, it should be reduced rather than being totally suppressed or eliminated.

✒ SORE THROAT AND TONSILLITIS

Both of these conditions can be helped with ferrum phos remedy. It is especially useful when the throat and face appear bright red and the patient has a powerful thirst for cold drinks.

Feverfew

Feverfew (*Tanacetum parthenium*) is known among herbal enthusiasts as the "migraine headache herb," and there are enough clinical studies to confirm that the leaf of this plant does help to prevent migraines. While herbalists have used feverfew to prevent and treat migraine headaches for centuries, it also has a rich history for the treatment of menstrual cramps, as a pain reliever during labor, and as a remedy that can help reduce fever. It has also helped treat arthritis, toothaches, and respiratory tract conditions such as asthma and bronchitis. Today, most people and practitioners use feverfew for migraine headaches and, to a lesser extent, for arthritis.

Feverfew grows up to three feet tall and is native to different parts of Europe. It is also grown commercially in North America.

Scientists aren't sure why feverfew can help prevent migraine headaches, but they do have theories. It's thought that the herb helps reduce the clumping of specialized cells in blood that form blood clots—the cells called platelets. Researchers believe that platelet aggregation leads to the release of inflammatory chemicals, which alters the way blood circulates through the brain. When platelets begin to aggregate in an abnormal way, the process is thought to cause biochemical imbalances with the neurotransmitter serotonin, and these imbalances, in turn, lead to migraine headaches. Feverfew seems to help prevent this chain reaction.

Also, feverfew contains significant amounts of the hormone melatonin. Low levels of melatonin have been held as a potential cause of migraine headaches.

Another theory about feverfew relates to a substance called parthenolide. Though it's just one constituent found in feverfew, some researchers consider parthenolide to be important in preventing migraines. However, more research needs to be done before anyone can be certain of the precise therapeutic effects of parthenolides.

Feverfew also inhibits arthritis and other inflammatory conditions. In all probability, this occurs because feverfew prevents the release of immune cells that cause problems when they reach a body joint and begin to cause inflammation. So the action of feverfew helps prevent joint and tissue destruction.

DOSAGE

I recommend the capsule form to patients. Look for a standardized extract that contains 0.3% to 0.7% parthenolides. Make sure the product also contains a base of the whole herb, since we don't know, for sure, which constituents of feverfew are the active components.

For the treatment of acute migraines, take 300 mg every 30 minutes to a maximum of four doses daily. If you notice improvement, continue on an as-needed basis without exceeding the four-a-day dosages.

While feverfew might help relieve acute migraine in some people, in my own experience I've found that it's a better preventive than treatment of migraines. The preventive dose that I recommend is 300 to 400 mg of the standardized capsule, taken daily. If you still get migraines, don't give up on the feverfew. You may need to take it for up to three months before it really begins to work as a preventive.

The tincture form can also be used. I recommend 30 drops per dose.

Though some people make a tea of feverfew, I've found that the tea doesn't contain the active ingredients that you need for best results.

As far as I know, you can also chew on feverfew leaves (although I have yet to meet someone who has done this).

Be aware that feverfew can take up to three months of use to be effective in preventing migraines.

WHAT ARE THE SIDE EFFECTS?

A very small percentage of feverfew users may experience digestive upset. Since this herb has some blood-thinning properties, you should check with your healthcare professional if you are already on blood-thinning medication or if you're taking migraine medication.

Also, if you're a woman who's pregnant or breast-feeding, be sure you're under the guidance of a knowledgeable practitioner before you start taking feverfew.

If you are one of the few people who decides to chew the leaves, do so with caution as mouth ulcers may occur.

FEVERFEW
RECOMMENDATIONS FROM THE NATURAL PHYSICIAN FOR . . .

ARTHRITIS

Feverfew can help relieve the pain of osteoarthritis and rheumatoid arthritis. Do not expect immediate pain relief, however, as it takes time for the anti-inflammatory action to kick in. I prefer to use feverfew in formulations that contain other natural anti-inflammatory supplements such as MSM, boswellia, turmeric, and bromelain. (If you're suffering from osteoarthritis, then glucosamine sulfate is a must, whether or not you also take feverfew.)

MIGRAINE HEADACHES

Some prescription medications can effectively relieve migraine headaches, but there's always the potential of drug toxicity and side effects, which don't occur with feverfew. I typically recommend feverfew along with other natural therapies such as treating food sensitivities, spinal manipulation, hormone balancing, stress reduction, and detoxification. These other therapies address the underlying causes of many migraines— and if one or more is successful, you might be able to stop taking feverfew. Otherwise, as one study has shown, the migraines may recur as soon as the herbal treatments are discontinued.

The effectiveness of feverfew is supported by some good clinical data. A 1998 study looked at 59 people who suffered migraine headaches. For the first four months of the study, subjects took a daily, regulated dose of feverfew in capsule form. (As usual in such studies, there was a control group for comparison.) Researchers found that daily treatment with feverfew led to a 24% reduction in the number and severity of migraine headaches. Also, symptoms of nausea and vomiting were improved. No side effects were reported from feverfew. It was interesting to note that 47% of the people in the study had already tried conventional migraine drugs without any improvement in the severity or frequency of migraines.

PAIN

Feverfew can be used in the treatment of many other types of pain. Some practitioners and herbalists prescribe it for toothaches, muscle injury, and other similar types of trauma.

Fiber

Want to look healthy on the *outside*?

Then you have to look healthy on the *inside*.

That's one of the fundamental premises of natural healing traditions. Of all the substances that help make your insides look healthy, the best is surely fiber. Fiber not only keeps your digestive tract healthy, it also helps create good health and vitality through detoxification.

Hippocrates, the "father of medicine," acknowledged the health benefits of fiber in the fifth century BC. Some 2,400 years later, an American entrepreneur by the name of Sylvester W. Graham picked up the cause, expounded heartily on the benefits of roughage in the diet, and created the company that produced the eponymous Graham cracker.

However, it was not until the 1960s that researchers seriously studied the role of fiber in the diet. Interest was piqued by studies showing that the native Africans who subsisted on a very high-fiber diet had a very low incidence of colon cancer, diverticulosis, gallstones, hemorrhoids, appendicitis, diabetes, and some forms of heart disease. Researchers concluded that there was a clear connection between consumption of high fiber and overall digestive good health. A 40-year study of 1,373 men conducted in the Netherlands has found that for every additional 10 g of dietary fiber consumed daily the risk for death from all causes dropped by 9% and coronary heart disease mortality was reduced by 17%.

BULKING UP FOR GOOD HEALTH

Also referred to as "roughage," fiber is the indigestible portion of plants that forms the bulk of stool. The human body does not secrete enzymes that break down fiber, and the roughage doesn't provide any calories, vitamins, or minerals. But having that undigestible matter in the digestive system is actually a benefit. As the fiber moves through, it acts like a broom, sweeping out the garbage and toxins that accumulate in our digestive tract. Without this cleansing effect we could not survive, as infection in our digestive tract would be rampant.

Fiber also helps control blood-sugar levels by slowing the rate at which the intestines release blood-sugar into the bloodstream. Even though it doesn't provide any nutrients directly to the body, certain types of fiber feed the friendly bacteria that live in your intestinal tract,

helping to speed digestion and preventing unfriendly microbes from causing infection.

For vegetarians, getting enough fiber is usually no problem. If you're eating a lot of vegetables, fruits, legumes, nuts, seeds, and whole grains, you'll be getting a full spectrum of various types of fiber. Studies have shown that many vegetarians have a lower risk of many chronic conditions such as heart disease and many types of cancers, compared with the general population.

For the average American who is *not* a vegetarian, fiber intake is usually far below what it should be. Most of us eat a dismal 11 to 20 g of fiber daily—and I'm sure there are many teenagers or college students living on fast food, soda, and coffee who get as little as 5 g of fiber daily. Yet, for optimal health and for the prevention of many diseases, we should all be getting 40 to 50 g daily.

BENEFITS GALORE

Fiber has many important, proven health benefits. Here are the top ten:

1. Decreases appetite and gives a feeling of satiety without increasing body fat or weight. This leads to weight loss.
2. Reduces fat absorption.
3. Reduces cholesterol.
4. Improves blood-sugar regulation.
5. Promotes bowel regularity.
6. Reduces the risk of certain types of cancer.
7. Binds and eliminates toxins.
8. Promotes healthy intestinal bacteria.
9. Promotes hormone balance.
10. Increases your intake of phytonutrients (many of which are found in the fiber portion of plants).

A Double Requirement

There are two main types of fiber that are distinguished by the way they react to water. "Insoluble fiber" is the kind that cannot dissolve in water—and this is the kind that "bulks up" in the intestine and acts like a broom, sweeping undigested or undigestible matter out of your colon. Insoluble fiber includes cellulose, the indigestible portion of plants. This type of fiber is found in the leaves of plants, in the peels and skins of fruits and vegetables, and in the coverings of whole grains.

Both wheat bran and psyllium seed are two excellent sources of insoluble fiber. While it does not dissolve in water, it does bind to water, which helps to bulk up the stool and prevent diarrhea. Insoluble fiber protects against diseases such as diverticulitis, irritable bowel syndrome, and possibly colon cancer.

The second category is "soluble fiber," the kind that dissolves in water. As soluble fiber passes through the digestive tract, it binds together bile acids and cholesterol, so they pass through without being reabsorbed. Oat bran, perhaps the best-known form of soluble fiber, has been shown to reduce cholesterol. But it's not the only beneficial source of soluble fiber. You can get similar benefits from dried beans, peas, rice bran, and barley.

One particular form of soluble fiber known as pectin is found in the outer skin and rind of fruits and vegetables. The skin of an apple contains 15% pectin, while an onion skin contains 12%. Pectin, like other forms of soluble fiber, lowers cholesterol levels by preventing the reabsorption of cholesterol in the gut.

Mucilages—found in the inner layer of nuts, seeds, grains, and legumes—is yet another kind of soluble fiber. Guar gum, the most common mucilage, is used as a thickening agent and stabilizer in commercial products such as salad dressing, ice cream, and skin creams. As with pectin, mucilage forms a gel in the digestive tract and slows the rate of blood-sugar digestion and absorption. This helps in the regulation of blood-sugar levels.

Flaxseeds contain a high amount of both soluble and insoluble fibers. One-quarter cup of flaxseeds contains 20 g of fiber. The water-soluble mucilage in flaxseeds is very soothing and healing to the digestive tract, helps to feed the good bacteria, and also has a natural laxative effect. Also a rich source of omega-3 fatty acids, flaxseeds contain hormone-balancing and cancer-protecting lignans.

FIBER SUPPLEMENTS

Many people benefit from taking fiber supplements. They may be helpful to you if you suffer from constipation, hemorrhoids, or digestive conditions such as irritable bowel syndrome (IBS), Crohn's disease, or ulcerative colitis.

When patients have these conditions, I generally recommend that they first try to increase their dietary intake of fiber before taking supplements. But when you just can't get enough fiber from your daily diet, supplements are extremely helpful.

Psyllium husks are often used because they absorb a lot of water and bulk up the stool, which improves elimination. Another good supplement is wheat bran, which is also a good insoluble source of fiber (but not helpful if you have a wheat sensitivity or allergy).

When you're selecting a supplement, make sure the product doesn't include sugar, artificial sweeteners, or artificial coloring. Any of these added ingredients may cause digestive upset. Whatever supplement you take, be sure to drink lots of water along with it. Otherwise, the supplement can "bulk up" inside your intestinal tract rather than passing readily through it, causing constipation.

EDIBLE GOOD HEALTH

There are many sources of dietary fiber, but, as you can see from Table 5, there is a wide variability in the content of fiber in servings of different foods. To get a good mix of soluble and insoluble fiber in your daily diet, here are some foods to consider:

DOSAGE

While adults should get 40 to 50 g of fiber daily, children need less. For a quick calculation of a child-appropriate dosage, just add five to the age of the child to get the number of grams of fiber the child should be taking. For example, a 10-year-old would require 15 g of fiber daily.

If you haven't been getting sufficient fiber in your diet, and want to work up to the optimum level, you should gradually increase your daily fiber intake. If you suddenly start taking more fiber, you may experience excessive bloating and flatulence—but this is less likely to happen if you raise your intake more slowly.

Whether you're taking supplements or just eating more fiber, make sure to drink plenty of water throughout the day. Try to get six to eight 8-ounce glasses so that the fiber doesn't "plug you up."

It's also helpful to get fiber from a variety of different sources. As you can see in Table 5, there are many common foods you can eat that are good sources of the various fibers. One simple technique is to make sure you are getting one or more fiber-rich foods with each meal. For example, if you can eat whole oat cereal for breakfast, you'll get both soluble and insoluble fiber—about twice as much as you'd get from cornflakes or Special K.

For lunch or dinner, have some broccoli or a green leafy salad. Whole-grain bread is good with any meal, as it provides plenty of insoluble fiber.

If you still find that your fiber intake is too low, then I highly recommend grinding up flaxseeds each day. You can get as much as 20 g of fiber from one-quarter cup of ground flaxseeds.

Fiber supplements should be used according to the containers' labels. They are generally available in powder or capsule form. I usually recommend psyllium, with a starting dose of 1 teaspoon or 2 capsules daily along with an 8-ounce glass of water. Over a period of six weeks, you can build up the doses until you're taking the amount of fiber that is necessary for the bowels to move. The maximum is typically 4 teaspoons or 8 capsules of supplemental fiber.

WHAT ARE THE SIDE EFFECTS?

You can avoid the gas and bloating if you steam or cook vegetables, then gradually switch to more raw vegetables (which have more nutrients and a higher concentration of enzymes) as your body adjusts to the increase in fiber.

Fiber supplements can inhibit the absorption of certain drugs and can "bind up" various minerals, also preventing absorption. This can be avoided, however, if you avoid taking fiber supplements at the same time as medications or vitamin/mineral supplements.

TABLE 5
Soluble and Insoluble Fiber

	SERVING SIZE	INSOLUBLE FIBER (G)	SOLUBLE FIBER (G)	TOTAL FIBER (G)
Fruits				
Apple	1	2.6	0.4	3.0
Banana	1	1.3	0.5	1.8
Blueberries	½ cup	1.9	0.2	2.1
Blackberries	½ cup	4.5	0.4	4.9
Grapes	10	0.5	trace	0.5
Grapefruit	½	0.3	0.4	0.1
Honeydew melon	½ cup	0.4	0.5	0.1
Peach	1	1.1	0.6	1.7
Raisins	¼ cup	1.4	0.2	1.6
Vegetables				
Artichoke (fresh, cooked)	1 medium	6.4	2.9	3.5
Beans (black, dry, cooked)	½ cup	2.7	2.8	0.1
Broccoli	½ cup	1.0	2.6	1.6
Brussels sprouts (frozen, cooked)	½ cup	2.8	3.2	0.4
Lentils (dry, cooked)	½ cup	2.8	2.9	0.1
Peas (green, canned, or frozen)	½ cup	2.8	3.1	0.3
Lettuce	½ cup	0.3	0.5	0.2
Spinach (canned, cooked, or raw)	½ cup cooked or canned, 2 cups raw	2.0	2.3	0.3
Vegetable soup (canned)	1 cup	1.6	2.2	0.6
Grains				
Bread (white or Italian)	1 slice	0.6	0.8	0.2
Bread, rye	1 slice	0.5	0.7	0.2
Bread, whole wheat	1 slice	2.2	2.5	0.3
Cereal, Total cornflakes	1 cup	0.8	0.9	trace
Cereal, Rice Krispies	1 cup	0.4	0.5	0.1

	SERVING SIZE	INSOLUBLE FIBER (G)	SOLUBLE FIBER (G)	TOTAL FIBER (G)
Cereal, Special K	1 cup	0.7	0.8	0.1
Cookies, oatmeal	1 large	0.6	0.9	0.3
Cookies, plain sugar	1	0.2	0.1	0.1
Crackers, Ritz	4	0.2	0.3	0.1
Muffin, blueberry	1 small	0.8	0.6	0.2
Oats, whole	½ cup	1.6	1.1	0.5
Pancakes	2	0.9	0.7	0.2
Rice, medium grain	½ cup	0.4	0.3	trace
Nuts				
Almonds, roasted	22 whole	2.5	2.4	0.1
Peanuts	30 to 40 whole	2.0	1.9	0.1
Walnuts	14 halves	1.1	1.0	trace
Legumes				
Beans (black, dry, cooked)	½ cup	2.8	2.7	0.1
Lentils (dry, cooked)	½ cup	2.9	2.8	0.1

FIBER

RECOMMENDATIONS FROM THE NATURAL PHYSICIAN FOR . . .

ᐱ CANCER

One of the benefits of fiber, especially insoluble fiber, is that it binds to cancer-causing substances so that they are excreted out of the body. Epidemiological studies demonstrate that if you have a diet high in saturated fats and low in fiber, you increase the risk of many different types of cancer, including colon cancer.

Of course, all these benefits can't be attributed to fiber. Fruits, vegetables, legumes, and whole grains—foods with the most dietary fiber—also contain vitamins, minerals, and phytonutrients, all of which are believed to be responsible for some of the protective effects against cancer. Lignans in flaxseed, for example, are phytonutrients that have a protective effect.

That said, it's evident that a high-fiber diet can be protective against certain kinds of cancer—especially colon cancer. This makes sense to me, as toxins are

(continued)

bound by fiber and removed through the stool. Also, when fiber is acted on by bacteria in the colon, it produces the substance butyric acid, which is known as a "short-chain fatty acid." Butyric acid is the main energy source for the colonic cells, and it's thought to be one of the mechanisms that helps dietary fiber prevent colon cancer.

Hormone-dependent cancers in women—such as breast, uterine, and ovarian cancers—seem to show up more often among women on low-fiber diets. Men on low-fiber diets seem to have a higher rate of testicular cancer.

Women on vegetarian diets have been shown to have up to 50% lower levels of free estrogen in their blood than women who eat meat and foods made from animal products. Insoluble fiber helps to bind and excrete excess estrogen. Researchers believe this may be one of the reasons why vegetarian women have lower rates of breast cancer.

☙ CHOLESTEROL

Many of the different forms of fiber help to reduce cholesterol levels. Pectin, as found in apples and other fruits, lowers total and LDL cholesterol. Similarly, the water-soluble fiber in oats seems to improve cholesterol levels. It contains a substance called beta glucan, which has been shown to lower cholesterol.

In 1997, the Food and Drug Administration (FDA) allowed oat bran to be registered and promoted as a cholesterol-reducing food. But studies on the effects of oat bran have produced somewhat mixed results. Some oat bran studies have been shown to produce very little improvement in cholesterol levels, while others show up to a 21% reduction in serum cholesterol. Researchers have found that as little as 18 g of oat bran fiber favorably affect the total and LDL cholesterol levels in men with mildly elevated cholesterol markers. (In most studies that produced benefits, people ate around 100 g of oat bran.) Guar gums have also been shown in animal and human studies to lower cholesterol markers. Psyllium has also been shown to lower cholesterol.

The body eliminates cholesterol through bile acids, which are produced by the gallbladder and released into the small intestine. Water-soluble fibers bind to the cholesterol in these bile acids so that they cannot be reabsorbed and are carried out with the stool.

☙ CONSTIPATION

Fiber bulks up the stool so that gravity and peristalsis (contractions of the smooth muscles of the digestive tract) pull down the stool. Insoluble fiber is most important as it pulls water into the large intestine, and with more liquid, you'll have softer stools and easier elimination.

Soluble fiber also contributes, to a lesser degree, to the weight and water content of the stool. Ground-up flaxseeds as well as vegetables are the best forms of fiber to relieve constipation. (Other major factors contributing to constipation are too little water consumption and not enough exercise.)

If it takes a long time for stool to move through the intestinal tract, there's a higher chance that toxins can be reabsorbed into the bloodstream.

The transit time, the length it takes to go from the mouth to the anus, is significantly reduced when you have a high-fiber diet. For example, cultures that consume a high-fiber diet (100 to 170 g per day) have a transit time of 30 hours. In comparison, the low-fiber American diet (10 to 20 g per day) has a transit time that exceeds 48 hours.

DIABETES AND HYPOGLYCEMIA

Water-soluble fiber is extremely important if you have diabetes or hypoglycemia. Foods such as oat bran, legumes, nuts, seeds, apples, and most vegetables slow down the release of blood-sugar from the intestine to the bloodstream.

In addition, dietary fiber has been shown to increase the cells' sensitivity to insulin, so additional fiber helps balance blood-sugar levels. (I also recommend guar gum for blood-sugar balance.) People with diabetes or hypoglycemia need to consume good portions of fiber with every meal. For someone with diabetes, I recommend 50 g of fiber a day.

IRRITABLE BOWEL SYNDROME (IBS) AND INFLAMMATORY BOWEL DISEASE (IBD)

If you have either of these digestive conditions, it's essential to pay attention to your dietary habits—especially fiber intake. A lack of dietary fiber creates an unhealthy environment in the digestive tract, setting the stage for digestive disease.

Besides helping with elimination, a good supply of insoluble fiber helps to feed the "friendly" bacteria that live in the colon and assist digestion. In fact, if you have IBS or IBD, there's a good chance you have a condition known as dysbiosis or bacteria imbalance, which can be detected by stool analysis.

I find most of my patients with these conditions benefit from increasing dietary sources of fiber, but I generally recommend steamed and cooked sources of vegetables. If you have IBS or IBD, you'll probably want to reduce or avoid wheat and other grain products because they tend to be irritating. Psyllium supplements, for instance, are helpful for some people with these digestive problems, but they can be very irritating to others.

If you want to try ground-up flaxseeds—which are generally well tolerated—start with a low dosage of 1 to 2 teaspoons with one tall glass (8 ounces) of water. If you don't experience discomfort, you can gradually increase the dosage over time.

Fish Oil

Gary's father had died at the age of 54. "It was a heart attack," Gary told me.

Now 44 himself, Gary almost felt as if he were living on borrowed time. He could hear the clock ticking.

"Gary, most cases of heart attacks can be prevented," I assured him. I also let him know he was doing the right thing—showing some concern about his heart health before anything happened. Most people, sad to say, wait until they've had a heart attack before taking the measures that they could and should have taken years before.

True, there are inherited factors that make some people more susceptible than others to heart attack—specifically, homocysteine and cholesterol levels just seem to be higher in some people than in others. But most heart attacks are due to diet and lifestyle factors.

Gary had done enough reading to be aware of that. It was one reason he wanted to get started on an aggressive program to keep his heart as healthy as possible.

Among the strategies we discussed were stress reduction, exercise, a series of lab tests, and, of course, diet and supplements. I emphasized the importance of omega-3 fatty acids found in fish, especially cold-water fish such as salmon, mackerel, herring, and sardines. Above all, I recommended fish-oil supplements to optimize the amount of these heart-healthy fatty acids. As part of a total strategy for heart health, the steady intake of fish oil could, potentially, add decades to his life expectancy. I also explained how fish oil was one of the best substances, out of the natural or pharmaceutical categories, to reduce inflammation in the body. Chronic inflammation underlies many chronic diseases.

OIL WELL

Among the essential fatty acids that we need to live, omega-3s are very important. These are fats that your body can't manufacture on its own, so they need to come from food sources or supplements.

While omega-3 is also found in flaxseed and flaxseed oil, the kind that you get from fish and fish oil has some unique properties that are not present in these other foods. The fish and fish oils are a direct source of two long-chain fatty acids known as EPA (eicosapentanoic acid) and DHA (docosa-

hexanoic acid), and both are very important for heart health.

Another reason doctors are confident about the benefits of fish oil is pragmatic. The vast majority of studies on essential fatty acids have been done on fish oils. The good news for flax oil is that recent research demonstrates flax oil can increase blood levels of good omega fatty acids. Other oils that contain omega-3 fatty acids include hempseed oil and macadamia nut oil.

Fish became more popular as a "healthy heart" food when researchers studied the Mediterranean diet—that is, the diet of many cultures around the Mediterranean during the 1960s in Crete, parts of Greece, and southern Italy. (There, as in many other cultures, the American diet has crept in, raising the rate of heart disease and other chronic diseases.) In the classic Mediterranean diet, people had many plant foods (vegetables, legumes, fruit, bread, pasta, nuts), lots of olive oil, and low to moderate amounts of fish, poultry, meat, dairy, eggs, and wine.

Nutritionists believe the consumption of fish was one of the key benefits of this diet, which resulted in a much lower incidence of obesity, heart disease, diabetes, and cancer. A four-year study of the Mediterranean diet found that people could reduce their risk of heart attack by as much as 70%.

SEA RATIONS

In a more direct study of fish consumption, a team of researchers who looked at mortality data from 36 countries confirmed that life expectancy is longer in those countries where people get a lot of fish in their daily diet. Men and women who eat more fish have a lower risk of early death from all kinds of illnesses, particularly stroke and heart disease.

Essential fatty acids form a group of hormone-like messengers known as prostaglandins. The omega-3 fatty acids as found in fish oil—helped along by the EPA and DHA in the fish—tend to decrease inflammation, thin the blood, and balance the immune system.

In the immune system, EPA appears to be particularly important for its anti-inflammatory effects, so it's helpful to people who have arthritis. DHA is critical for the proper development and function of the brain because your brain cells need it to transmit electrical impulses efficiently. It's not surprising, therefore, that a DHA deficiency can lead to memory, behavior, and learning problems.

Some studies have also indicated that supplementing infant formula with DHA can improve children's IQ. Interestingly, it's also important for mood regulation, and studies have shown that a deficiency can contribute to depression.

The DHA found in fish oil also appears to calm down hyperactive children. It's also required for proper retinal development for infants.

DOSAGE

The richest sources of EPA and DHA, however, are cold-water fish—particularly salmon, herring, anchovies, and sardines. Halibut, mackerel, and tuna also have omega-3s, but I recommend eating them no more than once per month due to concerns about possible mercury contamination.

In my opinion, wild fish are always preferable to farm-raised fish since farmed fish are often fed corn and grains, raising their omega-6 content. Also, instead of living far out to sea, farm-raised fish live near shore—and so are more likely to be contaminated with man-made toxins, such as PCBs (harmful compounds formerly used as insulating and cooling fluids, which are extremely slow to biodegrade). I recommend limiting consumption of farmed fish to no more than once a month. Supplements are sold in health-food stores and online in liquid or gel capsule form. The liquid provides a higher concentration per dose, is usually less expensive, and now is available flavored with lemon or orange to reduce the fishy taste. Even so, I find that most people prefer capsules, which have no taste.

For some people, fish oil (especially in liquid form) triggers unpleasant bouts of belching. To minimize this, take your fish oil with meals. If the problem persists, buy enteric-coated fish oil capsules—their harder casing keeps the capsule from opening until it reaches the small intestine, preventing the stomach gassiness that causes burping. Fish oil capsules often come in 1,000 mg doses—but this refers to the weight of the oil, not to the actual amount of DHA and EPA they provide. Check the label to see how many capsules you must take daily to get the standard dose of 500 mg to 1,000 mg of combined DHA and EPA. People with existing arthritis or cardiovascular disease may need up to 3,000 mg of combined EPA and DHA.

It is good to take vitamin E on the same day as fish oil. It prevents oxidation of vitamin E in the body and fish oil may lower the body's vitamin E levels.

WHAT ARE THE SIDE EFFECTS?

Some people who take fish oil experience digestive upset including burping—which can be disconcerting because you may burp a "fishy" smell. But you probably won't have that problem if you take the capsules with meals.

Also, some companies make specially

designed capsules that ensure the oil makes it into the small intestine before breaking down. Such claims are advertised so you might want to try their capsules to see whether their product alleviates the problem of burping or "fish breath."

Since fish oils also have a blood-thinning effect, check with your doctor if you are taking any blood-thinning medications.

You may have an increase in LDL cholesterol while supplementing fish oil (although not common). If a blood test shows your cholesterol count is on the rise, you can take a garlic supplement to help neutralize this potential effect of the fish oil.

Although people have relatively few and minor problems with the side effects of fish oil, there's a risk that the capsules can contain rancid oil. It's easy to check, however. Just cut open the end of a capsule. If the fish oil has gone rancid, you can easily smell the strong odor. You're better off getting a fresh bottle with new capsules.

Finally, check the label of any brand you buy to make sure the product was tested for contaminants such as heavy metals.

FISH OIL
RECOMMENDATIONS FROM THE NATURAL PHYSICIAN FOR . . .

🐟 ATTENTION DEFICIT DISORDER (ADD) AND ATTENTION DEFICIT/ HYPERACTIVITY DISORDER (ADHD)

Many school-age children have been diagnosed with ADD or ADHD, and their problems are sometimes related to nutritional imbalances. (Excess sugars and some additives in junk food have particularly been blamed.)

Essential fatty acids such as DHA are critically important for proper brain function, but—well, how many children do you know who eat fresh cold-water fish three times a week? When children aren't getting enough DHA and they're loading up on saturated fat, trans fatty acids, and omega-6 fatty acids from fast foods, the inevitable result is a fatty-acid imbalance.

DHA supplementation has been shown to decrease aggression while a child is under stress. The DHA in fish oil helps to improve the chemical balance in the brain while giving the general benefits of omega 3 fatty acid supplementation.

A small study involved nine children, ages 8 to 16, who had ADHD, which is characterized by inattention, hyperactivity, and impulsive behavior. Participants took high daily doses of fish oil, providing 8 g to 16 g combined of the omega-3 fatty acids *eicosapentaenoic acid* (EPA) and *docosahexaenoic acid* (DHA), for eight weeks. Researchers found the children's behavior improved significantly, as rated by a psychiatrist and parents.

I recommend that bottle-fed infants receive omega-3 supplementation, especially DHA, for proper brain and retina development. Breast-fed infants receive these critical essential fatty acids in the breast milk. I suspect that, before long, DHA supplementation will be required in all commercial baby formulas.

🐟 ARTHRITIS

Numerous studies with fish oil have been done on people with rheumatoid arthritis and the results have been very positive. For aggressive treatment using fish oil, take 6,000 mg daily. Some people need doses that are even higher, so talk to your health practitioner about the optimum dose if you have severe rheumatoid arthritis.

If the fish oil is helpful in reducing stiffness and pain, there's a good chance you'll be able to reduce the dosages of pharmaceuticals. Drug therapy for rheumatoid arthritis focuses on prednisone, methotrexate (also used for chemotherapy), and anti-inflammatory medications—all of which can have serious toxicity when used on a long-term basis. With fish oil, on the other hand, there's no toxicity, so it's a far more benign treatment than the classic pharmaceuticals. One study found that many patients were able to go off their anti-inflammatory drugs while supplementing fish oil and experienced no relapse in their rheumatoid arthritis. Researchers found that the fish oil had a balancing effect on the entire immune system.

And a new study in the *Journal of Biological Chemistry* showed that fish oil reduces the body's formation of chemicals called prostanoids, which in excess can promote inflammation.

It is recommended, as the result of studies, that a minimum daily dose of 3,000 mg EPA and DHA is necessary to derive the expected benefits, although I find not all my patients need this high a dosage. Once you start taking fish oil, you can expect to stay on it for at least 12 weeks before it begins to yield benefits. But after that, you can stay on it indefinitely.

Despite the many improvements you can get from fish oil, I do have to say it should be part of a total program when you're treating rheumatoid arthritis. It's also important to improve your diet and take steps to reduce the toxins in your body. I've seen the quickest results with detoxification programs when they also involved homeopathic remedies. But fish oil is a good long-term therapy for some people, and it can definitely help keep inflammatory conditions under control.

Although not so well studied, essential fatty acids found in fish oil are helpful to decrease the stiffness associated with osteoarthritis, the most common form of arthritis, where the cartilage has degenerated.

ASTHMA

The rate of asthma keeps increasing. Sadly, children's asthma is continuing to rise at an alarming rate. Environmental pollution and poor dietary habits are largely to blame.

Essential fatty acids in fish and fish oil help to suppress the inflammatory chemicals involved in this disease. Studies show that children who eat oily fish more than once a week have one-third the risk of getting asthma as children who do not eat fish or eat lean fish on a regular basis.

Fish-oil supplements are helpful for both children and adults with asthma. Again, the benefits of fish oil take months before the natural anti-inflammatory benefits begin to take hold.

CANCER

Omega-3 fatty acids are important for a healthy, well-functioning immune system. If you can get more omega-3 fatty acids in your diet and also take supplements, there's a good chance you can help protect yourself from certain types

(continued)

of cancers. Scientists now believe these EFAs may help prevent cancer and also slow or halt tumor growth, particularly of breast, prostate, and colorectal cancer cells. Though no one knows why, preliminary evidence suggests that omega-3s may also protect against leukemia, non-Hodgkin's lymphoma, and multiple myeloma (plasma cell cancer).

Animal studies have shown that fish oil can augment certain types of chemotherapy to fight cancer more effectively. Fish oil has also been shown to help treat cachexia, which is the loss of muscle mass and weight in cancer patients.

◦❧ CARDIOVASCULAR DISEASE

With many studies to back up its benefits, fish oil is often recommended as a preventative for heart and circulation problems. Along with the population studies showing that consumption of fish oil slashes the rate of cardiovascular disease, are literally hundreds of studies that support these observations. Fish oils reduce cholesterol and triglyceride levels and also act as a natural blood thinner, which results in the lowering of blood pressure. Omega-3s in fish oil help to prevent irregular heartbeat, lower blood-clot risk, and combat arterial plaque buildup. While the federal government traditionally has been slow to endorse supplement use, in 2004 its Agency for Healthcare Research and Quality expressed strong support for omega-3s, noting that "consumption of omega-3 fatty acids, whether from fish or from supplements, reduces all-cause mortality and improves various cardiovascular disease outcomes." A Greek study from 2005 showed that regular consumption of omega-3-rich fish

reduces blood markers of inflammation, including C-reactive protein and interleukin-6, which are known risk factors for heart attacks. In an Italian study, patients who received just 1 g per day of omega-3s during the critical three months following a heart attack reduced their risk of sudden death by an amazing 42%. The American Heart Association also recommends omega-3s and daily intake of at least 500 mg of EPA and DHA combined to prevent cardiovascular disease.

Fish oil has also been shown to prevent the reclosing of arteries after angioplasty. And it has also been shown to have a mild to moderate effect on regression of atherosclerosis (plaque in the arteries) in those with coronary artery disease.

◦❧ CHRONIC OBSTRUCTIVE PULMONARY DISEASE

More than 17 million Americans suffer from this group of serious breathing disorders that includes asthma, bronchitis, and emphysema. Smoking, as you might expect, is the factor that multiplies your chances of getting any of these diseases. But for smokers as well as nonsmokers, there are some benefits in eating fish as often as possible.

◦❧ COGNITIVE HEALTH

In a Swedish study published in 2006, patients in the earliest stage of Alzheimer's disease who took omega-3 supplements for 6 to 12 months had a slower rate of cognitive decline than those who did not take omega-3s. Alzheimer's disease involves brain inflammation, and omega-3 is a potent anti-inflammatory. Other studies suggest that omega-3s also have positive effects on mental well-being in healthy people, enhancing mood and increasing cognitive speed.

There are maternal and infant benefits, too. A small US study revealed that nine-month-old babies whose mothers supplemented with omega-3s during pregnancy displayed significantly better problem-solving skills, as measured by the ability to retrieve a toy covered by a cloth.

CROHN'S DISEASE AND ULCERATIVE COLITIS

Inflammatory bowel diseases such as Crohn's disease and ulcerative colitis can be helped by fish-oil supplementation.

In one study of ulcerative colitis, people who took fish-oil supplements (high in omega-3s) were able to cut their steroid medications in half. Again, I see fish oil as one component of a total natural-therapy program to address and alleviate these digestive conditions. Other measures include stress reduction, improving digestive capacity, and maintaining a healthful diet.

Herbal medicines and homeopathy are excellent therapies to help turn these conditions around without relying on pharmaceutical drugs that may have many damaging side effects.

DEPRESSION

The brain is 60% fat and requires essential fatty acids, especially DHA, to function properly. It has been shown that people deficient in DHA are much more likely to suffer from depression.

Consuming fish on a regular basis is a good way to prevent depression. I recommend concentrated DHA supplements for those already battling depression. Fish oil improves the outcome of pharma-

ceutical antidepressants. Fish oil also improves depression associated with bipolar disorder.

DRY EYE SYNDROME

Population studies suggest higher levels of omega-3 fatty acids decrease the risk of this disease.

ECZEMA

I have found that flaxseeds and flaxseed oil in combination with GLA work well for eczema. It also makes sense to consume cold-water fish rich in omega-3 fatty acids. Fish oil is also another option to treat eczema.

HIGH BLOOD PRESSURE

High blood pressure is one of the biggest risk factors for heart disease and stroke. Numerous studies have shown that fish oil reduces blood pressure. I find fish oil works best as part of a natural program—combined with stress-reduction techniques and a regimen that includes herbs such as hawthorn, minerals such as magnesium and calcium, along with the natural supplement CoQ10.

HIGH TRIGLYCERIDES

With high-dose fish oil, you can lower high triglyceride levels, which are an independent risk factor for heart disease by up to 50%. As a matter of fact, no drug can reduce triglycerides as well as high-dose fish oil.

INFLAMMATORY BOWEL DISEASE

I usually prescribe fish oil for those with Crohn's disease and ulcerative colitis.

(continued)

Studies have been mixed with regard to its benefit, but as part of an all-round natural anti-inflammatory protocol, I think fish oil is a good addition.

INSULIN RESISTANCE
The inability to metabolize carbohydrates effectively leads to high blood-sugar levels and a corresponding spike of the hormone insulin (the component that helps get the blood-sugar into the cells). As a result, many different biochemical reactions can occur, one of which is weight gain.

Clinical studies have shown that omega-3 fatty acids, such as those in fish oil, help improve the body's utilization of insulin. (It's interesting that an essential fatty acid can help *decrease* body fat!) This insulin-balancing effect is also important in relation to diabetes.

KIDNEY PROTECTION
People who receive organ transplants require extensive immune-suppressing drugs. These are needed to keep the body from rejecting the donated organ, but some of the drugs (such as cyclosporine) are so powerful that they can have life-threatening side effects.

In the case of patients who have had kidney transplants, however, it's been shown that they resume normal kidney function more quickly when omega-3-rich fish oil is supplemented. It appears that the fish oil actually protects the kidneys from the damaging effects of the immune-suppressing drugs.

LUPUS
Two pilot studies have shown fish oil to benefit people with lupus, an autoimmune condition where the immune system attacks its own tissue. For patients with lupus, I suggest eating cold-water fish regularly and supplementing with fish oil. It may take six months to a year before there's any improvement, but sometimes the benefits can be dramatic.

MULTIPLE SCLEROSIS
Dr. Roy Swank, the doctor who developed a natural protocol for multiple sclerosis (MS), recommended fish oil as well as flaxseed oil. In fact, Dr. Swank advocated that patients who have MS should eat fish three times a week or more. He was also a proponent of cod liver oil—one of the popular fish oils—as a daily supplement.

PAINFUL MENSES
Fish oil supplementation can reduce pain associated with menses, likely through its anti-inflammatory effect.

PSORIASIS
Several studies have shown that 10 to 12 g of fish oil daily can improve psoriasis. I routinely recommend fish oil and dietary fish as well as other natural therapies to improve this inflammatory condition.

SCHIZOPHRENIA
Some preliminary studies are showing that EPA and DHA may be helpful in the treatment of schizophrenia. More research needs to be done, but I would not be surprised to see these essential fatty acids become accepted as part of the routine treatment for schizophrenia. Dr. Abraham Hoffer of Victoria, Canada, has already demonstrated that a knowledgeable practitioner can provide a full-scale treatment of schizophrenia with nutritional therapies.

Flaxseed

"Dr. Mark, what can I do? My hair is falling out, my nails are peeling, and my skin is flaking because it is so dry!" The plea came from Rachelle, a 23-year-old university student.

My first step was to ask her about her usual daily diet and her digestion. She mentioned right away that she had chronic constipation, and wondered whether that could be somehow related to her dry-skin condition.

"Possibly," I replied. But after hearing what she ate on a daily basis, I found another factor that seemed even more important. It appeared that Rachelle had an omega-3 fatty-acid deficiency. Because she didn't enjoy the time and effort of cooking, she was eating about 90% of her meals in fast-food restaurants. Also, like many university students, Rachelle liked to eat out so she could socialize with her friends.

Her dry-skin problem could also be caused by low thyroid function—but once I ruled that out, I started Rachelle on flaxseed oil (*Linum usitatissimum* or linseed). Two months later Rachelle was a happier and healthier person. She said the first symptom to improve was the constipation. Instead of having a bowel movement every three days, it was now once daily. Her skin was less dry—and she was no longer losing hair the way she had been. Her nails, though still brittle, were starting to improve. Rachelle also noticed that her memory and concentration were better. (This made sense, as the brain needs a strong supply of essential fatty acids to function optimally.)

Given the success that Rachelle was experiencing, it was simple to make a recommendation at our next appointment. "Keep doing what you're doing," I advised. "Another month or two, and you will feel and look even better. Essential fatty acids take time to work. Sometimes, it's many months before you get the full benefits."

Obviously, this simple supplement had made a profound improvement in Rachelle's life. Ideally, she would have increased her intake of omega-3 fatty acids by eating more foods that were rich in it, such as fish, nuts, and some specific vegetables. Cutting down on the fried and fast foods rich in omega-6 oils and hydrogenated fats would have been a prudent choice as well. But, in reality, Rachelle wasn't about to change her lifestyle. Fortunately, she could get almost the same, optimum results just by taking 2 teaspoons of flaxseed oil every day.

As Mahatma Gandhi said, "Wherever flaxseed becomes a regular food item among the people, there will be better health."

CHANGING YOUR OILS

In an ideal diet, there's a balance between two kinds of essential fatty acids: the omega-3s (alpha linolenic) and omega-6s (linoleic). Most of us consume far too many omega-6 fatty acids (from red meat and vegetable oils) and not enough omega-3 fatty acids (from fish, flaxseed, some vegetables). Many experts feel the optimal ratio of omega-6 to omega-3 fatty acids is 4 to 1, while most people are getting these oils in a ratio that's about 20 to 1!

Many diseases are related to essential fatty-acid deficiency. The commercial processing of fats and oils has created an "essential fatty-acid crisis" for industrialized nations. These synthetic, rancid fats not only displace "good fats" in the body, but also have toxic effects on the immune and nervous systems.

More important than the total amount of fats is the *type* of fat we consume. Essential fatty acids such as those found in flaxseed are critical to the optimal health and functioning of all cells in the body, including brain cells. Essential fatty acids improve our cell walls, and this improvement has a direct effect on the functioning of the cells. Essential fatty acids influence the passage of nutrients and information that comes into a cell, and the elimination of toxic waste products. So, healthy cells equal a healthy metabolism and healthy body.

Flaxseed is a powerful disease-fighting food that most people desperately need. It has a history of more than 5,000 years of use. Records show that flax was cultivated as a food in ancient Babylon (3000 BC). Hippocrates (460–377 BC) recommended flax as a food to relieve intestinal discomfort.

THE GROWTH OF FLAXSEED

For centuries, flax has been a staple of Europeans' diets. No wonder the Latin translation of flax means "useful." There are nearly 100 different species of flax worldwide, and many of its health-yielding properties are now being acknowledged. Almost anywhere you go in North America, you can now find flaxseed breads or you can buy bags of flaxseed in bulk at health-food stores.

Flax has a very nutritious profile, containing vitamin A, some of the Bs, D, and E, carotene, lecithin, and many minerals. It also contains many different amino acids, the building blocks of protein. While it is not a complete protein source, it combines well with other protein foods, which means it ultimately helps you consolidate more protein in your body.

Well known as an excellent source of omega-3 fatty acids (alpha linolenic acid)—the type of "good fats" in which so many people are deficient—flaxseed oil helps pro-

tect against cardiovascular disease, cancer, arthritis, and many other chronic degenerative diseases.

But flaxseed oil has another attribute: an almost perfect balance of omega-3s with other kinds of fatty acids. Flaxseed has approximately 48 to 64% omega-3s, 16 to 34% omega-6s, and 18 to 22% omega-9 fatty acids. This type of fatty acid composition is an excellent fatty-acid balance.

In addition, flaxseed has some very powerful medicinal properties. It's an excellent source of insoluble fiber, which is the kind that helps out the digestive tract by forming the bulk of the stool and absorbing toxins. As an added bonus, flax also contains a second type of fiber, the soluble kind that dissolves in water and is absorbed in the digestive tract. Soluble fiber helps reduce cholesterol levels and regulate blood-sugar levels.

CONTENTS

One-quarter cup of flax contains approximately 20 g of total fiber, which is just about half of the recommended daily fiber requirement (doctors suggest 35 to 50 g daily). Flax also contains mucilage, a gel-like substance that soothes and heals the digestive tract. In addition, flaxseed helps feed the "good bacteria"—the kind that reside in the digestive tract, helping with digestion. It also has a natural laxative effect.

Flaxseed is also one of the top sources of a phytonutrient known as lignans. (Though wheat bran is also known for containing lignans, the amount in flaxseed is about 100 times what it is in wheat bran.) Found in the fiber part of flaxseed, lignans have many benefits, helping to fight cancer, viruses, fungi, and bacteria. Lignans also balance hormones, so it can relieve menopausal hot flashes.

Researchers are particularly interested in the anticancer properties of flax lignans. Research on animals and humans has shown that lignans have a protective effect against hormone-sensitive cancers such as breast, uterine, and prostate cancer. Lignans increase sex-hormone binding globulin (SHBG), which binds estrogen and helps to clear it out of the body. It also appears to block excessive stimulation of testosterone.

Lignans are broken down by the gut flora into two compounds known as enterolactone and enterodiol. These compounds interfere with the cancer-promoting effects of estrogen, especially breast cancer, which is probably a reason why vegetarian women have lower rates of breast cancer than non-vegetarian women. The omega-3 (alpha linolenic acid) has its own immune-enhancing and anticancer properties as well.

DOSAGE

✒ Flaxseed

There are various ways to consume flaxseed. If you're dealing with the actual seeds, you need to break the hard outer coating. One way is to grind them in a coffee grinder for about five seconds.

The typical adult dose is 1 to 2 tablespoons daily, but there's so much fiber in flaxseed that you may have digestive problems (including excessive flatulence) if you start with that much. If you're not already on a high-fiber diet, or if you're prone to digestive problems, I suggest you start with ¼ tablespoon daily and gradually increase the dosage.

Children can take 1 to 2 teaspoons of ground flax daily, but they, too, may need to start with a lower dose.

Make sure to always drink at least 8 ounces of water when you're taking ground-up flaxseed. The liquid is needed to help move the seeds through the intestinal tract. Alternatively, you can add the ground-up flaxseed to a shake, juice, or a glass of water to help it go down more easily.

Flaxseed is a good addition to salads and granola cereal and can also be used in baking. Try to take the flaxseed as soon as possible after grinding them up, because they start to oxidize as soon as they've been ground. The flaxseed oil starts to turn rancid with oxidation.

You can also let the whole seeds soak in water overnight, then take them the next day. The soaking softens them and makes them more digestible.

✒ Flaxseed Oil

The adult dosage for flaxseed oil is 1 to 2 tablespoons daily. Children can start at 1 teaspoon daily and the dose can be gradually increased unless the stools get too loose.

Flaxseed oil is also available in gel capsules, which work well if you don't want to taste the flax or take time to grind and/or soak the flaxseed. Unfortunately, the capsules are more expensive. You'll need to take nine to fourteen 1,000-mg capsules daily if you want to get the equivalent of 1 tablespoon of flaxseed oil.

When you're storing flaxseed oil, keep it away from light—preferably, in the refrigerator. I recommend buying small bottles of flaxseed, so the oil is always as fresh as possible. Make sure to check the expiration date on the bottle.

Fresh flaxseed oil has a characteristic nutty flavor, and if it goes rancid, you can tell at once by the smell. So as soon as you open a new bottle, give it a sniff to make sure the oil is fresh. Also, you should look for oil that's made from organically grown flaxseed to ensure that it isn't tainted with pesticides.

WHAT ARE THE SIDE EFFECTS?

People who have gallbladder problems, such as gallstones, may have trouble digesting flaxseed oil. That's because the gallbladder concentrates and releases the bile to help break down oils; if there's not enough bile, digestion is more difficult. This can be resolved if you start with a very small amount of flaxseed oil (1 teaspoon) and build up the dosage over time. Better yet, start by using ground-up flaxseed.

Another possible side effect is constipation if you don't drink enough water when you start taking flaxseed. One patient, for instance, called me with severe abdominal pain after taking ½ cup of ground flaxseed; but when I reminded her about taking more water, she recovered. (Having taken that much flaxseed, however, she needed to drink nearly ½ gallon of water during the next few hours!)

You should not ingest flaxseed at all if you have bowel obstruction.

A few patients have reported outbreaks of adult acne after starting flaxseed oil—but over time, their skin improved. The outbreaks were probably the effect of the body detoxifying and adjusting to the new balance of essential fatty acids.

The high-fiber content of flaxseed may interfere with the absorption of certain medications. If you're taking pharmaceutical doses on a regular basis, be sure to check with your pharmacist about possible interactions.

FLAXSEED

RECOMMENDATIONS FROM THE NATURAL PHYSICIAN FOR . . .

❧ ACNE

Omega-3 fatty acids help reduce skin inflammation and have a balancing effect on the production of sebum, the substance that forms pimples. The results are not immediate, however, and you may have to take flaxseed for several months before you begin to see benefits. However, it is worth taking on a long-term basis to keep acne under control.

Some cases of acne are related to poor elimination. Flaxseed or flaxseed oil help to keep the bowels regular and decrease systemic toxicity.

❧ ARTHRITIS

Omega-3 fatty acids as found in flaxseed oil help to keep the inflammatory pathways in the body in balance. It also works to keep joints "lubricated," which makes it especially helpful for osteoarthritis.

It may also help people who have rheumatoid arthritis, but the connection is more indirect. There have been a number of studies using essential fatty acids for rheumatoid arthritis, but the best results have been produced with high doses of fish oil—a direct source of eicosapentanoic acid (EPA), which has anti-inflammatory properties. If you take flaxseed, some of the alpha linolenic acid does get converted to EPA, but the amount of conversion varies with each individual—and conversion is further inhibited if you have a deficiency of the mineral zinc.

I recommend more than flaxseed oil for patients who have rheumatoid arthritis. You should also eat cold-water fish such as salmon, mackerel, and herring, and—for more aggressive therapy—supplement with a quality fish oil to further reduce pain and inflammation.

CANCER

Flaxseed is an excellent supplement to use for the prevention and treatment of cancer, primarily because of the hormone-balancing and immune-supportive effects of lignans.

Since one out of every eight women is likely to get breast cancer in her lifetime, I recommend flaxseed as a standard preventive for every woman who is concerned about this disease.

In breast cancer research, an increasing number of studies are suggesting that a form of estrogen known as 16 alpha-hydroxyestrone (toxic estrogen) needs to be balanced out with another form called 2-hydroxyestrone to lower the risk of developing cancer. Some plant nutrients can alter this ratio in a positive way, and so can flaxseed.

In one study, researchers compared the health of women who had diets that included flaxseed and, in some cases, wheat bran as well. Researchers found that flaxseed supplementation positively increased the urinary ratio in favor of the "good estrogen" 2-hydroxyestrone, while wheat bran had no effect. The significance of this study is that serious cancers such as those of the breast, uterus, and cervix may very well be prevented and to some degree treated with flaxseed and possibly flax oil lignan extracts.

The health of the prostate gland in men is also very much associated with essential fatty acid and hormone balance. Flaxseed, with its high lignan content, should be on the dietary list for any men who have enlarged prostates. It's a prostate-cancer preventive, and also useful as part of a comprehensive treatment for prostate cancer.

With its excellent fiber and lignan content, flaxseed has been shown to protect against colon cancer as well.

CHOLESTEROL AND HEART DISEASE

You can definitely lower your cholesterol and triglycerides by adding omega-3 fatty acids to your diet—but most of the studies that show the benefits of this therapy have been done with fish and fish oils. However, some research also shows that flaxseed has a similar effect of lowering cholesterol and LDL cholesterol (the "bad" kind).

While I haven't seen flaxseed oil make dramatic improvements in the blood profiles of patients, I think long-term use of flaxseed and flaxseed oil makes sense as part of a comprehensive nutritional approach for the balancing of cholesterol. The high omega-3 fatty acids in flaxseed have natural blood-thinning properties. This helps to prevent strokes and optimizes circulation to the heart and body tissues.

DIGESTIVE DISORDERS

What do irritable bowel syndrome (IBS), Crohn's disease, ulcerative colitis, and constipation all have in common? The answer—low fiber intake.

Not only is flaxseed an excellent way to increase the daily fiber in your diet, it's also a way to get the soothing mucilage that can help heal an inflamed and irritated digestive tract. In addition, flaxseed

(continued)

"feeds" the good bacteria, which are usually deficient in people who have these digestive problems.

In fact, flaxseed oil is a tried-and-true old European treatment for constipation in children and infants. Just a teaspoonful can get the bowels moving in short order.

ꙮ DRY SKIN

Dry skin, like eczema, is often a sign of essential fatty-acid deficiency—a fact that's acknowledged by most nutrition-oriented doctors. (Low thyroid is another possible contributing factor.)

If I put a patient on an essential fatty-acid supplement, such as flaxseed or flaxseed oil, his or her dry skin starts to improve.

ꙮ ECZEMA

Any kind of omega-3 fatty-acid supplementation, whether it comes from flaxseed or fish oil, can help treat eczema. Often, flaxseed oil alone is not enough. When parents bring their kids with eczema into my office, I always recommend increasing the fish in their diet and check for food sensitivities. When my own son began getting eczema on his cheeks, at the age of about 14 months, we increased the amount of fish in his diet and supplemented with an essential fatty-acid supplement that contained a high percentage of omega-3 fatty acids and some GLA from evening primrose. At the same time, we also cut the cheese and citrus fruit from his diet. Over the next four months, his cheeks cleared up nicely.

It's important to know that essential fatty acids take awhile to "kick in," so be patient and give them at least a few months to work.

ꙮ ENERGY RECOVERY

Athletes who train hard need extra amounts of essential fatty acids as well as many other nutrients. I recommend supplementing with flaxseed for quicker recovery from workouts. The flaxseed also helps to protect the immune system that can be weakened from exhaustive training.

ꙮ MEMORY PROBLEMS

The brain is 60% fat—and essential fatty acids are an integral component of this fat. Perhaps the most critical of these essential fatty acids is DHA, which is necessary for memory and learning. Since a certain amount of alpha linolenic acid from flaxseed is converted into DHA, this supplement can be a beneficial memory booster. Also, omega-3 fatty acids have an anti-inflammatory effect, which appears to be important for brain health.

ꙮ MENOPAUSE

Taking 40 g of flaxseed orally per day significantly reduces symptoms of hot flashes and night sweats in women with mild menopausal symptoms. This is believed to be due to the hormone balancing lignans.

ꙮ MULTIPLE SCLEROSIS

Essential fatty acid balance is one of the most important areas to focus on for people with this disease of the nervous system. People with multiple sclerosis (MS) may suffer from a multitude of symptoms that range from visual changes to muscle weakness, all related to deterioration of the tissue (the myelin sheath) that covers the nerves.

Dr. Roy Swank, a neurologist from

Portland, Oregon, has proven that a diet rich in essential fatty acids and low in saturated fat is key to the successful treatment of MS. Dr. Swank advocates that his patients with MS eat fish and supplement cod liver oil. For MS treatment, many practitioners find that flax-seed works as well as cod liver oil. Both are rich in omega-3 fatty acids.

Food-Sensitivity Therapy

One of the most misunderstood areas in medicine today is the concept of food allergies. One problem is that people confuse the term "food allergy" with "food sensitivity." Even health practitioners occasionally use the terms interchangeably—but they're quite different.

If you have a food allergy, you'll see some pretty obvious symptoms as soon as you eat the food that's causing the allergy. Those symptoms might be an outbreak of hives, sudden difficulty breathing, or even vomiting. If you get a conventional lab test, it will probably reveal the offending food that's causing an increased immune reaction. Common food allergens, for example, are peanuts and milk, both detectable in a lab test.

But apart from these distinct food allergies, people can experience food sensitivities that involve a whole different set of reactions. Symptoms of food sensitivity may include headache, bloating, cramps, diarrhea, nausea, runny nose, skin rash, mood changes, joint pain, and many other potential symptoms. In children, just the presence of dark circles under the eyes might be a sign of food sensitivities.

Unlike food allergies, evidence of food sensitivities may not show up in conventional testing. If a doctor orders a conventional skin-scratch test or blood test, it's quite possible nothing significant will show up, even though your immune system may be having an adverse reaction to a whole range of foods. Likely, you'll feel mystified because it's obvious that when you eat that certain food, an adverse reaction occurs—even though the lab test doesn't support what seems obvious.

The fact is, food sensitivities—also known as food intolerances—often do not show up on conventional allergy tests. Some people don't exhibit reactions to certain food items until two or three days have passed.

Because the tests are so unreliable in these situations, if you don't have life-threatening reactions to foods, I wouldn't even bother with a conventional food-allergy test. There's a good chance you'll make far more progress by using the information provided in this section. In addition, many holistic doctors and natural health practitioners are skilled in dealing with food sensitivities or intolerances.

SENSITIVITY SITUATIONS

Why do some people have these sensitivities in the first place?

There are several explanations. Usually—that is, in 80% to 90% of the cases—food sensitivities are "acquired." Only a small percentage appear to be genetic. If a patient is having a reaction to apples or bread, often this is a new development, something that he or she did not experience as a child.

One reason for the development of food sensitivities is that people eat the same 15 or 20 foods all the time. With so little variety in the diet, for some reason the immune system develops a sensitivity to the frequently eaten foods.

Think about your own diet. Chances are you have "standard" breakfast, lunch, and dinner meals that you eat almost every day. Even snacks are the same. Once your body begins to become sensitive to these foods—whatever the reason—that sensitivity actually increases the more you eat these foods.

Another contributing factor is that people's digestive systems tend to get weaker as they get older. The typical digestive system is subject to a wide range of weakening forces, including the Standard American Diet (SAD), stress, medications like antibiotics—and, with some people, alcohol and smoking.

Yet another cause with some people could be a condition that many health practitioners have identified as "leaky gut syndrome." A lot of people who have leaky gut syndrome are unaware they have it or what it is—but essentially, it's a condition that leads to maldigestion and poor absorption of food in the digestive tract. Food proteins do not get broken down efficiently enough, and larger-than-normal protein molecules get absorbed across the small intestine. The immune system "sees" these larger-than-normal proteins as foreign invaders and attacks them. In this sequence of counterattack, inflammatory chemicals are released in the body, resulting in many different types of physical and mental symptoms—all adding up to food-sensitivity reactions.

Other culprits include fungal overgrowth in the digestive tract such as *Candida albicans* or parasite infections, which wreak havoc on the health of the digestive tract and immune system.

APPROACHES TO CONSIDER

If you suspect you have food sensitivities but haven't tracked down what's causing your problems, there are some logical steps you can take to identify the foods you're reacting to.

One way to find the culprits is with the elimination/reintroduction diet. Begin by eliminating the most common causes of food sensitivity. These include cow's milk, wheat, sugar, chocolate, soy, citrus fruits, and peanuts. You should eliminate all of these from your diet for one to two weeks.

At the end of the period of total sanctions, begin to introduce one food at a time every two to three days and see if you notice a reaction. Do this until you have gone through all the foods.

True, two weeks may seem like a long time if you're on such a restricted diet. However, the elimination diet is quite accurate.

As an alternative approach, I more often recommend a modified version of the elimination diet that's less stressful. I've found that the foods people crave the most are also the foods to which they're most sensitive. So you might shortcut the deprivation process if you just eliminate the foods you crave the most. If you stop having symptoms such as runny nose, headaches, or bloating while you're off those foods, then you can assume those are the ones most likely involved in causing your sensitivities.

MORE HELP

Another popular technique that I work with is the use of electrodermal testing, also referred to as electroacupuncture testing. Developed by a German medical doctor decades ago, it involves the testing of the electrical resistance of the skin to whatever food you want tested. A current runs through the testing machine and through a probe, which touches the patient's skin. It doesn't cause any pain, but the machine picks up subtle bioelectric changes that are caused by the food.

Though electroacupuncture testing may sound like something out of a science fiction book, I've found that it works well, and at least one controlled study lends support to this type of testing. In the study, the test proved accurate and reproducible when compared against conventional tests.

Another testing resource are the laboratories that provide special blood tests for people who have food sensitivities or allergies. These blood tests measure immediate and delayed reaction to foods by measuring antibody response (IgE and IgG4) or other markers of immune reaction.

AVOIDANCE MECHANISMS

No matter what technique you choose to help identify your food sensitivities, there are some common ways to desensitize yourself from these foods. Here are the steps to consider:

1. Avoid the food you are being desensitized to for one to two weeks to give your immune system a break.
2. Increase the variety of foods you're eating. In fact, try to double the number of different kinds of foods you are eating regularly. This will not only help to prevent sensitivities, but will increase the spectrum of nutrients you get.
3. Take supplements that will help improve your digestive power. The better you break down foods, the less you're likely to react to them. Microbial-enzyme supplements can be taken with meals to aid your

digestion. The typical adult dose is two capsules with meals. Also, a probiotic supplement (contains *Acidophilus* and other good bacteria, as well as FOS, a type of sugar that feeds good bacteria) will help to replenish the good bacteria in your digestive tract, which aids in digestion and works to repair a "leaky gut." Herbs such as gentian root, dandelion root, and ginger also stimulate digestive function. Look for herbal digestive formulas that contain these herbs and take them with meals.
4. Take betaine HCl to increase stomach acid. I generally reserve its use for seniors (who have very low stomach acid) or those who do not respond to other digestive supplements.
5. Use constitutional hydrotherapy to strengthen the digestive system (see Hydrotherapy, page 258).

Beyond these treatments there are ways to specifically get desensitized to foods you react to. Homeopathic remedies can be used. For example, if you are sensitive to apples, you can take a homeopathic apple remedy that, over time, can desensitize your immune system. Look for homeopathic desensitization drops that have the name of the food on the label. Most of these remedies can be found in a health-food store or obtained from a homeopathic practitioner.

General strengthening of your overall health, what practitioners call "constitution," can reduce your susceptibility to food sensitivities. Homeopathy and traditional Chinese medicine are ideal ways to help strengthen the constitution. Consult with a practitioner for individualized treatment.

FOOD-SENSITIVITY THERAPY

RECOMMENDATIONS FROM THE NATURAL PHYSICIAN FOR . . .

✐ ATTENTION DEFICIT DISORDER (ADD) AND ATTENTION DEFICIT/ HYPERACTIVITY DISORDER (ADHD)

Many children with behavior and attention problems show some improvement when food sensitivities are treated. For instance, it's well known that sugar aggravates ADD and ADHD symptoms in some children.

✐ ALLERGIES

I have seen many patients who thought their allergy symptoms were due to something in the environment, but their symptoms cleared up after food sensitivities were treated. Though of course other factors can contribute to allergies, you may find that environmental allergies diminish or disappear entirely when a food sensitivity is treated.

✐ ARTHRITIS

Food sensitivities can cause flare-ups of many types of arthritis, especially rheumatoid arthritis.

✐ ASTHMA

With cases of asthma continually on the rise, especially among children, it makes sense to look at every possible cause. Food sensitivities are often associated with this condition, especially reactions induced by milk and wheat products. Artificial sweeteners and preservatives are suspect as well.

✐ AUTISM

Reactions to wheat and milk products have been reported to cause some cases of autism. Many aspects of a child's behavior may improve when these foods are removed from the diet. Some practitioners have noted great improvements in learning, behavior, and emotional responses. Since there are no conventional treatments for autism, it's always worthwhile to try dietary changes that might have a positive impact.

✐ AUTOIMMUNE CONDITIONS

Since food sensitivities affect the immune system, treating those sensitivities is just one way of taking some burden off an already-imbalanced system. Conditions such as multiple sclerosis and lupus can be helped to some degree with food-sensitivity therapy.

✐ BLOATING

Have you ever wondered why you sometimes feel bloated within seconds of eating certain foods? This is a food sensitivity reaction—and when you treat it, you'll probably have a lot fewer problems with bloating.

✐ BRONCHITIS

Chronic cases of bronchitis can be due to food sensitivities, especially in children. Children who have milk sensitivity are especially likely to get frequent cases of bronchitis.

✐ CANDIDA

I have many patients come to my office convinced that they have yeast (*Candida*) overgrowth in their bodies. Symptoms can include—among other things—mood swings, depression, digestive upset, weakened immune system, and skin eruptions. In many cases, their symptoms were actually due to food sensitivities and disappeared when they were given food-sensitivity therapy.

❧ CONSTIPATION

If you're eating lots of fiber but still suffer from constipation, it's quite possible your food sensitivities are causing the bowels to slow down. Wheat can often be one of the offending foods.

❧ DEPRESSION

Depression can sometimes be caused or worsened by a chemical imbalance due in part to food sensitivity. If chemical imbalance is a salient factor, it will improve if you have food-sensitivity therapy. Pay special attention to this therapy if you notice that your depression gets worse after meals (though this can also be a sign of hypoglycemia).

❧ DIARRHEA

If you have chronic diarrhea, it could be associated with regular consumption of foods that are causing negative reactions. Children, for instance, are often sensitive to fruit juices and react by getting diarrhea. (The symptoms might go away if you dilute the fruit juice with water or try various types of juices.)

❧ EAR INFECTIONS

Want to increase your child's chances by at least 50% of never getting another ear infection? Want to break that vicious cycle of antibiotic therapy? Then identify and treat the child's food sensitivities.

Foods such as cow's milk can cause fluid buildup in the middle ear. This pro-vides a perfect breeding ground for viruses and bacteria. Wheat, sugar, soy, and citrus fruits are also commonly involved.

❧ ECZEMA

Food sensitivities might eliminate the underlying cause of this condition (though you should also consider fatty-acid imbalances as a possible cause). Eczema is not a cortisone-cream deficiency: You're not treating the cause if you just stop the irritation and itching with an over-the-counter ointment.

❧ FATIGUE

There can be many causes of fatigue. A comprehensive protocol should also address diet and the role of food sensitivities.

❧ GALLBLADDER PROBLEMS

Dr. Jonathan Wright, a respected holistic medical doctor, states that in his experience most cases of gallstones do not need surgery. He reports that the patients in his care often recover from gallstones if their food sensitivities are addressed. By removing certain foods from your diet, you may be able to prevent inflammation of the bile duct.

❧ HEADACHE

Many people get headaches immediately after eating certain foods. My wife has that problem with tomatoes. Chronic migraine headaches can be caused by food sensitivities.

(continued)

🐦 HEARTBURN

Instead of popping antacids all day long to prevent or treat heartburn, it's a good idea to look at the role of diet. Food sensitivities might be a cause. Unless you have an underlying stomach infection, foods and stress are likely causing your symptoms—which may immediately improve when you identify the culprits.

🐦 HEMORRHOIDS

One of my colleagues in Portland, Oregon, Dr. Steve Gardener, has a practice devoted almost exclusively to the natural treatment of hemorrhoids. To avoid flare-ups, he says, just follow the procedures to identify your food sensitivities, then avoid the foods that are causing problems. Most common on his list are citrus fruits, tomatoes, wheat, and sugar. This agrees with my own observation of the common-problem foods.

🐦 HYPOGLYCEMIA

Reactions to food sensitivities can cause blood-sugar changes. If you suffer from hypoglycemia, investigate the role foods can be playing.

🐦 IMMUNE DEFICIENCY

Food sensitivities waste immune power. If you are prone to getting sick easily or have an illness (such as HIV or tuberculosis) that leaves you open to secondary infections, then food-sensitivity therapy is highly recommended.

🐦 INFLAMMATORY BOWEL DISEASE

Crohn's disease and ulcerative colitis can be greatly helped with food-sensitivity therapy. As you cut out the offending foods, you'll probably note a sharp decrease in the variety of digestive symptoms you're experiencing. I have seen some patients become symptom-free as a result of a change in diet.

🐦 IRRITABLE BOWEL SYNDROME

This is really another name for stress, poor digestion, and food sensitivities. Dramatic improvements are generally seen when the reactive foods are identified and treated.

🐦 PSORIASIS

Many people with this condition experience improvement with food-sensitivity therapy. Although I have seen mixed results, it's worth trying.

🐦 SCHIZOPHRENIA

Dr. Abraham Hoffer, a leading authority on the natural treatment of schizophrenia, has found that food sensitivities can be a major contributor to this disease. Wheat and milk are high on the list of common food offenders.

🐦 SINUSITIS

I have found chronic sinusitis often involves wheat and/or cow's milk allergy.

🐦 SKIN RASH

Any unexplainable skin rash can be a result of food sensitivities.

🐦 VAGINITIS

Chronic cases of vaginitis can be related in part to food sensitivities. Milk and sugar are commonly involved.

Garlic

It isn't hard for me to believe that garlic (*Allium sativum*) is one of the bestselling supplements in North America and Europe. I would estimate that half of all my patients over the age of 50 are taking garlic supplements, whether or not I've recommended it for them. But it's actually appropriate that so many people are taking garlic supplements or eating more garlic for their health, as it's one of the most well-researched herbs in the world.

Even my grandmother is a garlic-taking advocate. As a child, she got into the habit of eating raw garlic every day, and she continues the habit to this day. She says that whenever she feels a cold or sore throat coming on, she just eats more garlic and she doesn't get sick.

To date, more than 200 human studies and at least 800 animal studies have contributed to our understanding of the effects of garlic. Many of these studies have pointed to the conclusion that garlic is a powerful aid in the fight against heart disease and cancer—so, it's natural that so many people are motivated to use this clinically proven wonder herb.

Garlic has many extraordinary attributes both as a food and supplement. Garlic's main medicinal uses are for cardiovascular protection, as it improves cholesterol levels, lowers blood pressure, inhibits blood clots, and improves circulation. In fact, it is one of the premier herbs for protection against cardiovascular disease and infectious diseases as well as cancer.

GOOD BURN

A member of the lily family, garlic is in the same genus (*Allium*) as onion. The Latin translation of *Allium* means "hot" or "burning," and the word "garlic" translates to "spear plant." This refers to the leaves of the garlic plant that have a spearlike shape.

Garlic is a staple in the diets of many different cultures. It has long been recognized for its valuable medicinal properties. We know from Sanskrit records that are 5,000 years old that Middle Eastern people have long cultivated garlic and used it as a medicinal remedy. It was widely traded throughout the Middle East, and the Ancient Greek and Roman physicians relied on garlic to treat a host of conditions including low energy, parasites, respiratory ailments, and poor digestion. It also became an important part of traditional Chinese medicine.

In 1858, Louis Pasteur confirmed garlic's antibacterial properties. In both World Wars, soldiers relied on this herb's powerful antiseptic properties to help prevent gangrene. In fact, it was so widely used among Russian soldiers in World War II that it earned the nickname "Russian penicillin."

GOOD CONSTITUENTS

Garlic has had many different constituents identified. Raw garlic cloves contain a high amount of a sulfur-containing compound called alliin, as well as the enzyme alliinase. Garlic also contains amino acids, vitamins, and minerals such as selenium and germanium.

Allicin is broken down in the body into other compounds, including one called diallyl disulfide. Allicin, diallyl disulfide, and other "metabolites" (the products of metabolism) are responsible for garlic's strong smell and pungent taste as well as many of the medicinal benefits. But these series of metabolic conversions only occur when you eat raw garlic. Aged garlic extract is rich in water-soluble sulphur compounds such as S-allyl cysteine (SAC), S-allyl mercaptocysteine (SAMC), and S-methyl cysteine, and gamma-glutamyl cysteine derivatives. If you eat raw garlic, of course, the fragrance lingers for a long time. For that reason alone, many people prefer to take garlic supplements in a form such as ground garlic powder contained in a capsule.

DOSAGE

Raw garlic provides medicinal effects. Not many people chew raw garlic, but if you do, the recommendation is ½ to 1 whole clove daily.

More commonly, garlic is used in cooking, but as I've mentioned, some of the benefits are lost when garlic is heated.

To take the more conventional route, you can find garlic supplements in supermarkets and pharmacies as well as health-food stores, and they do have the distinct advantage of being odor-free. Capsules and tablets contain the ground powder, while soft gels are made up of garlic oil. Each form contains different active constituents of garlic and have various medicinal effects depending on the product. The type of garlic with

the most published studies is aged garlic extract.

Garlic potencies vary depending on the product. A typical dose is 600 to 900 mg daily. For aged garlic extract, take 600 mg one to two times daily.

WHAT ARE THE SIDE EFFECTS?

Garlic has no known toxicity. However, some people experience digestive upset from eating garlic or taking garlic supplements.

Garlic does have natural blood-thinning effects, so you should discuss its use with your doctor if you are on blood-thinning medications such as aspirin, Coumadin, and others. Also, if you are planning to have surgery, discuss your garlic use with your surgeon beforehand. He or she may advise you to cut down on the dose.

Breast-feeding mothers should be cautious about eating a lot of garlic or taking a lot of garlic supplements. Garlic can contribute to colic because it passes from the breast milk into the baby's intestinal system.

GARLIC

RECOMMENDATIONS FROM THE NATURAL PHYSICIAN FOR . . .

ANTIMICROBIAL EFFECTS

Garlic exerts a wide spectrum of antimicrobial activity against viruses, bacteria, fungi, and worms. I find that garlic usually works best to build immunity and prevent infections, rather than treating acute conditions—with the exception of respiratory tract infections like sore throat, bronchitis, and pneumonia. (A number of patients have told me that when they get an upper respiratory tract infection, they just load up on garlic and soon feel better.) Garlic is excellent on a long-term basis for those with an overgrowth of yeast in their systems and for women who have vaginal yeast infections.

People who have immune suppressive conditions, such as HIV/AIDS and tuberculosis, are at serious risk of developing secondary infections from many different organisms. Garlic is one natural option to help with protection from these infectious agents.

AORTA ELASTICITY PROBLEMS

Long-term use of garlic helps to protect the elasticity of the aorta. The aorta is a huge blood vessel that carries oxygenated blood out of the heart, branching out into other arteries to feed blood to the rest of the body. Stiffening of the aorta is associated with aging as well as with high blood pressure and cholesterol imbalances.

Elasticity is particularly important to help prevent an aortic aneurysm, a life-threatening event. (If the blood vessel wall weakens, losing its integrity and flexibility, there's a chance the aorta may burst.) Researchers who conducted a 1997 study of garlic's properties came to the conclusion that "garlic intake had a protective effect on the elastic properties of the aorta related to aging in humans."

BLOOD CLOTTING

Garlic has a direct effect on the blood's clotting activities. It is known to prevent the clumping of platelets, which are cells that cause blood clotting to occur. Excessive clumping (medically termed as aggregation) is linked to cardiovascular disease because it contributes to poor circulation.

Garlic also lowers fibrinogen, a protein that is involved in blood clotting, which is also highly associated with cardiovascular disease.

CANCER

Population studies have shown that garlic reduces the risk of cancer of the colon, esophagus, and stomach. One study looked at 41,000 American women and found that one or more servings a week of garlic was associated with a 35% decrease in the risk of colon cancer. It is thought that garlic's sulfur compounds are key in preventing these types of cancers by helping to control carcinogens (cancer-causing substances).

CARDIOVASCULAR DISEASE

Investigators at the Research and Education Institute (REI) at Harbor-UCLA

(continued)

Medical Center have found in a human study that AGE supplementation reduces or inhibits plaque formation in the heart's arteries. In a yearlong, double-blind, randomized clinical trial, researchers administered 1,200 mg of AGE to a group of patients who had a history of bypass surgery and were currently taking statin therapies. The control group received a placebo. Using electron beam tomography, researchers were able to evaluate artery health. After a year, the group taking aged garlic extract demonstrated a 67% slowing of calcified plaque in the coronary artery. This group also had a reduction in homocysteine and LDL cholesterol, with a tendency toward increased HDL cholesterol.

🐗 COMMON COLD

As you may have expected, garlic supplements have been shown to prevent the common cold when taken preventatively.

🐗 HIGH BLOOD PRESSURE

High blood pressure is recognized as one of the leading causes of heart disease, and garlic has been shown to have mild blood-pressure-lowering effects. Clinically, I would not rely on garlic alone to lower blood pressure. It should be used in conjunction with corrective changes in diet and lifestyle, and specific blood-pressure-lowering supplements such as hawthorn berry, ginkgo, magnesium, and calcium.

🐗 HIGH CHOLESTEROL

The most popular use of garlic is to protect against cardiovascular disease. Many studies have shown that garlic lowers total cholesterol, and scientists believe it does this by interfering with the manufacture of cholesterol in the liver.

More than 250 scientific studies have been published, most suggesting that garlic protects the cardiovascular system by lowering cholesterol and triglycerides, and inhibiting blood clots. In an overview of 16 prominent garlic studies, including a total of 952 people, researchers concluded that garlic lowered total cholesterol levels by 12% after one to three months of treatment. Eleven of the studies used dried garlic powder at a daily dosage ranging from 600 to 900 mg.

Garlic had a similar positive effect in the trials that looked at triglyceride levels, lowering health-threatening levels of triglycerides by as much as 13%, without having an adverse effect on the level of HDLs (the "good" cholesterol).

Other studies have shown that garlic can lower the LDLs ("bad" cholesterol) while also increasing HDLs. Garlic has also been shown in studies to reduce the oxidation of cholesterol, which is now recognized as a way to help control the development of heart disease.

I usually advise patients to take garlic for at least a few months. It takes at least that long, I've found, before garlic has a significant impact on cholesterol levels.

🐗 SYSTEMIC TOXICITY

Garlic is one of the best foods and supplements to use to promote detoxification. The high sulfur content helps the liver to detoxify various substances so that they can be metabolized and excreted from the body.

Gelsemium

Tori, a 29-year-old mother who had just come down with flu, described the muscle ache as being "like someone had beaten me."

She had other symptoms as well. "I have the chills and a little diarrhea. It was hard getting out of bed to get to your office."

But she was strongly motivated to come see me. Her daughter's birthday was just two days away.

Tori's appearance wasn't promising. Her eyes looked heavy and droopy. Even in the warm examination room, she kept on her jacket to ward off the recurrent bouts of chills.

But I was glad she'd come. I didn't know whether homeopathic gelsemium would help her recover in the requisite 48 hours. But I did know that if she took it, she'd be feeling a lot better by the day of the party.

I made my recommendation and, as I requested, Tori called me the next afternoon to report how she was feeling. She said that her chills had subsided, muscles were much less achy, and her energy had improved. I was happy to find out later that she had recovered well enough to host her daughter's birthday party.

Gelsemium is the homeopathic preparation of yellow jasmine. Most homeopathic practitioners know it as a major flu remedy. It is also a top remedy for fatigue and headaches. It's also the remedy commonly recommended by naturopathic and homeopathic physicians for neurological conditions such as multiple sclerosis and tremors. Gelsemium is also the most common remedy for stage fright.

As with every homeopathic remedy, there are specific symptoms that suggest someone will readily benefit from gelsemium. People requiring gelsemium tend to exhibit four symptoms, referred to as the four D's: dizziness, drowsiness, droopiness, and "dumbness." The last refers to the fact that the person feels too tired to concentrate. These symptoms help you pick this remedy whether a person has the flu or a more complicated illness such as chronic fatigue syndrome.

DOSAGE

For acute illness such as the flu, I recommend two pellets of 30C potency to be given two to four times daily. Lower potencies can also be used and may be effective with some people.

You usually don't have to take the remedy for more than two or three days. Practitioners often give one dose of a higher potency such as 200C, which is enough to help the body recover from acute illness.

For chronic health conditions such as chronic fatigue syndrome, I recommend a lower potency, such as 6C, taken one to two times daily. The pellets of this concentration can also be taken on an "as needed" basis, whenever they provide relief or improve your condition.

WHAT ARE THE SIDE EFFECTS?

As with most homeopathic remedies, side effects are not a concern. When I recommend gelsemium for acute illnesses, I find that it either helps or there is no effect at all. I do recommend, however, that anyone with a chronic condition such as multiple sclerosis or chronic fatigue syndrome consult with a homeopathic practitioner in addition to your regular medical doctor.

Gelsemium is safe to use with children without the worry of side effects.

GELSEMIUM

RECOMMENDATIONS FROM THE NATURAL PHYSICIAN FOR . . .

🐦 ANXIETY

You can take gelsemium if you have anxiety caused by anticipation of a future event, such as an exam or speaking (a *very* common concern!). This is the main homeopathic remedy for stage fright, especially when the fear is so intense that it causes diarrhea. If you find you actually tremble from anxiety about an upcoming event, then this is the best remedy. It's also helpful to take if you have anxiety about an upcoming plane flight.

🐦 DIARRHEA

Gelsemium is indicated for acute illness, such as the flu, where diarrhea occurs. It is a specific remedy for diarrhea caused by anxiety.

🐦 FATIGUE

Patients who have endured chronic fatigue for months or years may recover completely if they take this remedy. The person who needs gelsemium feels apathetic, weak (especially the legs), and wants to sleep all day. If you're so tired it's hard to keep your head up, I recommend this remedy. It is also used to help recover from jet lag.

🐦 FLU

Gelsemium is the most common remedy for the flu. If you do not know which homeopathic remedy to use, try gelsemium first. You'll probably get good results if you're feeling as if your muscles are bruised, you have a low-grade fever with no thirst, and you have chills that run up and down your back.

🐦 HEADACHES

This is an excellent remedy for the kinds of headaches that begin in the back of the head or neck and then radiate to your forehead. A unique symptom that suggests this remedy will help is if your headache improves after urinating. I also recommend taking it if your tongue and head feel heavy.

🐦 MONONUCLEOSIS

Gelsemium is a main remedy for mononucleosis and can help you cope with all the fatigue that goes with it. This remedy works well against viral infections like mono. It is also indicated in cases where a person has had mono at one time, but never felt well since then.

Gentian Root

"It just doesn't make sense, Dr. Mark," said Arthur a 40-year-old business executive. "For the past two years, I've been eating an excellent diet. I rarely have junk food. I avoid fast-food restaurants and stay away from red meat and sugar. My wife prepares almost all my meals. But I still have this problem with bloating."

Arthur described how, after a meal, he always had to undo his belt and unbuckle his pants. Along with bloating and gas, Arthur sometimes got abdominal cramps that were extremely painful.

"I've seen two different gastroenterolo-gists, and they can't find anything wrong," Arthur told me.

"How is your stress level—low, medium, or high?" I asked.

"It's low." He must have thought I looked skeptical, because he quickly added, "It really is. I had a lot of stress three to four years ago from my business, but things are great now."

Following our appointment that day, I had the lab do a comprehensive stool analy-sis for Arthur. We met later so we could go over the results of this and other tests.

I told him that the stool analysis showed he was not breaking down protein very effectively and he had some yeast over-growth in his intestine. Briefly, I explained that the "overgrowth" simply meant his body—or the undigested food in his intes-tine—was producing an overabundance of yeast that could potentially cause health problems.

"Why didn't those other doctors find this out?" Arthur asked.

"Well, the average stool test is pretty basic. The report leaves out quite a bit, unless the doctor asks for specific tests. In your case, the test was done by a lab we often use that specializes in stool analysis. So the test was very comprehensive."

"How did I get these problems?"

"Based on your history and this test, I think the stress you experienced three to four years ago took its toll on your digestive system. You said you never had digestive problems until a few years ago, suggesting to me that the problems began earlier, dur-ing that stressful period."

I went on to explain that when your body is under stress, you have less blood flow to the digestive organs and more to the brain and muscles. There's also less nerve stimula-tion, which affects the organs of the diges-tive tract. When digestive organs don't work at peak efficiency, you don't break food down so well.

"In your case, you're not breaking down protein very well. As a result it causes the digestive symptoms you are experiencing," I concluded.

"Why am I still having problems, even though I'm not stressed anymore?" asked Arthur.

"Even though your stress level is no longer a problem, your digestive tract has not recovered. We need to get your nervous system and digestive organs back into gear again. We can do that with natural medicines."

"Good. What should I take?" asked Arthur.

"I get really good results with herbal medicines, particularly one called gentian root. It stimulates the digestive organs to work more effectively. It's great for stimulating the stomach to produce more hydrochloric acid, which is mainly what breaks down protein. After a couple of months of taking gentian root, your digestive organs will be retrained to work more efficiently."

"That sounds great," said Arthur. "Now, what should I do about the yeast?"

"Don't worry about that. The yeast is feeding off the byproducts of poor digestion. Once we get your digestive system working better, the yeast will die off because it will have nothing to eat."

As Arthur went on a regimen of gentian root over the next two months, he noticed that his digestive symptoms were constantly improving. He no longer had to loosen his pants after he ate. A follow-up stool analysis, four months later, showed normal levels of yeast in his stool.

GETTING BETTER WITH BITTERS

The Bible makes several references to the health benefits of bitter herbs such as gentian root (*Gentian lutea* and related species). The plant grows wild in Europe and throughout Asia. In many cultures in these areas, people recognize the health benefits of gentian and other bitter herbs. They are used to help digest large or fatty meals, and to increase the digestive powers of the elderly or those with chronic disease. Gentian is considered to have cooling and drying qualities, which is significant to practitioners of Chinese medicine who help their patients "balance out" one body system by introducing food and herbs that have opposing qualities. (So someone with a warm constitution would benefit from the cooling effect of gentian root.)

Historically, bitters have always been taken in the form of liquid, so that one would taste the bitterness on the tongue. Gentian happens to be one of the most bitter substances known. According to Dr. Rudolf Weiss, "The bitter taste (of gentian) persists even in a dilution of 1:20,000. It is the most important of all European bitters."

It is believed that when bitter receptors on your tongue are stimulated, a reflex occurs that stimulates the vagus nerve. This nerve is known to stimulate the digestive organs to produce the enzymes necessary for digestion.

Studies have shown that gentian can also stimulate stomach function even if you don't actually put it on your tongue and taste it. This is an important issue for those who prefer to avoid the bitter taste and take gentian root in capsule form. I have used it in capsule form with good results.

One study involving 205 people found that gentian root capsules gave quick and dramatic relief of constipation, flatulence, appetite loss, vomiting, heartburn, abdominal pain, and nausea. Gentian is particularly good for improving stomach function.

DOSAGE

The recommended dosage is 10 to 20 drops in a small amount of water (2 ounces) or 300 to 600 mg of the capsule form taken 5 to 15 minutes before meals. With this "lead time," the digestive juices can begin to kick in before you start eating.

I have found that gentian can still be helpful to stimulate the digestive system when taken with or shortly after meals. It can also be taken in tincture formulas that mask the bitter taste.

Gentian works well in combination with other bitter herbs such as wormwood. It also works well with scutellaria, which relaxes the nervous system and stimulates stomach function.

WHAT ARE THE SIDE EFFECTS?

Gentian should be used with caution by those who have active ulcers, which can be aggravated by the herb.

Pregnant women and nursing mothers should also avoid it, since the effects on an unborn infant are not known.

GENTIAN ROOT

RECOMMENDATIONS FROM THE NATURAL PHYSICIAN FOR . . .

⌐ ANEMIA

Vitamins and minerals that are essential to your health can't be absorbed very well if your stomach acid is low. By boosting the action of your stomach acid, gentian root can help ensure that you don't suffer from some deficiencies—particularly from vitamin B12 and folic acid—which could conceivably cause problems like fatigue, poor memory, and poor circulation.

Also, the iron that comes from food is not absorbed very efficiently when your stomach acid is low. Gentian root improves the levels of acid in the stomach.

⌐ CANDIDA

Many people take drugs or supplements to kill intestinal Candida, which is an overgrowth of yeast. While there may be initial improvement if you take this approach, many people experience relapses.

I learned many years ago that most cases of intestinal yeast overgrowth are in large part due to poor stomach and digestive function. By using gentian, and thus improving digestion and absorption, you stop the development of metabolic toxins that feed the yeast. Once their food supply is cut off, they die.

⌐ CONSTIPATION

Aside from not having enough dietary fiber, water, and exercise, some people suffer from constipation because the digestive organs and colon are not receiving enough nerve and hormonal stimulation, and peristalsis does not occur. Gentian root has a tonic effect on the entire digestive tract.

Also, the stimulation of bile flow from the gallbladder improves stool movement through the intestines and colon.

(continued)

⚹ FOOD ALLERGIES AND FOOD SENSITIVITIES

Many cases of food sensitivities are the result of poor digestion, especially due to inadequate protein breakdown. I have found that gentian is a valuable, long-term treatment for food sensitivities.

⚹ HEADACHES

Gentian is often prescribed for people who get frontal headaches, especially when the headaches are related to eating.

⚹ INDIGESTION AND IRRITABLE BOWEL SYNDROME

Since gentian targets all the major organs of digestion, it can be used as a tonic for many digestive complaints. Europeans often use gentian or other bitters to prevent indigestion after eating large or rich meals. It's especially helpful to have gentian along when you're having a big holiday meal.

⚹ LOW APPETITE

Interestingly, gentian has been used as an adjunctive treatment for anorexia because it stimulates appetite. It is also good to use for people with chronic illnesses who have reduced appetite because of the disease or medicine they're taking.

I have prescribed gentian root to children who had flu or pneumonia, which are infections that often cause them to lose their appetite. Their appetite soon comes back with gentian—which is important for nutritional reasons.

Ginger Root

"I just got back from Mexico and I think I got poisoned!" said Ned, a patient of mine, over the phone.

"What do you mean?"

"For the past two days I have had watery diarrhea and now I have sore throat. I am feeling chills in my back as well. It must have been something I ate—or something in the water."

"Ah, the old Montezuma's revenge!"

Momentarily felled by the problem, Ned was staying with his sister-in-law in Los Angeles. The diarrhea was so bad that he didn't think he could make it into my La Jolla office, and asked me if I could recommend something that would be readily available.

"Have your sister-in-law pick up some fresh ginger root from the local grocery store," I suggested. "Cut a half-inch and steep it in one cup of water for ten minutes." I recommended that he drink one cup of the ginger tea every couple of hours. "That should help the diarrhea and sore throat."

The next day I had another call from Ned. "Ninety percent better," he reported. "Hard to believe I was getting ready to go to the emergency room yesterday!"

From what Ned was telling me, it wouldn't be necessary to see him. But I did make a recommendation for his next trip to Mexico: "Take along some *Acidophilus* and garlic supplements," I said, noting that it would prevent infection of the digestive tract. I didn't have to tell him to also keep some fresh ginger root on hand for just such an emergency.

NOT JUST FOR COOKIES

For centuries, ginger (*Zingiber officinale*) has been widely valued as a medicinal herb.

It is one of the most widely prescribed herbs by practitioners of Ayurvedic and Chinese traditional medicines. The botanical name for ginger is "zingiber," which, in Sanskrit, means "shaped like a horn." Technically speaking, the root is actually a rhizome, a stem that runs underneath the surface of the ground.

It's most commonly used to treat digestive disorders and arthritis in all the healing traditions. It is known as a warming herb, especially suited to people with "cold constitutions," and it's said to enhance circulation. Chinese herbalists use fresh ginger to "warm the lung and stomach."

Ginger is prescribed in Chinese medicine for the common cold, flu, coughs, vomiting, nausea and general digestive upset, and bleeding. It also reduces the toxicity of other herbs, so it's essentially an antidote to plants that might have side effects. Also, as Ned's case demonstrates, ginger can help protect an intestinal tract that has been ravaged by tainted or toxic food.

To practitioners of traditional Chinese medicine, every form of ginger root has certain distinct properties. Fresh ginger has a warming effect on the exterior of the body, while the dried ginger is apt to be recommended for warming the middle of the body.

One of the more intriguing Chinese medicine cures is quick-fried ginger, which is made by frying ginger until the surface is slightly blackened. Practitioners say this is the type that's effective for stopping bleeding and treating conditions that affect the lower abdomen.

Today, ginger is used by herbalists and physicians to treat colds, arthritis, digestive conditions, respiratory tract infections, headaches, motion sickness, and cardiovascular disease.

As with many herbs, ginger has many different active constituents. Dried ginger root contains between 1% and 4% volatile oils, which account for the strong taste and aroma. (The volatile oils include bisabolene, zingiberene, and zingiberol.) Two of the pungent principles—gingerol and shogaol—are believed to be responsible for a lot of the medicinal effects.

Ginger also contains proteolytic enzymes that help to digest proteins and reduce inflammation. Many commercial products are standardized to the constituent gingerol.

DIGESTIVE POWER

Ginger has the unique ability to improve many organs that are involved with digestion. Known as an "aromatic bitter," it tonifies the intestinal muscles and stimulates the digestive organs. It also stimulates secretion of bile from the liver and gallbladder, which helps digest fats. Ginger is also a well-known carminative, meaning that it can reduce gas and bloating.

ANTI-INFLAMMATORY

Ginger acts as a natural anti-inflammatory by inhibiting the release of prostaglandins and other chemicals in the body that promote inflammation and pain. Unlike nonsteroidal medications such as aspirin, it does not have the potential to damage the stomach, liver, and kidneys. For centuries, people used ginger as an anti-inflammatory without knowing how or why it worked. Modern tests have now proven the herb's anti-inflammatory powers.

CIRCULATION AND CARDIOVASCULAR HEALTH

Ginger promotes cardiovascular health by making platelets (cells responsible for blood clots) less likely to clump together. This preventive action allows the blood to keep flowing smoothly and helps prevent hardening of the arteries.

Studies have shown that this protective effect is achieved by inhibiting the formation of thromboxanes, substances that promote blood clotting. Other substances in ginger promote the synthesis of prostacyclin, a component that helps prevent platelets from "aggregating" or clumping together.

Animal studies have also shown that ginger improves the pumping ability of the heart.

DOSAGE

Fresh ginger root can be made into tea. It's also sold in capsules, tablets, and tinctures. I have found all these forms to work well.

The tea is relaxing and works well for digestive upset, as do the capsule and tincture forms. For the treatment of inflammatory conditions, I recommend a standardized capsule to get high levels of the active constituents that reduce inflammation.

The typical capsule dosage is 500 mg two to four times daily. If you're taking the tincture, I recommend 20 to 30 drops two to three times daily.

WHAT ARE THE SIDE EFFECTS?

Side effects are rare with ginger, though some people (my wife among them!) report heartburn after taking it. In the short term, pregnant women can take ginger for nausea and vomiting related to morning sickness. One to two grams appear to be safe and effective.

Ginger stimulates bile production, so some herbal experts recommend that you should avoid this herb if you have gallstones.

Although I have seen no human studies on drug interactions and ginger, it theoretically may cause a problem with blood-thinning medications such as Coumadin. So check with your physician before using high doses of ginger if you are on a blood-thinning medication.

One last piece of advice you may not find in many books is that ginger root by itself may aggravate those who are very warm-blooded. If you are the type of person who gets warm and sweats easily, then long-term use of ginger is not recommended just because it can cause discomfort by making you even warmer.

GINGER ROOT

RECOMMENDATIONS FROM THE NATURAL PHYSICIAN FOR . . .

🌿 ARTHRITIS

Many herbal medicine experts mention that ginger is effective in treating arthritis, but in day-to-day treatment of patients, I have not found this to be true. Ginger by itself does not usually provide substantial relief. That said, however, it can be helpful to some people as part of a comprehensive herbal formula, such as practitioners of Chinese herbal formulas have created for patients with a "cold constitution."

🌿 BLOATING AND FLATULENCE

Ginger is the remedy par excellence for relieving bloating and flatulence, which is the common result from the Standard American Diet (SAD). It reminds me of one lady who came up to me after a talk, looked around to make sure no one else was listening, and asked if there was anything I could recommend for her 36-year-old son who was having trouble with a lot of gas. It turns out this son was newly married, and his mother was worried that his flatulence would cause marital problems.

I recommended she give her son a bottle of ginger capsules to use with meals. Hopefully it rescued the young groom from some embarrassment—or possibly saved the marriage!

CARDIOVASCULAR DISEASE

Since ginger is a natural blood thinner, it promotes good circulation and therefore improves cardiovascular health. Animal studies show that it helps with the pumping action of the heart. To me, it is most beneficial as a synergestic herb—one that makes other herbs more effective rather than working by itself.

DIARRHEA

There's a specific type of diarrhea, called "cold diarrhea" in Chinese medicine, that ginger seems to help significantly. This is the kind that gives you a case of the chills as well as loose stools. (What's called "hot diarrhea," as you might expect, is the kind where loose stools are accompanied by a feeling of feverishness.)

HIGH CHOLESTEROL

In animal studies, ginger has been found to lower cholesterol levels in rats. Unfortunately, it doesn't show exactly the same effect in humans. But if you're taking ginger for other conditions, there is a possibility that it could also help lower your cholesterol.

MORNING SICKNESS

Ginger has actually been studied as a relief for severe morning sickness. In 19 of the 27 women who took ginger for nausea and vomiting, both symptoms became less frequent within four days of treatment. The dosage of ginger-root capsules was 250 mg taken 4 times daily.

Since publication of the earliest studies, which were done in 1990, many conventional doctors have started to recommend ginger root for morning sickness. (My wife's gynecologist and obstetrician, for instance, recommends it to her patients.) However, I don't advise that women take more than 1 g daily during pregnancy, and there's no reason to continue taking it after the morning sickness passes.

MOTION SICKNESS

Ginger has received a lot of attention for its ability to prevent and treat motion sickness. A study in 1982 revealed that ginger was superior to the drug Dramamine for reducing motion sickness. Not every study since then has supported this finding, but some excellent research done in 1994—involving 1,741 people—confirmed that ginger was indeed very effective in treating motion sickness.

The 1994 study was done with a group of people who were taking a whale-watching trip. Before boarding the boat,

(continued)

people were asked to take various kinds of motion-sickness remedies, ginger among them. (None of the passengers knew which remedy they were being given.) The study showed that 250 mg of ginger was just as powerful as the pharmaceutical medications, but without side effects such as drowsiness.

❧ NAUSEA AND VOMITING
Bad food, flu, chemotherapy, and surgical treatments are just a few of the possible causes of nausea and vomiting. No matter what the cause, however, ginger has been shown to be an effective remedy.

In two studies, ginger helped reduce nausea and vomiting in patients who had just undergone surgery where they received anesthesia. (Anesthesia makes some people very nauseated.) If you are scheduled to have surgery, talk with your surgeon about taking 1 g of ginger before and after surgery.

Ginkgo Biloba

Not long ago, a 45-year-old female patient came to me for the treatment of painful feet. Shawna had seen many doctors—and none had been able to explain the problem or give her an effective treatment.

As with all patients, I talked to her at length—not just about the pain in her feet but also about her lifestyle, her everyday habits, moods, family illnesses, and many other questions that, to some other listener, might have seemed totally unrelated to the pain in her feet. I did not for a moment doubt that the pain was "real." Nor did I doubt that her doctors had done the best they could to diagnose her problem. But something had been missed along the way—obviously, since the unresolved condition continued to aggravate her and cause intense discomfort.

I was struck, however, by one remark she made almost in passing—that her feet often "felt cold." Later on, when I examined her feet, that was the first thing I noticed. She wore practical shoes and thick socks, and she had been sitting in a warm room, yet when I felt her feet they were almost literally like icicles.

But something else was wrong as well, as I discovered when I took the pulse in her feet. Normally, of course, the doctor checks the pulse in your wrist or the side of your neck, where it's strongest. That's usually sufficient, since an MD usually checks for pulse rate. But what I was trying to measure was the *strength* of Shawna's pulse—and when I touched the part of her ankle where the arterial blood flows close to the surface, the area where the pulse should be strongest, I felt almost nothing.

Clearly, her feet were chilly because she had a circulation problem. The flow of warming blood to these extremities was so slight that it wasn't even doing its job of warming her feet from heel to toe. Quite likely, the lack of circulation could also account for the pain.

But what could I "prescribe" that would improve her circulation? Many pharmaceuticals are available, from the powerful blood-thinning agents that are injected into heart-attack victims to common, everyday, over-the-counter aspirin, with its milder blood-thinning properties.

What I recommended for Shawna, however, was a simple extract that comes from the leaf of a very ancient tree—ginkgo biloba.

She took 180 mg each day, in doses of 60 mg three times daily. We kept careful track of her progress during the next few weeks. The circulation to her feet steadily improved. The pain, as well as the chilliness, began to subside.

Shawna's feet were pain free at the end of two months. She continues taking ginkgo to this day—and has never had a recurrence of the chronic foot pain that originally brought her to my door.

What Shawna didn't realize at the time is that ginkgo biloba is one of the most all-around beneficial herbs that anyone could possibly take for his or her health. The power to cure cold feet is only one small fraction of its many powerful attributes.

A POWER PLANT

While ginkgo may well be the most widely publicized herb to come along in the past 50 years, the history of its healing powers certainly predates its current popularity. In fact, the Chinese have known about it and have used it for more than 3,500 years.

Ginkgo ranks among the top five herbs that I prescribe to patients on a daily basis. Millions of people around the world use ginkgo every day. In countries such as Germany and France, where doctors are accustomed to writing herbal prescriptions, ginkgo is among the most commonly prescribed medicines. European doctors use it to treat a wide range of conditions—from memory impairment, dizziness, and ringing in the ears (tinnitus) to headaches and depression. There are even more uses—as Shawna discovered—such as a blood mover for improved circulation.

If ginkgo trees could speak for themselves, some would give first-person accounts of Aztecs, Vikings, and the Battle of Hastings, since the grandparents of the species have lived as long as 1,000 years. Some reach a height of 120 feet, with a girth of 48 inches. Apart from longevity, ginkgoes boast venerable ancestors.

Fossil records show that the ginkgo is the world's oldest living species of tree. It's very hardy, able to thrive in extreme heat and cold, and to withstand the pollution of downtown Los Angeles or New York. It's also almost pest-proof: There doesn't seem to be an insect that can do serious damage to this hardy tree.

The leaves, the source of ginkgo medicinals, are fan-shaped and bilobed, resembling the maidenhair fern. The resemblance is so close, it's sometimes called the "maidenhair tree."

TURNING OVER AN OLD LEAF

Researchers in the 1950s, having heard of the medicinal powers of ginkgo leaves, began mashing and distilling the components in search of the so-called active ingredients—that is, the chemical compounds that seemed to have potential healing power. What are believed to be the key medicinal ingredients have now been identified. I know it would be rash to say these are *all* the active, healing constituents—certainly more will be discovered—but at least we're starting to understand how some of the ginkgo-leaf ingredients make important contributions to improved health.

While the active constituents are important, however, I remind people that it's best to use the whole herb rather than focus on one ingredient or component. Studies have shown that the whole herb plus standardized active constituents are more effective than just using the isolated active constituents.

The two groups of active components include flavone glycosides and terpene lactones. Quality ginkgo products are "standardized" to 24% flavone glycosides and 6% terpene lactones—which is a virtual guarantee that the products contain at least these proportions of those particular ingredients. Such products have the same proportion of these ingredients as the extract that's used in clinical studies.

POTENT CELL PROTECTOR

Flavone glycosides are types of bioflavonoids, the plant-based compounds that are found in oranges and other fruits and vegetables. With bioflavonoids, ginkgo has been blessed with the potent powers of an antioxidant. That means if you take ginkgo, you're less likely to suffer the cellular damage caused by free radicals—unstable molecules that are a result of metabolic activities in the body and environmental pollution.

Many researchers believe that ginkgo produces more antioxidant activity than many of the better-known vitamin antioxidants such as C, E, and beta carotene. Several studies have demonstrated that ginkgo exerts antioxidant activity in the brain, eyes, and cardiovascular system. This could easily explain why ginkgo seems to be effective in the prevention and treatment of diseases that affect those parts of the body—including Alzheimer's disease, strokes, cataracts, macular degeneration, and diabetic retinopathy.

Ginkgo bioflavonoids also protect blood vessels by strengthening and reducing inflammation of their elastic walls. So that's an additional benefit of this herb—significant in helping to relieve varicose veins and reverse the effects of cardiovascular disease.

KEEPING UP CIRCULATION

In addition to the bioflavonoids, ginkgo has another component, unique to this plant. A family of terpene lactones—specifically called ginkgolides and bilobalides—give ginkgo an extraordinary ability to increase circulation to the brain and extremities. The substances cause the blood vessel walls to relax and dilate, which permits increased blood flow. They also have what's called a "tonifying effect" on the venous system, allowing for the more efficient return of blood to the heart.

Ginkgo also has a natural blood-thinning effect. It helps to prevent blood platelets from sticking together—and platelets are the cells that form blood clots.

The way ginkgo improves circulation is particularly impressive. In one study where researchers measured the blood flow through capillaries in healthy adults, they found a 57% increase in blood flow among those who were regularly taking ginkgo. This finding is particularly important to seniors. As we age, we're more likely to have blockages in the blood flow that reaches the brain and other parts of the body. These problems are directly attributable to plaque buildup in the arteries. Ginkgo acts as sort of a bypass mechanism, helping the blood make its way through partially clogged arteries.

NERVE RENEWAL

The ginkgolides also help protect nerve cells from being damaged. This is important for people who are recovering from a stroke. In addition, some ongoing research will probably show whether ginkgo has the benefits that it's reputed to possess for people who are recovering from brain trauma. What's certain is that nerve cells need the kind of protection that ginkgo provides—particularly people (such as those with diabetes) who have problems with neuropathy (nerve disorder).

DOSAGE

As a standard dosage, I recommend a ginkgo extract standardized to 24% flavone glycosides and 6% terpene lactones. Dosages used in studies range from 120 mg to 360 mg daily. Most of my patients take 60 mg two to four times daily, for a daily total of 120 to 240 mg. The vast majority report beneficial results.

For severe cases, like early-stage Alzheimer's disease, I recommend that people take 240 to 360 mg daily.

If you start to take ginkgo for a particular condition or for general health, I suggest you continue taking it for at least eight weeks to assess its therapeutic effect. Most of my patients who take it to improve their memory or help their circulation (like Shawna, the woman who came to me with foot pain) notice the beginnings of improvements within about a month.

Ginkgo supplements are available in capsule, tablet, and tincture form.

WHAT ARE THE SIDE EFFECTS?

Doctors, researchers, and practitioners have noted very few adverse effects among people who take ginkgo. A small number—less than 1% of those who take it—have reported mild digestive upset.

Other rare side effects mentioned in the literature include headaches and dizziness. I've had very few patients who complained of these problems, and in those few cases, the side effects disappeared when I lowered the dosage.

One warning, however. If you're taking a blood-thinning medication such as Coumadin or aspirin, be sure to notify your doctor. These medications, like ginkgo, have a blood-thinning effect—and the cumulative doses might be more than you need. Your doctor can monitor how well your blood is clotting through regular blood work, by taking blood samples and testing them in the lab.

GINKGO BILOBA
RECOMMENDATIONS FROM THE NATURAL PHYSICIAN FOR . . .

❧ **ALZHEIMER'S DISEASE**

Ginkgo has shown to be of benefit in cases of senility and Alzheimer's disease. In fact, it has been approved for the treatment of Alzheimer's disease by the German government. While it's not a cure—none exists—ginkgo has been shown effective in delaying the mental deterioration that often occurs rapidly in the early stage of the disease.

A study done in 1994, involving 40 patients who had early-stage Alzheimer's disease, demonstrated that 240 mg of ginkgo biloba extract taken daily for three months produced measurable improvements in memory, attention, and mood.

Most of the patients I see do not have Alzheimer's, but they experience a general decline in short-term memory and concentration. Ginkgo is at the top of

(continued)

the list for safe and effective supplements I recommend. Plus, it is not overly expensive—about $12 to $16 per month at the dosage I recommend—so you won't break the bank if you take it regularly.

🐚 ATTENTION DEFICIT DISORDER (ADD)

Although I have not seen any studies on ginkgo and ADD, I have had parents tell me that it helps their children with concentration and memory with schoolwork. These are specifically children with memory and concentration problems—*not* hyperactivity.

🐚 CIRCULATORY DISEASES

Ginkgo is one of the best medicines in the world for improving circulation to the hands and feet. For this reason it's an effective treatment for intermittent claudication.

People who have intermittent claudication—which is really a circulatory problem—experience pain and severe cramping in the lower legs, particularly while walking. This condition is particularly prevalent among the elderly. Many clinical studies have shown ginkgo can help alleviate the condition in three to six months if you take daily dosages of 120 to 160 mg.

Ginkgo has also been shown to improve the condition of people who have Raynaud's disease, a condition where the hands or feet instantly turn blue if you just reach for something in the freezer or step outside on a cold day. (For some reason, women are much more likely than men to suffer from this condition.) Again, the problem is circulatory. I have frequently recommended ginkgo—

and achieved positive results—when patients were bothered by cold hands and feet.

Finally, people with diabetes are particularly prone to have poor circulation in their extremities. Supplementing with ginkgo is certainly beneficial.

🐚 DEPRESSION

Ginkgo is an effective natural antidepressant when the depression is related to poor blood flow to the brain. When blood flow improves, more oxygen and nutrients naturally reach the brain cells as well as extremities.

Ginkgo also improves the activity of neurotransmitters, the brain's chemical messengers. A study of elderly patients who took doses of 240 mg of ginkgo extract daily showed that many experienced significant improvements in mood after only four weeks. The improvements were even more dramatic after eight weeks of taking the same concentration of extract.

🐚 HIGH BLOOD PRESSURE

Ginkgo is one of the main herbs I recommend to patients who have hypertension or high blood pressure. It helps to relax the artery walls, thus reducing pressure within the blood vessels. A typical dosage would be 120 to 180 mg daily.

🐚 IMPOTENCE

Impotence occurs in the vast majority of cases because there's poor circulation to erectile tissue. Instead of recommending Viagra to patients with impotence problems, I usually start with a prescription of ginkgo biloba (and sometimes some ginseng as well). Ginkgo works very well, is much less expensive, and doesn't have any side effects—unlike Viagra.

Because ginkgo improves penile blood flow, it provides the physiological basis for an erection. In one study, 50% of patients treated for impotence using 60 mg of ginkgo per day regained potency.

I generally recommend 180 to 240 mg of ginkgo in the treatment of impotence. If ginkgo doesn't help, I'll have the patient tested for the hormones DHEA and testosterone. If these hormones are deficient, I'll recommend they be used in therapeutic dosages.

ᴥ MEMORY LOSS

Even if you don't remember things so well as you used to, the awareness of memory loss is not a signal of oncoming Alzheimer's disease or senility. Memory loss is quite common—and understandable, given the fact that we do tend to lose some memory capacity as we age and that we are quite susceptible to distractions.

"Cerebral vascular insufficiency" is a phrase that's often used to describe poor blood flow to the brain. Often, the problem gets worse as people get older because people gradually experience atherosclerosis—hardening of the arteries—which sharply decreases the efficiency of blood flow. Simply put, when the brain doesn't get enough oxygenated, nourishing blood, we're more likely to have memory loss. (Depression, as noted, can also be related to restricted blood flow.) Given its power to improve blood flow, ginkgo biloba is the treatment of choice. Once the brain cells get

the oxygen and blood-sugar needed to help them function properly, memory improves. Clinical studies have confirmed that significant change can occur in as little as 8 to 12 weeks. Ginkgo extract has been shown to help cognitive function in elderly people with age-related memory impairment as well as healthy middle-aged adults.

ᴥ PMS

For women who experience cramping, pain, and breast tenderness around the time of their periods, ginkgo may also provide some benefits. I have been surprised to learn that these typical symptoms of PMS might respond to ginkgo. Studies have shown that ginkgo can be helpful in alleviating breast tenderness and fluid retention.

ᴥ RADIATION EFFECTS

After the Chernobyl nuclear accident in 1986, Russian scientists tried a wide variety of treatments to help workers and residents who had been exposed to radiation. Researchers discovered that ginkgo helped combat the effects of radiation. It was found to be a potent agent in fighting free-radical damage to the cells, providing the same antioxidant benefits that help protect normal body cells from the effects of rapid aging.

ᴥ RAYNAUD'S SYNDROME

Ginkgo extract has been shown to decrease the frequency of the painful attacks that often occur with this condition.

(continued)

🐦 RINGING IN THE EARS (TINNITUS)

Studies have been done to test the effectiveness of ginkgo in relieving the condition known as tinnitus, which is simply ringing in the ears. Results have been mixed. I feel it is worth trying if there's the possibility that tinnitus is the result of poor circulation. Sometimes the condition is related to the fact that insufficient blood is reaching the inner ear. In other cases, however, tinnitus occurs when people are exposed to excessive noise—and in those cases, ginkgo doesn't seem to help very much.

Ginkgo can be helpful if you've had acute hearing loss as a result of pressure changes or sound trauma. Even if you don't know the factors that have contributed to loss of hearing, taking this herb might produce some positive effects.

🐦 STROKE

Ginkgo is valuable both in the immediate treatment of stroke and in helping stroke victims during the months or years of recovery. One of the keys to the prevention of stroke is keeping the blood thin. Again, the objective is to improve circulation so sufficient blood gets to the brain. New research is also showing that therapeutic doses of antioxidants may be an important treatment for strokes. As I mentioned, ginkgo provides antioxidant activity as well.

Many doctors who are oriented toward holistic medicine—treatment of the whole patient rather than a single "problem"—often recommend ginkgo to people who are particularly susceptible to a stroke. Among those who need to take special care are anyone with a personal or family history of high blood pressure, atherosclerosis, diabetes—particularly if you're a smoker or if you've had a previous stroke. But remember: Many doctors prescribe pharmaceutical blood-thinning medications after a stroke, so if you're taking one of these, you need to talk to your doctor and have some blood work done before you start taking ginkgo, too.

🐦 VERTIGO

Studies show that ginkgo can improve symptoms of vertigo and equilibrium disorders.

🐦 VISION

Ginkgo is also useful in the prevention and treatment of macular degeneration and diabetic retinopathy. If left untreated, both conditions can result in blindness. Macular degeneration, often associated with age, is the result of nerve degeneration in the particularly sensitive light-receptor cells of the eye. Diabetic retinopathy is a serious eye disease that can lead to blindness.

Ginkgo has been shown to be helpful in both conditions. I also recommend ginkgo as part of a natural treatment for cataracts.

Ginseng

"I have been taking ginseng for about two months. Shouldn't my energy be better by now?"

An electrician who was used to working long hours on an irregular schedule, Will had been taking regular doses from a bottle of ginseng that his wife picked up at the pharmacy. Both of them had read that ginseng was a good energy booster, and Will was expecting to see some improvement.

"It depends on a few things," I replied. "We have to figure out what was causing your low energy. But I'll also need to know what kind of ginseng you're using, and the quality of the ginseng product."

Will had the bottle with him. I glanced at the label, then set it aside while I got a more thorough history. I also ordered some blood work.

Later, I returned to the subject of ginseng.

"I'll bet you've been feeling more irritable and restless since you've been taking the ginseng from that bottle," I speculated.

"That's true!" Will looked startled. "How did you know?"

"You have been taking Chinese ginseng, also called *Panax* ginseng. This can be quite a warming and stimulating herb. You told me that you get warm and sweat very easily. Based on your constitution, Chinese ginseng is not very compatible. It is too warming and stimulating for you and I would have expected that it would aggravate your symptoms."

Like many people who buy off-the-shelf ginseng, Will's wife had no idea there were different types of ginseng, and of course she didn't have a clue what would be best for her husband.

I briefly described the characteristics of each of the most common kinds—Chinese, Siberian, and American.

"You would do much better on Siberian or American ginseng instead of Chinese," I told him. "Because you are so physically active and warm, I am going to recommend the American ginseng."

Two weeks later, Will reported that the switch to American ginseng had the desired effect. He had noticed a distinct improvement in his energy level.

I recommended that he stay on a regular dose as long as it produced the desired effects—improving his energy levels and decreasing the effects of stress at work—and he continued to do so.

GOOD ROOTS FOR ATHLETES

All three types of ginsengs can be used to enhance athletic performance, but Chinese and Siberian ginsengs have produced the best results in research tests.

Chinese ginseng has been shown to increase endurance and quicken recovery time after workouts. A placebo-controlled, double-blind, 20-week trial with male athletes supplementing 200 mg of a standardized Chinese ginseng extract found that it increased performance significantly.

In a study of Siberian ginseng, 12 male athletes were given either the herb or a placebo. Athletes who took Siberian ginseng showed a 23.3% increase in total exercise duration and stamina as compared with only 7.5% among those who were taking a placebo. Athletes who take Siberian ginseng generally notice improved performance and quicker recovery from workouts and competition.

HUMMING WITH GINSENG

Fatigue and stress are universal health problems, and ginseng has a well-earned reputation for addressing both. But the situation with my patient Will is quite typical of what happens when people don't know which kind of ginseng to select.

All varieties are what we call "adaptogens," herbs that essentially help the body to adapt to changes in environment and resist the effects of stress. This term was first used by two Russian scientists to describe the effects of Chinese ginseng and later to its relative, Siberian ginseng. Here's how these adaptogens can help your body cope with the effects of stress and also help with energy production—each in its own, unique way.

🦉 Chinese Ginseng (Panax ginseng)

The Chinese translation for ginseng is "root of man," and the root of this plant is what's used to make the herbal medicines that are so widely used throughout China and Southeast Asia. The "grandparent of ginsengs," and possibly the most well-known herb in the world, is *Panax ginseng*. This comes in two types: white and red. White ginseng is the dried root, and is more cooling and less stimulating than the more potent form of red ginseng, which is steamed and cured (dried over a fire or in the sun). These types of *Panax* have had numerous common names including Asian ginseng, Korean ginseng, Red ginseng, and Ren-Shen.

The word *Panax* is Latin for "panacea"—appropriately enough, as this type of ginseng is highly revered by the Chinese for its health-enhancing effects. The *Panax* variety used to grow wild in China, Japan, Korea, and the eastern portion of Russia; now it's widely cultivated for commercial use in Asia, the United States, and Canada.

Chinese herbalists will tell you that the root of the wild plant is more potent than the cultivated kind. But wild ginseng is now so rare that you'd have to travel to China or Korea on a wild-root chase to find it—and you'd probably end up paying thousands of dollars if you tried to buy the real thing. In my experience, the commercially grown varieties work fine, as long as the herbal preparations are taken appropriately.

Panax ginseng has been used for more than 5,000 years in traditional Chinese medicine. Historically the elderly seized upon it as a rejuvenating tonic. Among its "tonic" effects, *Panax* improves sexual function, increases energy and vitality, helps speed the recovery from illness, and even slows the aging process.

In the not-so-distant past, traditional Chinese herbalists wouldn't even prescribe ginseng for younger people. They recommended "saving" this potent medicine for the elderly. Today, however, *Panax ginseng* is prescribed by Chinese herbalists for anyone who suffers from shock or collapse, heart palpitations, insomnia, or forgetfulness. It's also used to strengthen the lungs—particularly for people with asthma, for improving digestive function, and for combating diabetes. (While it can help type 1 or type 2 diabetes, I mainly recommend it for type 2.)

The exact mechanism of how Chinese ginseng works is not completely understood. Animal and human studies have shown that it supports and strengthens the function of the adrenal glands. These are sometimes called stress glands because they produce stress hormones that enable the body to respond to stress, danger, or threats.

Panax ginseng has a balancing effect on the stress hormones, and it improves the cells' ability to "burn" oxygen as fuel, thus improving energy production and enhancing physical performance. In addition, it helps muscles utilize glycogen, which is the "stored" form of blood-sugar or glucose.

A group of compounds known as ginsenosides are thought to be responsible for many of the therapeutic effects of Chinese ginseng. The ginsenosides Rg1 and Rb1 have been most intensively studied. Rg1 has been shown to stimulate brain and central nervous system activity, allowing increased energy and improved intellectual performance. Rb1 has been shown to relax brain activity and lower blood pressure. So, these two constituents represent both sides of the "adaptogenic" properties of Asian ginseng.

Other ginsenosides, as well as polyacetylenes and polysaccharides, activate the immune system and also prompt anticancer activity. Undoubtedly, other active constituents of ginseng are still to be discovered.

Today, Chinese ginseng is commonly recommended for fatigue, immune enhancement, improved mental alertness, cardiovascular disease, and diabetes. It also serves as a sexual tonic, an athletic-performance enhancer, and a "soother" that helps fight stress. Holistic doctors also recommend it to lower high cholesterol, provide support for the immune system if someone is undergoing chemotherapy and radiation, and for the control of anxiety and depression.

Although there have been at least 400 published studies on Chinese ginseng, the vast majority of experimental work was done on rats. However, researchers are beginning to undertake more human studies.

❧ Siberian Ginseng
(Eleutherococcus senticosus)

When it was reported that a Russian Olympic athlete had taken supplements of Siberian ginseng to improve his endurance and speed his recovery from training, many athletes from other countries took notice. This type of ginseng—or eleuthero, as it's sometimes called—is hardly a novelty. It has long been used by the Siberian people to enhance their quality of life and to reduce their susceptibility to infections.

Though this isn't the same species as Chinese ginseng, it's popular in many of the same countries where *Panax* is used, including northern Korea and Japan. It's been used for more than 2,000 years in China as a tonic for energy and vitality, as well as to prevent respiratory tract infections, cold, and flu.

The Russian medical doctor I. I. Brekhman, the researcher who coined the word "adaptogen," completed many studies of the medicinal effects of Siberian ginseng—paralleling his investigations of *Panax*—in the 1940s and 1950s. He was interested in eleuthero because he could see that its properties were similar to those of *Panax*, though the Siberian variety is more economical to grow commercially. Intensive research continued on Siberian ginseng for the next 30 years.

Eleuthero appears to be the perfect adaptogen. In addition to being a favorite with many athletes, it has also been used by Russian cosmonauts to improve energy and help adapt to their new environment—and by many other Russian workers who appreciate its energizing powers. Interestingly, after the Chernobyl accident, many Russians within range of the fallout area were given Siberian ginseng to counteract the effects of radiation.

While there have been more than 1,000 studies on *Eleutherococcus*, most are in Russian. As with *Panax* ginseng, Siberian ginseng seems to support adrenal gland function and oxygen utilization by the cells. Though Brekhman and other researchers have identified similar healing properties in both the Chinese and Siberian forms, the known active constituents of Siberian ginseng are completely different from those found in Chinese ginseng. The active constituents of Siberian ginseng that have received the most attention are a group of saponins known as eleutherosides.

While there are many different eleutherosides, the forms known as B and E have received the most attention. Siberian ginseng also contains polysaccharides, which are believed to help support immune function.

One of the nice things about Siberian ginseng is that it has a neutral temperature—that is, taking it doesn't necessarily make you warmer or chillier. It seems to be well tolerated by many people, and it can be taken for extended periods of time.

🌿 American Ginseng (Panax quinquefolius)

In contrast to Siberian ginseng, which has a neutral temperature, and Chinese ginseng, which is warming and more stimulating, the species known as American ginseng is a cooling herb.

Panax quinquefolius—the genus and species name of American ginseng—translates as "five-leafed *Panax*." Indigenous to North America, it grows wild in forests of northern and central United States, as well as parts of Canada. It is also commercially grown in the United States, China, and France. Historically, Native Americans such as the Iroquois and Cherokee used American ginseng for a wide variety of medicinal purposes. They used it to treat fevers, improve digestion, heal wounds, and ease menstrual problems. It was also used to relieve shortness of breath.

American ginseng was imported by China in the 1700s and became a highly esteemed herb in the vast formulary of Chinese botanical medicines. Today, most American ginseng still travels from the United States to China, though a small amount is raised in Southeast Asia. Despite the lively export business, it wasn't until lately that the healing benefits of American ginseng were recognized on its home continent.

Chinese doctors value the herb because it's more cooling than Chinese ginseng and can be applied to more health conditions. During hot summer weather, Chinese physicians prescribe it regularly as a cooling tonic.

Despite the differences between American and Chinese ginseng, there are some striking similarities as well. Their appearance is similar, American ginseng being a smaller-looking version of the Chinese root. Also, both these ginsengs need to mature for four years before the roots are ready to be harvested. (Chinese ginseng is best between the fourth and sixth years.)

Both the American and Chinese versions contain similar, active constituents—namely, ginsenosides, which support adrenal gland function. However, the ratio and types of ginsenosides are different. American ginseng contains much more of the Rb1 group, which are less stimulating than the Rg1 group found in Chinese ginseng. The Rb1 ginsenosides in American ginseng are believed to give off nerve-relaxing, anti-inflammatory, antifatigue, fever-reducing, blood-pressure-lowering, pain-relieving, and digestive-tonic properties.

When I recommend either herb to patients, it's often for similar health problems. Both can decrease the effects of stress, and both types of herb help to support the immune system. But because it contains more Rb1 ginsenosides, American ginseng is considered to be the superior herb for treating digestive problems, especially ulcers. It is much better suited for the person who gets warm easily, is "uptight," but not suffering from burnout. Chinese ginseng, by contrast, is preferred for people who are chilly, totally exhausted and depleted, and feeling burned out.

Siberian ginseng is somewhere in the middle, just as its temperature is in the middle range between Chinese and American. Siberian ginseng is for people who are still fairly healthy and need extra support to help combat the effects of stress, athletes being a prime example.

DOSAGE

❧ Chinese Ginseng

I recommend using a product that is standardized between 4% to 7% ginsenosides. The dose is 100 mg two to three times daily.

Be sure to check the label of any product you purchase. On the standardized extract label, it will say *Panax ginseng* C. A. Meyer. This refers to a specific type of Chinese ginseng and the one used in most studies. It was named by C. A. Meyer in 1843 to differentiate it from other ginsengs native to China and North America.

If you can't find the standardized version, I recommend consulting with a reputable Chinese herbalist to make sure you get a quality product and take the proper dosage. *Panax ginseng*, like the other ginsengs, is typically taken for three weeks straight. Some herbalists recommend taking a break every four to eight weeks before resuming its use.

❧ Siberian Ginseng

In most studies where Siberian ginseng has been proven effective, people take 8 to 10 mL of an alcohol extract two to three times daily.

I have also seen good results with a standardized capsule extract containing 0.4% eleutherosides at a dosage of 300 mg taken two to three times daily. For long-term use, I typically have people take Siberian ginseng for four weeks before taking a week off. You can repeat this cycle as often as necessary, as long as you continue to get benefits from the ginseng.

❧ American Ginseng

There is currently no ideal standardization recommended by researchers or herbalists. In my experience, the most effective dosage is 1,000 to 2,000 mg daily of the capsule or 30 to 60 drops (1 to 2 mL) of the tincture taken two to three times daily.

WHAT ARE THE SIDE EFFECTS?

❧ Chinese Ginseng

If you overdose on Chinese ginseng, you may detect symptoms of anxiety and insomnia, as I've witnessed with a few patients. Also, be cautious with this herbal remedy if you have high blood pressure.

Women should not take Chinese ginseng during pregnancy unless they're under the guidance of a practitioner of Asian medicine. (Sometimes, it's helpful to a woman in pregnancy, but its use needs to be monitored by a practitioner.)

I recommend staying away from any other stimulants, including caffeine, when you're taking Chinese ginseng.

Women who have heavy menstrual flow or fibrocystic breast syndrome should avoid this herb unless they have the guidance of a practitioner of Asian medicine.

It is best to not take *Panax ginseng* before bedtime.

❧ Siberian Ginseng

People rarely have side effects from Siberian ginseng, though I've had patients who have trouble sleeping when they take it just before bedtime.

The German Commission E says people with high blood pressure should not use this herb. (I don't agree, since I've seen studies showing that Siberian ginseng can reduce high blood pressure.)

In general, I would caution against taking Siberian ginseng before bedtime, and I recommend that it should be avoided during pregnancy.

🪶 American Ginseng

Side effects to American ginseng are uncommon. Similar to the other ginsengs, some people who are sensitive may notice too much stimulation and require a lower dos-

age—so I recommend that people avoid taking it before bedtime.

At least one study has demonstrated that American ginseng may lower blood-sugar levels, and the authors of that study concluded that people should take it with meals. This would make even more sense for people with diabetes—but if you have diabetes, be sure your doctor knows you're taking it.

Like the other ginsengs, the American variety should not be taken during pregnancy unless you're under the care of a doctor or practitioner who knows how and when to recommend it.

GINSENG

RECOMMENDATIONS FROM THE NATURAL PHYSICIAN FOR . . .

🪶 AGING

Nothing can stop aging, of course, nor is it a "health problem" like arthritis or diabetes. Nevertheless, there are certain herbs with adaptogenic qualities that can be reasonably classified as "anti-aging herbs"—and two types of ginsengs are among the best. Studies show that the Siberian and *Panax ginseng* have a balancing effect on stress hormones. Prolonged, high levels of hormone such as cortisol have been shown to accelerate aging as do the relative deficiency of hormones such as DHEA. Balancing of these hormones with ginseng is a safe way to slow down the aging process.

In addition, all three types of ginseng have been shown to have good antioxidant activity, which is also thought to slow the aging of cells. (The ginsenosides in Chinese and American ginseng are particularly effective.)

The ginsengs have proven themselves to restore vitality. Of course, vitality is a subjective feeling that is hard to quantify with lab tests, but in controlled clinical trials, people taking ginseng (without their knowledge) reported feeling more vital and full of energy than people who were taking a placebo. There are also ways to measure energy in terms of physical response. In one trial with 49 elderly people, the results demonstrated that 1,500 mg of *Panax* (red) ginseng improved coordination and reaction time as well as increased alertness and energy.

🪶 ASTHMA

American ginseng is a good tonifying herb for the lungs and benefits some people with asthma and allergies. It is best used under the guidance of a natural healthcare practitioner.

❧ CANCER

Ginseng may have protective effects against cancer. One Korean study found that those taking *Panax ginseng* had approximately half the risk of cancer as those in the control group who did not take it. They found that the preventive effects seemed to apply to all types of cancer, not just one kind.

In a study of one type of ginsenoside, researchers showed that this component of ginseng had a suppressive effect on the growth of prostate cancer cells.

A Chinese study suggests ginseng improves survival rates and quality of life for breast cancer patients. Published in the *American Journal of Epidemiology*, this population study of 1,455 breast cancer patients in Shanghai found those who used ginseng (average of 1.3 g of root material) before or after a breast cancer diagnosis experienced benefit. All of the women in this study received at least one type of conventional breast cancer treatment such as chemotherapy or radiation. Researchers found women that had taken ginseng regularly before the diagnosis had a higher overall survival rate than pre-diagnosis non-users (88.6% versus 80%), and a higher disease-free survival rate (83.8% versus 77.4%). Quality of life was also improved among the women who started ginseng after the diagnosis.

Another study compared the effects of American ginseng and estrogen on breast cancer cells. Estrogen was shown to increase the proliferation phase of cancer cell formation while American ginseng decreased the cell proliferation phase and had no adverse effect on breast cancer cells.

Russian and German cancer clinics commonly use Siberian ginseng to reduce the side effects of chemotherapy and radiation and to improve immune function. One Russian clinic studied the effects of Siberian ginseng on 80 women undergoing chemotherapy and radiation treatment for breast cancer. Half of the women received Siberian ginseng and the others received no additional treatment. Women who took the Siberian ginseng had a significant reduction in side effects.

Natural healthcare practitioners often report benefit in people receiving chemotherapy treatment and Siberian ginseng. Apparently, the ginseng helps to normalize the ratio of white blood cells in the body.

Much more research needs to be done in this area, but ginseng should at least be considered for the complementary treatment of cancer, and certainly to help protect anyone who's receiving chemotherapy and radiation treatments.

❧ DIABETES

A study done by the University of Toronto in early 2000 found that American ginseng reduced blood-sugar levels in people with type 2 diabetes. It was also found that ginseng significantly reduced blood-sugar levels when taken 40 minutes before patients with diabetes were injected with a glucose solution—but not when the ginseng was taken at the same time as the injection.

In a double-blind, placebo-controlled study, 36 type 2 diabetic patients were treated for eight weeks with *Panax ginseng* (100 or 200 mg) or placebo.

(continued)

Researchers found 200 mg daily decreased fasting blood glucose levels and hemoglobin A1c (HbA1c)—a marker of long-term glucose control in patients with type 2 diabetes.

If you have diabetes, and your doctor is in agreement, I recommend taking ginseng 40 minutes before your meals.

❧ FATIGUE

Historically, as I've mentioned, Chinese ginseng was used to help improve fatigue and restore vitality to those who were chronically tired, especially the elderly. Different studies have shown that the various ginsengs can improve fatigue, presumably through their benign action on the adrenal glands. When your adrenal glands function more efficiently, your body uses oxygen and stores energy more effectively. The result is increased energy.

I've found that the ginsengs can be helpful to restore energy levels, though that doesn't mean it's fast-acting. In people who have chronic fatigue, it can take weeks before improvement begins to show. But by strengthening adrenal gland function with ginseng, people with chronic fatigue are less likely to suffer relapses.

❧ HEART FAILURE

In one Chinese study, doctors looked at the effects of Chinese ginseng on heart function. Selecting 45 patients who had suffered heart failure, doctors gave one group the heart drug digoxin, a second group was given Chinese ginseng, and the third received Chinese ginseng plus digoxin. (None of the groups, of course, knew which treatments they were actually getting.)

The most significant improvements occurred in groups two and three. The combination of Chinese ginseng and digoxin had the best results of all. The authors of the study stated that this drug–herb combination was safe and effective.

❧ IMMUNE SYSTEM PROBLEMS

German research has shown that Siberian ginseng increases immune function, particularly the activity of lymphocytes, the bodies that combat infection. Chinese ginseng has also been shown to improve immune function.

❧ MEMORY PROBLEMS

A few human studies show that Siberian and Chinese ginsengs improve mental function, including both memory and concentration. It is now accepted that high, prolonged levels of the stress-hormone cortisol destroy brain cells and can cause memory problems, and it's possible that additional stress even contributes to the development of Alzheimer's disease.

It's quite possible that ginseng, with its hormone-balancing, stress-reducing effect, also improves mental function. Perhaps memory and concentration improvements might be the result of better circulation and increased brain oxygenation, which is another benefit of ginseng.

❧ MENOPAUSE SYMPTOMS

All three types are used by naturopathic doctors and herbalists to reduce menopausal symptoms.

❧ REDUCED LIBIDO

I have not seen any good human studies of lowered sexual desire, but my patients report that they've gotten some benefits, especially from Chinese and Siberian ginsengs. The Chinese species can be helpful for both men and women. The Siberian, in my view, mainly helps men.

Herbs such as the ginsengs and tribulus (puncture vine) are a good first line of treatment for people with low libido, and I'd certainly recommend any of these before resorting to hormone replacement.

In younger males, Chinese ginseng can sometimes be too stimulating and the sex drive actually increases to the point of excess. The Chinese who are familiar with traditional treatments have great respect for the ability of Chinese ginseng to improve libido and sexual performance, especially among aging men.

STRESS

The ginsengs are, without question, the best possible herbs to combat the effects of stress. Of course, exercise and proper nutrition are also essential—and prayer is a proven stress-reliever. But along with these measures, ginsengs allow you to be more proactive in reducing the effects of stress on the body.

TOXINS

Siberian and Chinese ginsengs have been reported to help the body deal with toxins. Both have also been shown to protect against the side effects of radiation exposure.

Glandulars

Thousands of years ago, people would eat the organ of an animal with the hope that the healthy organ would treat the corresponding diseased organ in the human body. For example, if you had liver disease, why not eat a cow's liver to help recover? The practice was so common that the traditional Chinese doctors introduced "glandulars" into their herbal medicine formulas. In fact, glandulars have been part of their formulas for more than 4,000 years.

Today, glandulars are still used as nutritional treatments for the prevention and treatment of disease. The term "glandulars" refers to supplements that are available to "tonify" and support the function of the major organs of the body.

Julieta, a 31-year-old teacher, came to my clinic to consult with me for help with her thyroid. She had been experiencing symptoms of fatigue, PMS, weight gain, and chilliness for the previous two years. Her doctor ran many lab tests, including a "thyroid panel"—that is, a complete examination for thyroid problems—but all the tests proved negative. Believing that there was nothing physically wrong with Julieta, her doctor simply told her to get more rest. He surmised that the stress of teaching was likely the cause of her symptoms.

After my initial exam of Julieta, I asked her to take her body temperature each morning for five days in a row. The temperatures she reported were on the low side of normal, averaging about 97.4 degrees Fahrenheit rather than 98.0 to 98.6 degrees. I recommended that we put Julieta on a nutritional protocol that included two kinds of glandulars: thyroid and adrenal extracts. The idea behind this treatment was to nourish and stimulate her glands so that they would work more effectively.

Julieta had what holistic doctors call "subclinical" symptoms of thyroid and adrenal insufficiency. That is to say, her hormones are not so low that they showed up as abnormal on standard lab tests, but on the other hand they weren't high enough to be at optimal level.

The adrenal glands and thyroid gland work in tandem to help control the body's metabolism—that is, the way it burns energy. Those glands also help the body adapt to stress.

Julieta felt her energy begin to improve within a few weeks after she started the glandular therapy. I recommended that she stay on the glandulars for at least three months. After two months of use her temperature had increased to an average of 97.8 degrees. The nighttime chills were less of a problem, and she felt that her PMS symptoms were beginning to improve.

THE BEST OF THE BEASTS

The glandular preparations sold in the health-food market have usually been purified to adjust the concentration of cells from the animal's organ or to ensure that there's no contamination. The most reliable and safest source of glandulars, from most reports, are New Zealand sheep. These sheep reportedly have the lowest amount of contamination from hormones, antibiotics, pesticides, and other undesirable chemicals.

Of course, there are other sources as well, and some companies use bovine (cow) as the source for their glandular products. Using such products raises the specter of contamination with the virus that causes Mad Cow disease, a deadly infection of the brain, and few people think that taking a glandular is worth that kind of risk. Nonetheless, there has not yet been a case of infection resulting from glandular products sold in North America. (Britain has been the most-publicized location of Mad Cow disease.)

I have not seen any solid scientific evidence to explain how glandulars work. It is thought that the amino acids and polypeptides (chains of amino acids) are absorbed through the small intestine and exert either a stimulating effect on the organ being treated or have a minor, hormone-altering effect. It has also been postulated that the amino acids are incorporated into the gland cells' DNA and then act to help regenerate the cells. In addition, very small amounts of hormones may still be left intact in the glandular extracts.

Also, some practitioners have suggested that glandulars act like a crude form of homeopathy—that is, "like cures like." That's a possibility, but, at this point, we can only say that the scientific mechanisms of glandulars are still unknown. What we do know is that many doctors and health practitioners have seen successful outcomes when they treated patients with glandulars.

DOSAGE

Glandular products, like most supplements, have various potencies. However, the general adult dosage is 1 to 2 capsules or tablets taken two to three times daily. Both tablets and capsules have the same effect. But the greater your body weight, the higher the dosage you'll need.

It is best to take glandulars between meals, although they're almost as effective when you take them with food. Some people begin to see positive results after a few weeks, but for others, glandular therapy may take several months or more.

WHAT ARE THE SIDE EFFECTS?

A small percentage of people get digestive upset from glandulars. If that happens, try taking the supplements with meals instead of between meals.

People who take adrenal glandular extracts tend to have the most problems with other side effects, such as headaches, heart palpitations, anxiety, and insomnia. Generally, the side effects will diminish or stop entirely if you reduce the dosage. For people sensitive to supplements and medicines, it is always best to start at a low dosage—one capsule or tablet daily—and build up to a higher dosage over time.

Of course, glandulars are not compatible with vegetarianism since all are made from animals. But there is an alternative to animal-derived glandulars in homeopathic preparations of the glandulars known as isopathy or organopathy. These homeopathic preparations are effective with some people, and they're compatible with a vegetarian diet.

There are a variety of different organ-specific glandulars available. Following are some of the common ones, with their recommended uses.

GLANDULARS

RECOMMENDATIONS FROM THE NATURAL PHYSICIAN FOR . . .

ADRENAL

Adrenal glands, located on the top of each kidney, are the organs that help us survive stress. They secrete a variety of hormones including epinephrine (adrenaline), cortisol, DHEA, and others.

Adrenal glandulars are used for people who are "burned out," either from too much physical activity or from emotional stress. Excess secretion of one kind of hormone—such as cortisol—may create an imbalance. That gives an opportunity for other illnesses to set in.

People with chronic fatigue syndrome may benefit from adrenal extracts. These extracts are also recommended for chronic inflammatory illnesses such as rheumatoid arthritis, lupus, and ulcerative colitis. By supporting stress-hormone production, the adrenals keep inflammation to a minimum.

However, I don't advise anyone to use adrenals as substitutes for prescription medications such as prednisone (cortisone). Rather, they're an excellent supplement if you're coming off prednisone

and other steroids, helping to ensure that the adrenals do not become "lazy."

You may also need adrenal support if you have allergies or asthma. Women can benefit from adrenal glandulars during menopause, when the ovaries quit producing hormones and the adrenals have to "take up the slack."

Other nutrients that act synergistically with adrenal glandulars include pantothenic acid, vitamin C, zinc, licorice root, and the ginsengs. All of these related therapies help to support adrenal function.

LIVER

Liver glandular is used to support the detoxification properties of the liver. I have recommended them in cases of hepatitis and cirrhosis. They can also help with the liver detoxification process.

OVARY

Since the ovaries are responsible for the production of hormones as well as

(continued)

ovulation, good ovary function is critical to hormone balance. I have seen women who have hormone imbalances respond very favorably when they were given ovarian glandulars for PMS, menopause, and ovarian cysts.

✦ PANCREAS

The pancreas is responsible for producing and secreting enzymes that break down food in the small intestine. A different section of the pancreas produces hormones such as insulin and glucagons that control blood-sugar levels. I have mainly seen pancreatic glandular used for people with chronic pancreatitis (inflammation of the pancreas) with modest results.

✦ PITUITARY GLAND

The pituitary gland, located in the brain, releases many different hormones that help regulate other hormones in the body. For example, the pituitary hormone LH signals the ovaries to ovulate every month. It also secretes a hormone called TSH (thyroid stimulating hormone), which signals the thyroid gland to release thyroid hormone.

I have mainly used pituitary glandular to increase the activity and metabolism of the thyroid gland. There are many hypothyroid products available that contain pituitary and thyroid glandulars together, which makes a lot of sense.

✦ SPLEEN

A fist-size organ located underneath the left ribs, the spleen is a filter for blood cells. It's also an important part of the immune system because it produces white blood cells and destroys bacteria and other microbes.

When I've recommended spleen glandular, it's usually for people who need immune-system support, especially if they have had their spleen removed. According to naturopathic physician Michael Murray, the spleen produces two immune-enhancing compounds known as tuftsin and splenopentin. Since these compounds are important to the vital functioning of the immune system, Murray says, "Spleen extracts should probably be viewed as a necessary medicine for people who have undergone a splenectomy."

✦ TESTICLES

The testicles produce the hormone testosterone, which is responsible for a man's sex characteristics. Testicular glandular—often labeled as orchic glandular—is typically used for conditions such as low libido, impotence, and poor sperm production (infertility). (The Chinese used to use tiger testicle and tiger penis in herbal formulas to increase sexual performance in elderly men—but sale of these formulas is now, thankfully, outlawed to protect the tiger population. Bovine glandular, from bull testicles, is generally used instead.)

✦ THYMUS GLAND

The most well-studied glandular is the thymus, which is located just behind the breastbone. The thymus gland in the human body is responsible for the production of T-lymphocytes, especially in children. Anyone who needs extra immune support may benefit from thymus.

Because it appears to have a balancing effect on the immune system, thymus extract is particularly recommended for people who have cancer, HIV, rheumatoid arthritis, and allergies. Some chiropractors and naturopathic doctors say they've seen very good results when they gave thymus extracts to children who were getting recurring ear and throat infections.

THYROID GLAND

It is amazing the number of patients who have been diagnosed with low thyroid. There are many more who have subclinical hypothyroidism—that is, a slight deficiency of thyroid that is too small to detect, yet has an impact on health.

Lack of exercise, stress, emotional traumas, hormone imbalance (among estrogen, progesterone, pituitary hormones, and adrenal hormones), and environmental toxins have a lot to do with the pandemic of low thyroid.

Thyroid glandular can work well for mild cases of hypothyroidism. Many women who have been newly diagnosed with low thyroid by their doctors assume they will need to begin a medication such as Synthroid, the most commonly prescribed pharmaceutical for hypothyroidism. But thyroid glandular is another option.

For more severe cases I recommend Armour Thyroid—a thyroid prescription medication that's rarely prescribed by nonholistic doctors. Armour Thyroid contains thyroid glandular as well as thyroid hormones. I find it works better than Synthroid in most cases because it has a glandular effect, which Synthroid does not have. Also, it contains a wider spectrum of thyroid hormones than Synthroid.

Because thyroid glandular contains very little thyroid hormone, you might have to take it quite a while before you begin to see benefits. I have had patients who feel better in a week with thyroid glandular supplementation, but more often, it needs to be taken for months to get the full benefit.

Glucomannan

"I can only eat so many vegetables with a meal. I know I need the fiber to help lower my blood-sugar and cholesterol levels. Any suggestions?" asked Brian, a 48-year-old executive with type 2 diabetes.

"As a matter of fact I do. What you really need is a soluble type of fiber that slows down sugar absorption from your foods and binds up cholesterol. Let me tell you about glucomannan . . ."

When you read the fiber chapter in this book (page 172), you will see there are two main types of fiber. Insoluble fiber as found in leafy greens, for example, does not dissolve in water and acts like a broom sweeping undigested material out of the colon and promoting bowel elimination. On the other hand, soluble fiber, such as that found in glucomannan, dissolves in water and acts like a sponge, expanding and making one feel full. It also binds cholesterol, so it is not absorbed from foods, and slows the rate of glucose digestion and absorption in the digestive tract.

Glucomannan is a type of soluble fiber from the root of the Asian konjac plant. An analysis of 14 studies published in the *American Journal of Clinical Nutrition* demonstrated it was effective for treating blood fats, elevated glucose levels, body weight, and blood pressure.

DOSAGE

For weight loss, the typical adult dosage is 1 g taken 30 minutes to 1 hour before each meal. For type 2 diabetes and high cholesterol, study dosages have ranged between 4 and 10 g taken before or with meals. Take glucomannan with a glass of water. You can take it as either a powder mixed with the water or as capsules. For the powder, ¼ teaspoon equals 1 g glucomannan.

WHAT ARE THE SIDE EFFECTS?

Since glucomannan expands when it comes in contact with water, don't take tablets. They are more likely to swell up in the throat and be a choking hazard. Those prone to flatulence or bloating should start with about 500 mg daily for a week and increase this amount over several weeks to 2 to 8 g (2,000 to 8,000 mg) daily.

GLUCOMANNAN
RECOMMENDATIONS FROM THE NATURAL PHYSICIAN FOR . . .

🐦 CHOLESTEROL AND TRIGLYCERIDES

Studies have shown that use of glucomannan supplements can lead to significantly decreased total cholesterol, LDL (bad) cholesterol, and triglycerides (fat)—which cause increased risk of heart attack.

🐦 CONSTIPATION

A study published in the *Journal of the American College of Nutrition* found that glucomannan supplements promoted frequency and ease of bowel movements 30% more than a placebo. When mixed with water or gastric fluids, glucomannan forms a gel-like mass in the gut, creating a sense of fullness and diminishing appetite. Because it takes up space, it causes carbohydrates to be absorbed at a slower rate over a longer period of time and slows the movement of food from the stomach to the upper intestine.

🐦 DIABETES, PRE-DIABETES, AND INSULIN RESISTANCE

Glucomannan supplements may help lower and maintain a normal blood-sugar level. In the 14-study analysis, glucomannan was found to decrease fasting blood-sugar by an average of 7.4 mg/dL, about a 6% decrease if your blood-sugar level is 126 mg/dL (the number that indicates diabetes).

🐦 HIGH BLOOD PRESSURE

A *Diabetes Care* study found that glucomannan led to a 7% decrease in systolic blood pressure (the upper number) after two to three weeks.

🐦 WEIGHT MANAGEMENT

Glucomannan is the nutritionist's secret to help with weight loss. In an *American Journal of Clinical Nutrition* analysis, supplement use led to an average 1.7-pound weight loss in studies lasting about five weeks (a greater loss than that provided by a typical low-calorie diet). Another study, in *Medical Science Monitor*, showed that people who combined glucomannan with a low-calorie diet sped up the process—and lost that much weight weekly.

Glucosamine

Can glucosamine combat osteoarthritis?

More than 40 million Americans would urgently like to know the answer to that question. That's the number of people—most over the age of 45—who have osteoarthritis, the most common of nearly 100 different forms of this widespread problem.

Fortunately, the answer is yes. Osteoarthritis is the form that glucosamine is tremendously effective in treating.

More than 7 million people visit their doctors every year to seek relief from the swollen and stiffening joints that are caused by arthritis. A degenerative disease, osteoarthritis is characterized by the breakdown of joint cartilage—the spongy, cushioning tissue that protects the ends of the bones. Bones rub against each other when cartilage breaks down. The pain can be intense. Movement is usually restricted. Other common symptoms include tissue swelling and crepitus (creaking of joints), and feeling very stiff in the morning.

This type of arthritis mainly occurs in weight-bearing joints, such as the hips, knees, and spine. But people get it in their finger joints as well—which makes sense, since the fingers are in such constant use.

The exact cause of osteoarthritis is unknown, but researchers have seen an association with many other common health problems. This type of arthritis is associated, for instance, with obesity—which makes sense, since the joints have to carry excess weight. It's also associated with aging (joints are simply "wearing out") and with joint damage (the result of sports injuries, for instance). There also seems to be a genetic factor, because you're more likely to have osteoarthritis if a close relative has had it.

From my own observations, I'd say there are other associated factors as well. Biomechanics can be part of the problem, because it seems as if people are more likely to develop arthritis if they have flat feet or if the spine is out of alignment. Other factors that seem to contribute are poor digestion, high concentration of toxic substances, food sensitivities, hormonal imbalances, and nutritional deficiencies (if you're not getting enough vitamins, minerals, or essential fatty acids, for instance).

FROM PAIN TO RELIEF

Several well-designed studies have proven that glucosamine sulfate and other forms of glucosamine are just as effective as standard drug therapy for relieving the symptoms of osteoarthritis—and, in some cases, the supplement is even *more* effective than conventional medicines.

In a number of double-blind studies, researchers have demonstrated that glucosamine sulfate can be beneficial for people with osteoarthritis. Many of these studies compared glucosamine sulfate head-to-head with standard NSAIDs (nonsteroidal anti-inflammatory drugs), the pharmaceuticals that are often prescribed to reduce pain by reducing inflammation. Glucosamine was shown to produce better long-term results than these conventional medicines.

For example, in one four-week study, scientists compared glucosamine sulfate (1,500 mg daily) to ibuprofen (1,200 mg daily). All the people in the study had osteoarthritis affecting their knees. The ibuprofen group experienced pain relief faster—but by the end of the second week, the people who were taking glucosamine were getting just as much pain relief as those in the ibuprofen group.

There were drawbacks to taking ibuprofen, however. Those in the ibuprofen group experienced significantly more side effects—35%, as opposed to just 6% in the glucosamine group.

Other trials support the benefits of glucosamine. In a study that involved 252 doctors and 1,506 patients, each patient was given 1,500 mg of glucosamine sulfate every day for about seven weeks. When asked to judge the improvement in their patients, the doctors reported "good" results for about 59% of the patients and "sufficient" improvement in an additional 36% of them. Both doctors and patients rated glucosamine sulfate as being significantly more effective than previous treatments, which included NSAIDs, vitamins, and cartilage extracts.

Glucosamine is not a pain reliever, per se, so in general it doesn't work as swiftly as conventional drugs. But in the long run, I've found it relieves pain just as effectively as NSAIDs.

BETTER BUILDING MATERIAL

This supplement has another asset as well. Glucosamine helps rebuild cartilage or, at least, prevent further loss of cartilage. In this respect, it's quite different from the commonly used drugs, which tend to combat pain and can actually increase cartilage degeneration.

The body naturally manufactures its own glucosamine, but apparently our ability to produce the substance begins to wane as we age. (One theory holds that nutritional deficiencies may be a contributing factor.) When the body does not produce as much glucosamine as it once did, supplementation is in order.

Most glucosamine supplements are made from chitin, which comes from shellfish. It has an absorption rate of 90% to 98%, so most of the supplements' ingredients are effectively incorporated into the joint cartilage.

There are additional benefits when you take these supplements in the form of glucosamine sulfate. Glucosamine sulfate stimulates the repair and growth of proteoglycans, an important component of cartilage. Also, the sulfur portion of this complex is thought to stabilize joint tissue and cartilage. In this respect it's like SAMe—the one other supplement I recommend to help the body build more cartilage.

DOSAGE

The typical adult dosage is 1,500 mg daily. But the optimum dosage depends to an extent on body size and weight. For people who are overweight, I usually recommend 2,000 mg daily to achieve full benefits.

Of the different types of glucosamine available, I prefer glucosamine sulfate for two reasons. First, most studies have been done with this supplement, so we know how well it's absorbed and how well it works. Second, as I've mentioned, the sulfur content helps ligaments and tendons as well as cartilage. It should be noted that glucosamine hydrochloride has also been shown to be effective for osteoarthritis. Vegetarian forms of glucosamine are also available.

WHAT ARE THE SIDE EFFECTS?

Glucosamine sulfate is extremely safe. On rare occasions, some people get mild, digestive upset accompanied by diarrhea. Even these symptoms tend to go away if you take glucosamine with meals.

Some people who are allergic to sulfite and sulfates wonder whether it's safe for them to take glucosamine sulfate. My answer is always yes. Glucosamine sulfate contains the mineral sulfur, which is a normal constituent of the body, while sulfites and sulfates are preservatives.

Similarly, I've been asked about adverse effects by people who take sulfa drugs. But with these medications, too, the source of the drugs is different from the mineral sulfur found in glucosamine sulfate. Even though the name suggests sulfur, this is a completely different chemical from glucosamine sulfate.

People who are allergic to shellfish some-times worry that the chitin in glucosamine supplements comes from shellfish. But the usual allergic reaction is caused by the protein found in shrimp and crabmeat, not from a reaction to the shell material. There have been no reports of severe reactions to glucosamine sulfate. (If you are concerned, however, you can test a small amount on the tip of your tongue while in the presence of your doctor before taking a regular dose.) Vegetarian glucosamine is now available for those who are allergic to shellfish or require a kosher form.

GLUCOSAMINE

RECOMMENDATIONS FROM THE NATURAL PHYSICIAN FOR . . .

✒ OSTEOARTHRITIS

In my view, given the risk of osteoarthritis that faces most of us, this is one of those supplements that nearly everyone over age 45 should be taking. Glucosamine sulfate is a superior long-term treatment for osteoarthritis, far outweighing the power of conventional medications such as aspirin, the NSAIDs such as Tylenol, and commonly prescribed steroids. All of these pharmaceuticals only mask the pain while cartilage degeneration continues. (In fact, there's evidence that NSAIDs and aspirin actually destroy cartilage by suppressing the cells and enzymes that should help to build it!)

As for the side effects of medications, it is a well-known fact that long-term use of a steroid like prednisone can damage the body's tissue, bone, immune system, and joints. Also, people who are committed to long-term use of NSAIDs and aspirin run the risk of kidney and liver damage. Aspirin is also one of the leading causes of hospitalization for bleeding stomach ulcers.

Given all the benefits of glucosamine, and the deleterious side effects of so many medications, it's a possible solution for anyone with chronic arthritis problems. It can be used by people who have diabetes or blood-sugar imbalances such as hypoglycemia. It's also safe for people who have high blood pressure. (However, I recommend sodium-free glucosamine sulfate products for anyone concerned about sodium intake.)

If you begin with a 1,500-mg dosage of glucosamine sulfate, you may be able to cut back after a while. It really varies, depending on the individual. Some of my patients are able to cut back to 500 mg daily after a few months of taking 1,500 mg, while others regress after cutting back their dosage and have to resume the higher level. Studies show that benefits wear off after a few months if you completely discontinue glucosamine supplementation.

(continued)

If you're already taking anti-inflammatory medications, it's safe to take glucosamine sulfate as well. In fact, I have many patients who do this all the time. Just be sure to let your doctor know you will be using this supplement. Chances are your doctor will be able to decrease your medications after eight weeks of use.

Ever since the publication of *The Arthritis Cure*, people have asked about the benefits of taking glucosamine sulfate and chondroitin sulfate together. In my experience, I've found that most people do well by just supplementing with glucosamine sulfate—and there have been fewer studies on the chondroitin sulfate. Occasionally, however, when I have a patient who doesn't respond as well as I would like to glucosamine sulfate, I'll also recommend a combination with chondroitin sulfate—and sometimes the two, taken together, produce a better effect.

There's certainly no harm in trying the combination (though cost may be a consideration). The daily dosage recommended for chondroitin sulfate is 1,200 mg.

Other supplements may be beneficial as well. For some patients I recommend MSM and SAMe in addition to glucosamine sulfate. You may also want to consider taking antioxidants such as vitamins C and E, selenium, and lipoic acid, or natural herbal anti-inflammatories such as bromelain, boswellia, and cat's claw. To help relieve pain—and possibly improve the condition of cartilage—you can apply ointments that contain MSM or capsaicin.

Goldenseal

"I don't want to take antibiotics, but all this mucous congestion in my nose and throat is driving me crazy. If I weren't in another state right now, I'd be headed for your office to see you."

Jonathan, a patient of mine, was calling me from his cell phone between sales calls. Was there anything he could pick up at a nearby health-food store that would help him get through the next few days?

"Pick up some goldenseal," I advised. "Take twenty drops mixed in a quarter cup of water, three to four times a day for the next few days. But if you don't feel better after a few days, you'll have to see a local doctor to make sure the infection is not getting worse," I added.

Three days later, Jonathan called to leave a message with my receptionist. He was doing 80% better. His message?

"Thanks!"

GOING FOR THE GOLDENSEAL

We have the Native Americans to thank for a lot of our current knowledge of goldenseal (*Hydrastis canadensis*). The Cherokee, Iroquois, Crow, Seminole, Blackfoot, and other tribes used goldenseal for many different medicinal effects, including respiratory tract infections, eye infections (eyewash), skin cancer, skin disorders (acne, wounds, ulcers), pelvic bleeding, and liver disease. This knowledge was passed on to pioneers, who used the popular herbal medicine for many different ailments. Eventually, a Jesuit priest collected the advice in a single volume that was published around 1650.

Among eclectic physicians and homeopaths in the 1800s, goldenseal was often recommended as a digestive stimulant and tonic for the mucous membranes. It is one of the few North American herbs that can positively affect these two systems of the body simultaneously. When I recommend goldenseal, it's usually for one or both of these benefits.

Goldenseal is a bitter-tasting herb. In herbal medicine, bitters are known to stimulate digestive secretions, which is helpful if you have a weak digestive system. In many European countries it's common to take some "bitters" before meals as a time-honored method of improving digestion and elimination. (Dandelion and gentian root are also favored as bitters.)

When the "bitter receptors" on the tongue are stimulated, there's a reflexive reaction from the nervous system that stimulates the digestive organs such as the stomach, liver, gallbladder, and pancreas. So if you take goldenseal before your meals, over time it will help build up the power of the digestive system. A small dose of 5 to 10 drops is all that is needed to stimulate digestion.

MORE MUCUS

As a tonic for the mucous membranes, goldenseal provides benefits to many different areas of the body—the sinuses, respiratory tract, digestive tract, urinary tract, and vagina. Herbalists have stated that goldenseal has an "alterative action" on the mucous membranes. That means it literally alters the action of the membranes, stimulating the secretion of more mucus when there is not enough.

As a fluid that helps keep things flowing, mucus is an important part of the immune-system response to allergies and infection. It transports immunoglobulin A (IgA), which binds to foreign invaders and helps block infection. By stimulating secretions that produce extra IgA, goldenseal helps carry away viruses or bacteria that could cause infections.

That stimulating effect only lasts for a day or so, however. After that, goldenseal has a drying effect. This makes it effective for combating sinusitis, sore throats, bronchitis, pneumonia, colitis, vaginitis, and urinary tract infections.

Goldenseal is often referred to as a natural antibiotic, but this description is somewhat misleading. It hasn't been proven to directly kill bacteria. It does, however, contain very small amounts of a group of constituents known as alkaloids, including berberine, hydrastine, and canadine. These are considered the active substances, and often, they're the constituents that are tested.

THE BERBERINE FACTOR

There has been a lot of research on berberine, but usually in the form of berberine sulfate, which is much more concentrated than the amount present in goldenseal. Berberine sulfate has been shown in test-tube studies to have antimicrobial power, so it can help wipe out many bacteria, fungi, and parasites. But no one's sure whether the berberine in goldenseal has the same antimicrobial power as the more concentrated form that's found in berberine sulfate. In fact, berberine is poorly absorbed when it comes from goldenseal.

My thought is that goldenseal may have a direct "killing" effect on microbes if it's applied directly to certain tissues. If you use it as an eyewash, for instance, it actually helps block infection—and it may have a similar effect on the mucous membranes if you take it in tincture form for a sore throat. But whatever its power as a microbe-killer, goldenseal definitely stimulates IgA secretion, so it optimizes the immune response against pathogens.

In traditional Chinese medicine—where the energy of each herb is considered—goldenseal is regarded as a cooling herb. Bacterial infections tend to cause "heat," in the view of Chinese practitioners, and that heat is best treated with the application of cooling herbs.

Without question, goldenseal is one of the more popular medicinal herbs, but this has had an unfortunate ecological impact. Due to the tremendous demand for herbal supplements by the public, goldenseal has become endangered in a number of different states. As a result, some suppliers are cultivating goldenseal in an attempt to meet retail demand.

There are some good alternatives if goldenseal is unavailable. First on my list is Oregon grape root, which contains berberine along with a number of alkaloids not found in goldenseal. Like goldenseal, Oregon grape root also works to improve digestion and fight infections, and I actually prefer it for the treatment of acne. I find it works quite well, especially when combined with burdock root and hormone-balancing herbs such as vitex. Other goldenseal substitutes include coptis, also known as gold thread, and barberry.

DOSAGE

There is no agreed-upon standardization for goldenseal, so the concentrations of alkaloids like berberine will vary.

Most people take goldenseal in the form of a tincture or capsule, though you can also drink goldenseal tea. The typical adult dosage for acute infections is 15 to 30 drops of the tincture, or one 500-mg capsule taken three to four times daily. As a digestive stimulant, I recommend you put 5 to 10 drops of the tincture in a glass of water and drink it before meals.

To make an eyewash, dilute 10 drops of tincture in ½ ounce of saline solution and place 2 drops in each eye three to four times daily.

Many people use a combination of goldenseal and echinacea to combat infections.

Goldenseal is generally used for a limited time, so my usual recommendation is to continue using it until the condition improves. For acute infections this may be a week or so, and for digestive tonification, up to a few months.

WHAT ARE THE SIDE EFFECTS?

If you take too much goldenseal, it can dry out mucous membranes or cause irritation along the digestive tract. Also, some people get heartburn and digestive upset unless they take it with meals.

It is best to not use goldenseal in the beginning stages of a cold. If you take too much at the onset of a cold, it can suppress mucus formation, and you need as much mucus as possible for a healthy immune response.

Don't take goldenseal during pregnancy. Alkaloid-containing herbs or drugs may cause harm to the baby or cause miscarriage.

Some authors state that long-term use of goldenseal can destroy good bacteria in the body, but this claim has not been supported by any studies. Research findings have shown that the active ingredient berberine—when tested apart from goldenseal—doesn't destroy beneficial bacteria.

GOLDENSEAL

RECOMMENDATIONS FROM THE NATURAL PHYSICIAN FOR . . .

ACNE

The hair follicles secrete an oily substance called sebum. When sebum gets blocked up and infected with bacteria, the result is acne. Goldenseal is sometimes found in acne formulas. Perhaps it fights bacteria, though that's unknown. In any case it helps stimulate a sluggish liver and improve digestion, which are underlying causes of some cases of acne. So goldenseal may be worth a try, though, as mentioned, I've found that Oregon grape root generally works better.

COMMON COLD

It is best to not use goldenseal in the first stages of a cold so that mucus can flow freely. However, it can help to clear up the end stages of a cold where there is excess mucus. If you have just started to have cold symptoms, wait a day or two before you take goldenseal to fight it.

Similarly, if you have a case of the flu, I don't advise taking goldenseal right away. Wait a couple of days—after that, it can help speed your recovery.

DIARRHEA

Goldenseal does help with many cases of bacteria. In studies, berberine sulfate (one of the active substances in goldenseal) has been shown to kill different bacteria such as *E. coli*.

DIGESTIVE DISORDERS

Goldenseal stimulates the digestive organs so that food can be broken down and assimilated more effectively. It can be used for irritable bowel syndrome,

Crohn's disease, and ulcerative colitis. Because goldenseal helps stimulate a sluggish liver and gallbladder, it assists your body in breaking down fats more effectively.

EYE INFECTIONS

Goldenseal works well for eye infections. Be sure to dilute it with a sterile saline solution before applying it topically to the eyes.

PARASITES

Many herbalists and natural doctors use goldenseal in a blend of herbs—including wormwood, garlic, and coptis—to eradicate parasitic infections.

RESPIRATORY TRACT INFECTIONS

The most popular use for goldenseal here in North America is for respiratory tract infections, including sore throats, bronchitis, and pneumonia. It works best when there is excess mucus—but for a serious infection like pneumonia, you will need the advice of a doctor. I have treated strep throat using goldenseal and other herbs effectively, but I do not recommend you do this by yourself.

URINARY TRACT INFECTIONS

Goldenseal has a history of use for urinary tract infections. I like to use it in formulas with herbs such as echinacea, uva ursi, horsetail, and marshmallow.

Green Tea

"Darla, it's pretty simple. You need to cut down on the amount of coffee you're drinking."

Darla, the 55-year-old owner of a jewelry store, had just told me she was drinking about nine cups a day. Clearly, all that caffeine was contributing to her insomnia and anxiety. Though she valued coffee for its stimulating effect, it was also contributing to her fatigue—because the "caffeine high" was invariably followed by plummeting energy levels. Another, unrecognized side effect was going on in her skeleton. By drinking a lot of the caffeinated beverage, she was excreting more calcium than normal whenever she urinated. All that coffee was speeding the hidden process of bone loss or osteoporosis.

Like many coffee drinkers, Darla questioned how she could possibly give it up, or even reduce her consumption. "Caffeine is what keeps me going during the day," she told me. "I *can't* give it up!"

"Well, there's a way you can still get in some caffeine without causing damage to your body. It's called green tea," I replied.

Darla had heard about green tea. She had a few friends who drank it occasionally. "But I've never tried it," she confessed.

Briefly, I described its assets. Green tea has many antioxidants that help provide protection against heart disease and cancer—and it also helps the liver with detoxification. With about half the amount of caffeine as coffee, green tea provides a reasonable energy boost, without the sharp ups and downs so often experienced by coffee drinkers.

I suggested that, over time, Darla could reduce her coffee intake to a couple of cups in the morning. "The rest of the day," I suggested, "have green tea instead."

"If you think it's important, I'll give it a try," replied Darla.

Over the next few months Darla was able to cut down her coffee consumption to the recommended two cups per morning, shifting to green tea the rest of the day. (A number of her friends and coworkers also adopted this change.) Darla noticed almost at once that her insomnia and anxiety improved.

TEA FOR YOU

Green tea (*Camella sinensis*) comes from the same leaves that are used to make oolong and black tea—but, compared with those, green tea undergoes the least amount of processing.

To make green tea, the fresh-picked leaves of *Camella sinensis* are lightly steamed or sometimes lightly pan-cooked. This process inactivates enzymes that would otherwise degrade the tea and reduce the antioxidant activity. The green tea leaves are then rolled and dried.

By comparison, oolong tea is allowed to partially oxidize, which gives it a stronger taste but interferes with its antioxidant activity. Black tea is allowed to oxidize even more, by exposing the rolled-up leaves to air until they're oxidized to black. This gives black tea the strongest flavor of all three, but the long drying time reduces the antioxidants because of the oxidation that occurs.

THE GREENING OF AMERICA

Millions of people drink green tea every day—but until recently, most green-tea consumption seemed to be confined to the Far East. Among the Chinese, for instance, green tea is actually held in high esteem. Almost 90% of the Chinese population has at least one cup of green tea every day.

While Chinese records mention the use of tea as a medicinal beverage around 300 BC, it has also been popular in Japan and India. Made popular by emperors in these countries, it eventually became the drink of choice at almost all social and spiritual gatherings. In the early 1600s, Dutch traders brought green tea to Europe, and from there the beverage made its way (via the Dutch and English) to America.

In the United States, it's probably most popular in its cold form—that is, iced green tea. But you can now find green-tea extract supplements in many supermarkets, health-food stores, and pharmacies.

POWERING UP WITH POLYPHENOLS

The group of antioxidants that have helped give so much fame to green tea is known, collectively, as polyphenols. Polyphenols prevent free radicals (unstable molecules) from damaging body tissues and genetic material inside the cells. These phytonutrients are even more powerful than the vitamins most commonly taken as antioxidants—vitamins C and E.

Diseases such as cancer, heart disease, and many other chronic conditions are linked to the damage caused by free radicals, so any antioxidants that help prevent this damage will also help guard against these diseases. In fact, every aspect of aging is associated, in part, with various kinds of free-radical activity.

When the green tea polyphenols go to work in your body, they offer some powerful protection against the ravages of free radicals. Polyphenols contain flavonoids such as catechin, epicatechin, epicatechin gallate, epigallocatechin gallate (EGCG), and quercetin. Of all these, EGCG appears to have the strongest antioxidant and anticancer activity. The polyphenols have been shown

to have a protective effect on vitamin E, helping to maintain vitamin E levels in the body rather than allowing it to become depleted.

Green tea also contains vitamins C, D, K, and B12. It has ample supplies of minerals, too—including calcium, magnesium, chromium, manganese, iron, copper, zinc, molybdenum, selenium, and potassium.

Green tea enhances the liver's ability to detoxify and also protects liver cells from damage. It helps the liver process carcinogens.

DOSAGE

🐾 Tea Form

To prevent disease and maintain wellness I recommend two to three cups of green tea daily. This approximates the average green-tea consumption of three cups a day that people drink in many Asian countries. (Many of the population studies of green tea have been done in Asia, so this consumption is considered the minimum standard for producing benefits.) Each cup of green tea contains 50 to 100 mg of polyphenols.

Many companies now offer organic green tea, which ensures that it has not been contaminated by pesticides or other chemicals. Decaffeinated green tea is also available, in case you happen to be sensitive to caffeine.

🐾 Supplement Form

Green-tea extract is available in capsules or in whole-food formulas. If you're getting a supplement, check the label for standardization. Look for formulas standardized between 80% to 90% polyphenols and 35% to 55% epigallocatechin gallate. The typical capsule dosage is one 500-mg capsule taken one to three times daily.

The supplemental form of green tea usually has the caffeine removed.

WHAT ARE THE SIDE EFFECTS?

Regular, caffeinated green tea can cause the usual effects associated with caffeine, such as irritability, insomnia, nervousness, and tachy-cardia (fast heart rate). The longer the tea is steeped, the higher the amount of caffeine. Of course, if you're concerned about caffeine or don't like the side effects, you can always choose decaffeinated green tea instead.

GREEN TEA
RECOMMENDATIONS FROM THE NATURAL PHYSICIAN FOR . . .

✎ CANCER

Green tea provides protection against some of the organic processes that increase your risk of cancer. The strong antioxidant activity of polyphenols helps to protect the DNA against damage, thus providing some protection for the critical genetic material in every human cell. The polyphenols also block the formation or reduce the cancer-causing activity of nitrosamines—that is, nitrites and nitrates. These are the agents in processed meats such as hot dogs, bacon, and ham that are associated with an increased risk of stomach cancer. Researchers have found that if you want the most protective effect of this kind, you should drink green tea before any meal that might contain nitrites and nitrates. (You'll get some benefits from drinking the tea afterward, as well, but it's more effective if you drink it before your meal.)

Lastly, green tea polyphenols prevent certain enzymes (specifically, cyto-chrome P450) in the liver from activating carcinogens during the detoxification process.

Most of the excitement about the cancer-prevention properties of green tea has come about because of population studies. In general, it's been found that in populations of people who con-sume green tea on a regular basis, people have a much lower incidence of cancer than in populations where people drink other kinds of tea or none at all. In Japan, for example, researchers have noted sig-nificantly lower cancer rates. In large part, they feel, that's attributable to the high consumption of green tea.

One study looked at 472 women in various stages of breast cancer (labeled I, II, or III, depending on how far the can-cer had progressed). Increased green-tea consumption was associated with a decreased risk of lymph node metastasis in premenopausal women with stages I and II cancer. The researchers also found that if women with these stages of breast cancer consumed five cups a day of green tea on a long-term basis, they were more likely to be in remission six months later when the follow-up study was done.

Vanderbilt University researchers exam-ined the link between green tea and the risk for colorectal cancer in 69,710 Chinese women, ages 40 to 70. Participants were interviewed about their tea-drinking habits at the start of the study and again two to three years later. During six years of follow-up, 256 women got colorectal cancer. Conclusion: Women who drank green tea at least three times weekly for at least six months had a 37% lower risk for colorectal cancer than those who drank less green tea. The more tea consumed, the lower the risk. Drink one or more cups of organic green tea daily to guard against colorectal cancer.

Green tea appears to target some specific cancers. Researchers say that it may help protect against breast, prostate, esophagus, stomach, colon, lung, skin, liver, bladder, and ovarian cancers. It also seems to help guard against leukemia and oral leukoplakia.

Summing up their recommendations, a group of Japanese researchers concluded that green tea is potentially beneficial to anyone who takes it to help prevent cancer. "We suggest drinking green tea may be one of the most practical methods of cancer prevention available at the present," the Japanese team concluded.

CARDIOVASCULAR DISEASE

It seems the French drink red wine to prevent heart disease while the Japanese drink green tea to prevent heart disease. Meanwhile, North Americans don't seem to drink anything that prevents heart disease.

Cholesterol is one of the factors involved with heart disease. Animal studies have shown that green tea polyphenols, especially EGCG, prevent cholesterol from being absorbed from food into the body. By resisting absorption, you also reduce the risk of heart disease and other kinds of circulatory diseases that are so closely associated with high cholesterol.

A study of 1,371 Japanese men showed that a high consumption of green tea (more than 10 cups daily) was associated with lower total cholesterol levels. This quantity of green tea actually raised the level of HDL, which is "good cholesterol," while sharply lowering the concentration of lower LDL or "bad cholesterol."

Green tea was also shown to reduce the oxidation of LDL cholesterol, which is implicated in the initial development of atherosclerosis.

Also, green tea has natural blood-thinning properties. Doctors in China use high-potency green tea extracts for this purpose. (Blood thinners help lower high blood pressure and reduce the risk of stroke.)

DETOXIFICATION

While helping to support the liver—your body's chief detoxifier—green tea also prevents the formation of cancer-causing substances. I recommend using green-tea extract as part of a detoxification program, or simply drink the tea on a regular basis so that toxins do not build up in your body.

Wisely, many whole-food supplements—often dubbed "green drinks"—contain green-tea extract in their formulations.

DIGESTIVE HEALTH

According to *The Green Tea Book*, "Green tea promotes a healthy digestive tract by altering the intestinal environment to make it favorable to the growth of the friendly bacteria and less favorable to the growth of undesirable bacteria."

One Japanese study demonstrated that a special green-tea extract improved the levels of the good bacteria *Lactobacilli* and *Bifidobacteria* in nursing home

(continued)

patients. It also lowered the levels of certain kinds of potentially harmful bacteria.

✦ TOOTH DECAY

Green tea contains small amounts of fluoride that can help prevent tooth decay. Animal and human studies have shown that the polyphenols found in green tea prevent the growth of bacteria that cause cavities and plaque. In one study with human subjects, researchers discovered that green tea polyphenols decreased plaque deposits even when the volunteers just took the green tea, without bothering to brush or floss their teeth.

✦ WEIGHT LOSS

Most people know that caffeine is a stimulant, but not everyone realizes that this stimulant can help promote weight loss. I am not an advocate of using caffeine products as a "quick fix." The supplements themselves are not a shortcut to weight loss. But some preliminary research has shown that green tea can help stabilize blood-sugar. Indirectly, then, green tea might help promote weight loss by preventing insulin spikes from occurring. As long as insulin doesn't shoot up, you're less likely to store excess fat. But so far, we still aren't sure that green tea can really prevent these spikes. Also preliminary studies on green tea extracts are showing benefit in fat metabolism. Two recent studies have found that a beverage containing green tea extract enhanced exercise-induced loss of abdominal fat. More research needs to be done.

Guggul

Mention the condition "high cholesterol," and most natural healthcare practitioners will think of the herb guggul (*Commiphora mukul*), often referred to as guggulipid.

Cholesterol imbalance is one of the major risk factors for heart disease which, in turn, is the leading cause of death in the United States. With this in mind, the promise of guggul is obvious. It offers a safe and effective alternative to cholesterol-lowering drugs.

In several well-designed human studies, guggul has been shown to lower the "bad markers" of cardiovascular disease, such as total cholesterol, LDL, and VLDL cholesterol. Simultaneously it increases the level of the "good marker" HDL cholesterol.

Guggul has a storybook history. In the 1960s, an Indian researcher read about the medicinal effects of guggul in the ancient Ayurvedic medical text called *Sushrutasamhita*. This classic text described the effectiveness of guggul for the treatment of obesity and disorders of fats. Inspired by the text, researchers began to conduct studies to determine the effects of guggul on animals that had heart disease. The early animal studies showed that guggul resin significantly reduced high cholesterol and offered protection against atherosclerosis.

During the next four decades, in numerous trials with people who had high cholesterol, guggul extract proved to be a potent herbal therapy, helping to reduce not only high cholesterol but also triglycerides. Studies show it to be as effective—or even more effective—than many cholesterol-lowering drugs. It's much safer, too. It is approved by medical authorities in India as a lipid-lowering drug.

A TREE GROWS IN BANGLADESH

Guggul is a small, thorny tree native to India and Bangladesh. The resin is extracted from underneath the bark where yellow fluid oozes out. Guggul resin contains a mixture of lipid steroids termed guggulipid, which exerts the cholesterol-lowering and anti-inflammatory effects.

Within guggulipid are guggulsterones. Guggulipid also contains other compounds that exert a synergistic effect.

In traditional Ayurvedic medicine, guggul is indicated as a potential cure for arthritis, diabetes, gout, and skin disorders. It's also recommended to improve immune function, appetite, and digestion. Since it's been reputed to help prevent dental problems, it's also used as a mouthwash.

Guggul reduces cholesterol by "prompting" the liver to metabolize or "burn up" excess cholesterol. It also inhibits the cholesterol that's produced by the liver.

Animal studies show that guggulsterones stimulate the thyroid gland, so it may also be helpful for people who have low thyroid. It's an interesting connection between this thyroid effect and the metabolism of cholesterol. It's known that low thyroid function leads to reduced cholesterol metabolism by the liver—so thyroid stimulation would theoretically reduce cholesterol levels. There's ample evidence for this, since thyroid hormone medications reduce high cholesterol when given to people who have low thyroid function.

Guggul extracts also prevent platelet aggregation—the clumping of platelets that can lead to blood clotting—so it may prevent strokes.

In general, I favor this type of treatment over pharmaceutical, cholesterol-lowering drugs. I've found that the pharmaceuticals carry the risk of liver toxicity, so even though they may help reduce the risk of heart disease, they can aggravate other health problems.

DOSAGE

For cholesterol and triglyceride reduction, I recommend 500 mg of a 5% guggulsterone standardized extract three times daily. This is equivalent to 25 mg of guggulsterones three times daily.

An equivalent dosage that some products contain is 1,000 mg of a 2.5% guggulsterone standardized extract taken three times daily. Researchers recommend the extract be taken for at least four weeks before reevaluating blood cholesterol and lipid levels. I find it may need to be taken for two to two and a half months before reasonable improvements are seen with lab testing.

I typically recommend that guggul be taken in combination with other cholesterol-balancing supplements such as niacin (*Inositol hexaniacinate*) and garlic. In Canada a supplement known as Policosanol is very effective as well.

WHAT ARE THE SIDE EFFECTS?

Guggulipid has been shown to be nontoxic, but a small percentage of people experience minor digestive upset when they take it. It should not be used during pregnancy or by women who have heavy uterine bleeding. You probably shouldn't use it in combination with cholesterol-lowering pharmaceutical medications either, though the interaction with such drugs hasn't been studied in detail.

Those on thyroid medication should be especially monitored while taking guggulipid (and should be monitored even if *not* on guggulipid).

GUGGUL
RECOMMENDATIONS FROM THE NATURAL PHYSICIAN FOR . . .

ACNE

One study found guggul extract was comparable to the drug tetracycline for the treatment of cystic acne.

ATHEROSCLEROSIS

Animal studies have shown that guggul extract both prevents and reduces existing atherosclerosis. More studies are needed before we know for sure that the herb holds the same benefits for humans.

CHOLESTEROL AND TRIGLYCERIDES

As mentioned, guggulipid extract has been shown to decrease LDL, VLDL, total cholesterol, and triglyceride levels while increasing the protective HDL cholesterol. One 12-week study demonstrated that 1,500 mg of guggulipid had average reductions in serum cholesterol of nearly 22%, while triglycerides were reduced about 25% in people who took it regularly.

Another scientific study involving 233 people with elevated cholesterol or triglyceride levels (or both) showed that guggulipid worked better than the cholesterol-lowering drug clofibrate. People taking guggulipid had the added benefit of seeing some improvements in HDL, the "good cholesterol"—an effect that wasn't in evidence with the pharmaceutical. As for the length of time the benefits lasted, it was about the same—approximately 20 weeks—for those who took the herb and those who took the drug.

As researchers have identified some very specific types of high cholesterol, they have conducted studies to see which types are best treated with guggulipid. One study showed that guggulipid works best for people who have high-cholesterol readings of the type IIb (increased LDL, VLDL, and triglycerides) and type IV (increased VLDL and triglycerides).

OSTEOARTHRITIS

Studies have shown that guggul can improve pain associated with osteoarthritis.

Gymnema Sylvestre

"My doctor told me that I need to lose 25 pounds. He told me to quit eating at McDonald's and get more exercise. And if I don't improve my blood-sugar levels over the next two months, my doctor says I'll have to go on drugs for diabetes."

Stephen, a new patient, was obviously chagrined at the program his doctor had outlined for him. To me, it sounded like pretty sound advice—though of course I didn't like the idea of diabetes drugs any better than Stephen did.

"That's good, basic advice," I assured him. "But I'd like you to get on a more thorough program. You're 35 years old. That's pretty young to be having type 2 diabetes. If you do what I suggest, I think we can get your blood-sugar levels back in the normal range. Type 2 diabetes can be completely reversed with proper nutrition and exercise. Throw in effective herbs and nutritional supplements, and your progress will be even better."

Stephen's lifestyle is fairly typical. Like a very large segment of the US population, he's ready to admit that he probably watches too much TV, and eats too many sweets and white bread. Most of his exercise is turning the steering wheel of his sports car.

Not surprisingly—given this general lifestyle pattern—the statistics on type 2 diabetes have become alarming. In recent years, the largest increase among those who have "adult-onset diabetes" occurs in people ages 30 to 39.

To help Stephen, I gave him a more detailed diet plan than he'd gotten from his doctor. If he followed my recommendations, he would be eating a lot of complex carbohydrates, getting more of his protein from quality sources, and consuming more essential fatty acids. I also asked him to restrict simple carbohydrates such as breads, pastas, and sugar products.

Recognizing that he needed some kind of regular exercise program, Stephen started walking 20 minutes a day. He also followed my supplement recommendations, including daily doses of the herb gymnema sylvestre. This herb helped Stephen to control his appetite for sweets. It was just one of the tactics we used to help bring his blood-sugar levels under control.

TAMING THE SWEET TOOTH

Also known as gurmar, or "sugar destroyer," gymnema sylvestre has been embraced by many physicians who practice Ayurvedic medicine. Somehow, it has the ability to block the taste of sweetness, so it helps to stave off the "craving for sweets" that leads to overeating of simple-carbohydrate foods.

Gymnema grows in the forests of India and has been used by local healers and Ayurvedic physicians for the treatment of blood-sugar imbalances for more than 2,000 years.

Gymnemic acids are thought to be the important active constituents in gymnema. But this herb contains other important components as well, including resins, saponins, stigmasterol, quercitol, and the amino-acid derivatives betaine, choline, and trimethylamine.

A number of mechanisms seem to be activated when gymnema goes about its business of balancing blood-sugar. Two animal studies found gymnema extracts doubled the number of insulin-secreting beta cells in the pancreas and returned blood-sugars to almost normal. Gymnema also increases the activity of enzymes responsible for glucose uptake and utilization.

WATCHING WHAT HAPPENS

Since the 1930s, scientists have been trying to figure how gymnema can provide botanical therapy for types 1 and 2 diabetes.

In a controlled study, a standardized gymnema extract was given to 27 people with type 1 diabetes, all receiving a dose of 400 mg daily for periods ranging from six months to two and a half years. Thirty-seven of the other people in the study continued to take the usual insulin therapy without the addition of gymnema. Among those who took the herbal extract, researchers found that insulin requirements fell off dramatically. In addition, there was a statistically significant decrease in the blood-sugar marker that tests long-term blood-sugar. Those in the control group showed no significant decreases in blood-sugar or insulin requirement.

In another study, 22 people with type 2 diabetes were given 400 mg of gymnema extract every day for 18 to 20 months while they also continued to get their usual medication for hypoglycemia. Average blood-sugar levels improved significantly in this group, along with another sugar-related blood factor (glycosylated hemoglobin). Results also showed that there was an increase in pancreatic release of insulin among the people who got gymnema. People in the study were able to reduce their medication, and five were able to discontinue their drugs entirely.

As these studies show, gymnema has the ability to make quite an impact on blood-sugar metabolism. It is even more effective when combined with exercise and proper diet.

Several animal studies have also confirmed the blood-sugar lowering effect of gymnema sylvestre.

Dosage

A therapeutic dose of an extract is standardized to contain 24 to 25% gymnemic acids. I usually recommend 400 to 600 mg daily of the capsule form. I typically have patients take divided doses throughout the day before or with meals.

Gymnema also works well in combination with other blood-sugar balancing herbs such as bitter melon and fenugreek.

What Are the Side Effects?

No side effects have been reported, but researchers have not established whether this herb is absolutely safe for pregnant women.

Be cautious using this herb if you're taking pharmaceutical medications (oral hypoglycemics or insulin) for diabetes. The combination of gymnema and these medications can lower blood-sugar levels to potentially risky levels. If you're already taking diabetes medications, it's extremely important to work with a physician before supplementing with gymnema because the physician needs to closely monitor blood-sugar levels. In many instances, your doctor will need to lower the dosage of the pharmaceutical medication you are on.

GYMNEMA SYLVESTRE
Recommendations from the Natural Physician for . . .

❧ DIABETES

Gymnema can be effective for people who have either type 1 or type 2 diabetes, although I mainly recommend it for type 2.

❧ INSULIN RESISTANCE

When there's a high level of blood-sugar, the body produces more insulin, which is the hormone that helps shuttle blood-sugar into the cells of the body. But as too much insulin is produced, the body's cells become resistant to it—hence, the term "insulin resistance." When that happens, blood-sugar remains high.

Many people who have insulin resistance gain weight, no matter what their diet. Gymnema may help. It improves the cells' uptake of blood-sugar and helps the body utilize it.

❧ SYNDROME X

The term "Syndrome X" describes a whole cluster of health problems that increase the risk of diabetes and heart disease. (Many older Americans, as you might expect, show many of the symptoms of Syndrome X.) Insulin resistance is the underlying factor in this condition. As a result, people who have Syndrome X often show signs of glucose intolerance, obesity, high blood pressure, and elevated levels of cholesterol and triglycerides.

Since gymnema helps improve blood-sugar uptake and utilization, it is the herb I recommend for Syndrome X.

Hawthorn

Hawthorn is truly a superstar when it comes to the heart and cardiovascular system. Millions of people can benefit from the medicinal effects of this herb, including anyone who suffers from high blood pressure, coronary artery disease, angina, or heart arrhythmia.

Since cardiovascular disease is the number one killer in this country, hawthorn is a crucial treatment when it comes to herbal prevention and natural treatment of this pandemic disease. Chances are high that nearly all of us will suffer from one or more of these heart-related conditions by the age of 60—so you might also think of hawthorn as the anti-aging herb for the heart.

ONE FOR THE HEART

I love to prescribe hawthorn to patients. Most people begin feeling much better, almost from the first instant they take it. The herb improves oxygenation, and thus has an immediate, beneficial impact on energy levels. In addition, it improves blood flow through the coronary arteries (the vessels that supply blood to the heart), increases strength of heart contractions, prevents plaque buildup in the arteries, relaxes blood vessels so that blood flows more efficiently, and helps prevent pressure buildup inside the arteries. No wonder so many European doctors and North American "natural doctors" prescribe hawthorn on a daily basis. As far as I am concerned, every cardiologist should be recommending this lifesaving heart tonic to patients.

Many parts of the plant—leaves, flowers, and berries—are used medicinally, although most extracts are mainly from the berry. Researchers have found that the active ingredients in this herb seem to be a group of flavonoids that provide unique benefits to the cardiovascular system. A leading characteristic of these powerful flavonoids is their incredible ability to improve blood flow to the heart.

Hawthorn is the premier cardiotonic in European herbal medicine, meaning that it's often prescribed simply to support normal heart functions.

DOSAGE

Practitioners commonly use standardized extracts of 2.2% flavonoids or 18.75% procyanidins. In many of the studies where patients showed the greatest improvement, researchers were administering between 160 and 900 mg daily of the capsule extract.

With serious heart conditions like congestive heart failure, it's important for anyone taking hawthorn to get the benefit of its therapeutic effects as quickly as possible. For those taking it in tincture form, I have seen good results with doses of 30 to 60 drops three times daily.

The tea form is also available, but I prefer to use capsule or tincture with my patients. (I have no experience with haw-thorn tea.)

WHAT ARE THE SIDE EFFECTS?

While there are no adverse side effects, haw-thorn does provide one bonus—it enhances the heart drug digitalis, making it more potent. The herb may also increase the effectiveness of beta blocker drugs that are used to treat high blood pressure.

If you're being treated for a heart-related condition by a conventional doctor, be sure to let your physician know if you're also taking hawthorn, because it has a mild blood-thinning and diuretic effect. With close monitoring by your doctor, you may be able to use a lower dosage of the pharma-ceutical medications—which is an advan-tage, because so many of them have side effects.

HAWTHORN
RECOMMENDATIONS FROM THE NATURAL PHYSICIAN FOR . . .

☙ ANGINA

Angina pain, according to patients, is like having your heart squeezed until it hurts. The pain can be brought on by stress, but it might also be caused by a shortage of oxygen reaching heart tissue. That's one thing that happens when you have arte-riosclerosis, more commonly known as hardening of the arteries.

I have seen hawthorn help numerous patients with angina. For the most severe conditions, I recommend taking haw-thorn in combination with the herb cac-tus (*Cereus grandiflorus*).

In a three-week study that confirmed the benefits of hawthorn for people with angina, researchers demonstrated that daily doses of 180 mg had a significant effect on blood flow to the heart. Though 78% of these people had "abnormal" endurance readings before the study, those who took hawthorn quickly showed a 25% improvement in their exercise tol-erance—whereas those in a control group (who received no hawthorn) showed no improvement at all. The conclusion I drew from this study is that a simple

supplementation program of hawthorn can make an incredible difference in oxy-genation to the heart and help treat the underlying cause of angina.

☙ ARRHYTHMIA

Almost anyone who has a mild case of heart arrhythmia can be helped with haw-thorn. Better yet, in my view, is a combi-nation that includes not only hawthorn but also the supplement coenzyme Q10, L-carnitine, and the mineral magnesium.

☙ CONGESTIVE HEART FAILURE

Researchers have focused on congestive heart failure in most of the studies on hawthorn. Symptoms of this condition include shortness of breath, poor exer-cise tolerance, fatigue, elevated heart rate, and swelling of the ankles (edema). This is the result of a loss of efficiency in the body's one and only blood-pumping organ, the heart.

But the problem doesn't originate in the heart itself. Rather, it's caused by

(continued)

arteriosclerosis, the condition where plaque buildup in the arteries prevents adequate blood flow into the heart, or from long-term high blood pressure.

For CHF, hawthorn comes highly recommended by the German Commission E, which evaluates the effectiveness of a wide range of herbs. This official government agency based its recommendations on a number of supportive studies. One high-quality study, for example, showed that eight weeks of hawthorn extract supplementation improved heart function and symptoms in people who had a moderate degree of congestive heart failure. In another study, researchers learned that hawthorn extract is just as effective as the drug catopril, a pharmaceutical medication that's custom-designed for people with high blood pressure who are prone to congestive heart failure. Among those who had a moderate degree of congestive heart failure, hawthorn reduced heart rate and improved exercise tolerance.

The latter study, which was done with 900-mg daily doses of hawthorn extract, demonstrated that the potency of hawthorn is roughly equal to that of heart medications. But unlike the pharmaceuticals, hawthorn doesn't create unwanted side effects. However, it should be noted that all studies with hawthorn have found benefit for CHF.

❧ HEART ATTACK RECOVERY

I routinely prescribe hawthorn to people who have a history of a heart attack. Of course, having been in and out of the hospital, and under the care of conventional doctors, these are people who are already taking their share of medications

such as the blood thinner Coumadin or common aspirin. Frequently these medications are prescribed by cardiologists to help prevent a second attack.

A good case can be made for hawthorn supplementation as an adjunct to drug therapies. But hawthorn is more than a good assistant. It does something the pharmaceuticals can't accomplish— increases circulation to the coronary arteries. Since these small arteries feed the heart muscle, they're critical to the health of this organ. It's when your heart tissue isn't getting sufficient blood flow that a heart attack is most likely to occur.

Hawthorn by itself only has some of the healing properties that are needed for complete recovery. So in addition to this herbal supplement, I typically recommend others as well to heart attack survivors—including natural vitamin E, coenzyme Q10, magnesium, L-carnitine, and a host of antioxidants.

As long as your physician knows you're taking natural supplements that may have a mild blood-thinning effect, you can probably continue taking pharmaceuticals as well as the supplements. I have not had any drug–herb interaction problems among patients who took both.

❧ HIGH BLOOD PRESSURE

Hawthorn alone is a good treatment for high blood pressure, but I see even better results when it's combined with ginkgo, viscum, dandelion leaf, and valerian.

Hawthorn has a mild diuretic effect, which reduces the amount of water in the blood, thus reducing blood volume and blood pressure. Hawthorn also relaxes blood vessel walls, which also helps lower blood pressure.

Horse Chestnut

Most patients who have varicose veins have read all about the possible remedies, and they've tried a number of pills and powders. So the question I'm most frequently asked is this: "If you had to pick one supplement for varicose veins, which one would it be?"

The list of possibilities is fairly extensive. I've had good results with ginkgo, grape seed, bilberry, hawthorn, witch hazel, Pycnogenol, and vitamin C. But at the top of my list is horse chestnut.

As the baby-boom generation continues to age, conditions like varicose veins will receive more attention from the medical and natural health communities. This condition occurs when the minuscule valves in veins begin to weaken. Instead of supporting the flow of blood that's making a return trip to the heart, the tiny valves allow a backwash that results in pooling. This leads to the engorgement of veins, especially in the legs where gravity is exerting a strong, downward pull.

Varicose veins are not harmful, but people occasionally have a problem with a related symptom called thrombophlebitis, where veins become painfully swollen and inflamed. With this condition—commonly called phlebitis—there's a risk of blood clot formation, a potentially serious situation.

Fortunately, the seeds of horse chestnut (*Aesculus hippocastinum*) produce a tonic effect on veins—and, indeed, on the entire circulatory system. In addition, horse chestnut has natural anti-inflammatory properties, so it's also helpful for the treatment of swelling and edema, bruises, arthritis, and backaches.

While the seeds are the seat of the horse chestnut's power, I don't recommend eating them. Before they're ready for human consumption, the seeds must be specially processed to remove harmful, naturally occurring components.

THE ROOTS OF CHESTNUT LORE

As with many of today's popular herbs, horse chestnut has a rich history in Europe. As a matter of fact, the main active constituent that has been identified, called aescin, is a registered drug in Germany. German doctors recommend it for edema and muscular injuries, and it's also given by injection for head trauma. Not surprisingly, the German Commission E—a government body that holds responsibility for herb testing—has approved horse chestnut for the condition called "venous insufficiency," which simply means lack of blood flow through the veins. The commission also endorses the herb for nighttime leg cramps, swelling, and itching of the legs.

Horse chestnut is native to Asia but can also be found throughout the United States and Europe. The seeds come from the fruit that is picked each September.

Horse chestnut has an interesting mechanism of action. The active constituent aescin helps strengthen the vein walls and valves, as well as capillaries. Aescin also decreases the permeability of the tiniest blood channels, the capillaries, by preventing key enzymes from breaking the walls of capillaries. Research has shown that these enzymes are at much higher levels in people with varicose veins—presumably causing a faster breakdown of capillary walls—so aescin helps put the brakes on this process.

Horse chestnut also improves circulation and reduces edema by promoting fluid drainage from the tissues into the capillaries. This is important, since excess fluid in the tissues accumulates around and in the veins—and when the veins become distended, they're a less efficient circulation mechanism.

Finally, horse chestnut contains small amounts of a blood-thinning agent called Coumadin. When blood becomes thinner, it flows more easily and swiftly, which helps explain why this herb helps to improve circulation and relieve congestion.

DOSAGE

I recommend patients use a standardized capsule of horse chestnut at the same dosage used in clinical studies, which was 600 mg daily. This is equivalent to 100 mg daily of the active constituent, aescin. Topical gels containing horse chestnut are also available.

WHAT ARE THE SIDE EFFECTS?

Side effects are rare. A small percentage of people get digestive upset, and some patients have reported skin itching and headaches. Since horse chestnut has a natural blood-thinning effect, be sure to check with your physician if you're on blood-thinning medications or have any kind of bleeding disorder. If you have concerns about such conditions, you can always use the horse chestnut gel, applied directly to the surface of the skin (rather than taken internally).

HORSE CHESTNUT

RECOMMENDATIONS FROM THE NATURAL PHYSICIAN FOR . . .

🐎 BACK PAIN

European doctors use horse chestnut for the relief of back pain. Though I don't have any experience using it for this condition, I have treated people with the homeopathic form called aesculus. (Aesculus is specific for pain that radiates to the low back and hips.)

🐎 HEMORRHOIDS

Hemorrhoids are really a collection of varicose veins that are distended and protruding. Horse chestnut is a popular herb that's often recommended by naturopathic doctors and herbalists to shrink hemorrhoids and alleviate pain and itching.

🐎 VARICOSE VEINS

Most of the research with regard to horse chestnut has been focused on varicose veins. One study of 240 people found that horse chestnut was just as effective as the treatments most often used in conventional medicine—combining compression therapy (heavy, elastic, custom-fitted stockings) with daily doses of a diuretic (a medication that reduces body fluids by increasing the need to urinate).

In my own practice, I have seen good results in people with mild to severe cases of varicose veins. It's especially recommended in severe cases, because varicosity can lead to thrombophlebitis. I also recommend horse chestnut for people who have had vein surgery, so that the varicosities do not return.

Huperzine

One of the great memory boosters is huperzine, also known as qian ceng ta and Chinese club moss. Practitioners of Chinese medicine have used huperzine for centuries as a diuretic and anti-inflammatory. About 20 years ago, a Chinese scientist discovered that a certain alkaloid (an organic compound containing nitrogen) in huperzine known as huperzine A (HupA) could improve brain function. This discovery sparked dozens of clinical studies, some still ongoing, at research institutes in China and the United States.

HupA improves memory and slows general age-related cognitive decline. It can even slow down mental decline in early-stage Alzheimer's disease patients—although, like the pharmaceuticals available, it is not a cure.

HupA's cognitive benefits are due mainly to its effects on acetylcholine, a neurotransmitter critical for normal thinking, memory, and attention. These mental processes falter when acetylcholine production diminishes and/or when an enzyme called acetylcholinesterase (which normally breaks down unused acetylcholine) becomes overactive, degrading the much-needed acetylcholine.

HupA appears to inhibit activity of acetylcholinesterase, thereby sparing the available acetylcholine. This is also how pharmaceuticals for Alzheimer's work—but several human clinical trials have shown HupA to be even more effective than the drugs donepezil (Aricept) and tacrine (Cognex). Animal studies have shown that HupA further supports cognitive function by protecting brain cells from damage caused by free radicals (harmful negatively charged molecules), toxins and/or lack of oxygen (for instance, from poor circulation or stroke). It may also work by reducing formation of beta amyloid (a protein that forms lesions in the brain tissue of Alzheimer's patients).

DOSAGE

For intermittent problems with short-term memory, take 100 mcg HupA daily. After eight weeks, people under age 55 may lower the dosage to 50 mcg daily. People who are older may benefit from staying on HupA indefinitely at a dose of 100 mcg twice daily. For those with more severe memory problems, such as early-stage Alzheimer's disease, 200 mcg twice daily is appropriate.

WHAT ARE THE SIDE EFFECTS?

HupA generally is considered safe. Side effects, though uncommon, may include nausea, diarrhea, dizziness, and loss of appetite. Before starting HupA, discuss it with your doctor. If you take medication for Alzheimer's disease or other psychiatric diseases, you should not use HupA, because it might worsen the drugs' side effects. If you are dissatisfied with Alzheimer's medication, ask your doctor about discontinuing the drug and trying HupA instead.

HUPERZINE

RECOMMENDATIONS FROM THE NATURAL PHYSICIAN FOR . . .

🐦 ALZHEIMER'S DISEASE

An interesting multicenter, prospective, double-blind, parallel, placebo-controlled, and randomized study included 103 people with Alzheimer's disease. Fifty people were given 200 mcg huperzine while 53 patients were given a placebo for eight weeks. All patients were evaluated with various types of standard testing. Approximately 58% of those treated with huperzine A showed improvements in their memory, cognitive, and behavioral functions, compared to a 36% improvement with placebo. No severe side effects were found.

🐦 COGNITIVE FUNCTION

HupA has also been shown to benefit memory in middle school children when supplemented for four weeks. I have found that it works to improve memory for people of all ages.

🐦 DEMENTIA

Huperzine may benefit those with senile dementia. One placebo-controlled study found significant improvement after two to four weeks of treatment. Larger studies are needed but this is one natural substance worth considering for this condition.

Hyaluronic Acid

"The joint formulas I have taken, which mainly revolve around glucosamine sulfate, haven't worked for me like they have for most of my friends," exclaimed Larry, a 61-year-old carpenter with osteoarthritis in his knees.

"Well, I guess we should take a different approach. I have also seen good results with the supplement hyaluronic acid. And interestingly it has shown good results in helping those with arthritis of the knees. You should feel less stiffness and pain over the course of six to eight weeks," I explained. Sure enough, Larry did notice obvious improvement in his symptoms within the time frame I predicted.

Hyaluronic acid (HA) is a naturally occurring substance in the body. It is formed by the union of two carbohydrates known as D-glucuronic acid and N-acetyl glucosamine (called a disaccharide unit) strung together in a very long linear chain of identical disaccharide units (a polysaccharide). HA is an intricate component of many connective tissues of the body, including the joints, skin, and eyes. It is also found in blood vessels and the umbilical cord. A deficiency of HA is thought to contribute to premature aging and disease in these tissues

HA is a key component of synovial fluid, the clear fluid that functions as a lubricant in joint cavities. Your joints (such as the knees and elbows) are covered by a membrane known as the synovial membrane. Its function is to form a capsule around the ends of the bones and secrete synovial fluid to prevent friction and degradation of the joints and bones. This is similar in effect to the lubrication of oil in moving car parts. In addition, the synovial fluid also acts as a shock absorber and transports nutrients within the joint. Cartilage, the main shock absorber of the joint does not contain blood vessels. Therefore, synovial fluid is critical for the transport of nutrients required for cartilage healing and regeneration and the removal of waste products. Lastly, HA is an actual component of cartilage and is required for healthy cartilage formation. It is important for retaining water in cartilage. During the progression of the two main types of arthritis, known as osteoarthritis and rheumatoid arthritis, synovial fluid breaks down into smaller units and decreases in its lubricating and shock-absorbing abilities, and cartilage degrades due to inflammation and water loss. HA works to counteract both of these effects.

HA is not new in the field of medicine. In 1997, HA injections were approved in the United States for patients with osteoarthritis of the knee. Examples of trade names include Hyalgan, Supartz, Orthovisc, and Synvisc. Common side effects include pain at the site of injection, skin rash and bruising, and joint pain and swelling. HA is considered to be an alternative treatment for those who want to delay knee replacement surgery or for those who cannot tolerate anti-inflammatory and pain medications commonly used with osteoarthritis. Studies on HA for osteoarthritis of the knees are mixed. I have spoken with some patients who feel the injections were effective in reducing their symptoms. HA is also used by veterinarians for the treatment of osteoarthritis in animals.

The shots cost about $230 per injection. Insurance may or may not cover the cost, depending on your policy. HA can be supplemented alone but also works well in tandem with classic arthritis-fighting supplements such as glucosamine, chondroitin, methylsulfonylmethane (MSM), fish oil, and S-adenosylmethionine (SAMe).

One of the first studies to demonstrate that HA is absorbed effectively into the bloodstream and the joints was presented at the 2004 Experimental Biology Conference. Researchers gave rats and dogs one oral dose of HA that was radio labeled (chemically joined with a radioactive substance), allowing the substance to be tracked with diagnostic imaging. The HA was absorbed into the animals' bloodstreams and distributed to their joints. We can assume similar absorbability with humans in light of positive studies conducted in people with arthritis.

HA is also used for supporting healthy skin. Collagen is the glue of connective tissue that holds its structure together and maintains elasticity and skin tone. HA supports collagen production and is critical for maintaining moisture in the skin cells and between cells.

DOSAGE

The oral dosage for HA varies depending on the type of product used. Be aware that some products are labeled as collagen, which contains HA. Studies done on a form of HA known as hydrolyzed type II collagen used 1,000 mg daily. I commonly use the oral form in doses of 1,000 to 2,000 mg daily.

WHAT ARE THE SIDE EFFECTS?

Side effects with the oral supplement are not common. The topical form may rarely cause skin irritation.

HYALURONIC ACID
RECOMMENDATIONS FROM THE NATURAL PHYSICIAN FOR . . .

❧ ANTI-AGING AND OTHER SKIN REPAIR

HA is commonly used in the injection form as a medical treatment for wrinkles, lines, and depressions from acne, scars, and lip enhancement. The injections normally need to be repeated in six to nine months to maintain their benefit, although this is a longer lasting effect than collagen injections. Examples of FDA-approved injectable skin fillers include Hylaform and Restylane. Both of these HA gel injections should be administered by trained cosmetic surgery professionals. For more mild cases, the supplemental form can be tried both orally or as a topical ointment available from health-food stores. In preliminary studies, HA has been shown to inhibit the enzyme in the skin and connective tissue called hyaluronidase, which degrades wrinkle-fighting hyaluronic acid. It also stimulates production of fibroblast, the cells that produce collagen, which is important in reducing wrinkles and lines.

❧ ARTHRITIS

HA can be used for both osteoarthritis and rheumatoid arthritis. One small study included 16 patients with osteoarthritis of the knee or hand who were taking COX-2 inhibitors or other non-steroidal anti-inflammatory drugs. Eight patients received two 1,000 mg hydrolyzed type II collagen capsules daily and eight were given a placebo. After two months of treatment, the group receiving the collagen reported significant improvement in pain, range of motion, and swelling—whereas the placebo group showed no significant changes.

❧ BRUISING

I have found HA to be helpful for patients who have thin skin and easy bruising from the use of prednisone, a drug used as a powerful anti-inflammatory. HA likely strengthens the connective tissue so it is more resilient to trauma.

Hydrotherapy

"My chest hurts, especially when I breathe in. I also have a lot of mucus coming up, which makes me cough even more. I don't want to see my family doctor. I know she will give me antibiotics."

Sherry was speaking from experience. The year before, she'd had several courses of antibiotics for various infections—and each time, she'd suffered the side effects of yeast infections and bloating. This time, she wanted to make sure she tried the alternatives if she could.

"You can help me, right?" asked Sherry.

"Let's see what is going on with you and then I will let you know what I can do," I replied.

I listened to her lungs, then ordered X-rays and blood work. The results confirmed my suspicion that Sherry had bacterial pneumonia. She was 39 years old, and I would have considered her a healthy individual, except that she got bronchitis or pneumonia a couple times every winter. But if she continued to get antibiotics for these problems, I felt there was a real risk that she would eventually get a bacterial infection that couldn't be fought off with conventional antibiotic medications. She, too, knew about this risk, which was why she'd asked me to treat her with natural medicine.

But the need for treatment was urgent and immediate. Bacterial pneumonia is a serious condition, and we had to bring it under control right away.

To Sherry's question of "What next," I proposed an aggressive treatment protocol. Perhaps the most important part of the plan would be constitutional hydrotherapy.

HOT AND COLD

Naturopathic doctors have used constitutional hydrotherapy for more than 100 years. Essentially, it means alternating heat and cold by applying water-soaked towels over the chest and back.

I was quite sure that constitutional hydrotherapy would increase Sherry's white blood cell count, which would enhance her body's natural ability to fight off the bacterial infection. At the same time, the treatment with hot and cold would be likely to reduce congestion and inflammation of the lungs by improving circulation. I also prescribed an herbal formula and homeopathic remedy to accompany the hydrotherapy treatments.

Sherry's husband helped her with the hydrotherapy treatment at home.

Sherry returned to the clinic for follow-up visits at three-day intervals. Sherry noted that after a hydrotherapy treatment, she was able to cough up mucus that seemed to be deep in her lungs. When she had therapy in the evening, she noted that it also enabled her to sleep better that night.

Sherry was showing evident improvement at each visit. Nine days into the therapy, she had returned to work and felt that she was close to being her old self.

WATER TREATMENTS— WITH GUIDANCE

I would never recommend that anyone try to treat bacterial pneumonia without the help of a physician, and I know many medical doctors who might think I was crazy to recommend hydrotherapy for Sherry. Then again, many doctors who readily prescribe antibiotics are not completely informed about the powerful natural healing therapies that can be very effective in fighting many kinds of disease.

Hydrotherapy simply refers to the use of water for healing. The actual treatments can take many forms. Steam inhalation and a wet sauna are forms of hydrotherapy. So are baths or hot tubs, and hot and cold applications with towels, compresses, or gel packs. Some practitioners use colonic hydrotherapy, which means "flushing out" the colon with sterile water to remove toxic or harmful substances.

Hydrotherapy is very common in European countries. Even in the United States, however, many health spas have extensive hydrotherapy programs. There are many medical doctors as well as naturopathic physicians who advocate various forms of hydrotherapy treatments for certain conditions.

The healing powers of water have been recognized for thousands of years. Hydrotherapy treatments were certainly well known to Ancient Egyptians and Babylonians. The Greeks and Romans emphasized the importance of baths and the healing power of natural springs.

WATER EXPLORER

If any single individual were to be described as the founder of this therapy, it would have to be Vincent Priessnitz, who lived from 1799 to 1852. Born a peasant in a small European mountain village in what was the former Czechoslovakia, Priessnitz observed how an injured animal instinctively headed for a nearby creek when it had an injury. The cold, flowing water healed its injuries.

Priessnitz experimented with different forms of hydrotherapy on injuries he sustained when he was working on the family farm. When he was 17 years old, Priessnitz was run over by a wagon carrying a heavy load of wood. A local surgeon evaluated his internal injuries and pronounced them untreatable. He seemed convinced that Priessnitz would never recover.

Undeterred by his surgeon's evaluation, Priessnitz went home and set his broken ribs by pressing his abdomen against the arm of a chair, then covered the injured ribs with cloths that were moistened with cold water. Ten days later, he had resumed his place on the farm with his previous rounds of chores.

Duly impressed with the effectiveness of his own self-treatment, Priessnitz became a strong advocate of hydrotherapy, using the treatments with the sick and injured who came from far and near for treatments. His fame spread until medical authorities became jealous of the popularity and success of his practice. But their efforts to get him to halt his practice were futile, even when they resorted to legal means. In the view of the court, Priessnitz was just making use of a natural substance, water, and was not using medicine.

In one instance, when a patient was called as a trial witness, the judge asked specifically who had helped the patient. The patient replied, "They have all helped me. The doctors, the apothecaries, and Priessnitz. The former helped me to get rid

of my money, and Priessnitz, to get rid of my illness."

Eventually, Priessnitz's critics were muted by his record of success with such patients. In the end, the Austrian Emperor gave Priessnitz a gold medal for civic merit, the highest mark of distinct in Austria.

TAPPING INTO HYDROTHERAPY

As I have noted, there are many different types of hydrotherapy. The one I recommend most frequently, known as constitutional hydrotherapy, was taught to me by Dr. Jared Zeff of Portland, Oregon. Dr Zeff, in turn, had inherited his knowledge and ability from older generations of naturopathic doctors.

Constitutional hydrotherapy benefits the whole body. Among the many benign effects of this type of therapy, it helps to produce the following results:

- Optimizes circulation
- Detoxifies and purifies the blood
- Enhances digestive function and elimination
- Tonifies and balances the nervous system
- Stimulates and enhances the immune system

Constitutional hydrotherapy is best done with an assistant, who is needed to lay the wet towels on various parts of the body and replace the towels as they cool. The usual sequence of events is as follows:

1. Lie in bed on your back.
2. The assistant covers your bare chest and abdomen with two thicknesses of towels that have been placed in

hot water and wrung out. (If it's a child who's being treated, rather than yourself, you need to make sure the water is tolerably warm. Before you give a full-scale treatment, be sure to place a small section of the towel on the child to make sure the cloth isn't too hot.)

3. The assistant should cover the wet, hot towels with a dry towel.

4. Blankets go on top of the dry towel. Once you're bundled up, the towels and blanket should stay on at least five minutes.

5. After five minutes, remove the hot towels and replace them with a single thickness of a thin towel that has been run under cold water and then wrung out. (There should still be some moisture left in the towel.)

6. Place the cold towel on the bare chest and abdomen. Cover with a dry towel and blankets. Leave the towel on for 10 minutes, which is about how long it takes to reach body temperature. (If it takes longer than that to warm up, leave it on longer and don't make the towel so cold or wet next time.)

7. Your assistant may have to take off the cold towel (depending on what part of your body it covers). After it's off, turn over and lie on your stomach.

8. Repeat the same procedure on your back while lying on your stomach—following five minutes of hot towel treatment with 10 minutes under a thin, cold towel.

The contrast between hot and cold is the effective part of this therapy. Heat dilates the blood vessels, while cold initially constricts and then dilates them. The alternating dilation and contraction creates a pumping action that improves circulation through the superficial and deep blood vessels.

DOSAGE

I recommend one or two treatments daily if you have an acute condition. For a chronic condition, once a day is sufficient. After each treatment, drink at least 8 ounces of purified water and rest for at least 15 minutes.

If you're giving treatments to an infant, be sure to follow the guidelines of a natural or holistic doctor.

Do not eat large meals before a hydrotherapy treatment.

WHAT ARE THE SIDE EFFECTS?

Hydrotherapy is not recommended if you have an asthma condition. Also, it should only be done with the guidance of a naturopathic or holistic doctor if you're pregnant or have diabetes.

HYDROTHERAPY

RECOMMENDATIONS FROM THE NATURAL PHYSICIAN FOR . . .

🐦 ARTHRITIS

Constitutional hydrotherapy is effective for all types of arthritis. It improves circulation and reduces inflammation of the joints. It also addresses the underlying cause of many cases of arthritis such as toxicity and poor digestion. Local applications of hot and cold, or alternating hot and cold, help to soothe and relieve pain.

🐦 BRONCHITIS AND PNEUMONIA

Hydrotherapy is one of the best therapies for respiratory tract conditions. If you apply alternating hot and cold directly over the bronchial area, you may be able to see very rapid results.

🐦 CANCER

The stronger your immune system, the greater your ability to resist cancer. Hydrotherapy helps your immune system in a number of ways: aids detoxification, improves digestion, and stimulates immune-cell activity. This therapy also helps with lymphatic drainage that is so important for a healthy immune system.

I advise patients who have cancer to use constitutional hydrotherapy as part of a comprehensive program coordinated by the doctor who's overseeing the treatment. It does not interfere with any conventional treatments such as chemotherapy or radiation.

🐦 DETOXIFICATION

You cannot be healthy in today's world without efficient detoxification. Constitutional hydrotherapy stimulates circulation through the liver and kidneys to eliminate toxins. It also brings blood flow to the skin to help with the toxin-elimination process. In addition, it improves digestion and, therefore, elimination.

If you're already on a detoxification program, I advise adding constitutional hydrotherapy as part of the therapy. As a matter of fact, some naturopathic doctors get amazing results by detoxifying people with hydrotherapy combined with dietary changes.

🐦 DIGESTIVE CONDITIONS

When hydrotherapy is applied to the abdominal area, there's a great increase in circulation to the digestive organs, including stomach, intestines, colon, liver, gallbladder, and pancreas. The improved circulation helps to heal inflamed or damaged tissues, promotes better function of the digestive organs, and improves elimination through the colon. I commonly recommend it for the following digestive conditions:

- *Constipation.* Hydrotherapy helps normalize the messages that travel from the nerve centers to the colon and digestive organs. It helps to stimulate and balance peristalsis— the wavelike contractions that move stool through the colon.

- *Crohn's disease, ulcers, and ulcerative colitis.* Tissues are inflamed and damaged with these diseases. I have seen a lot of people with these problems have long-term improvements from constitutional hydrotherapy. If the condition is serious, it may take months of treatments to heal the damaged tissues, but consistent treatments are almost invariably effective.

- *Irritable bowel syndrome.* Often, this condition is the result of stress combined with poor digestion. Hydrotherapy helps to tonify the system, which usually produces good improvements. This therapy is also good for treatment of acute symptoms associated with irritable bowel syndrome, such as abdominal pain, gas, and bloating.

FEVER AND INFECTIONS

Constitutional hydrotherapy stimulates the white blood cells, increasing their number and their activity. This makes it an excellent therapy for fevers and infections. As a matter of fact, the fever may increase slightly, and temporarily, with hydrotherapy treatments, a sign the immune system is "kicking in." Soon after, the fever drops below where it started, a sign that the infection is calming down.

HEADACHES

Chronic headaches can be greatly improved or relieved with constitutional hydrotherapy. People suffering from toxicity, maldigestion, and poor liver function are most helped with this therapy. A more effective treatment for acute headaches is foot hydrotherapy.

While there are different versions of foot hydrotherapy, I've found the following sequence to be effective:

At the onset of a headache, place your feet in a bucket or tub of hot water. (The water should be as hot as possible, but still tolerable to the touch.) Then place a cold cloth on your forehead or an ice pack on the back of your neck.

With this combination of hot and cold, your body diverts blood flow to the feet and away from the head, thus reducing head congestion. The treatment can also be helpful for sinusitis.

SKIN CONDITIONS

The skin is the largest organ of elimination. Therefore, internal toxicity often shows up on the skin. Such is often the case with chronic skin rashes and eczema. I have seen constitutional hydrotherapy help to clear up long-standing cases of skin rashes.

Hypericum

"Since I had that root canal a few days ago I have this intense shooting pain through my upper right jaw. Anything that you recommend?" a friend of mine inquired.

"Yes, the best thing to take is homeopathic hypericum," I replied. Two hours later after taking the hypericum my friend's pain had vanished.

Many people are surprised to find that the homeopathic remedy hypericum is made from the popular botanical St. John's wort, a natural antidepressant. Even in the botanical form, which is undiluted, St. John's wort (also known by its botanical name, *Hypericum perforatum*) can be applied topically or taken internally for nerve pains related to crushing injuries or burns.

Homeopathic hypericum is convenient to use and works very quickly for nerve injuries and related pain. It is commonly used for injuries to areas where there is a rich nerve supply such as the head, eyes, teeth, tongue, tailbone, fingers, and toes. The classic symptom this remedy helps is sharp, shooting pains.

DOSAGE

A potency of 30C is commonly available in health-food stores, although you can use whatever potency is available. Dissolve two pellets of hypericum in your mouth every 15 minutes for the relief of physical trauma. Two to three doses should give noticeable improvement and can be continued for approximately three days. A single dose of a 200C or higher can also be very effective. This remedy can be used in conjunction with pain medicine and can be alternated with homeopathic arnica (see page 33) for injuries where soft tissue and nerves are affected.

WHAT ARE THE SIDE EFFECTS?

Side effects are rare. Generally this remedy works or has no effect at all. There is usually no in-between effect. If you have no improvement after a few days of using hypericum, stop using it.

HYPERICUM

RECOMMENDATIONS FROM THE NATURAL PHYSICIAN FOR . . .

❧ DENTAL PAIN

Hypericum is an excellent treatment for nerve pain as the result of dental work. I recommend you have this homeopathic on hand to use if needed after such procedures, including dental surgery.

❧ INJURIES

Any injury that causes nerve pain and damage may be helped by hypericum.

These could range from a finger caught in a door to a concussion causing headaches. Hypericum is also very specifically used by homeopathic practitioners for injuries to the tailbone and spine, which are rich in nerve supply.

Ignatia

———

"Dr. Mark, I am so stressed-out! With all the things going on at my job and with my kids, I'm embarrassed to say that my husband and I are having problems again. I just don't know if I can handle it anymore."

These were the words of Jacqueline, a patient whose family I had consulted with over the years. In the past, I had helped her children with various health problems. Now Jacqueline felt the time was right to get her own health in order.

During Jacqueline's visit, she described herself as a caring person whose feelings are hurt very easily. She takes her work and home life quite seriously—perhaps too seriously, as she admitted. As a result, she suffered from tight shoulder and neck muscles, which could trigger excruciating tension headaches.

"I get very moody," she observed, when I asked her to talk about her emotions. She went on to say that she would occasionally lose her temper with her kids or husband over trivial matters that had never bothered her in the past. Jacqueline often felt like crying, sometimes for no apparent reason, and she spoke of "walking around with a lump in my throat." Even in our first interview, I noticed that from time to time, she would sigh heavily as if she was trying to bear up under a great load of stress.

Jacqueline's situation is hardly unique. Many women feel themselves in similar situations, with similar reactions. My prescription, in these cases, is the homeopathic remedy ignatia.

In fact, many women and men in our society would benefit from taking ignatia (*Ignatia amarus*), along with using a number of stress-reduction techniques. Frequently prescribed by homeopathic physicians for the effects of stress, it's especially effective when people are suffering grief of any kind. This could be grief from the death of a loved one, grief from a turbulent relationship or divorce, or grief from some kind of misgivings.

The connection between stress and grief is obvious. Anyone who's grieving has all sorts of stored emotions that may cause her to "tighten up." These emotions can be expressed in many different ways—crying, mood swings, or tightening muscles. All these factors contribute to what homeopathic physicians call an ignatia state.

But there may be other factors as well. I often find the person requiring ignatia to be a perfectionist. Living in an imperfect world leads to easily hurt feelings and a lot of disappointments. The feelings of disappointment and grief are suppressed, which leads to a very interesting ignatia symptom—the sensation of a lump in the throat.

As strange as it may sound, many patients requiring ignatia have said almost exactly the same thing—that they felt a "lump in the throat." Now, whenever I hear of this characteristic symptom, the remedy ignatia immediately comes to mind.

But there's another unique symptom that suggests the need for this remedy—sighing.

I realize that no conventional doctor would ask a patient, "Are you sighing a lot?"—but we all recognize, and know intuitively, that sighing is a very real expression of an emotion. As I have learned in Chinese medicine, symptoms of suppressed grief often show up in the lungs, with sighing being an outlet for this contained grief.

By the way, Jacqueline responded very nicely to ignatia. After only two days she felt "calmer" and in the following two months, her muscle tightness greatly decreased and that "lump in the throat" feeling went away. She felt that she was now in more control of her feelings and that the ignatia definitely was helping.

DOSAGE

The typical dosage for ignatia is to take a 30C potency twice daily for a week or longer, or until the user has experienced substantial relief of symptoms. When symptoms have been acute, most people notice a difference in one or two doses. Homeopathic practitioners often give a single dose of 200C or higher in the belief that it will have a deeper effect. I have noticed that some patients respond better to a higher potency of ignatia.

WHAT ARE THE SIDE EFFECTS?

Ignatia has no side effects at all with some people. If it's not helpful, however, you can simply stop using it. If you have questions about whether or not you should use ignatia in the first place, you'll want to consult a homeopathic practitioner.

A JAW-DROPPING REMEDY

One of the most dramatic cases of homeopathic healing I have ever seen involved a 30-year-old patient of mine, Laura, who had a severe case of TMJ. As a matter of fact, it was so severe her doctor was recommending jaw surgery. In an attempt to forego surgery, Laura was getting regular chiropractic, massage, and acupuncture treatments. All gave her temporary relief, but no permanent escape. A few hours after each treatment, her jaw muscles would tighten up again and the unbearable pain would set in.

After taking her case, I found out that she and her husband were very stressed about having children. Laura had an emotionally traumatic history of miscarriages. Many people who have TMJ can trace the onset to some physical trauma like a car accident. But in Laura's case, the TMJ problem began about the same time as her first miscarriage.

Coincidence? Perhaps, but even so, I felt ignatia was worth trying.

Five minutes after Laura took her first dose of ignatia 30C, she noticed improvement of her TMJ discomfort. She called me immediately, very excited about the improvement. Of course, I simply recommended that she continue taking it as needed.

Over the next week, Laura found that she had to take ignatia a few times a day to prevent the muscle tightness and TMJ from flaring up. But about two weeks later, after receiving a number of encouraging reports from her, I got a panicked call.

"The remedy is not working any more. My TMJ is killing me!"

"All right," I replied. "I want you to take the 200C potency of ignatia and call me back in 30 minutes."

After about a half-hour of suspense, Laura called to say the higher potency was effective. Triumphantly, she announced that the TMJ pain went away in about five minutes after taking the stronger dose.

Miraculously, Laura has only had to repeat the high-potency ignatia a couple of times in the ensuing five years. I spoke to her much less frequently, but at last report, she was no longer suffering from TMJ syndrome.

IGNATIA

RECOMMENDATIONS FROM THE NATURAL PHYSICIAN FOR . . .

ANXIETY

I commonly prescribe ignatia to my patients with anxiety. It works particularly well for those who are stressed easily and have problems with tight muscles of the neck and shoulders.

DEPRESSION

Ignatia works quite nicely to relieve depression when it comes on after a grief or disappointment. A common example is a person who is suffering in a relationship where things are not going well, and depression sets in from the suppression of grief. Ignatia helps to release the suppressed grief and relieve some of the symptoms of depression.

GRIEF

Ignatia remedy comes in handy when grief occurs suddenly, in unforeseen circumstances. If a loved one has died suddenly, people may ask me what kind of natural therapy can help ease the shock and pain of the moment. Ignatia is the first remedy to try. Obviously, it will not take away all the emotions that naturally accompany a tragedy. But for those who are very sensitive, who have a hard time coping, it helps reduce that "heart pain." With ignatia, you can avoid the use of tranquilizing and antidepressant medications.

Many practitioners of homeopathy, as well as psychologists and counselors, have observed that patients who are undergoing counseling for deep-seated emotional traumas recover more quickly when they are also given the indicated homeopathic "grief" remedy like ignatia. I have seen this with patients who have made little improvement with various counselors over the years. When given ignatia, they make dramatic changes in their outlook on life.

Ignatia works to help remove emotional blockages. For example, I remember one 44-year-old patient, Minnie, who had a bad case of multiple sclerosis (a serious condition where the immune system attacks the body's nervous tissue). Minnie related to me that her condition had started right after her divorce four years previously. Although she had tried various natural and conventional therapies, her condition was getting worse.

Based on the fact that her illness began after the trauma of her divorce, I prescribed ignatia. Two weeks after taking ignatia, Minnie came to see me, as she was feeling very emotional. She found herself crying a lot and losing her temper more than usual. My comment to her was "Great!"

"What do you mean, great?" she shot back. "I feel like an emotional basket case. I haven't felt like this in years!"

"This is probably similar to how you

(continued)

felt during your divorce," I suggested. After a moment's hesitation, she agreed.

"That's an excellent sign," I went on. "You need to heal emotionally before you can heal physically."

The intensity of Minnie's symptoms began to diminish over the next week. She felt a commensurate increase in her energy level, another sign the remedy was working.

Over the next two months, her muscle weakness and visual problems ceased to be a problem, and during the next three years, Minnie lived without symptoms of multiple sclerosis. Apart from taking repeated doses of ignatia during times of severe stress, she takes no other medicines.

🐦 HEADACHE

As most of us have learned by experience, stress contributes to the most common type of headache, known as a tension headache—an experience of pain that patients sometimes describe as a "vice tightening around their head." Tension headaches are related to tight neck and shoulder muscles.

Since ignatia helps to reduce the effects of stress, and also reduces muscle tightness, it's a remedy worthy of consideration any time you have a tension headache. It

is particularly indicated when the headaches occur on the left side of the head.

🐦 MUSCLE SPASM

If you're prone to muscle tightness as the result of stress, the tightness usually occurs in the neck and shoulders. Ignatia, as well as massage, works nicely to prevent the tightness and muscle spasms in this area.

In addition, ignatia can save a lot of trips to the chiropractor. My wife, who is also a naturopathic physician, treated one woman who had chronic, severe fibromyalgia, a painful condition of the muscles and joints. After my wife administered one high-potency dose of ignatia, the woman discovered that her symptoms were alleviated—permanently!

🐦 PMS

Premenstrual syndrome can be greatly helped by ignatia. It is indicated when symptoms of crying, mood swings, and jealousy come out during the premenstrual days.

🐦 TMJ SYNDROME

This is not something you will find in too many books, but I have found ignatia to help a number of patients who have temporomandibular joint disorder (TMJ), a painful condition of the jaw joint.

Ipecacuanha

"I might need to go home soon. I woke up this morning feeling nauseated, and it hasn't gone away. Do you have a homeopathic that can help me?" asked Val, the office manager at our clinic.

"Sure, but are you pregnant?" I asked half-jokingly.

"No, I'm not. It feels like I may be coming down with the flu," replied Val.

"Here you go. Take two pellets and let's see how you do over the next 15 minutes," I said.

As I walked by the front desk five minutes later, Val stopped me.

"It's amazing," she said. "The nausea is all gone. Can it work that fast?"

"Yes, homeopathics can be pretty incredible," I said.

"They really can be. What was the one you gave me?" inquired Val.

"It's called ipecac."

"Isn't ipecac used to make people throw up?"

"Regular ipecac is used for that; but homeopathic ipecac has the opposite effect. It relieves nausea and vomiting."

The next day, Val reported that she had felt fine for the rest of the evening.

ROOTS FROM THE NEW WORLD

Ipecacuanha is the homeopathic preparation from the leaves of the ipecacuanha shrub from Brazil. The leaves of this shrub have a bitter, nauseating taste. Thus, it has been used in Brazil since 1648 as an emetic (to make people throw up to expel ingested poisons). The standard medicine is found in medicine kits and in pharmacies. The homeopathic has the opposite effect, and helps to relieve nausea and vomiting.

Homeopathic ipecacuanha, referred to by homeopaths as ipecac, is the main remedy for nausea and vomiting, no matter what the cause. This could be the result of the flu, as in Val's case, or intestinal problems that result from spoiled food, bronchitis, or a condition where there is marked nausea and/or vomiting such as from a migraine headache.

Ipecac is also commonly recommended for women who have nausea associated with pregnancy. In addition, I've recommended it as a remedy for hemorrhaging—such as uterine hemorrhage—as well as for bronchitis and asthma.

As with any homeopathic remedy, physicians look for certain key symptoms. In the case of homeopathic ipecac, the telltale symptom is constant nausea that is unrelieved by vomiting. But there may be another symptom as well—the tongue looks clean despite constant vomiting.

This is definitely a remedy that belongs in every first-aid kit.

DOSAGE

Dissolve two pellets of the 30C potency (or whatever potency you have on hand) in your mouth every 15 minutes for the relief of symptoms. Two to three doses should be sufficient for acute cases.

NOTE: The dosage is the same for all age groups.

WHAT ARE THE SIDE EFFECTS?

There is no concern about toxicity or side effects with homeopathic ipecacuanha. As with any homeopathic remedy, take it as needed for relief of symptoms.

IPECACUANHA

Recommendations from the Natural Physician for . . .

🌊 **ASTHMA AND BRONCHITIS**

Ipecac is useful for a rattling cough that is accompanied by gagging and vomiting resulting from increased mucus. These symptoms might indicate a case of bronchitis or asthma. Symptoms are worse at night, when eating, and when in a warm room. The person feels better in the open air, after coughing up mucus, and being in a cool room.

Homeopathic ipecac is a common remedy for childhood asthma.

🌊 **HANGOVER**

Ipecac can help reduce the nausea and vomiting that occur the "morning after" indulging in too much alcohol.

🌊 **HEMORRHAGE**

Ipecac is a good remedy for uterine hemorrhage or heavy menstrual flow, accompanied by nausea and vomiting.

🌊 **MIGRAINE HEADACHE**

The severe nausea and vomiting caused by migraines can be alleviated with ipecac. The headaches tend to be on the left side. It's most likely to be effective if you have a migraine headache that makes you want to remain still and if you feel better with fresh air.

🌊 **MORNING SICKNESS**

Ipecac is one of the main remedies to help relieve the classic nausea and vomiting that some women get during pregnancy. The nice thing about homeopathic ipecac is that there is no risk of side effects that would harm the baby.

Ipriflavone

"Here is what I am taking."

Mary, a 55-year-old restaurant owner who had come to see me about her osteoporosis, lifted a supplement-filled plastic bag to my desk. As I watched in wonderment, she methodically arranged 21 bottles of supplements single file along the edge.

"Is that *all?*" I asked, when she had added the last bottle to the row.

Mary looked chagrined at the note of awe in my voice. "I've been looking forward to this day. I really have no idea what I should or should not be taking. The trouble is, I read a whole lot of health magazines, and I have a friend who works in a health-food store. Adding up all the advice I get from one place or the other, well—" She paused, waving her hand. "Here's where I am."

Reading the formulations on each bottle, I made some notes, then asked, "Suppose you could reduce the number of supplements from twenty-one to five? Would you do it?"

"Wouldn't that be nice!" She hesitated. "But I want to make sure I'm not missing anything. I saw what my mother went through when she had a hip fracture in her 70s. She was never the same after that. I know a lot of women who worry about osteoporosis, but it seems to be a particular problem in our family. I don't want to end up with a hip fracture like my mother did."

In principle, Mary was absolutely right to be concerned about her osteoporosis. A recent bone-density study showed that she was below average for her age, and she had the beginnings of osteoporosis (decreased bone density).

But her supplement program was out of control. As I told Mary, I would help her simplify that program, but at the same time, I wanted to add one important supplement to it. "It's called ipriflavone," I said.

"It sounds like something all women such as me should be taking," Mary observed.

"Probably," I replied, "and it can help men's bones, too."

A MASTER BUILDER

Ipriflavone increases the activity of the cells that form fresh bone. At the same time, it decreases the activity of bone cells that aid in the destruction of the bone. This supplement also raises the levels of a hormone that helps to increase the amount of new bone that's constantly being created by a healthy body.

So ipriflavone really has two effects. It helps *maintain* bone density, and, when it's combined with calcium and other substances in your body, it does even more—it helps to *increase* bone density.

Ipriflavone is still being scrutinized, and not all studies support its effectiveness. For instance, as this book was going to press, a negative study about ipriflavone appeared in the *Journal of the American Medical Association* indicating that ipriflavone combined with calcium was no better than a placebo in slowing bone loss. However, as with most drug or supplement studies, it is common to have a certain percentage of

studies that are not favorable. In general, clinical studies over the past 15 years on ipriflavone have been positive. More than 150 studies of its safety and effectiveness, in both animal and human studies, lend support to its use.

In fact, the use of ipriflavone is likely to become more prevalent. One out of every three women in North America develops osteoporosis, and researchers expect that the percentage of Americans with osteoporosis is going to continue to climb steadily as baby boomers move into their elder years.

An estimated $7 to $10 billion each year are spent treating the complications that arise from this disease—such as the hip fracture that Mary's mother endured. Broken bones are debilitating when they happen to older people. Statistics show that after a hip fracture occurs, approximately 15% of patients die within one year. (Often, the problem is some complicating factor, such as a blood clot that's related to prolonged immobility.)

Ipriflavone is an isolated copy of an important chemical found in soy, called isoflavone daidzein. First discovered in 1930, ipriflavone has been widely studied in humans, though it really didn't become widely used until the mid 1990s.

BARRING BREAKDOWNS

Bone continually remodels itself. Bone cells are constantly being eroded by cells called osteoclasts, while new bone is being formed with the help of other cells called osteoblasts. The key to good bone health? Just replace as many or more bone cells than are lost.

But, of course, that replacement and rebuilding process requires assistance. That's where ipriflavone comes in.

Ipriflavone has been found to have its

own receptor site on immature osteoblasts—the bone-building cells. It directly stimulates the activity of these cells, which in turn promote bone-cell formation. And ipriflavone does not have an estrogenic effect. That's an advantage, because estrogen produces a number of side effects and has been shown to increase the risk of breast cancer as well as other kinds of cancer.

In one study, 15 postmenopausal women were given ipriflavone or a placebo. Various hormones, including estrogen, were measured after a single oral dose of 600 or 1,000 mg, and after 7, 14, and 21 days of treatment with 600- or 1,000-mg doses. By the end of the study, there was no elevation of estrogen among any of the women. Clearly, the ipriflavone did not have the effect of increasing estrogen levels.

Studies do show that ipriflavone acts synergistically with estrogen to normalize calcitonin secretion. In other words, it helps open the pathway for more active bone growth.

DOSAGE

I recommend ipriflavone be supplemented at 600 mg daily. This is the same dosage used in the osteoporosis studies.

It's important to note, however, that calcium was given to many of the people who participated in the studies, so the bone-strengthening benefits were really the result of dual supplementation.

Take ipriflavone with meals to enhance absorption. For maximum effectiveness, I always recommend taking it with other vitamins and minerals known to play a role in bone metabolism. Calcium, magnesium, and vitamin D are the most important. But there are other important supplements as well, including zinc, silicon, manganese, vitamin C, vitamin B6, boron, vitamin K,

vitamin B12, and folic acid. All these can be found in bone-building formulas offered by many companies, so you don't have to purchase them separately.

WHAT ARE THE SIDE EFFECTS?

In general, ipriflavone appears to be very safe. In a study that was launched in 1997, researchers showed the long-term safety of ipriflavone for periods ranging from 6 to 96 months, when the supplement was taken by 2,769 people.

The most common side effect is digestive upset, but this symptom is likely to go away if you take ipriflavone with food. Other symptoms observed, to a lesser extent, included skin rashes, headache, depression, drowsiness, and rapid heartbeat (tachycardia). A small percentage of people, when tested, showed minor abnormalities in liver, kidney, and blood, but the abnormalities were quite minor and they rapidly disappeared.

I advise caution with ipriflavone, however, if you're taking the drug theophylline for asthma. In one case, someone who was already taking theophylline had excessive levels of this substance in her blood when she started taking ipriflavone along with her regular asthma medication. Animal studies have found that ipriflavone may inhibit certain liver enzymes that break down theophylline, leading to higher-than-normal blood levels.

For anyone who's had kidney failure, I advise close monitoring before supplementing with ipriflavone, although it appears to be safe in those with mild kidney disease. Researchers recommend lower doses (200 to 400 mg daily) in patients with more advanced renal failure. Further study is required to determine absolute safe dosages for those with kidney disease.

Lymphocyte levels should also be watched by a doctor. In one study of 132 women who were taking ipriflavone, 29 of the women in the group developed a reduction in lymphocytes, a type of white blood cell that is an integral component of the immune system. According to some researchers, the reduction in lymphocytes in this study is not clinically significant. However, to be safe your doctor can measure your lymphocyte levels with a simple blood test every six months to make sure your levels are within normal ranges. Optimally, blood work would be done at the onset of starting ipriflavone and every six months thereafter.

IPRIFLAVONE

RECOMMENDATIONS FROM THE NATURAL PHYSICIAN FOR . . .

➤ HYPERPARATHYROIDISM

In this condition, high levels of parathyroid hormone cause calcium to be withdrawn from the bone and cause elevated levels of blood calcium. As a result, bone health suffers from calcium loss. One study showed that 1,200 mg of ipriflavone daily resulted in significant reduction of bone turnover. Researchers interpreted this to mean that there was increased bone formation among those who took ipriflavone.

➤ KIDNEY FAILURE

Ipriflavone is not a supplement for the treatment of renal failure. It may, however, be of value if someone is losing bone minerals because of kidney failure (known as renal osteodystrophy). One study of 23 people on kidney dialysis with decreased bone mineralization due to renal failure were given ipriflavone (400 to 600 mg daily) and observed for a period of one to nine months. Researchers found evidence that there was significantly less breakdown of bone and significant increases in bone formation. No adverse side effects were reported. But I would want to see more research before recommending ipriflavone for anyone with a kidney condition.

➤ OSTEOPOROSIS

There have been more than 60 human studies in the past 10 years, many of which are double-blind and placebo-controlled—meeting the standards for scientific validity.

The most significant study I've run across involved 100 postmenopausal women between the ages of 53 and 65, whom researchers tracked for a full year. Each woman received 200 mg of ipriflavone three times a day after meals. They were also given 1,000 mg of calcium daily. Ninety women completed the study, and the results indicate that bone-mineral density was increased by 2% after six months and 5.8% after 12 months!

During that time, pain symptoms also decreased and mobility improved. Only three women dropped out of the study because of problems with digestive upset. This study is even more remarkable when its outcome is compared with what happens with other kinds of drug therapies. Most pharmaceutical drugs only slow down the loss of bone, and usually, when calcium is added as a supplement, the rate of bone loss increases,

(continued)

but the calcium supplement doesn't help increase bone density. Researchers came to the conclusion that ipriflavone was the decisive factor in improving bone density.

Researchers have explored in a number of studies the possibility of combining ipriflavone with estrogen for the treatment of osteoporosis. Some of these studies have, indeed, shown that bone density improves more significantly when people get a combined dose of ipriflavone and estrogen. With the combination treatment, it's feasible to take lower doses of estrogen—which is a benefit, since that may reduce the risk of estrogen-related cancers.

For example, in one controlled, one-year study, 83 postmenopausal women were divided into three groups. The first group received neither estrogen nor supplements; the second received estrogen; and the third got ipriflavone along with estrogen. At the end of the 12 months, those who got the combination treatment showed a significant increase in bone-mineral density. Though bone density decreased or increased only slightly in the other groups, it was up 5.6% among those who had a combination of estrogen and ipriflavone. These results have been supported by other human studies as well.

Ipriflavone can also help women who have had their ovaries removed (ovariectomy). Typically, the removal of the ovaries results in rapid bone loss because there's a sharp decrease in hormone production. A study of 32 women who had recently had ovariectomies showed that ipriflavone appeared to protect them from sudden bone loss. In the study, the women received 500 mg of calcium and 600 mg of ipriflavone daily for 12 months.

➴ OTOSCLEROSIS

There are sometimes small but significant changes in the structure of one of the bones involved with hearing—a very tiny structure called the stapes. This condition leads to gradual hearing loss, the condition known as otosclerosis. It's sometimes accompanied by another type of hearing problem, tinnitus, which is essentially "ringing in the ears."

Otosclerosis can be treated surgically, and a hearing aid can help compensate for some hearing loss. To find out whether ipriflavone could help this condition in some way, researchers tried a small study of patients who had tinnitus due to otosclerosis.

All the patients also had stapedectomies—that is, removal of the inner ear bone. People in the ipriflavone study received 200 mg of the supplement four times daily. Supplementation began three months before the operation, then continued at the same dosage for three months afterward. During the preoperative phase, tinnitus was stopped in four of nine patients. (Only one out of seven in the placebo group experienced relief of tinnitus.) Postoperatively, all patients in the ipriflavone group, but only 50% of the patients in the placebo group, experienced relief of tinnitus.

Though researchers can't explain why the ipriflavone was beneficial in this study, it will almost certainly lead to further exploration.

➴ PAGET'S DISEASE

This is a disorder of the skeleton where bone turnover is increased to an abnormal rate. As a result, bones develop in abnormal ways, people have more fractures, and some of those with Paget's disease have severe bone pain. Almost 3% of people over the age of 40 have this disease, though the cause is unknown.

When doctors studied 16 patients who had this disease, they found that ipriflavone supplementation reduced the evidence of bone breakdown—which means the "turnover" was slowed. Bone pain was also reduced. Dosages used in the study were 600 to 1,200 mg daily.

Iron

Iron has paradoxical qualities. It can be a healing therapy, but it can also be toxic, causing illness. A simple health-giving goal is to get the most out of iron and avoid the potential risks.

We need iron to live. It enables our red blood cells to carry oxygen to the cells. It also is involved in different enzyme reactions, one of which is to produce energy. However necessary, though, it can create problems if you get too much iron in supplements or if you suffer from a genetic condition like hemochromatosis—which means, simply, that your body absorbs abnormally high amounts of iron. An excess of iron definitely causes side effects, and researchers think it's also connected with certain diseases. There's some evidence that there is a correlation between excessive iron levels and increased risk of heart disease and cancer.

There are two sources of dietary iron, referred to as heme and nonheme. Heme iron is found in animal products and is the form that our bodies absorb most efficiently. Nonheme iron is found in plant foods and is not absorbed as well.

Your body stores iron in the liver, spleen, and bone marrow.

SOME IRONIES

Though it's easy to get iron in the diet or in supplements, iron deficiency is the most prevalent type of nutrient deficiency in the United States—and it has consequences. Iron-deficiency anemia, as the name implies, is a direct result. If you have this kind of anemia (there are other kinds as well), your red blood cells lose some of their capacity to carry oxygen. From that microscopic change in transport capabilities, you can end up with a whole range of serious problems, including fatigue, poor memory and concentration, learning problems, paleness, increased menstrual loss, and weakened immunity.

Symptoms of chronic, severe iron deficiency are even more pronounced. Some people get a condition called pica, a craving for substances, such as dirt, ice, or pencils, that have no nutritional value. Cracks in the corner of the mouth, or cheilosis, is another common problem. People with severe deficiency may also develop spoon-shaped fingernails and toenails.

There are serious consequences of iron deficiency in children. Studies show that approximately 9% of all children in the United States between the ages of 12 months and 36 months have iron-deficiency anemia. The prevalence is higher among children living at or below poverty level, and it's also higher among black or Mexican-American children.

When children are iron deficient, they may have delayed physical growth, slow mental development (as evidenced by lower IQ scores and poor short-term memory), and behavioral disturbances such as hyperactivity and problems with social interaction. Unfortunately, if the iron deficiency continues beyond age five, these changes can be irreversible.

Growth spurts in children and teenagers can lead to an increased demand for iron and thus iron-deficiency anemia.

Severe iron deficiency also has consequences for adults. Among women, iron deficiency can lead to prolonged menstrual bleeding. For adults of either sex, if you frequently feel tired, or if you can't sustain activity for a prolonged length of time, these symptoms of fatigue may be due to iron deficiency.

BLOOD BOTHERS

The question is, how do we become deficient in iron in the first place?

The most common cause for adults is blood loss. For women this is mainly due to heavy menstrual flow. A vicious cycle occurs when a menstruating woman is anemic, because the iron-deficiency anemia actually leads to even more bleeding. In some cases, the bleeding is continuous, not just cyclical. So a woman with this condition needs to raise her iron levels and get the anemia improved to correct the underlying cause of the heavy menstruation. But the underlying problem—and what leads, ultimately, to iron deficiency—could be a hormone imbalance.

Shelly is a good example of what women can go through with this condition. A 22-year-old college student with a four-year history of heavy menstrual bleeding, Shelly had become severely anemic. I could see indications of that, even before I did an examination. Her face was pale and she had purple circles under her eyes. Suspecting iron deficiency, I checked the inside of her eyelids—which were as pale as her face—and felt her hands, which were chilly.

Shelly's medical doctor had put her on high doses of iron tablets. Though she was taking 600 mg a day, the therapy wasn't helping. In fact, these large doses of iron caused severe constipation. Her cyclical menstrual flow had been heavy, but with the addition of large doses of iron, it turned into continuous bleeding that was uninterrupted throughout the month. It was not heavy every day, but there was always some blood loss.

Her doctor had then recommended the next, usual step in conventional medicine: prescribing a birth-control pill to help regulate Shelly's menstrual cycle. These pills, however, gave her severe migraine headaches, and she stopped using them—whereupon her doctor told her that the only option left was a hysterectomy. At that point, Shelly knew she wanted to try other resources, and upon the advice of a friend, she came to see me.

The first lab test revealed immediately that the anemia was very severe. I switched her over to 50 mg a day of a more absorbable form of iron. I also asked her to take other nutrients to help build her blood—among them, vitamin C (which improves iron absorption), folic acid, and vitamin B12. Finally, I gave her homeopathic ferrum phos 6x and the herb vitex for hormone balancing.

Things did not improve overnight, but over the next two months, Shelly could feel that progress was being made. She felt more energetic. I continued to do the lab work necessary to monitor her blood—and the results showed a steady increase of iron. After three months of treatment, the bleeding was under control. We were eventually able to get her off the iron and other supplements, and she made a full recovery.

MINDING YOUR IRON MINE

Good sources of iron include beef, organ meats, and eggs. Good plant sources include lima beans, tofu, legumes, kelp, green leafy vegetables, whole grains, brewer's yeast, pumpkin, and nuts.

It's important to keep in mind that the iron you get from meat is much more easily absorbed than the kind that comes from plant foods. Approximately 30% of heme iron (from meat) is absorbed while only 2% to 10% of nonheme iron (from plant foods) makes its way into your cells. This does not mean that people living on a vegetarian diet are destined to become iron deficient. You can get all the iron you need without eating meat. On a vegetarian diet, however, it's important to get plenty of iron-contributing plant foods or to supplement your diet with a well-absorbable form of iron.

How much iron do you need on a daily basis? Following is the recommended daily allowances (RDA) for iron. While some people may need more than these recommended daily amounts, they are usually adequate.

Dietary Reference Intake

0 to 6 months: 10 mg

6 to 12 months: 15 mg

1 to 10 years: 10 to 15 mg

11 to 18 years: 10 to 18+ mg

18+ years (male): 10+ mg

18+ years (female): 18+ mg

50+ years (female): 10+ mg

Pregnant/lactating: 30 to 60+ mg

Whether or not you show physical, external signs of iron deficiency, your doctor should give you a regular blood test for iron. The test is quite simple, and children, in particular, should be screened regularly. It also makes sense for your doctor to run a ferritin test, which measures the amount of stored iron in the body.

LINKS AND CAUSES

Iron deficiency is often a problem in pregnant women. The growing baby uses much of the mother's iron stores and so she is prone to iron-deficiency anemia, which can lead to complications if the condition isn't identified and treated. The rate of premature delivery is twice as high for a mother who has iron-deficiency anemia, and the birth weight of the newborn tends to be much lower. Infants who are born prematurely are also much more prone to iron deficiency than those who reach full term.

Among men who have iron deficiency, the most common cause is what's known as chronic occult bleeding—the medical term for internal bleeding. (Women may have chronic occult bleeding as well, though it's a less common cause of iron deficiency than menstrual bleeding.) Adults of either sex may have bleeding in the gastrointestinal tract, related to polyps or ulcers, or by hemorrhoids. Internal bleeding may be associated with drugs that irritate the gastrointestinal lining, such as aspirin. There's also a risk that the bleeding can be caused by cancer.

Among infants and children who have iron deficiency, the main cause is obvious—lack of iron in the diet. But there's another, lesser-known cause: The consumption of cow's milk may cause gastrointestinal bleeding.

Some people simply don't absorb iron as efficiently as they need to. In some cases, particularly among the elderly, the problem is low production of stomach acid. Similar problems can arise if you take a lot of antacids, because the antacid neutralizes stomach acid.

DOSAGE

Since dosages depend on the severity of iron deficiency, you should work with a nutrition-oriented doctor when supplementing iron so that it can be monitored correctly. A typical adult dosage is 25 mg of elemental iron taken twice daily, but you'll probably need higher dosages if you have severe anemia. I recommend taking the iron supplement with meals to avoid digestive upset.

Iron supplements can be absorbed on an empty stomach and some studies show that it has a higher absorption taken this way. Vitamin C enhances the absorption of iron so it is prudent to take a couple hundred milligrams with every dose of iron. I commonly recommend homeopathic ferrum phos 6x and the herbs yellow dock and nettles for blood building as well.

There are some supplements that can interfere with the absorption of iron, including calcium carbonate, magnesium, and zinc—so don't take them at the same time you're taking iron. Antibiotics can also interfere with absorption: If you have a prescription, take it as recommended, but wait at least a couple of hours before you take iron. Plant foods have phytates, which can

also decrease absorption, so you'll get more benefit from the iron supplement if you don't take it immediately before or soon after a meal.

Some iron supplements are much more well-absorbed than others. I recommend that you avoid taking iron sulfate (ferrous sulfate), which is commonly prescribed by conventional physicians. It is not well absorbed, it irritates the digestive tract, and it also causes constipation.

Constipation is probably the worst for pregnant women. Pregnant women are often given a cheap, prenatal vitamin containing iron sulfate as a way to help prevent iron-deficiency anemia, and the supplement worsens constipation problems. (It can also contribute to other health problems during pregnancy such as headaches and hemorrhoids.) When giving iron to pregnant women, I recommend other forms that are more absorbable and that don't produce so many side effects.

Good forms of supplemental iron include iron citrate, iron glycinate, iron succinate, and iron fumarate. The form of the supplement should be clearly indicated on the label.

I do not recommend taking a multivitamin that contains iron. If you're not iron deficient, the extra iron may cause oxidative damage and liver toxicity. If you are iron deficient and need that extra iron supplement, then you don't want to be taking it along with other minerals that might impede its absorption. Depending on the brand of multivitamin, you can usually find one that's iron free.

WHAT ARE THE SIDE EFFECTS?

Current research is showing that excessive levels of iron in the body promote oxidative damage. Researchers believe that high iron levels increase the risk of heart disease, cancer, and possibly other serious conditions. More definitive research is being done in this area.

You should avoid iron supplementation if you have hemochromatosis, a genetic condition where there is increased iron absorption from the diet.

Iron poisoning can be very serious for children. If you're taking iron supplements, be sure to keep them in a secure cabinet where children can't reach them. An overdose of iron can lead to digestive tract damage, nausea, vomiting, liver failure, and possibly death. Iron is the most common cause of accidental poisoning in children.

IRON

RECOMMENDATIONS FROM THE NATURAL PHYSICIAN FOR . . .

ATTENTION DEFICIT/HYPERACTIVITY DISORDER (ADHD)

Have your child checked for iron-deficiency anemia, which can worsen symptoms of ADHD. If your child's iron level is low, then studies show supplementation can help improve some symptoms.

FATIGUE

Many people believe they should take iron supplements if they have fatigue, but that's only true in some cases. While fatigue can be a major symptom of iron deficiency, lack of the mineral is only one possible cause. If your fatigue has another cause, but you start taking iron anyway, the supplement can actually make your fatigue worse.

IRON-DEFICIENCY ANEMIA

Obviously, it makes sense to take iron supplements if you know for sure you have this condition. Be patient, though, because it may take months for more severe iron deficiencies to be brought back to the normal ranges. If you're seeing a conventional medical doctor for this condition, be sure to ask about the more absorbable forms of iron supplements—that is, iron citrate, glycinate, succinate, or fumarate.

LOW THYROID

Iron deficiency may impair the body's ability to manufacture thyroid hormone. Have your doctor check your iron status if you have low thyroid. If you do need iron, make sure you don't take it along with your thyroid medicine. Iron can interfere with thyroid-hormone absorption—but that will be less of a problem if you take the iron supplement at a different time of the day.

PREGNANCY

I generally recommend iron be taken during pregnancy to prevent iron-deficiency anemia. The usual dosage is 25 to 30 mg of elemental iron daily—that is, the usual adult dosage—which is perfectly adequate for pregnant women as long as they don't have anemia. Prenatal vitamins contain iron. Again, look for formulas that do not contain ferrous sulfate, which is constipating.

(continued)

RESTLESS LEG SYNDROME

Iron deficiency in the elderly may cause restless leg syndrome. Supplementation can help improve this condition. Note, however, that other minerals may also be lacking—particularly zinc, calcium, and magnesium—so you may need additional supplementation to help the condition.

Juicing

It doesn't take a rocket scientist, as they say, to figure out that anyone can make delicious, refreshing, and nutritious drinks by squeezing fresh fruit and vegetables until their juice pours out. But beyond the good taste, there are proven rewards for health and vitality.

Today, more people than ever are benefiting from the healing power of juices. What is so great about juicing? Well, it's a way to get vitamins, minerals, enzymes, and phytonutrients all in one drink that happens to be "highly absorbable." What that means is, when you get your nutrients in this form, they're readily incorporated through your digestion into your bloodstream, and from there to the cells of your organs and tissues.

Studies show that most people consume woefully small amounts of fruits and vegetables in their daily diets. Yet, nutritional experts and researchers keep turning up evidence that our bodies can get a lot of protection from these same plant foods, if we just eat enough of them. The beauty of juicing is that it gives us a different way to get these life-enhancing nutrients in a very concentrated and tasty form, without carrying around bushel baskets of fruits and vegetables each day.

TURNING ON THE JUICE

The typical juicer extracts the juice and expels the pulp or fiber. This makes juice easy to digest and assimilate. You can completely control taste by varying the ingredients you put in. But there's a downside to using this type of juicer. When you extract the fiber, you're leaving something out that's essential for digestion and for assimilation of the nutrients.

Fiber slows down the rate at which your body absorbs sugar, taking it from the digestive tract and pouring it into the bloodstream. If you don't have the fiber that helps control that assimilation, you could end up with a blood-sugar imbalance. For this reason, I recommend that you drink juice with meals: The fiber and bulk in your food helps with the blood-sugar regulation.

But I also advocate using a juicer that doesn't remove fiber or a blender. One common example is b Vita-Mix. I mention this machine in particular because it uses the whole plant—pulp as well as juice—blending the fruit or vegetable into a juice that has fiber as well as liquid. Having the pulp and juice all blended together really makes an appetizing drink—almost a meal in itself.

Of course, you can also buy packaged juices. These juices are great if no sweeteners have been added (the label will tell you), but even the "purest" of packaged juices aren't as healthful and nutritious as fresh juices. That's because pasteurization destroys enzymes, and oxidation destroys some of the nutrients. (Oxidation is essentially a speeding up of the ripening process, and it accelerates as soon as organic material—like fresh food—is crushed and exposed to air.)

People who have heard about juicing sometimes ask me whether they can get the same benefits from "whole-food supplements," that is, freeze-dried and packaged supplements that are created from the original juices. You'll find these supplements in the form of "green drinks" in many health-food stores. The reference to "green" in the label usually indicates that these supplements contain plant material with high nutritive content such as wheatgrass, barley grass, chlorella, and spirulina. But the label shouldn't be taken too literally, as many formulas contain other plants, such as carrots, beets, and various herbs, that are not green.

The advantage of these formulas is that they are ready to be used and require little effort to prepare. They include a blend of vegetables, fruits, and herbs that would be hard to cram into a single fresh drink—so you get the benefit of a wide variety of food extracts. The drawback, of course, is that the green drinks aren't made up of fresh foods, so you do lose some of the nutritive value of fresh juices. But they are helpful, easy, and convenient—and you can get green drinks in powder or capsule form.

One of the major reasons I recommend juicing for patients is that it helps them to detoxify. The phytonutrients, vitamins, minerals, and enzymes in juices work at the cellular level to promote detoxification, and they also help detoxify the liver. I estimate that the vast majority of the population could benefit from concentrated foods that promote detoxification.

DETOXING JUICING RECIPES

There are many different juicing recipes that help to promote detoxification. Following are a few that I recommend:

Fresh Juicing

In this formula the carrots provide a blend of carotenoids and the apple contains vitamin C and other nutrients. The burdock root, or beet, works to promote bile flow and liver detoxification.

2 medium-size carrots

½ apple

stick of burdock root or 1 small beet

Start with one glass daily with a meal; you can drink more than 1 cup daily if you desire.

Natural Physician Shake

1 to 2 cups rice milk (calcium-enriched)

1 banana

½ to 1 cup blueberries

probiotic (*Acidophilus*) containing 2 to 4 billion organisms

1 tablespoon flaxseed oil or essential fatty-acid blend such as flaxseed and evening primrose oil

2 digestive enzymes such as papain and bromelain

1 scoop soy or whey protein powder

Mix in a blender.

This is a particularly good shake for people on the go. Rather than skipping breakfast in the morning, if you can take a few minutes to put this blend together, you'll have more energy throughout the day. It also helps normalize your appetite, so you're less likely to get hunger pangs or food cravings during the day. This blend is also good to take before or after workouts.

Bring It On

Following is a formula I make with my Vita-Mix several mornings a week. It provides a super helping of vitamins, minerals, and phytonutrients.

1 cup baby spinach

¼ cup celery

¼ cup green or purple cabbage

½ medium apple (remove core)

1 cup carrots

1 sliver (1 tablespoon) beet

2 cups water

Combine all the ingredients in a blender and blend until thin.

Makes two servings. One serving equals ½ cup fruit and 1¼ cups vegetables.

Green Drink

Many different formulas labeled as "green drinks" can be purchased at health-food stores and some pharmacies. I use a formula (all organic) that mainly consists of the "super green foods" such as wheatgrass, barley grass, alfalfa, spirulina, chlorella, and kelp. It also contains carrot juice, dandelion root, milk thistle, Siberian ginseng, pineapple extract, milk thistle, and natural sweeteners such as mango and ste-via. I like to mix this powder in a glass of 3 parts apple juice and 1 part water.

The combination of supergreen foods and detoxifying herbs such as milk thistle and dandelion root has helped many patients as part of a detoxification program.

WHAT ARE THE SIDE EFFECTS?

Since juices can contain a lot of sugars, even if no sweeteners have been added, they can be hard on blood-sugar levels. As I've mentioned, that's why I recommend taking them with meals that slow sugar absorption or using a Vita-Mix to ensure that the fiber is included in the drink.

Green drinks that contain spirulina and chlorella are good for people with blood-sugar problems as they contain a high amount of protein. Some people need to build up the amount of juice they are drinking gradually, as it may cause detoxing reactions such as skin eruptions, headaches, or digestive upset.

Make sure to use organic fruits and vegetables whenever possible, and wash the foods thoroughly before juicing. Remove seeds and pits before juicing—particularly apple seeds, which contain the poisonous substance cyanide. Do not juice carrot tops, which contain toxic substances.

K

Kava

Minnie, a 44-year-old business executive, was facing a stressful time at work, but she had already dismissed the idea of using sedatives to control her anxiety and insomnia. She had taken a prescription sedative several years before that had made her feel "all doped out."

"I'm not going to take that again," she told me. "It's hard to get things done when you're taking medicine that makes you feel like a zombie."

Nonetheless, Minnie still felt she needed some help to cope with stress, and a friend had recommended the herb kava. Before taking it, she wanted to know whether, in my view, it would be helpful for her.

"I'd like to give it a try if you think it would help me," she said. "But before I do, I want to make sure it's safe."

In all honesty, I could tell her that I had seen many people benefit from the use of kava. The benefits depended not only on the individual, but also on the dosage used and the quality of the extract.

As I took a more thorough history on Minnie, I realized she had other problems besides insomnia associated with her anxiety. She frequently got headaches and suffered from neck and shoulder tension that were obviously brought on by stressful conditions at work.

I agreed kava (or kava kava) would be very worthwhile for her to try. She was not currently taking any pharmaceutical drugs

for her anxiety, so it was feasible for her to start kava right away. (With many drugs used to treat anxiety, phobia, or depression, it's essential to decrease dosages slowly, with advice and monitoring from the prescribing doctor.)

"Kava will be a good alternative to a pharmaceutical for the next couple of months to help you with all the stress and anxiety," I observed. "You'll probably find that it helps for those bouts of insomnia that you sometimes experience from work-related stress. It may also help with the neck tightness and headaches you get. I have successfully recommended it for those same problems with other patients."

I also let her know that kava's safety record was almost perfect.

"It is just as effective as common anti-anxiety medications, but without causing problems like poor concentration and drowsiness." But I also encouraged her to accept a broader program of treatment. "Keep in mind though that kava is not a replacement for stress-reducing techniques like exercise and prayer." If I was going to recommend kava for Minnie, I also wanted her to pursue the other kinds of self-treatment as well.

A GIFT FROM THE ISLANDS

Kava (*Piper methysticum*) has a unique history. The natives of the South Pacific islands (Fiji, Tonga, Samoa, Vanuatu, New Guinea, and Hawaii) have used kava for thousands of years. Inhabitants of these islands mainly used it as a ceremonial drink and to increase sociability.

Though kava is relaxing, it doesn't create side effects, apart from the mild euphoria that some people experience. Tea-drinking tribesmen report trancelike states and greater clarity of thought. The Greek translation of kava is "intoxicating." The root was and still is ground up by natives and soaked in coconut milk or water.

Interestingly, Captain Cook and his crew discovered kava during his voyage to the South Pacific in 1768, but it wasn't until the early 1860s that kava was available on the European market. In the United States, Kava gained popularity after World War II for its calming properties. I noticed the popularity of kava began to soar in the American health-food market in 1996 and 1997, probably because of all the media play it was getting. It seemed to become an overnight success as a natural stress, anxiety, and depression reliever.

Kava has a number of different constituents that are thought to have effects on various parts of the brain and nervous system. Animal studies have shown that kava influences GABA (gamma-amino-butyric acid) receptors. GABA is a neurotransmitter, which promotes relaxation, and whole kava extracts appear to have a strong interaction with them. Although there are active constituents called kavalactones in kava, the whole herb has a greater effect than the constituents, so it seems reasonable to assume that this complex herb has more than one set of active constituents.

Kava has been shown to affect the part of the brain that influences emotions, known as the amygdala. It also prevents the hormone norepinephrine from initiating a stress response. The herb relaxes the muscles and reduces pain. It's been shown in laboratory studies to have some properties that are similar to those of antiepileptic drugs.

DOSAGE

For stress and anxiety, I recommend the standardized capsule form with a base of the whole herb. This form has worked well with my patients, and it's been used in many studies.

The dosage is 70 mg of kavalactones two to three times daily. Remember that many products are labeled in total milligram amount and then a standardized extract percentage is given. For example, a 250-mg capsule containing 30% kavalactones contains 75 mg kavalactones.

For insomnia, I recommend 2 capsules (usually 500 mg) one-half hour before bedtime. The dosage for muscle relaxation is 70 mg of kavalactones three times daily. If the tincture form is used, I recommend 20 to 30 drops in water three times daily.

(**INTERESTING NOTE:** One typical bowl of kava drink—as consumed by the Polynias—contains approximately 250 mg of kavalactones. It's customary to consume many bowlfuls at one sitting.)

Kava is best used for short-term use (up to three months). I have not seen any reports that show it is harmful if used longer than three months. However, long-term studies have not been done.

WHAT ARE THE SIDE EFFECTS?

The kava supplements purchased in North America are quite safe, with no side effects. When studies were done with the original kava drink, researchers found that some people occasionally suffered from an upset stomach, but none of my patients have had these side effects from the normal doses I've recommended.

It is assumed that some ingredient is present in the drink form that is not found in the capsule or tincture form. Some members of Captain Cook's expedition reported that they got a scaly skin rash and eye irritation from drinking kava, especially in large amounts, but the effects went away when they stopped drinking. This side effect has not been reported with the supplement form. Perhaps the extraction process removes the ingredient that causes the side effects.

Although no problems with pregnancy have been reported, I recommend that you avoid kava if you're pregnant or nursing, since we don't have any good studies about the effects on the fetus. Also, I advise that you don't combine kava with alcohol, mood-altering pharmaceutical medications such as antidepressants, or antianxiety medicines. In fact, if you're on any medications at all, consult with a doctor first before using kava. There have been cases of liver toxicity reported with kava but the results of these are questionable. Nevertheless, I recommend avoiding kava if you have liver disease.

If you are a first-time user of kava, I would advise you to try it in a situation where you don't have to drive. Though kava probably won't impair your driving ability, it never hurts to be on the safe side. I advise against using kava when you have to operate heavy machinery.

KAVA
RECOMMENDATIONS FROM THE NATURAL PHYSICIAN FOR . . .

🐚 ANXIETY

Many patients have reported that they felt reduced anxiety while using kava. The anxiety-relieving effects are borne out by studies.

One placebo-controlled study looked at 101 people with anxiety who were given an extract of kava three times daily (approximately 70 mg of kavalactones per dose). Psychological tests were given before, during, and after the study. Researchers found that kava was superior to the placebo for short- and long-term effectiveness, and most people improved within two months.

Kava was well-tolerated and side effects were very rare among the people in the study. As a matter of fact, more people on the placebo dropped out than those on kava. There were no physical side effects or adverse reactions among those who took kava.

In other studies, kava was shown to reduce stress as well as anxiety, and it proved to be just as effective as an anxiety-reducer as the antianxiety drug oxazepam. Also, in the comparison of the drug with the herb, researchers found that people who received kava had a greater reduction in fear and psychosomatic nausea and vomiting than those who were taking the drug.

Not surprisingly—given these studies—more and more doctors and psychiatrists are incorporating kava into their practice.

🐚 DEPRESSION

Herbalists and naturopathic physicians often include kava in formulas for the treatment of depression. I have not found it to be as effective as St. John's wort. It is, however, an excellent complement to St. John's wort and other herbs and nutrients that are typically used for depression.

HEADACHES

I have found kava to be the most effective for tension-type headaches. Kava can prevent or alleviate tension headaches by helping to relax the muscles in the neck.

INSOMNIA

Kava is one of the better herbs to use for insomnia. It does not cause that "hangover feeling" that some people get the following morning when they've used pharmaceutical sleep aids the night before. It is a good option for someone who experiences grogginess or a hangover effect from the herb valerian.

Kava is best used on a short-term basis for insomnia, as it does not really address the underlying cause. Many natural-health insomnia formulas include kava as a principal ingredient.

MUSCLE TENSION AND SPASMS

In a clinic where I used to practice, a chiropractor and I both recommended kava to patients to help them reduce muscle spasms and tightness. We found that patients reported very good results, especially when their ailments were the result of stress or accidents.

PAIN

Many people report that kava helps to reduce pain, but I have found that its effects are usually minimal. However, it can help to relieve pain indirectly by reducing the spasms that cause some kinds of muscle pain.

PANIC ATTACKS

Several patients have told me that kava helps to ward off panic attacks if taken near the onset of the attack. For some patients with this disorder, I recommend the herb as a preventative. I recommend their taking kava regularly throughout the day (two times daily) to prevent an attack. This helps prevent acute attacks, but it's most effective when combined with counseling and homeopathic treatment.

Lachesis

Dr. Constantine Hering, a botanist and homeopath, was researching plants in Europe in 1828. He heard the legend about a gigantic, venomous snake known as the bushmaster (*Lachesis muta*) that lived in the bushes in tropical Latin America. According to natives, the bushmaster snake's venom was so deadly that a single drop could kill a person. In addition, the snake had a reputation. According to people who lived in the region, the bushmaster was not only very aggressive, it was also extremely protective of its territory.

When Hering traveled to Latin America, he offered to pay some of the local natives if they would help him catch the deadly bushmaster. His offer was universally declined. In fact, the natives thought Hering was crazy. Why would anyone want to capture this dangerous snake?

Among homeopathic researchers, however, there was logic in Hering's pursuit. If a bushmaster's venom could cause the symptoms of a deadly disease, perhaps the same substance—diluted to almost-invisible amounts—could be made into a homeopathic remedy that would cure human diseases when the victims had similar symptoms.

Hering steadily increased his offers of payment until the natives finally relented. A hunt for the bushmaster ensued, and one was finally captured. As Hering was extracting some of the venom, however, a few drops landed on his exposed skin. According to onlookers, he keeled over, unconscious, and was out cold for nearly 20 minutes. When he recovered, he had no memory of what had happened to him.

Returning to his home country, the United States, Dr. Hering continued to do research with lachesis venom, fully persuaded that it would be effective as a homeopathic remedy. Today, thanks to Dr. Hering's unrelenting efforts, lachesis is not only an accepted homeopathic remedy but one of the most important remedies in the homeopathic pharmacy for treatment of hormonal imbalances such as PMS and menopause, as well as circulation disorders.

PERSONALITY TYPES

Like other homeopathic remedies, lachesis has proven to be most effective with people of a particular personality type—specifically, those who are most intense and suspicious. Their aggressiveness is the result of pent-up anger, and they seem ready to lash out at somebody else at a moment's notice—not unlike the bushmaster.

Sometimes, they're very possessive, keeping close tabs on the people in their lives and yearning for material possessions. If you try to come into their territory, look out, for they will attack (another characteristic of the jungle snake). If they don't get you in the heat of the moment, they will, for they long for revenge.

Jealousy and envy also characterize people needing lachesis. They may lash out physically, but more often, they're talkers, and they use verbal abuse to get out their frustrations. If you're in a large group of people and one of them is particularly loquacious, you know that's probably the lachesis personality. When you try to get a word in edgewise, the lachesis individual is likely to cut you off because he or she wants to be heard and knows what is right. Even when you say you have to leave, it's quite possible the lachesis type won't even get the hint. This type of person may keep talking right in your face even as you're placing your hand on the door to leave.

There are other characteristics as well of someone who requires this remedy. This type of person will never wear a turtleneck, for instance, because he or she can't stand to have anything around his or her neck—just as the person can't bear to have anyone touching him or her. Again, I think of the snake itself, which always tries to protect its own neck.

One last interesting note about the lachesis personality type is that the person has a fear of snakes!

IN THE BLOOD

Lachesis, like all the snake remedies, has a pronounced effect on the circulatory system. The venom from the bushmaster snake acts to prevent blood from clotting, which is what normally stops blood flow. Without blood clotting, a person can't stop bleeding. But the mild homeopathic dose will not cause such a dire reaction, so it's sometimes prescribed for circulation problems. For example, massive purple blood clots that cause excruciating pain during a woman's menstrual cycle can be relieved with this venom remedy.

It also contains neurotoxins that cause a person to freeze up if he or she is bitten by the snake. Used in the mild dose of a homeopathic remedy, lachesis can have the beneficial effect of causing constriction of some blood vessels. It's valuable for hemorrhage conditions, such as an abnormally heavy menstrual flow or even something like a retinal (eye) hemorrhage. A woman in menopause, who is experiencing severe hot flashes, can get much-needed relief. Lachesis is also one of the best remedies for the heart, improving conditions such as heart palpitations.

A person who needs lachesis is someone who tends to have left-sided symptoms. I remember Jessie, a 58-year-old patient of mine, who came to see me for the natural treatment of her arthritis and headaches. She had arthritis. I wouldn't usually treat arthritis with lachesis, except in her case, the physical symptoms were on the left side. For example, it was only her left knee and left wrist where her arthritis occurred. In addition, she had headaches, and these primarily afflicted her in the left temple.

There was another clue—body temperature. Those requiring lachesis tend to have a higher body temperature than most people. Even though it was winter, Jessie wore light clothing that seemed to keep her quite comfortable.

For all these reasons, I prescribed lachesis for Jessie's conditions. Over the next three months, the lachesis totally eliminated Jessie's headaches, and her arthritis improved tremendously.

DOSAGE

For the treatment of long-term conditions I prefer to use low dosages of lachesis, such as potencies of 6C that can be taken two to three times daily for a few weeks—and, thereafter, on an as-needed basis. A much higher potency, 30C, is commonly available at health-food stores and pharmacies, but if you're taking 30C, try it one or two times daily for just a week or two to see if your symptoms improve. I recommend taking it regularly for one week, then on an as-needed basis after that.

You can take 200C potency for certain acute conditions, but don't take more than one dose.

WHAT ARE THE SIDE EFFECTS?

As with other homeopathic remedies, side effects are not a real concern. If the potency or frequency are too high, you might get a temporary aggravation of symptoms. But symptoms will return to normal if you just stop the remedy.

LACHESIS
RECOMMENDATIONS FROM THE NATURAL PHYSICIAN FOR . . .

If you suffer from any of the conditions listed below, lachesis is worth trying. I find it invaluable for women's health problems such as PMS, menopause, menstrual cycle abnormalities, ovarian cysts, and left-sided headaches. I also find it works better than hormones for some menopausal symptoms.

ALCOHOLISM

Anyone with a history of alcoholism certainly needs counseling, but some people are helped by homeopathic remedies as well. The "lachesis personality type"—that is, someone who might be helped by lachesis treatments—is the person who tends to become violent when drinking. This includes verbal as well as physical violence. The person who swears and makes wild accusations while under the influence of alcohol is usually a lachesis type.

ASTHMA

Lachesis is especially effective in people who have the type of asthma that's worst when they first wake up from sleep or when they're in a warm room—but the asthma improves when someone is cold. If you have asthma that wakes you with

a suffocating feeling, lachesis might help. It's "very indicated," according to homeopathic physicians, when the asthma starts after feelings of jealousy.

EAR INFECTIONS

Lachesis is a main remedy for left ear infections in children. The child has severe ear pain and feels hot. The left ear is all red and feels better with cold applications. If your child has a left-sided earache, then lachesis is worth trying and usually works quite well.

ENDOMETRIOSIS

Lachesis can be quite helpful and sometimes curative when a woman's endometriosis symptoms match the remedy. Lachesis helps to balance the hormones, which are almost always a root problem in this condition.

HEMORRHAGE

Lachesis is one of the main remedies to use for hemorrhage or when you have a susceptibility to hemorrhage. I typically use it when a woman says she's been having heavy menstrual cycles and blood clots that have a purplish color.

❧ HYPERTENSION

As mentioned, lachesis can be used to help the circulatory system. Many practitioners have found that it helps reduce high blood pressure.

❧ HYPERTHYROID

Lachesis is indicated for hyperthyroid, especially in the early stages. I recommend it if the person has flushes of heat and heart palpitations. Sometimes these symptoms are accompanied by left-sided thyroid gland pain.

❧ MANIC DEPRESSION

Many cases of manic depression have been reported to be helped with lachesis. For this condition, however, you will need the supervision of an experienced doctor.

❧ MENOPAUSE

Lachesis is one of the five most common remedies used in menopause. I recommend it if you have hot flashes, heavy uterine bleeding, and increased feelings of suspiciousness and jealousy. Menopausal women who benefit from lachesis often have one uncharacteristic symptom: Unlike many women in menopause, the sex drive usually stays very high for those requiring lachesis.

❧ MIGRAINE

This remedy is the main homeopathic for left-sided migraine headaches. Recently, a woman came to me for the natural treatment of migraine headaches. When she told me these headaches usually began on the left side, I immediately recommended lachesis, which is an excellent nondrug treatment, especially for prevention of these types of headaches. It balances the hormones and normalizes circulation. The patient told me she was pregnant when she started to develop these headaches, but lachesis is so safe that a woman can use it during pregnancy.

❧ OVARIAN CYST

Lachesis is the main remedy for left-sided ovarian cysts. Gynecologists are baffled when their patients who have had ovarian cyst problems for years take a homeopathic remedy like lachesis and the ultrasound shows they have disappeared! But seeing is believing! I have seen many chronic, painful cases cured with this remedy.

❧ PMS

Symptoms of irritability, jealousy, and depression are relieved with lachesis. One peculiar symptom that differentiates it from other remedies is that menstrual cramps disappear once the flow begins.

❧ SHINGLES

Painful, burning blisters that pop up on the left side of the body respond to lachesis.

❧ VARICOSE VEINS

Lachesis is one of the best remedies for varicose veins that have a purplish discoloration and look like they could burst at any moment.

L-carnitine

L-carnitine is a substance that's involved in the transportation of a particular kind of fatty acids into the mitochondria (energy factory) of cells. It's often called "carnitine"—which is the same thing.

Think of it as part of the transport system that shovels coals into the fire for burning. The "burning of fats" by the mitochondria is important, as this process fuels the energy that reaches your heart cells and your muscle cells.

Because carnitine is such an integral part of this fueling process, it's particularly valuable as a preventative and therapeutic supplement. If you have a problem related to energy production, carnitine can come to the rescue. Because it helps get energy to the heart muscles, it also assists with several cardiovascular conditions.

Other conditions that seem to benefit from supplementation of L-carnitine include anorexia, chronic fatigue, hypoglycemia, male infertility, and muscular myopathies. Also, L-carnitine is showing promise for premature infants, dialysis patients, and HIV-positive individuals.

You have three sources of carnitine. First, the body manufactures carnitine from the amino acid lysine. But there are other important substances involved in this process as well. These include methionine, SAMe, magnesium, vitamin C, vitamin B6, niacin, and iron.

You can also get carnitine in your diet. Meat is the major dietary source. Carnitine comes from animal protein—with red meat being the richest source.

Plant foods, unfortunately, contain little or no carnitine, which is a cause for concern if you're a strict vegetarian. But fortunately, there's a third possible source of carnitine that can be used by vegetarians and others.

The supplement form of L-carnitine is available and commonly recommended by nutrition-oriented doctors.

DEFICIENCY NOTICE

L-carnitine deficiencies do occur, though some cases are more severe than others. There are a number of possible causes, such as:

- *Genetic defect.* Due to some genetic defect that prevents the body from synthesizing carnitine, some people simply don't get enough.
- *Deficiency of certain amino acids.* If lysine and methionine are missing—or if either one is lacking—you'll have a problem getting adequate carnitine.
- *Deficiency of "cofactors."* I have already mentioned the other substances required for synthesis of carnitine, including SAMe, magnesium, vitamin C, vitamin B6, niacin, and iron. These are called cofactors, and if any of them are missing, you may have problems assimilating carnitine.
- *Strict vegetarianism.* Since there's no carnitine in plant foods, supplementation is required.
- *Formula-feeding babies.* Most infant formulas do not contain carnitine, which is naturally present in breast milk.
- *Liver or kidney disease.* When the liver or kidneys aren't functioning properly, your body can't produce adequate carnitine. People with kidney disease receiving dialysis are almost certain to need supplementation.
- *Severe infections*, such as chronic bronchitis.

- *Increased metabolic stress,* such as the kind caused by heavy physical exertions or chronic disease.
- *Intestinal malabsorption.* If you've had a portion of the small intestine removed (a resection), you'll need carnitine supplementation.
- *Side effects from medications.* Some people will have an increased need for carnitine when they're taking certain kinds of medications.

There are a number of leading signs of carnitine deficiency. I always suspect it when patients report muscle fatigue and cramps. If their lab tests show a deficiency of carnitine in the tissue and red blood cells, I know supplementation will be necessary.

If there's a severe chronic carnitine deficiency—that is, over a long period of time—one may see symptoms of low blood-sugar, fatigue, and nervous system disorders. Also, tests will show that the transport of fatty acids is impaired—a condition called impaired lipid (triglyceride) metabolism—resulting in an increase in triglycerides. That's because carnitine is required to shuttle fatty acids into the cells.

When the condition is chronic, fatty acids are likely to accumulate in the muscles and liver. The heart muscle is affected. This buildup of fats in the muscles causes progressive muscle weakness. So a chronic deficiency of carnitine can lead to serious conditions related to the heart, such as cardiomyopathy and congestive heart failure. It can also contribute to liver enlargement (hepatomegaly) and brain swelling (encephalopathy).

Children appear to be very susceptible to carnitine deficiency. I'm particularly concerned about infants who only get infant formula. Most of these formulas do not contain L-carnitine. In susceptible children, this may hinder their growth and development.

DOSAGE

I typically recommend an adult dosage of 1,000 mg taken two to three times daily. You can take higher dosages, up to 2,000 mg per dose—but it appears that this is the maximum that can be absorbed and utilized at one time. For this reason, I recommend divided doses—taken several times during the day if necessary—rather than large single doses.

If you have heart disease, consider a formula that contains L-carnitine in combination with CoQ10. This is a powerful supplement combination for treatment of a number of related conditions including cardiomyopathy, angina, or congestive heart failure. I recommend the L-carnitine form—which is the designation of most of the carnitine supplements. The D,L carnitine form is also available, but I don't recommend it, as it is not biologically active and can cause side effects.

NOTE: I have only seen the L-carnitine form in health-food stores and pharmacies.

WHAT ARE THE SIDE EFFECTS?

Carnitine is a very safe supplement. Occasionally, people get digestive upset, but if you reduce the dosage or take carnitine with your meals, you can usually resolve the problem.

Don't supplement with carnitine if you're taking the respiratory stimulant drug pentylenetetrazol.

L-CARNITINE
RECOMMENDATIONS FROM THE NATURAL PHYSICIAN FOR . . .

🍂 ANGINA

Several studies have shown that L-carnitine is effective in the treatment and prevention of angina. In a well-controlled scientific study of men and women taking L-carnitine, researchers found that 22% of angina patients given L-carnitine became angina-free during the study. That was more than twice the percentage of those in the placebo group—that is, the ones who were not taking L-carnitine. Those taking carnitine also experienced increased exercise tolerance. When doctors did follow-up electrocardiogram tests, they found that the patients taking L-carnitine showed evidence that there was less restriction of blood flow in their arteries.

Another study looked at what happened when scientists gave L-carnitine supplementation of 2,000 mg daily to 100 randomly selected patients with stable angina over a six-month period. The carnitine was given in addition to the therapy already started. Researchers found improvements in a number of important indicators of heart health. Those receiving L-carnitine were found to be more likely to have their cardiac medications reduced.

I find that carnitine, in addition to CoQ10, vitamin E, magnesium, hawthorn berry, and cactus (*Cereus grandiflorus*) are excellent for the prevention of angina.

🍂 ANOREXIA

In patients with anorexia nervosa, the combination of carnitine and vitamin B12 accelerates the gain of body weight and helps normalize gastrointestinal function.

Anorexia is best treated by a specialist, but nutritional support has proven helpful to many. With L-carnitine, people have a resource that helps them fight fatigue and improve mental performance.

The combination of B12 with carnitine has been proven helpful for infantile anorexia. It appears nutritional support with supplements such as carnitine, B12, as well as zinc are important to include as nutritional support to hasten the recovery process. But again, you'll need the help of a specialist before giving treatment to an infant.

🍂 ARRHYTHMIA

Double-blind studies have shown that carnitine supplementation helped patients to receive lower dosages of their antiarrhythmic drugs, indicating that carnitine has a beneficial effect.

🍂 CARDIOMYOPATHY

Children with this form of heart disease and who had carnitine deficiency responded favorably to carnitine supplementation. Along with CoQ10, it should be used with anyone who has cardiomyopathy to improve heart performance.

🍂 CHRONIC FATIGUE SYNDROME

One of the challenges with chronic fatigue syndrome is that it can have many different causes. Among the possible causes are viral infection, digestive disturbances, nutritional deficiencies, adrenal burnout, and hormone imbalances.

I find nutritional supplements such as carnitine act as complementary treatments to more primary treatments such as detox-ification and homeopathic treatment. This observation is supported by one study that showed clinical improvement in 12 of 18 people with chronic fatigue syndrome.

CONGESTIVE HEART FAILURE

Nutrition-oriented doctors routinely rec-ommend carnitine to patients with conges-tive heart failure. This is a condition where the heart is failing to pump out efficiently.

In one study, 21 people with conges-tive heart failure were given 1,000 mg of carnitine twice daily for 45 days along with conventional drugs. The participants showed improvements in levels of triglyc-eride and cholesterol, heart rate, edema, and breathing. Supplementation also allowed for lower daily doses of digitalis.

DEFICIENCIES FROM DRUG INTERACTIONS

Anticonvulsant drugs such as phenobarbi-tal, valproic acid, phenytoin, and carbam-azepine significantly lower carnitine levels. So does the drug pivampicillin. If you're on any of these medications, you should talk with your doctor about supplementing with carnitine to prevent deficiencies.

L-carnitine may prevent heart compli-cations in people with cancer who receive interleukin-2 immunotherapy and the chemotherapy drug adriamyacin. And it appears to also have a protective effect on the cell mitochondria for people with HIV using the drug zidovudine (AZT).

DIABETES

L-carnitine supplementation makes sense for people with diabetes who are predis-posed to cardiovascular and neurological disease.

DOWN'S SYNDROME

Although Down's syndrome is a genetic condition, one 90-day study found that ALC supplementation was beneficial in improving visual memory and attention in children who had the syndrome.

HEART ATTACK RECOVERY

L-carnitine has been helpful for people recovering from a heart attack. One study of 160 people who recently suffered a heart attack showed significant improve-ments in blood pressure, heart rate, angina attacks, and other markers of heart function. The dosage used in the study was 4,000 mg of L-carnitine, taken in divided doses throughout the day. Studies have also shown that victims of heart attacks are more likely to survive if they take carnitine supplements during the next 24 hours.

With such positive results, supple-ments like carnitine really should be rou-tinely prescribed for heart attack victims. It only makes sense as carnitine helps the heart produce energy so that it can func-tion more effectively.

HIV

A few studies have shown that carnitine supplementation can be helpful in improving the immune status (CD4 and CD8 counts) in people with HIV.

KIDNEY DISEASE

People undergoing dialysis for kidney disease are often deficient in carnitine. Supplementation helps to reduce triglyc-eride levels while increasing the good HDL cholesterol.

(continued)

🐟 LIVER DISEASE

Carnitine helps metabolize fatty acids in the liver. In people with liver cirrhosis it has been shown to reduce triglycerides, increase the good HDL cholesterol, and decrease elevated liver enzymes. It works to reverse fatty liver disease caused by alcohol.

🐟 MALE INFERTILITY

Carnitine is required to help improve the motility and number of sperm. Supplementation of L-carnitine can improve sperm quality in some patients with idiopathic asthenospermia (defective sperm motility of unknown cause).

Researchers provided 100 patients with 3,000 mg daily of L-carnitine for four months and found improvements in all assessed parameters of sperm motility, as well as an increase in the total sperm count. Other nutrients that I recommend to increase sperm count and motility include vitamin C, arginine, CoQ10, vitamin B12, vitamin E, and zinc.

🐟 PREMATURE INFANTS

Carnitine appears to be important to supplement to the mother if it is suspected or known that a premature delivery is inevitable. Carnitine is involved with the activation of surfactant, a substance that promotes proper function and maturation of the infants' lungs.

One study showed that women have healthier babies who are less likely to have respiratory distress syndrome if the expectant mothers are given carnitine along with the drug betamethasone during the prenatal period. The trial showed how the combination of supplement and pharmaceutical can reduce both the incidence of respiratory distress syndrome and the mortality of premature newborns. In the trial, some mothers were just given the prescription drug, while others got carnitine as well. For the mothers who took both, the incidence of respiratory distress syndrome among the infants was about half of that for the drug-only group. For mothers who took carnitine, the mortality rate of infants was 1.8%, while it was 7.3% for mothers who took the betamethasone alone.

🐟 WEIGHT AND FAT LOSS

In seniors, L-carnitine is involved in promoting lean muscle mass. In a study involving 66 centenarians, participants were divided into two groups. For six months, one group took 2 g of L-carnitine once a day and the other took a placebo. The study authors concluded that the L-carnitine helped to reduce body fat and increase muscle mass.

Ledum

Years ago, my mother got a needle biopsy for a breast lump that her doctor had discovered. My mother anticipated some pain from the procedure and when she asked my sister whether there was any way to avoid the aftereffects, my sister approached me with the question. "Mark, is there anything we can give Mom to help with the pain from her biopsy?"

"Yes. Give her a couple doses of ledum right after the procedure," I said.

After the biopsy—which proved to be negative—my sister gave Mom the ledum (*Ledum palustre*), a homeopathic remedy specific for puncture wounds. My mother said that in the following days she could not feel any pain where the needle was inserted.

In my view, surgery clinics and medical offices would serve their patients well if they would just make ledum available to patients. Every time a person gets an injection or gets blood drawn, a dose of ledum can help reduce the pain and speed tissue healing.

Ledum is the homeopathic preparation of an herbal preparation from wild rosemary, a small shrub. It is commonly recommended by homeopathic practitioners as an acute remedy for bites, stings, and wounds. It is also a good arthritis remedy.

DOSAGE

A few doses of the 30C potency or a single dose of 200C is helpful for acute situations that require ledum. Chronic cases like arthritis are generally treated with a 6C or 30C potency a couple of times daily.

WHAT ARE THE SIDE EFFECTS?

None of my patients have suffered from any side effects from taking ledum.

LEDUM
RECOMMENDATIONS FROM THE NATURAL PHYSICIAN FOR . . .

⁓ ARTHRITIS

Linda was a 53-year-old patient of mine who was consulting with me for natural treatment of multiple health problems. One of her most immediate concerns was the arthritis she suffered in her left foot. Chiropractic and acupuncture had helped slightly, but the pain was really concerning her.

Upon further examination, I found that the foot looked bruised, and Linda told me that it also felt hot at times. We discovered that ice water made the foot feel better, at least temporarily, whereas warm applications worsened the pain and inflammation. All these key symptoms suggested that ledum would be the best remedy.

Within one week of beginning the treatments, Linda felt what she described as "70% improvement!" Over the next few months, Linda reported that the pain in her left foot was almost gone.

Ledum is one of the remedies to consider when arthritis occurs in the feet and ankles. It is also one of the better remedies to use to treat flare-ups of gout.

⁓ BRUISES

Ledum is useful for bruises to the soft tissues, similar to arnica. I find it helpful for patients who get bruised from blood draws in the clinic. It helps reduce the pain and swelling the same day, often within a matter of minutes.

⁓ MOSQUITO BITES

I have recommended ledum on several occasions for people who react strongly to mosquito bites. Some people have very sensitive skin, and they get large, boil-like, itchy, painful lesions from normal mosquito bites. For them, I recommend mixing a couple pellets of ledum (any potency such as 6C or 30C) with water in a spray bottle. In a mosquito-infested area, it's best to spray the solution on the skin

(continued)

every hour. The itching will be more bearable, and the bites will not flare up so badly.

Ledum can also be used for relief from bee stings, especially the kind that are relieved by cold applications.

🐟 PUNCTURE WOUNDS

Before the creation of the tetanus vaccine, practitioners used to give ledum to prevent wound infections. In addition to cleaning a wound, you can help prevent infection by taking a dose of ledum for faster tissue healing.

But whether or not there's a risk of infection, ledum can be a pain-reliever for puncture wounds. I remember taking it myself when I received a vitamin B12 injection that was administered by a colleague of mine, Dr. Steve Nenninger. This was in his early days of practicing medicine—and both of us were just beginning to develop our skills as physicians. I felt a tremendous amount of pain after the injection. Fortunately, one dose of ledum quickly relieved this intense, sharp pain.

🐟 SPRAINS

Ledum is often given after a sprain, such as an ankle sprain. I typically use it if arnica does not reduce the swelling and discomfort in the ankle.

Licorice Root

By the time Ray, a 44-year-old salesman, came to see me for the treatment of his peptic ulcers, he had already spent two frustrating years trying to relieve his stomach pain with many different types of medications and natural remedies. Again and again he tried new pills, capsules, and formulas, each of which seemed to work for a while before gradually losing its effectiveness, leaving him to relapse into agony.

In the long list of remedies he'd taken, however, I discovered that one—the most effective of all—was conspicuously absent. This gave me the clue I needed to help him attack his problem. Besides having Ray reduce his coffee intake and increase his exercise as part of a stress-reduction program, I prescribed licorice root (DGL form). He was to chew two capsules at least 15 minutes before each meal every day.

The result? On the very next visit he reported his ulcer was healed! I knew better, of course. Even though he felt much, much better, it takes longer than two weeks to declare a complete victory over an ulcer, so I recommended that he continue using DGL for another four weeks.

Now, after six months, Ray still shows no sign of relapse.

THE ALL-PURPOSE REMEDY

In my experience, licorice root is the most versatile of all the herbs. Native to both Asia and the Mediterranean, it has been used by practitioners of Ayurvedic and Chinese medicine for more than 5,000 years.

In fact, close to 50% of all Chinese herbal formulas contain licorice root. The ancient Chinese texts say it can suppress coughs and moisten the lungs, relieve spasms, and soothe the digestive tract. It is also called a "harmonizing" herb. This means that it helps other herbs to work more effectively to reduce their toxicity when used in a formula.

Licorice also helps detoxify the liver, supports the adrenal glands (your body's major guardians against stress), balances the hormones, and has powerful anti-inflammatory effects.

IMMUNITY BOOSTER

Licorice contains two substances, glycyrrhizin and glycyrrhetinic acid, that have been shown in animal studies to increase the body's supply of one of nature's most powerful antiviral agents: interferon. Interferon helps to keep viruses from reproducing and stimulates the activity of other beneficial immune cells, as well. That's probably why licorice root is found in so many Western, Chinese, Japanese, and Ayurvedic formulas for treating infectious disease.

Licorice root is highly regarded among European physicians as one of the top herbal medicines for combating viral hepatitis. They use the intravenous form for the treatment of both Hepatitis B and C.

DELICIOUS DETOXIFIER

The Chinese have found through many centuries of using licorice that it reduces the toxicity of other herbs, so they add it to many of their remedies. For example, traditional Chinese herbal formulas containing ma huang (containing the chemical ephedrine, which helps open respiratory passageways but can also cause stimulant effects, such as fast heartbeat, sweating, and anxiety) almost always contain licorice root, which helps to prevent these unwanted side effects.

(**NOTE:** The Chinese species of licorice root is *Glycyrrhiza uralensis*. I find it works very similar in action to the kind used in North America—*Glycyrrhiza glabra*.)

DOSAGE

For most conditions, I recommend taking licorice in tincture, capsule, or tablet form.

As a tincture, take 10 to 30 drops two to three times daily. As a capsule, take 1,000 to 3,000 mg daily.

DGL comes in tablet form. Chew one or two tablets (380 mg per tablet) 20 minutes before meals or take between meals.

TREAT OR TRICK?

The Greek translation of *licorice* is "sweet root" or "sweet wood," and it's aptly named. The sweetness of licorice root is 50 to 100 times that of sugar! But oddly, the one place you won't find any licorice root is in American licorice candy, which actually contains anise oil and simple sugars like glucose and fructose, and artificial dyes, sweeteners, and preservatives that can wreak havoc with the brain. The active constituents that real licorice is known to contain include glycyrrhizin, glycyrrhizinic acid, glycyrrhetinic acid, flavonoids, sterols, amino acids, coumarins, and volatile oils.

Unfortunately, most of the licorice root imported to the United States is used as an additive in tobacco products, since it is sweet and soothing. (I doubt tobacco manufacturers included it to reduce the toxicity of the more than 100 toxic chemicals found in cigarettes.) The Europeans and Chinese, on the other hand, do give licorice root to their children as a healthy substitute for sugar candy.

WHAT ARE THE SIDE EFFECTS?

High dosages of licorice root (3,000 mg daily of the powdered extract or more than 100 mg of the constituent glycyrrhizin) taken over many days can have effects similar to those associated with the hormone aldosterone. These include sodium and water retention, and potassium loss, which can lead to high blood pressure. I occasionally saw this problem occur when practitioners began recommending very high dosages of licorice root for adrenal burnout and chronic fatigue (which it can help).

Overall, I feel the risk of developing high blood pressure from using licorice is greatly exaggerated. Historically, herbalists have used this root in formulas for thousands of years. The trick is to use it in small amounts.

I do hear the occasional story of someone who feels that taking small amounts of licorice root has caused an increase in his or her blood pressure. This is perfectly possible for people who are very sensitive to licorice root or are low in potassium. As a matter of fact, anyone concerned about high blood pressure should increase his or her intake of potassium-rich foods (bananas, orange juice, vegetables, etc.) and decrease the intake of sodium-containing foods (table salt, canned foods, and restaurant foods). Using table-salt substitutes, which usually contain potassium, can help reduce sodium intake. Multivitamins also contain potassium.

Unless instructed to do so by a natural healthcare practitioner, people who have kidney failure and hypokalemia (low potassium blood levels) should avoid using licorice root. Likewise, pregnant women and people with high blood pressure should use it with caution and under medical supervision. Whole licorice extract should not be combined with digitalis and diuretic medications. Taking only the DGL extract (for ulcers) eliminates most of the potential risk for high blood pressure.

LICORICE ROOT

RECOMMENDATIONS FROM THE NATURAL PHYSICIAN FOR . . .

✒ COUGHS

Licorice is an excellent herb to use for coughs, both wet and dry. Licorice has a moistening and soothing effect for dry coughs. It also has a direct cough suppressant effect and is a common ingredient in throat lozenges.

✒ DETOXIFICATION

Licorice is one of the herbs to consider when undergoing a detoxification program. As I mentioned, it helps support the liver and should be considered along with herbs like milk thistle and dandelion root. It also works to heal a damaged digestive tract, which is key to long-term detoxification success.

✒ ECZEMA AND PSORIASIS

Creams containing glycyrrhetinic acid are used to treat inflammatory skin conditions such as eczema and psoriasis. Its effect is similar to that of topical cortisone, and some studies have found it more effective. However, I do not recommend topical treatments (whether natural or pharmaceutical) as the main therapy for skin conditions, as they can simply mask a symptom without treating its underlying cause (e.g., food sensitivities, poor digestion, nutritional deficiencies, etc.). Topical treatments are fine, as long as you also address the internal imbalances that are creating the symptom.

FATIGUE

People who experience high levels of stress for long periods of time can suddenly find that their adrenal glands can no longer produce balanced levels of stress hormones, such as DHEA, pregnenolone, and cortisol. As a result, fatigue, poor memory, blood-sugar problems, decreased resistance to illness, and hormonal imbalance can occur.

Some doctors immediately recommend using hormone replacement, and in some cases this is necessary. However, it is worth trying a gentler approach, using supplements such as licorice root, especially to balance out cortisol levels. A typical adult dosage would be 1,000 to 2,000 mg of licorice root extract taken daily for two months or longer.

Other supplements that work synergistically to treat this condition include adrenal glandular, ginseng, pantothenic acid, vitamin C, beta carotene, and zinc. In more serious cases, hormones such as DHEA, pregnenolone, and even cortisol may need to be used.

HORMONE IMBALANCE

Licorice is one of the better hormone-balancing herbs. It appears to have a balancing effect between estrogen and progesterone, and reduces excess testosterone levels. It is commonly included in formulas for PMS and menopause.

INFECTIONS

As mentioned earlier, licorice root is very good for the immune system. The soothing and anti-inflammatory effect of licorice makes it especially good for respiratory tract infections.

INFLAMMATION

Licorice has potent anti-inflammatory properties. Glycyrrhizin is an important constituent that improves the effects of cortisol in the body (powerful anti-inflammatory and antiallergy effects), without the side effects seen with pharmaceutical anti-inflammatory agents such as prednisone. It also inhibits the formation of prostaglandins, which are substances in the body that cause inflammation.

INFLAMMATORY BOWEL DISEASE

Licorice root is often included in formulas designed to heal conditions such as Crohn's disease and ulcerative colitis.

MOUTH SORES

Mouth sores, also called aphthous ulcers, can be helped by licorice root. One study of 20 people found that a DGL mouthwash improved the symptoms of 15 of the participants by 50% to 75% within one day, and completely healed the sores within three days.

ULCERS

One of the most popular uses of licorice extract is for ulcers of the digestive tract. The recommended form is DGL. It has an interesting mechanism of action: It stimulates cell growth of the stomach and intestinal linings, increases the natural mucous lining of the stomach, increases blood flow to the damaged tissues, and decreases muscle spasms.

In a single-blind study of 100 people with peptic ulcers, participants took either DGL (760 mg three times daily) or the medication Tagamet (cimetidine).

(continued)

Both groups showed equally significant healing of ulcers after 6 and 12 weeks, demonstrating that DGL is as effective as pharmaceutical medications for this condition. Another study of 874 people also demonstrated that DGL was as effective as antacids and the antiulcer drug cimetidine in persons with duodenal ulcers.

More important, DGL actually works to heal ulcerated tissues instead of simply suppressing stomach acid in the way antacids and drug medications do. Remember, with insufficient stomach acid, you cannot digest proteins, minerals, and other nutrients very efficiently. Stomach acid also acts as a natural barrier that keeps bacteria, parasites, and other microbes from penetrating the digestive tract.

Lo Han

Lo han, also known as lo han kuo or luo han gu, is the fruit of the *Momordica grossvenori* plant, a member of the cucumber family. It grows in the mountains of southern China. For several centuries, the fruit has been used by practitioners of Chinese medicine to treat dry coughs, sore throats, skin conditions, and digestive problems, and to calm the nervous system. From the dried fruits, the Chinese people make tea, juice, soup, candy, and cake.

Lo han kuo is said to be 150 to 300 times sweeter than sugar. It contains no sugar or calories, and it is safe for people with diabetes or hypoglycemia (low blood-sugar). It does not lose its sweetness when heated, so it can be used in baking and cooking. The FDA has approved lo han as a generally regarded as safe (GRAS) food ingredient. There is no known toxicity with this fruit extract.

The lo han kuo products I have used resemble maple syrup in flavor and leave no aftertaste. The active constituents responsible for their sweetness are known as mogrosides.

DOSAGE

Supplemental lo han is available in powder and liquid form in health-food stores. Use as directed on the container, as concentration and potency vary among products.

WHAT ARE THE SIDE EFFECTS?

I have not seen any literature finding any common side effects.

LO HAN
RECOMMENDATIONS FROM THE NATURAL PHYSICIAN FOR . . .

✎ WEIGHT LOSS AND OBESITY
Lo han is an excellent choice as a natural sweetener that has no calories.

Lomatium

Scientists are in a race to find drugs that can eradicate bacteria, which are becoming more and more resistant to antibiotics. They are also frantically looking to develop drugs that fight off viruses as well, especially in light of HIV, Ebola, herpes, hepatitis, and the ever-changing strains of the flu.

Scientists are looking increasingly to the plant kingdom and reviewing the historical use of plants as medicines to fight off invading microbes. One of these plants is lomatium.

Lomatium (*Lomatium dissectum*) is an herb that has been known about for almost a century, but has been used by only a small percentage of natural healthcare practitioners. Recently, it has become more popular as a commercial immune-system enhancer to fight off pathogens such as viruses, bacteria, and fungi.

For almost a decade, I have been using lomatium for my patients, and quite often with extraordinary results. It ranks with some of the other well-known immune-system herbal therapies such as echinacea and astragalus.

Lomatium grows in British Columbia, Alberta, southern California, New Mexico, Colorado, eastern Oregon, eastern Washington, Idaho, and the Columbia Plateau. It is also referred to as desert parsley.

A HEALING INDIAN ROOT

Once again, we have the Native Americans to thank for our present use of lomatium. Historically, it was one of the most important medicinal plants used by several tribes of the western United States.

Lomatium was used to treat infections of the respiratory and urinary tracts, as well as of the eyes. The species used by the Native Americans and the one still popular today is *Lomatium dissectum.* They would also eat the shoots and roots. For medicinal use, a decoction was made by boiling the root in water. This decoction was also used topically for sores, rashes, and cuts. A poultice of lomatium was used for swellings, joint pain, and sprains.

One of the interesting historical notes about lomatium is that it was used by Native Americans during the Spanish flu epidemic of 1917–1918. This is the epidemic that killed more than 22 million people worldwide, and more than 500,000 people in the United States. A doctor noticed that Native Americans in the Nevada desert were recovering from the Spanish flu. He found they were boiling and ingesting lomatium root. He learned how to use the herb from them and began using it, as did other doctors who saw similar healing effects from using lomatium. However, the interest in lomatium dramatically decreased after the epidemic ended.

Several earlier in vitro studies have shown lomatium to have direct killing effects on many different types of bacteria and fungus, including *Candida albicans.* It is also believed that phytochemicals found in lomatium have the ability to inhibit viruses from replicating. Studies have shown these phytochemicals to be effective against DNA and RNA viruses—two major categories of viruses.

Practitioners of natural medicine find lomatium root effective against several types of viruses including Epstein-Barr, herpes, flu, common cold, cytomegalovirus, and *Condyloma acuminata* (genital warts).

DOSAGE

Lomatium is available in tincture form. I recommend taking 30 drops (0.5 mL) every two to three hours for acute infections. For chronic viral infections, I recommend 0.5 mL or 500 mg twice daily. I use lomatium in formulas that contain herbs such as echinacea, astragalus, reishi, and licorice. It also combines well with herbal cough formulas for a more aggressive treatment.

WHAT ARE THE SIDE EFFECTS?

The only side effect to be aware of is that a very small percentage of users will develop a measleslike rash. The rash is not serious, and will disappear after a few days if you stop taking lomatium.

LOMATIUM
RECOMMENDATIONS FROM THE NATURAL PHYSICIAN FOR . . .

🐦 COMMON COLD AND FLU

One of the most common uses of lomatium is for colds and flu. I have found it to have one of the strongest antiviral effects of all the herbs I have used. When taken at the onset of a cold or when you feel the first flu symptoms coming on, you'll find that it can greatly decrease the severity of symptoms. Also, you're likely to get over these viral infections more quickly: I have seen patients with severe cases of the flu show great improvement within 24 hours of taking lomatium.

🐦 EPSTEIN-BARR

This virus is noted for causing mononucleosis as well as some cases of chronic fatigue syndrome. Practitioners find that lomatium is one of the best herbs to use to eradicate this virus. (It is certainly a better protocol than the traditional one, which is generally bed rest.)

🐦 HERPES AND GENITAL WARTS

Lomatium is popular for the natural treatment of herpes—both the kind that occur on the mouth (type 1) and genitals (type 2). It's also effective as a treatment for genital warts. Again, this herb appears to have a direct effect of blocking viral replication as well as assisting the immune system's antiviral weaponry. It is taken internally in both cases.

People with herpes find that if they take lomatium at the first symptoms of an outbreak, it helps to suppress the outbreak or reduce its severity. Those with genital warts should use lomatium only with the supervision of a physician.

🐦 RESPIRATORY TRACT INFECTIONS

Lomatium was used in the past for bronchitis, pneumonia, and even tuberculosis. Today, naturopathic physicians frequently use it in a blend of herbs for respiratory tract ailments.

🐦 URINARY TRACT INFECTIONS

Lomatium can be used by itself or in combination with herbs that are specific for urinary tract infections, such as uva ursi and goldenseal.

Lycopodium

George, a 44-year-old lawyer, came to see me for treatment of chronic digestive problems and fatigue.

"No matter what I eat, I produce tremendous amounts of gas," he said. He went on to describe how difficult it was for him at work, where he had trouble restraining himself when he was meeting with clients. "At my desk," he added, "I have to loosen my belt and pants because of the abdominal pressure from the bloating."

Fatigue was also a problem, though he didn't know whether or not it was related to digestion. "It is getting more and more difficult for me to get up in the morning. Then, I get tired at 8 p.m., so it's difficult to stay awake. My wife is upset over my lack of sociability. I also find that I'm very irritable with my secretary and short tempered with my family."

I recommended lycopodium.

It worked wonders for George. Over the next couple of months, his flatulence and bloating were greatly improved; he felt more energy upon awakening, and although he still had a short temper, his wife commented that he seemed more patient.

AN EARTHY SOLUTION

Lycopodium, the homeopathic dilution of club moss, is one of the best homeopathic remedies for digestive problems. It is prescribed specifically for bloating and distension of the abdomen that is relieved by passing gas and burping.

People requiring lycopodium usually have very large appetites, and eating makes the bloating and gas worse. They find that warm drinks have a soothing effect on the digestive system, while cold drinks do not. It is also one of the more common remedies for heartburn.

People who respond well to lycopodium tend to have a strong craving for sweets. Another peculiar problem is that many of their symptoms worsen between 4 p.m. and 8 p.m., as was the case with George and his fatigue. Patients often say their digestion is fine until evening, and then it acts up.

There's another symptom, too, that could indicate a need for lycopodium. Physical problems tend to occur on the right side of the body. For example, one patient of mine had chronic headaches that always occurred in the right temple area. Lycopodium cleared up this chronic problem for her.

The mental profile of someone requiring lycopodium is unique and fits a lot of people in our "power hungry" society. These people want to be in control. Often, they are people who act bossy, arrogant, irritable, and domineering. (The typical schoolyard bully would benefit from lycopodium.)

DOSAGE

The typical dosage is 30C potency twice daily for the relief of acute symptoms such as gas or bloating, or right-sided headaches. Long-term treatment is best done with a lower potency, such as 6C, taken two to three times daily.

WHAT ARE THE SIDE EFFECTS?

Side effects are not a concern with lycopodium. If you are not sure whether you should use it, consult a homeopathic practitioner.

LYCOPODIUM

RECOMMENDATIONS FROM THE NATURAL PHYSICIAN FOR . . .

❧ ARTHRITIS

Typically, lycopodium is helpful for arthritis that is alleviated with warm applications and that affects joints on the right side of the body.

❧ COLITIS

Lycopodium has an amazing ability to heal the digestive tract. It has helped many people who have digestive problems such as colitis, Crohn's disease, and irritable bowel syndrome (IBS).

❧ HEADACHES

Whenever a patient complains of a right-sided headache, I immediately think of lycopodium as a possible remedy. The headache may be worse between 4 p.m. and 8 p.m.

❧ HEPATITIS

Lycopodium also has an affinity for the liver. It is one of the main remedies to use for liver problems such as hepatitis.

❧ IMPOTENCE

Lycopodium is the main homeopathic remedy for impotence and premature ejaculation. It is well indicated when the sexual problems of the man are psychological in origin, due to low confidence. I have seen this remedy help several of my male patients.

❧ OVARIAN PAIN

Right-sided ovarian pain is an indication for lycopodium. Women with ovarian cysts respond well to this remedy. It not only takes the pain away, but also helps in preventing the cysts from developing again.

❧ RESPIRATORY TRACT INFECTIONS

Right-sided respiratory tract infections often require lycopodium. This includes asthma, bronchitis, pneumonia, and sinusitis. I treated a one-year-old child who was having trouble breathing at night. On listening to his lungs through a stethoscope, I discovered that he had congestion in the right lobe only. I recommended lycopodium—and the treatment was successful.

Lysine

I was summoned to the phone.

"Dr. Mark, it's Rick calling. I'm on vacation in Hawaii and my mouth started breaking out with cold sores yesterday. I hope there's something you can recommend to clear them up. It feels awful and looks like the start of a bad outbreak. I haven't had a case like this in years."

"Go to a pharmacy or health-food store," I said, "and pick up the supplement lysine. Take 1,000 mg three times daily between meals. Get started right away, and it should help clear things up pretty quickly."

Then I recalled how much Rick liked to party. I was forced to add, "By the way—try to keep away from alcohol for the next few days."

"I'll get the lysine right away. Thanks, Dr. Mark."

(I noticed he didn't acknowledge my request to watch his alcohol intake—but I think he'd heard me nonetheless.)

The next time I saw Rick, he told me that the lysine had helped to keep the cold sore outbreak at bay. A few large cold sores did pop out, but they healed up quickly in four days. He also mentioned that this particular outbreak was significantly less intense than what he had experienced in the past.

LOOKING AT LYSINE

Lysine—also called L-lysine—is an essential amino acid. This means you must consume it in your diet as your body cannot synthesize it or make enough of it to function properly. Actually, the bacteria in the gut produce amino acids, including lysine in very small amounts. This amino acid is highly concentrated in muscle tissue.

Foods high in lysine include chicken and wild game, cottage cheese, and wheat germ. Most fruits and vegetables, except for avocados, contain little lysine.

Lysine is involved in many different metabolic activities in the body. It is required for growth, particularly in children. It is thought to be important for bone health, and some consider it a supplement for the treatment and prevention of osteoporosis.

Lysine helps to fight lead toxicity. It is required for the body's synthesis of carnitine, an amino-acidlike substance that's particularly essential for good heart function.

The primary use of supplemental lysine is to prevent or treat herpes outbreaks. A lysine deficiency can impair the immune system. It is one of the amino acids that are depleted from the body when it is under stress. People who have Parkinson's disease, hypothyroidism, kidney disease, asthma, and depression have been found to have low levels of lysine.

DOSAGE

A typical dosage is 13,000 mg for the acute treatment of herpes outbreaks (both type 1 and type 2). Lower dosages are used by some practitioners for the prevention of outbreaks, usually 500 to 1,000 mg daily.

A number of nutrients help your body absorb and use lysine. Among the nutrients involved in this process of lysine metabolism are niacin, vitamin B6, riboflavin, vitamin C, glutamic acid, and iron. Interestingly, B vitamins and vitamin C are commonly recommended for the treatment of herpes as well.

WHAT ARE THE SIDE EFFECTS?

Lysine is well tolerated. Studies have shown that people can take up to 8,000 mg without any problems. However, taking high doses of lysine for long periods of time may deplete the levels of the amino acid arginine.

Lysine should not be taken at the same time you're taking antibiotics.

LYSINE

RECOMMENDATIONS FROM THE NATURAL PHYSICIAN FOR . . .

☙ HERPES

Lysine is a common treatment for people suffering from herpes outbreaks. Research on the herpes virus showed that in a culture dish, the amino acid arginine stimulated growth of the virus while the addition of lysine inhibited growth.

A study was conducted on 45 patients who experienced frequent herpes outbreaks. They received 312 to 500 mg of lysine for two months to three years. The dosage was increased to 800 to 1,000 mg for acute outbreaks, and foods high in the amino acid arginine—such as chocolate, various kinds of seeds, and nuts—were restricted. This therapy reduced the frequency of outbreaks and greatly accelerated the recovery from acute outbreaks.

Another study found that 1,200 mg of lysine significantly reduced the recurrence of herpes simplex outbreaks. Lysine is effective for both oral and genital herpes. I recommend that persons with herpes reduce their intake of foods containing arginine during acute outbreaks. These include chocolate, nuts, seeds, peanuts, and grains (wheat).

☙ OSTEOPOROSIS

Animal studies have shown that lysine deficiency increases calcium excretion. While lysine deficiency is rare, it is theorized that a low-grade deficiency may lead to bone loss. Lysine is used by the body to form collagen, an integral component of bone. More research is needed to see if lysine supplementation would be helpful for increasing bone density.

M

Maca

"My hot flashes, fatigue, depression, and low libido have been a problem for more than a year. I have tried other supplements to treat these symptoms but have had little help. I want to avoid using hormones since my mother had breast cancer," explained Julie, a 51-year-old nurse.

I reassured Julie by replying, "I have the perfect option for you. It's been shown in studies to help all the symptoms you are having problems with. It's also herbal so you don't need to worry about taking hormones. Have you heard of maca?" I asked. I went on to tell Julie about the traditional use of maca root by Peruvians over the centuries, as well as modern studies done on it. Six weeks after taking maca, Julie reported that her symptoms had improved greatly.

Maca (*Lepidium meyenii or peruvianum*) is a great choice for treating perimenopause and menopausal symptoms. It is also used, in men and women, for improving adrenal gland function to support energy, combat stress, and strengthen libido.

Maca is cultivated as a vegetable crop in the Andes Mountains of Peru and has been for at least 3,000 years. The root of the maca is shaped like a large radish. It is a cousin to other cruciferous plants, such as cauliflower and Brussels sprouts. Peruvians traditionally boil or roast the maca root or grind it into flour for baking. However, despite maca's popular description as a "super food," in this country you won't see it in food form.

Instead the root is dried and ground into a fine powder. It is then distributed primarily in capsules, although you can also buy the powder to blend into beverages or sprinkle on foods.

In addition to healthful fiber, complex carbohydrates, and protein, maca provides numerous minerals, including calcium, magnesium, phosphorous, potassium, sulfur, iron, zinc, iodine, and copper; vitamins B1, B2, C, and E; nearly 20 amino acids, including linoleic acid, palmitic acid, and oleic acid; and various plant sterols, natural cholesterol-lowering agents. All of these nutrients have been shown to promote health in a multitude of ways.

DOSAGE

I recommend 1,000 to 2,000 mg of the extract form in capsule or tablet. For the powder form that can be mixed in a drink or shake, the dosage is 3 to 6 teaspoons daily. I have patients take maca supplements for three months, then stop using it for one or two weeks, and continue on this alternating regimen as needed for symptom relief.

WHAT ARE THE SIDE EFFECTS?

Maca is generally considered to be safe, based on the centuries of use by Peruvians and modern clinical data. Breast cancer patients taking tamoxifen or other estrogen blockers, or women who have had breast cancer, should discuss the use of maca with their doctor. Men and women taking thyroid medication should also be monitored by their doctor while using maca, as it may increase thyroid activity. Pregnant or breastfeeding women should not take maca.

MACA
RECOMMENDATIONS FROM THE NATURAL PHYSICIAN FOR . . .

🍃 ADAPTOGEN

Like the herbs ashwagandha, licorice, and ginseng, maca is an adaptogen. It boosts the body's ability to resist, deal with, and recover from emotional and physical stress. Maca helps to support energy and endurance levels without acting as a stimulant. It also improves memory and mood. Animal and in vitro studies have also demonstrated various other benefits. These include promoting cartilage growth (as demonstrated in animal studies), better blood-sugar control, healing ulcers, lowering LDL cholesterol and triglyceride levels, reducing prostate enlargement, and improving liver function.

🍃 MALE FERTILITY

A small study published in the *Asian Journal of Andrology* yielded some interesting results, indicating that maca also improves male fertility. Nine men, ages 24 to 44, received either 1,500 mg or 3,000 mg maca per day. Compared to tests done at study outset, semen analysis performed at the end of the four-month study demonstrated that maca increased semen volume, sperm count, and sperm motility at both dose levels. These results were not related to increases in testosterone or other hormones.

🍃 MALE LIBIDO

Folklore has long held that maca improves the sex drive of men and mod-

ern research has confirmed this. One double-blind, randomized study published in the journal *Andrologia* examined the effect of maca on sexual desire in 57 men, ages 21 to 56. Subjects took either placebos or 1,500 mg or 3,000 mg maca. After 4, 8, and 12 weeks, participants reported on their sex drive levels. Placebo users experienced no change in libido, whereas the men taking either quantity of maca reported heightened sexual desire starting at 8 weeks and continuing throughout the 12-week study. Blood tests showed that maca did not affect the men's levels of the hormones testosterone or estrogen. This is one of maca's virtues—it doesn't change hormone regulation in men. Its enhancing properties are attributed primarily to amino acids and sterols, among other substances.

🍃 OSTEOPOROSIS

There is preliminary evidence that maca extract improves bone density in women. Presumably this is due to its hormonal balancing effects.

🍃 PERIMENOPAUSE AND MENOPAUSE

What was once a Peruvian female menopause secret is now available to American women. Maca is a wonder botanical for women experiencing menopausal symptoms such as hot flashes, night sweats, low libido, anxiety, depression, fatigue, and many others.

Modern research has demonstrated the hormone-balancing effects of this Peruvian wonder. In a study published in 2006 in the *International Journal of Biomedical Science*, researchers at five sites in Poland focused on 124 women, ages 49 to 58, in the early stages of menopause. One group of women took placebos while the other group supplemented with 1,000 mg maca, twice daily for three or four months. Compared to placebo users, those taking maca experienced significant reductions in frequency and severity of menopausal symptoms, particularly hot flashes and night sweats. They also reported that maca reduced nervousness, mood swings, interrupted sleep pattern, fatigue, stress, headaches, and depression, and increased libido.

Interestingly, blood tests showed that maca reduced follicle-stimulating hormone, which normally increases during menopause and is thought to be one cause of symptoms such as hot flashes and night sweats. Study authors speculate that the maca stimulates the regulatory mechanism responsible for optimizing ovarian function and estrogen secretion, significantly increasing estradiol (estrogen). It appears, then, that maca offers a safe and effective way to reduce menopausal symptoms—and is unlikely to increase a woman's risk for breast cancer, heart disease, and stroke (as does hormone replacement therapy), since it does not put foreign estrogens in the body. And for all the maca consumed by Peruvian women, it certainly doesn't appear to increase breast cancer risk. As a matter of fact, breast cancer is not one of the leading causes of death in Peruvian women.

Magnesium

Fifty-six-year-old Gina said she often had muscle cramps and spasms during the day, but they were worse at night.

"My doctor can't find anything wrong," she continued. "My blood work didn't show anything out of balance. I was told to take some calcium, but it hasn't been helping."

"Does your calcium supplement also contain magnesium?" I asked.

"No, my doctor didn't mention anything about magnesium," she replied.

"That's likely to be the problem," I said. "Calcium and magnesium both help to relax the muscles. Some people with muscle spasms respond better to higher levels of magnesium, while some respond better to calcium. In any event, both should be taken, as both are commonly deficient.

Also, you need magnesium for your bones as well."

An extra 500 mg of magnesium did the trick for Gina. Within three days, her muscle cramps and spasms subsided, and she found that she slept better as well.

THE MIGHTY MINERAL

Magnesium is the second most abundant mineral in the cells after potassium. Sixty percent of the body's magnesium is found in the bones, while the muscles contain approximately 27%; and the rest is found in the tissues and blood. The body maintains a narrow range of magnesium blood levels, and will draw it from the bones if blood levels are low.

Magnesium is required as a cofactor for hundreds of enzymatic reactions. This includes energy production, lipid and protein synthesis, nerve impulses, muscle contraction and relaxation, and bone formation by helping to regulate calcium metabolism.

It is also necessary for the cardiovascular system. It is required for heart function and relaxes blood vessel walls, so blood pressure is reduced.

MISSING MAGNESIUM

Most children and adults do not get adequate amounts of magnesium in their diets. They tend to eat processed foods, and processing destroys the magnesium content. Only a small percentage of the population eats whole grains, legumes, nuts, and green leafy vegetables on a regular basis.

A magnesium deficiency can cause many different symptoms. These include muscle cramps, spasms, and weakness; fatigue; irritability and personality changes; confusion; loss of appetite; poor coordination; and cravings for sweets.

Conditions or diseases associated with a magnesium deficiency include high blood pressure, kidney stones, insomnia, premenstrual syndrome, hair loss, swollen gums, and reduced heart function.

Aside from poor diet, factors that could cause magnesium deficiency include digestive disorders (such as malabsorption or chronic diarrhea), kidney disease, use of diuretics, diabetes, and alcoholism.

Medications known to deplete magnesium include digoxin, corticosteroids, birth-control pills, theophylline, and warfarin.

Standard blood tests do not pick up a magnesium deficiency until it is very severe, usually after a serious condition has developed. Therefore, symptoms and diet analysis help to determine if there is a magnesium deficiency.

DIETARY REFERENCE INTAKE

0 to 6 months: 50 mg

6 to 12 months: 70 mg

1 to 10 years: 150 to 250 mg

11 to 18 years: 300 to 400 mg

18+ years: 300 to 400 mg

Pregnant/lactating: +150 mg

DOSAGE

I recommend for most adults 400 to 500 mg of magnesium daily. You can meet this goal by taking a multivitamin and/or a calcium/magnesium complex or bone health formula.

I recommend that children take 250 to 500 mg daily. These supplements should be taken with meals.

When someone needs a very high dosage of magnesium (such as a person with fibromyalgia), then magnesium may be taken by itself. Magnesium glycinate is a good form to use for a high dosage (750 mg or higher) as it is less likely to cause diarrhea. Otherwise, magnesium citrate or other chelates are well absorbed.

Vitamin B6 and magnesium work synergistically in many different enzymatic reactions.

WHAT ARE THE SIDE EFFECTS?

The most common side effect is loose stools or diarrhea. This tends to happen when the dosage is above 500 mg. I find some people need to start at a lower dosage (such as 250 mg) and slowly increase the amount over a few weeks until they reach their desired therapeutic dosage. Magnesium chloride, sulfate, carbonate, and oxide are more likely than magnesium glycinate and magnesium citrate to cause this problem.

People with kidney and heart disease should not use a magnesium supplement unless instructed to do so by a physician. It should not be taken at the same time as the drugs Fosamax, cimetidine, ranitidine, and tetracycline; these substances should be taken a few hours apart.

MAGNESIUM
RECOMMENDATIONS FROM THE NATURAL PHYSICIAN FOR . . .

ANGINA

This is a heart condition where a person feels a heaviness or squeezing sensation in the chest, often accompanied by a feeling of suffocation. In this condition there is a lack of blood flow and oxygen to the heart tissues, or spasm of the coronary arteries. Magnesium is important as it helps relax and dilate the arteries that feed the heart. Nutritional doctors also use magnesium intravenously for this condition. I find the oral supplement works best when taken in conjunction with CoQ10, L-carnitine, hawthorn berry, L-arginine, vitamin E, and other targeted support for the heart.

ARRHYTHMIA

Magnesium is often recommended for those with heart arrhythmias. It can reverse the condition in some people. I also recommend CoQ10 and calcium as well. If you are taking medication for heart arrhythmia, you must check with your doctor before using a magnesium supplement.

ASTHMA

Magnesium promotes the relaxation of the bronchial muscles. Using a magnesium supplement helps to reduce the incidence of asthma attacks.

Doctors have found that an oral supplement does not help in an acute asthma attack. However, if a doctor gives it intravenously, magnesium may be effective in relieving an acute asthma attack.

CARDIOMYOPATHY AND CONGESTIVE HEART FAILURE

When someone has cardiomyopathy, the heart is weakened by a viral infection or some other cause. Cardiomyopathy can lead to congestive heart failure—a condition in which the heart fails to pump blood adequately. Magnesium helps to support energy production and improve the pumping action of the heart.

One study showed that persons with congestive heart failure who had normal levels of magnesium had longer survival rates than those with lower magnesium levels.

DIABETES

Magnesium, along with vitamin B6, is important for the proper functioning of insulin so that glucose can get into the cells properly. A meta-analysis conducted by researchers from the Karolinska Institute in Stockholm assessed the association between magnesium intake and the risk for type 2 diabetes. The study of 286,668 adults found that for every 100-mg increase in magnesium intake, the risk of

(continued)

developing diabetes decreased by 15%. That is the equivalent of the amount of magnesium in four slices of whole-grain bread, 4 cups of cooked oatmeal, 1 cup of beans, ¼ cup of nuts, or ½ cup of cooked spinach. Magnesium may protect against diabetes by improving insulin sensitivity.

It also helps to prevent complications of diabetes such as heart disease and retinopathy. (It has also been shown that children with insulin-dependent diabetes have lower levels of magnesium than other children.)

FATIGUE

Magnesium is involved in the production of energy; it helps to prevent and treat fatigue. Studies have shown magnesium to benefit those with chronic fatigue syndrome.

FIBROMYALGIA

I routinely recommend magnesium along with calcium to help patients with this disorder affecting the muscles and joints. It helps to reduce muscle soreness and tightness, as well as relieve other symptoms such as fatigue and insomnia. The dosage I recommend for fibromyalgia is 500 to 1,000 mg taken in divided doses throughout the day.

GLAUCOMA

This is an eye condition in which there is increased pressure within the eyeball. If left untreated, blindness can result. One study showed that a dose of 141.5 mg taken twice daily for one month improved the visual fields of people with glaucoma.

HEARING LOSS

Oral supplementation of magnesium has shown to prevent hearing loss for people exposed to loud noise.

HIGH BLOOD PRESSURE

Studies have shown magnesium to be helpful in the treatment of hypertension. I always recommend it along with the mineral calcium and CoQ10. It seems to help for long-term treatment of hypertension.

KIDNEY STONES

Most kidney stones are composed of calcium oxalate. Magnesium makes calcium more soluble in the urine, and thus inhibits the formation of calcium-oxalate crystals. One study examined 55 people with recurring kidney stones who were given 500 mg of magnesium daily for up to four years. The study showed that 85% of these people remained stone-free compared with 41% of a group of people who did not receive magnesium supplements.

Taking vitamin B6 in conjunction with magnesium works even better as it aids in oxalate metabolism. I recommend 500 mg of magnesium citrate and 50 mg daily of B6 for the prevention of kidney stones.

MIGRAINE HEADACHES

Magnesium is helpful for the prevention of migraine headaches for some people. Those who suffer from chronic migraine headaches should supplement 500 mg of magnesium daily.

MITRAL VALVE PROLAPSE

Magnesium has been shown to be helpful for this condition. It should be taken with

L-carnitine and CoQ10 by anyone who has mitral valve prolapse.

OSTEOPOROSIS

Many researchers feel that magnesium is as important for the prevention and treatment of osteoporosis as is calcium. Remember, magnesium is of critical importance for the proper utilization of calcium by the bones. Magnesium should be part of a comprehensive supplementation protocol. A dosage of 500 to 1,000 mg daily is recommended.

PREGNANCY

Studies have shown magnesium to be helpful in preventing preeclampsia, a condition characterized by increased blood pressure, fluid retention, and protein in the urine. Preeclampsia can cause fetal growth retardation and premature delivery. Magnesium is often given intra-venously for treatment when this condition is acute. I recommend that all pregnant women take a magnesium and calcium supplement.

PMS

Magnesium levels have been shown to be lower in women with PMS than in those without this condition. One double-blind study found that 200 mg per day of magnesium supplementation allevi-ated PMS symptoms such as breast ten-derness, abdominal bloating, weight gain, and swelling of the extremities. Another study found that magnesium was effective in relieving premenstrual mood changes.

Magnesium is one of the cofactors required for estrogen metabolism. An imbalance between estrogen and pro-gesterone is one of the main theories as to why PMS occurs.

Maitake

Maitake has long been valued in Japanese medicine as a health mushroom. In Japanese, *maitake* means "dancing mushroom." Traditional Japanese medicine use of maitake is as an adaptogen, a substance that helps the body adapt to stress and "balance out."

Maitake has a track record of modern research that can be traced back to the early 1980s when microbiology and mycology expert Dr. Hiroaki Nanba, from Kobe Pharmaceutical University, was studying the properties of different medicinal mush-rooms. In his analysis he found that maitake had greater antitumor activity than other mushroom extracts and that it was effective when given orally. This led to Dr. Nanba's patented and published work on the mai-take fractions known as D and MD fraction. The MD fraction is his most recent advance-ment and is available commercially in the United States. It is a special type of immune-stimulating polysaccharide known as beta 1,6 glucan. The MD fraction has the ability to directly enhance the damaging activity of natural killer and cytotoxic T-cells, which attack tumor cells. Maitake seems also to combat cancer cells by protecting healthy cells from becoming cancerous, helping to prevent cancer metastasis, and slowing or stopping cancer cell growth.

I spoke in person with Dr. Nanba at a convention in Anaheim, California, about his interesting research and have been using his extract with patients for years. I most commonly use maitake for the complemen-tary treatment of cancer.

DOSAGE

For immune support, take 0.5 to 1 mg of MD or D fraction per two pounds of body weight per day.

WHAT ARE THE SIDE EFFECTS?

This mushroom extract is quite safe. It should be avoided in people with organ transplants using immunosuppressive agents.

MAITAKE

RECOMMENDATIONS FROM THE NATURAL PHYSICIAN FOR . . .

🐌 COMPLEMENTARY CANCER TREATMENT

Maitake is one of the relatively few natural products for which there is human data for cancer treatment. For example, a trial of cancer patients in stages II, III, and IV, ages 33 to 68, examined the effects of oral maitake. Data was collected under the cooperation of their medical doctors in Japan, and cancer regression or significant symptom improvement was observed in 58.3% of liver cancer patients, 68.8% of breast cancer patients, and 62.5% of lung cancer patients. Overall, maitake is most indicated for breast, prostate, liver, and lung cancers.

Maitake may help reduce the side effects of chemotherapy. In a study of 455 people at Japanese hospitals researchers found that combining maitake with chemotherapy was very helpful in reducing side effects such as lost appetite, vomiting, nausea, hair loss, and leukopenia (deficiency of white blood cells). These symptoms were ameliorated in 90% of the patients, and pain reduction was reported by 83% of the patients.

🐌 DIABETES

Small clinical studies in people with type 2 diabetes found that maitake was statistically significant in reducing blood glucose levels. The study involved a maitake standardized to a component called SX fraction.

Melatonin

"I just can't get to sleep," said Glen, a 59-year-old retired pilot.

"What therapies have you tried for your sleep problems?" I asked.

"My doctor prescribed many different drugs. Most didn't help, or if they did, it was temporary. With a couple of them, I couldn't handle the side effects—like feeling hung over in the morning."

Glen went on to name some natural remedies that his chiropractor had suggested, including kava and valerian.

"I also tried acupuncture," Glen continued. "That worked well for my back, but did nothing for my sleep."

"Well, you certainly have tried a lot of remedies. What about melatonin?"

Though Glen had heard of it, he hadn't tried it.

I explained how it works.

"Melatonin is a hormone produced by a gland in your brain that is released when it's dark, in the night, and it promotes sleep."

"How well does it work?" asked Glen.

"It's like everything else—it works for some people, and not for others. But overall,

I have found it to be reasonably effective. Since it is a hormone, I use it when other natural therapies aren't helping. However, I would say it's a heck of a lot safer and usually more effective than sleeping pills."

"I'm ready to try it," said Glen.

It was a few days before Glen called, but when he did, he reported that he no longer had a problem sleeping. Melatonin had done the trick.

FOR THE REST OF IT

Melatonin is a hormone produced by a pea-sized structure called the pineal gland, located in the center of the brain. Interestingly, it was once thought that the pineal gland had no function. Today, we know that the melatonin released by this gland helps to set the rhythms of waking and sleeping. Taken as a supplement, melatonin has been used as a potent antioxidant as well. For some people, it reduces jet lag.

Some preliminary research suggests that melatonin can strengthen the immune system, play a role in the prevention and treatment of cancer, and help people recover from heart disease. It is also recommended by some holistic doctors for people who have HIV and chronic infections. In addition, it is thought by some researchers to have "antiaging" properties.

THE DARK SIDE

Melatonin synthesis is stimulated by exposure to darkness, while it's suppressed by exposure to light. When light enters the eye, it activates a series of signals that are transmitted to the pineal gland, which cuts back on production of melatonin. In darkness, however, the eye sends a contrary signal, activating melatonin production.

Melatonin is actually produced from the amino acid tryptophan. Tryptophan is converted to a chemical called 5-hydroxytryptophan (5-HTP), then to the neurotransmitter serotonin, and finally into melatonin.

There are several substances that can decrease your body's production of melatonin. These include alcohol, aspirin, caffeine, and ibuprofen. The presence of nicotine also depresses melatonin production, so you have a problem if you smoke regularly. A number of prescription medications also reduce melatonin production, including beta blockers, calcium channel blockers, and tranquilizers.

Stress-reduction techniques such as prayer and meditation increase your body's level of melatonin.

Melatonin is found in foods such as oats, sweet corn, rice, ginger, tomatoes, bananas, and barley.

Some research has indicated that melatonin levels decrease as we age, but not all the studies are in agreement. I don't think all elderly people should take melatonin, but I do know it's helpful to some. It can greatly improve sleep quality.

Not surprisingly, shift workers have been particularly interested in melatonin. Working the night shift is hard on the biological rhythms of the body, because it's difficult to get proper sleep during the day when the sun is out. Melatonin has been particularly helpful for people who work the "graveyard shift." By regularly taking melatonin just before the "sleep time" in the morning, their biological rhythms and sleep patterns usually improve. Usually, it takes about a week for complete adjustment to take place.

DOSAGE

As with any hormone, it is best to use the lowest possible dosage to get the desired effect. This is especially true when using it for insomnia.

I find that a dose of 0.1 to 0.3 mg may be all that is needed to promote sleep for those with insomnia or for people using it to regulate sleep cycles as a result of time-zone changes (jet lag) or shift work. Some users will require higher dosages up to 3 mg, or occasionally 5 mg.

Dosages of 20 to 50 mg and higher are prescribed for immune-system enhancement and for the treatment of cancer. These high dosages should only be taken with a physician's guidance.

Melatonin is available in capsule, tablet, and liquid forms, as well as in time-release and sublingual forms.

Vitamins B3 and B6, and the minerals calcium and magnesium are important for melatonin synthesis. Many of my patients report that taking calcium or magnesium (or both) in the evening improves their sleep.

WHAT ARE THE SIDE EFFECTS?

Melatonin appears to be a safe hormone with relatively little toxicity, but unfortunately, there have not been good, long-term human studies.

Because it hasn't been adequately tested, I don't advise pregnant women or nursing mothers to take melatonin. If you're a woman who's trying to conceive, you'll want to avoid melatonin because high dosages have been shown to suppress ovulation.

It should not be used with children—again, because the long-term effects are not known.

People taking steroid medications such as dexamethasone and cortisone should avoid using melatonin unless a doctor prescribes it. Also, people with autoimmune diseases or cancer should use it only under the guidance of a doctor.

MELATONIN
RECOMMENDATIONS FROM THE NATURAL PHYSICIAN FOR . . .

❧ AGING
Researchers feel that melatonin may help prolong youth through several mechanisms such as reducing free-radical damage of cells, improving immune-system function, normalizing circadian and biological rhythms, improving sleep and repair, and through the stimulation of growth-hormone production.

More research needs to be done before we can say for sure that melatonin has an "anti-aging effect," but it seems to be promising.

❧ BENZODIAZEPINE WITHDRAWAL
Taking melatonin has been shown to help seniors with insomnia with benzodiazepine withdrawal.

❧ CANCER
Melatonin is recommended by some cancer specialists, though they usually advise taking it in conjunction with chemotherapy or radiation. It's thought to be helpful for treatment of various cancers, especially breast, prostate, lung, and skin. It also appears to have an antiproliferative effect on certain kinds of hormone-dependent cancers, helping to prevent the spread of those cancers to other organs or parts of the body. The antiproliferative effect seems to

apply to estrogen-dependent breast cancer and androgen-dependent prostate cancer.

Also, melatonin has been shown to increase the efficacy of chemotherapy and reduce the toxicity of the treatments.

CLUSTER HEADACHE

One study found supplementing 10 mg melatonin orally every evening helped to reduce the frequency of episodic cluster headaches.

HIGH BLOOD PRESSURE

Italian researchers reported in the *American Journal of Hypertension* that melatonin reduces nighttime blood pressure in women with hypertension. This randomized, double-blind study involved 18 women, ages 47 to 63. Nine of the women had normal blood pressure and another nine had hypertension. Participants received a three-week course of a slow-release melatonin pill (3 mg) or placebo one hour before going to bed. They were then switched to the other treatment for another three weeks. Blood pressure readings were tracked at the beginning and end of each treatment period. Of the women taking melatonin, 84% had a decrease in blood pressure as compared to 39% of those taking placebo. Previous studies have found similar results with men with untreated hypertension and people with type 1 diabetes.

INSOMNIA

Many studies have shown that melatonin is effective for those with insomnia, both in young adults and the elderly. It has also been shown to improve the sleep quality of people with chronic schizophrenia. I advocate the use of melatonin to help wean people off addictive benzodiazepine drugs that are used for insomnia.

Melatonin has been shown to help normalize the sleeping patterns of blind people. Since the pineal gland is light sensitive, blind people are often "out of sync" with the usual patterns of wakefulness during daylight hours and sleepiness at night. By pacing the way they take melatonin, they can adjust so they don't suffer from daytime sleepiness.

Low doses of melatonin are often the most effective. It should always be taken at night.

JET LAG

If you need to choose between melatonin and pharmaceutical sleeping pills for fighting jet lag, I'd recommend the melatonin. Sleeping pills may help one fall asleep but they do not help reset the body's clock. Also, sleeping pills can be addictive and cause drowsiness.

To combat jet lag, take melatonin one hour before your normal bedtime, in the time zone where you'll be landing. Several studies have demonstrated melatonin is effective for jet lag.

RADIATION EXPOSURE

Melatonin may become a common therapy for the prevention and treatment of radiation exposure. One study found that it protected human white blood cells 500 times more effectively than the potent antioxidant (DMSO) that was used for comparison.

(continued)

❧ SMOKING CESSATION

Melatonin supplementation for smokers has been shown to improve subjective symptoms of anxiety, restlessness, irritability, depression, and cigarette craving over the 10 hours following ingestion of melatonin.

❧ TARDIVE DYSKINESIA

This is a condition characterized by involuntary, repetitive movements from the use of certain pharmaceutical medications such as antipsychotics. Supplementing 10 mg daily may decrease symptoms by 24 to 30% after six weeks of treatment.

❧ THROMBOCYTOPENIA

This is a condition where the clotting cells of the blood—known as platelets—decrease below normal. There is evidence that supplementing melatonin can improve thrombocytopenia associated with cancer and treatments commonly used for cancer.

Mental Imagery

"Part of our treatment for your anxiety will be to imagine yourself in a beautiful, pleasant environment with a calm setting. Think of a place you have been before, where the atmosphere was very calming to you. A couple times a day, or when you feel your anxiety coming on, I want you to sit and envision yourself in this place. Take some deep, slow breaths and really see yourself in this place within your mind."

Thirty-year-old Allison had long been seeking an alternative treatment for her anxiety disorder. Though she had experienced the limitations of pharmaceutical medications, I wasn't sure whether she was quite ready to accept the practice I was suggesting—mental imagery—as the answer to her problems.

But whatever her unspoken skepticism, it vanished when she began using the technique I described. She soon found that this technique helped to keep her anxiety at bay. During times of stress, she could feel the anxiety coming back. That's when she would go off by herself to a quiet place and use mental imagery to relax and calm herself.

MENTAL FIX

Mental imagery is simply envisioning what you want something to be. In the health field, the practice of using mental imagery for healing has become well accepted. Much evidence has turned up in the field of oncology—the study of cancer—showing that cancer patients tend to live longer, and certainly have a better quality of life, if they are associated with programs where mental imagery is regularly practiced.

Some leading cancer clinics such as Cancer Treatment Centers of America, a national chain, have mental imagery programs available to patients. The term most often used to describe these programs is "mind–body medicine," or, in more scientific terms, "psychoneuroimmunology." "Psycho" refers to thought, emotions, and mood; "neuro" refers to the nervous system; and "immunology" refers to the immune system. So the translation of "psychoneuroimmunology" means the effect of the mind on the nervous system and immune system.

Your thoughts and feelings affect the chemistry of your nervous system and ultimately all the cells in your body, including the immune system. Studies have proven what many have always believed for ages. Yes, the thoughts in our minds and the images that we *bring* to mind do have direct effects on the cells of our bodies.

In one study that included 10 men and 10 women, researchers explored the effects of visualization, or mental imagery, on immune-system response in people who had depressed white blood cell counts. When white blood cells are "depressed," it means the body is more susceptible to the invasion of some disease. The patients in this study had a variety of health problems ranging from cancer and AIDS to viral infections.

When the patients in the study used mental imagery, their white blood cell count (the measurement of improved health) showed significant increases over a 90-day period.

A HEALTHY PRACTICE

Mental imagery isn't just for the sick. If it can have such a positive effect on health, that's ample reason to recommend it to those who are healthy. Using mental imagery can be a powerful way to maintain health and prevent illness.

How do you go about this? Well, picture in your mind what you want to look like and how you want to feel. The first time you try this imagery, it may seem like a mere exercise and you may well wonder how it will ultimately shape your future health and vitality. But with repetition, it does.

I saw a good example of this positive effect when I recommended mental imagery to a friend of mine, Jason, who had suffered many years ago from recurring bronchitis and pneumonia. After a long bout of pneumonia had left him feeling depleted and unwell, he started to find out whether he could use mental imagery to "turn the corner." During

quiet periods of reflection, he told himself he would never get pneumonia again. He envisioned his lungs and respiratory system becoming impervious to infection.

Treating this almost as an experiment, Jason did nothing else to materially improve his health. He didn't start taking new supplements, nor did he change his diet and lifestyle. Nonetheless, he discovered that just the change in his mental outlook made a very significant difference. From that day to the last time I saw him—very recently— he has not had any recurrence of pneumonia or bronchitis.

DOING IT YOUR WAY

Whatever illness you may have, you can picture "in your mind's eye" your body recovering.

When you practice mental imagery, try to get as detailed as you can. For example, if you have osteoarthritis of the knees, see your cells creating new cartilage in the knee joints. Also, envision yourself with less pain and with greater mobility.

If you have high blood pressure, envision yourself in a calm and serene environment. Then see your blood vessels relaxing and the pressure decreasing within the blood-vessel walls.

When you're using mental imagery, it's also good to use your other senses to make the positive images as real as possible. For example, if you picture yourself relaxing on a beach in Hawaii, then also smell the salt spray of the ocean, feel the warmth of the sun on your skin, and hear the waves on the shore.

Many different mental-imagery techniques are advocated by different specialists. If you want help learning the process, you can find psychologists, hypnotherapists, counselors, pastors, and doctors who specialize in mental-imagery practices. But it's also something you can train yourself to do. Of course, whether you see a specialist or teach yourself, the day-to-day exercise of mental imagery is up to you. But the evidence is steadily mounting that this is one of the most effective healing techniques we know about.

Milk Thistle

Most people in the United States have an overabundance of toxins in their bodies, and their livers are overburdened.

Take a hard look at the toxins in our environment, and the reasons for these health problems are hardly a mystery. According to the US Environmental Protection Agency, an estimated 2.2 billion pounds of environmental toxins were released into the environment between the years 1987 and 1994—and that's just counting industrial waste. If you also add over-the-counter and prescription medications that we consume, along with the additives in many food products, our bodies are dealing with a staggering number of chemicals that we're not equipped to handle.

Hence, the need for milk thistle (*Silybum marianum*). At one time or another, nearly everyone can benefit from this potent herb that has the power to protect and revitalize the liver, our major organ of detoxification.

SIZING UP THISTLE

Milk thistle has been used for its medicinal properties for more than 2,000 years. Over the span of those two millennia, herbalists have come to admire the beneficial effect it can have on the liver and gallbladder. In Germany, where doctors routinely prescribe herbal treatments, it's one of the favored treatments for liver problems. That may be news

to many people in the United States, but even here, it's getting increasing attention among health practitioners and the general public.

The "milk" in the name refers to the white sap that leaves markings on the leaf—but it also has the prickly, spiny appearance of a typical thistle. It grows wild in parts of Europe, Russia, Asia, and North Africa. English colonists brought it to North America.

It's the milk thistle seeds that have medicinal properties. The seeds contain a group of flavonoids that are collectively known as silymarin. Within this group are silibin, silidianin, and silychristin.

A COMPLEX SUBJECT

All the flavonoids in the silymarin complex have the combined power of antioxidants that can prevent free-radical damage from the toxic substances that enter the liver. Silymarin has been found to be 10 times more potent an antioxidant than vitamin E, the single vitamin most renowned for its antioxidant power. It's silymarin that has the unique ability to slow down the rate at which the liver absorbs toxic substances.

Additionally, milk thistle is one of the few substances that can increase the glutathione content of the liver. This is important as glutathione, one of the body's most important antioxidants, is critical for efficient detoxification. Milk thistle also increases the levels of another potent antioxidant known as superoxide dismutase (SOD).

Milk thistle stimulates the regeneration of liver and kidney cells. This makes it valuable for conditions such as hepatitis, fatty liver, and cirrhosis of the liver. Treatment with milk thistle is essential for anyone who has been poisoned by eating the deathcap mushroom (*Amanita phalloides*). In 49 reported cases where people with deathcap poisoning received an injectable form of milk thistle (silibin), physicians reported full recovery—even when treatment came as late as 36 hours after the poisoning occurred.

Milk thistle extract also has been shown to stimulate kidney-cell regeneration.

Milk thistle is also one of the better herbs for stimulating the flow of bile, which is essential to good digestion. For this reason, it's helpful for improving the digestion of fats and also helpful in improving bowel elimination.

DOSAGE

I recommend one take a 200- to 250-mg capsule of a standardized extract (80% to 85% silymarin) three times daily. This is equivalent to 480 to 600 mg of silymarin daily.

If you suffer from digestive problems, then take it 15 minutes before or with a meal. A special form of milk thistle bound to phosphatidylcholine, known as Phytosome, has been shown to increase absorption. The dosage for the tincture form is 20 to 30 drops three times daily.

WHAT ARE THE SIDE EFFECTS?

The only major concern with milk thistle is that a very high dosage can cause loose stools due to increased bile flow. If you have a sensitive digestive system, start with one capsule and gradually increase the dosage. If you experience loose stools or diarrhea, then cut back on the dosage.

MILK THISTLE

RECOMMENDATIONS FROM THE NATURAL PHYSICIAN FOR . . .

🦢 ALCOHOL AND DRUG ADDICTION RECOVERY

When recovering from addiction, the liver is working overtime to cleanse the tissues and regenerate its own tissues—and milk thistle helps with both these processes. I also find that it helps to improve mood and energy levels, which are essential in the recovery process.

🦢 ALLERGIES

If you have chronic allergies, especially multiple-chemical sensitivity, you may respond well to milk thistle. It enables the liver to process environmental allergens more effectively.

🦢 CIRCULATION

Herbalists and naturopathic doctors historically used milk thistle for the treat-

ment of hemorrhoids and varicose veins. Blood is continually flowing through the liver, and if you have a "sluggish liver" that doesn't process blood very efficiently, it tends to back up in the rectum and in the veins of the legs. In theory, at least, improved liver function and metabolism also improve the rate at which venous blood returns to the heart, so there's a reduction of hemorrhoid and varicose vein problems.

I have not used milk thistle by itself for these conditions, but I do, at times, incorporate it into a comprehensive protocol.

🦢 CIRRHOSIS

Cirrhosis refers to severe liver damage. Liver tissue can be scarred by the effects

(continued)

of alcoholism, drugs, or liver infections such as hepatitis. When blood tests demonstrate elevated liver enzymes, it's an indication that liver scarring or cirrhosis has probably occurred.

In a well-controlled study of 105 people with cirrhosis, researchers compared those who took 420 mg of silymarin with those who (unknowingly, of course) were taking a placebo. After an average of 41 months, it was found those in the placebo group had almost twice the mortality rate as those in the silymarin group. While the researchers acknowledged that milk thistle does not cure cirrhosis, this study provided compelling evidence that silymarin can improve the survival rate of people with this disease.

CONSTIPATION

The stimulation of bile secretion by milk thistle improves elimination. For people who eat enough fiber, get enough fluids, yet still have sluggish bowel movements, I recommend milk thistle supplementation to help increase bile flow.

DEPRESSION

One of the traditional ways to help alleviate depression is by improving liver function—which makes sense, when you consider the liver influences the biochemistry of the body as it metabolizes hormones and neurotransmitters. In traditional Chinese and naturopathic medicine, physicians and acupuncturists regularly incorporate milk thistle with other therapies that are designed to improve liver function.

DETOXIFICATION

Everyone can benefit from detoxification. A month or two of milk thistle supplementation "does a liver good"—and, of course, the results are even better when supplementation is combined with a good program of diet and exercise. There are benefits for the immune system, as well, since it is not as burdened with toxins.

In fact, I'd be wary of any detoxification formula that does *not* contain milk thistle. It does such a superior job that most high-quality detoxification supplements will include it as one of the main ingredients in a formula.

DIABETES

A study published in *Phytotherapy Research* reported that milk thistle reduced blood-sugar levels in people with type 2 diabetes. Fifty-one diabetic men and women (ages 40 to 65) took either 200 mg of *silymarin* (milk thistle extract) three times daily before meals, or a placebo, along with their regular diabetes medication. After four months, the average fasting blood glucose level (the amount of sugar in the blood eight hours after your last meal) fell by 15% in the silymarin group, compared with an increase of 13% in the placebo group. Silymarin users also had significant reductions in blood lipid levels that are markers of cardiovascular diseases, including total cholesterol, LDL "bad" cholesterol, triglycerides, and liver enzyme levels. Participants taking placebos had no changes in blood lipid levels. No side effects were reported.

GALLSTONES

Since milk thistle improves bile flow, it decreases the saturation of cholesterol in bile. (High cholesterol saturation in bile is what leads to gallstone formation.) That

said, I'd advise caution for those diagnosed with moderate to large gallstones.
Use milk thistle or other bile-stimulating
herbs under the guidance of a healthcare
professional.

HEPATITIS (VIRAL)

Silymarin has been shown to be effective
in the treatment of acute and chronic
viral hepatitis. In a study of chronic viral
hepatitis, silymarin not only lowered elevated liver enzymes, but liver cell damage was also reversed as demonstrated
by a liver biopsy.

I have had numerous patients with hepatitis B and C who responded favorably to
milk thistle supplementation. I've found it
helps to normalize or lower elevated liver
enzymes. Just as important, the patient
looks better and feels more energetic.

With such encouraging results, I think
milk thistle treatment will become much
more widespread. It is estimated that 3.9
million Americans and up to 3% of the
world's population are infected with hepatitis C, and conventional medical treatments with alpha interferon are often
unsuccessful.

In addition to milk thistle, there are
other safe and effective supplements
that I consider better options for long-
term treatment of hepatitis C. Among
the others I recommend are licorice root,
reishi, and selenium.

HORMONE IMBALANCE

Although not thought of as a hormone-
balancing herb, milk thistle can give indirect benefits by improving liver function
and metabolism of hormones. This makes
it helpful for conditions such as PMS or
even prostate enlargement.

INDIGESTION

One of the many functions of bile is to
digest fats. When patients tell me they
get indigestion only after eating fried or
fatty foods, I know their bile production
is deficient. I recommend taking milk
thistle several times daily, with meals, for
a few months.

LIVER PROTECTION

I recommend milk thistle supplementation to those who require long-term use
of prescription medications. Such medications can damage the liver, and milk
thistle seems to provide some protection
from this side effect.

In a double-blind, placebo-controlled
study of 60 people, researchers found
that silymarin protected against the
long-term use of drugs used for mental
illness. The benefits came with doses of
800 mg per day of silymarin. There was
evidence that these doses reduced the
blood levels of MDA (malon-dialdehyde),
which is the "marker" that shows the liver
has been damaged by long-term use of
psychotropic drugs.

I also recommend milk thistle to anyone who's exposed to toxins in the work-
place. A classic example would be a
welder, who is exposed to smoke and
other contaminants.

People who can't quit smoking may
be able to limit the liver damage by supplementing with milk thistle.

I commonly recommend milk thistle
extract for those undergoing chemotherapy or radiation treatments for cancer.
Metabolic waste products are produced
by these treatments, and the liver must

(continued)

metabolize the waste before it can be safely eliminated.

✍ SKIN CONDITIONS
Chronic cases of skin rashes, acne, eczema, and even some cases of psoriasis greatly improve when people take milk thistle. While improving the liver's detoxification ability, milk thistle helps remove toxins from the bloodstream, which can, in turn, help prevent skin eruptions. This is why it is sometimes referred to as a "blood cleanser."

MSM

I remember one of my professors in medical school saying that if you can't relieve a patient's pain quickly, the patient will not be coming back to your office.

It's true.

No one wants to experience pain—and when you're afflicted with it, all you want is relief. Yet chronic, ongoing pain is a major problem for many people. It's been estimated that one-third of all Americans have to deal with it, often as the result of disease.

I can't claim that the supplement called MSM will help everyone. But I do know we're fortunate to have it around. It's one of those breakthrough supplements that, for many people, works very effectively to reduce pain and inflammation.

MSM is the abbreviation for methylsulfonylmethane. It was originally discovered when research was being done on DMSO—dimethylsulfoxide, a related compound that was known to alleviate pain. One problem with DMSO is that it has a very strong and disagreeable odor.

MSM doesn't have the odor problem and it seems to be just as effective as DMSO—or even more so. Most of the research on MSM has been done by Dr. Stanley Jacob of Oregon Health Sciences University in Portland and Dr. R. Lawrence of UCLA in California. Both have treated many thousands of people who are afflicted with painful conditions with DMSO and MSM.

In their book, *The Miracle of MSM*, they report that MSM can deliver numerous benefits, including:

- Pain relief
- Reduced inflammation
- Increased blood flow
- Control of overactive nerve impulses
- Reduced muscle spasms
- Softening of scar tissue

In addition, MSM has an antiparasitic effect—that is, it helps to resist the invasion of unfriendly parasites. It also has a normalizing effect on the immune system, which means it's useful in treating autoimmune diseases like rheumatoid arthritis and lupus.

MSM is a component of many foods, including green vegetables, and it's a natural part of living organisms, including plants and animals. As the name implies, MSM is a source of the mineral sulfur.

The body uses sulfur for many different functions. It is an integral component of amino acids, the building blocks of protein. Amino acids are essential in numerous biological functions, from building enzymes, hormones, and immune cells to building tissues like the skin and hair.

Sulfur is particularly important for the three sulfur-containing amino acids methionine, cysteine, and cystine. It's also an important mineral for detoxification. Food sources of sulfur include meat, eggs, poultry, fish, and milk. Plant foods that contain sulfur include garlic, onions, broccoli, cauliflower, cabbage, legumes, and sunflower seeds.

Pain Control Without Side Effects

MSM is not the only supplement that has powerful, direct, anti-inflammatory and pain-relieving effects. Others that I recommend are bromelain, turmeric, boswellia, and white willow. But I would have to say that none of these are as quick in their pain-relief action as MSM.

While some medications are just as fast-acting as MSM, most pain and anti-inflammatory medications cause serious side effects. For example, aspirin is one of the leading causes of ulcers, and can damage the kidneys and liver. It also accelerates cartilage destruction.

Other NSAIDs (nonsteroidal anti-inflammatories) are known for their side effects. Research has shown that corticosteroids such as prednisone have been associated with emotional disturbances, osteoporosis, liver and kidney toxicity, weight gain, and suppression of the immune system. Long-term use of such pharmaceuticals can sometimes be worse than the disease itself.

MSM provides relief of pain and inflammation without causing damage to the body. This has enabled many people to work with their doctors to reduce or totally eliminate the use of pain medications.

MEDIA TREATMENT OF MSM

On one edition of *Larry King Live*, the talk show host was interviewing a panel of experts about natural treatments of arthritis. One of those experts was Dr. R. Lawrence, who advocated the use of MSM.

When a caller asked if MSM could be used for a child who had rheumatoid arthritis, Dr. Lawrence replied that it would be fine to try the supplement with the child, but certainly less than an adult dose.

A medical expert from CNN, who was also on the panel, said he could not agree with this recommendation. According to the CNN expert, the use of MSM was not supported by enough studies. Then the CNN medical expert went on to say that the standard steroid treatment would be the best option for this child.

Unfortunately, the discussion moved on before it was thoroughly explored. But I found myself cringing at the thought that if the parents took this advice, their child would be deprived of a nontoxic supplement that millions of people have used—a supplement, further, that was recommended by medical doctors like Lawrence and Jacob, and which had no proven side effects. In exchange, the child would probably be given many doses of steroids, whose side effects are established to be profound and long-lasting.

A Case of Arthritis

Joe was one of the many patients whom I have treated for arthritis—and his story is a good example of what MSM can do.

When I first saw Joe, he could not walk

without limping. There was no mystery about the cause of his pain. For years, he'd endured osteoarthritis that was progressively getting worse, and in recent days, the arthritis in his left knee had flared up. The pain was almost unbearable.

Though only 55, Joe wondered how much longer he would be mobile—and he envisioned having a knee transplant in the not-too-distant future. He had been on a regimen of painkillers prescribed by his doctor, but he stopped taking them when he discovered they caused ulcers and other digestive problems.

When I told Joe that many of the medications he had used in the past may actually accelerate the degeneration of cartilage in his joints, he replied, "Oh great. Why didn't my doctor tell me that?"

Though not particularly overweight, Joe was a large man, weighing 210 pounds, and he needed a higher-than-usual dose. I started him on 4,000 mg of MSM, taken daily in tablet form, and also recommended topical applications of MSM as a cream. Within two days Joe noticed a dramatic reduction in his knee pain.

For the next two months, Joe continued with the high dosage of MSM, then—at my recommendation—reduced to a maintenance dosage of 2,000 mg daily. The pain, he reported, was "80% improved," and he said there was noticeable improvement in his mobility.

I later added glucosamine sulfate to his protocol to help rebuild his knee cartilage. Some researchers believe that MSM helps to rebuild cartilage, which is possible because it has chemical properties that help to incorporate fluid in the joint tissue. But I wanted to ensure that Joe was also taking a supplement that would help reverse the deterioration of knee cartilage.

DOSAGE

For preventative purposes, I recommend 1,000 to 2,000 mg daily. When using it for therapeutic purposes (e.g., pain relief) the dosage varies depending on body weight, sex, and individual need. Usually, somewhere between 3,000 to 8,000 mg is effective. I typically have patients start at 3,000 mg and gradually increase the dosage until they begin experiencing relief. Most find they begin to feel a lot better when the range is somewhere between 3,000 and 5,000 mg. MSM is available in capsule, tablet, crystal, lotion, cream, or gel. If you're taking the crystal form, be sure to add it to water for dilution, as the crystal is very bitter tasting. Or you can take it with juice to make it more palatable.

It is best to take MSM with meals to avoid the chances of stomach upset. I tell people to avoid taking MSM before bedtime because the supplement can keep you awake. Lignisul MSM is the brand of MSM used in clinical studies.

WHAT ARE THE SIDE EFFECTS?

Most people experience no side effects from MSM, though there have been some reports of digestive upset on high doses. A few people are sensitive to MSM, and have stomach upset, cramping, or diarrhea—so I recommend people start at a lower dosage and then gradually increase the dose every few days. This helps the body adjust to the MSM and reduces the chance of side effects.

If you do have an adverse reaction, you'll probably find that the symptoms go away if you reduce the dosage or—if necessary—stop taking MSM.

I am commonly asked if people allergic to

sulfites or sulfa antibiotics can use MSM. The answer is yes. Sulfites and sulfa antibiotics don't have the same chemical makeup of MSM, which contains the mineral sulfur.

For children, I start with a very small dose of MSM. The gel or cream is particularly good to use with children for joint or muscle injuries.

The authors of *The Miracle of MSM* state that the supplement is safe to take during pregnancy, but I concur with their recommendation that a pregnant woman should consult with a physician first before using it.

Although it has not been studied, the authors also caution against using MSM in conjunction with blood-thinning medications such as heparin. If you are on a blood-thinning medication, consult with your doctor before using MSM.

MSM

RECOMMENDATIONS FROM THE NATURAL PHYSICIAN FOR . . .

⁓ ALLERGIES AND ASTHMA

Some patients have reported that MSM calms down pollen allergies. I certainly see many patients in the San Diego area with these problems, reacting to year-round influxes of different kinds of pollen. I haven't found that MSM is a cure for these allergies, but it effectively reduces the symptoms.

With its natural, antiallergy powers, MSM is also useful for asthma, which is often triggered by pollen allergies. People with chronic sinusitis may be helped because this, too, is a condition often associated with allergies.

Dr. Jacob also reports that MSM has helped reduce food-allergy symptoms in the people he has treated.

⁓ ARTHRITIS

While MSM is particularly effective for treatment of osteoarthritis, it can also be used to take care of rheumatoid and other types of arthritis.

I find that most people with osteoarthritis who take MSM supplements notice a decrease in their pain within two to three weeks. Some report improvements within a day or two, especially when the cream or gel is applied to affected joints.

Small clinical studies have been done on MSM. In one of these, reported in the *International Journal of Anti-Aging Medicine*, 16 patients ranging in age from 55 to 78 were randomly assigned to two groups. All of the patients had degenerative joint disease and had chronic severe pain. When researchers compared the outcome of people taking 2,250 mg daily of MSM with those who were getting a placebo, it was found that those taking MSM reported more than 80% improvement after six weeks. By comparison, those taking the placebo had less than 20% improvement.

⁓ AUTOIMMUNE DISEASES

MSM can offer a lot of pain relief to people with autoimmune conditions such as rheumatoid arthritis, lupus, scleroderma, and interstitial cystitis. While the supplement is not a cure, it does help many people manage the inflammation caused

(continued)

by these diseases and allows them to lead more normal lifestyles.

The supplement works even better when you take the precaution of combining it with nutritional changes and some natural therapies like homeopathy or acupuncture. With MSM supplementation, many people have lowered anti-inflammatory or steroid medications. This of course needs to be done under the supervision of a doctor.

One of the outspoken fans of the supplement MSM was the late actor James Coburn, who had rheumatoid arthritis for many years. He claimed that MSM made a dramatic improvement in his arthritic pain.

❧ FIBROMYALGIA

We still don't know what causes the painful muscle condition known as fibromyalgia, but my own clinical experience has shown that natural therapies work quite well for most people. Ongoing treatment with natural therapies is a far better long-term approach than trying to deal with the problem by administering megadoses of drugs. MSM is one of the supplements I recommend to help reduce the muscle pain.

❧ HAIR AND NAIL HEALTH

People report that MSM improves the strength and sheen of their hair, and also helps to preserve harder, shinier nails. In one study, 21 patients were assessed by a certified cosmetologist under the direction of a medical doctor, then given supplements, and finally, assessed again at the conclusion of the study. Both the patients and investigators were unaware of whether the "supplements" they received were actually MSM or placebo pills with no active ingredients. Dosages

were 3,000 mg daily of Lignisul MSM.

Those given supplemented MSM, evaluated by the cosmetologist, had shown significant improvement in hair health while those on placebo showed few or no changes. Participants as well as the investigators could see clear improvements in those who used MSM.

A similar study, done with dosages of Lignisul MSM, showed similar improvements in nail health. The 11 patients in the study, the examining cosmetologist, and the investigators were unaware of which patients had received MSM and which got placebos. When the study was done, and nails were measured for length, thickness, luster, and general appearance, those receiving MSM had shown significant improvement. The overall improvement rate was near 80%.

❧ HEADACHES

MSM helps to reduce muscle spasm and tension, so it is helpful to prevent tension headaches.

❧ HEARTBURN

MSM helps to relieve heartburn in some people, though researchers haven't yet discovered why it helps. MSM is certainly a better option than antacid medications that might provide temporary relief but also reduce the important stomach acid needed to digest food.

❧ MUSCLE AND SPORTS INJURIES

MSM is one of the best sports-injury supplements to use. It is the arnica of nutritional supplements. Apply it as a cream to sprains, strains, or other athletic injuries. It helps to reduce muscular soreness after workouts and competitions.

Multivitamins

Years ago, patients would customarily ask me if a multivitamin was really necessary as part of their preventative health program. Today, after all the current studies that have been released regarding nutritional deficiencies, many people understand that they are at risk for such deficiencies. Regular use of multivitamin supplements is much more common.

For optimal health, people need to consume certain amounts of vitamins and minerals on a regular basis. The recommended daily allowance (RDA) has been used as a guideline since 1941. The goal of the RDA is to reduce the incidence of diseases that occur as a result of severe nutritional deficiencies.

A classic example is scurvy. Once the scourge of sailors and arctic explorers who had to go long periods without any sources of vitamin C (such as fresh fruits and vegetables), scurvy has virtually been eliminated because vitamin C is so easy to get under normal conditions. If you get at least the RDA of vitamin C, it's a virtual guarantee that you'll never have a problem with a vitamin-C-deficiency problem such as scurvy.

The criticism of the RDA by nutrition-oriented doctors like me is that it often does not promote optimal health or take into account the nutritional requirements of each individual. While the guidelines may be adequate for most people, some require higher daily amounts of certain vitamins and minerals than the amounts designated as "acceptable" in the RDA guidelines.

For example, people who have homocysteinuria (a genetic condition where the amino acid methionine is converted to the potentially toxic compound homocysteine), have a much greater risk of heart disease and stroke. These people need higher amounts of vitamins B6 and B12 and folic acid to prevent the buildup of this toxic metabolite. Following the RDA guidelines will not work for most people with this condition.

OTHER FACTORS

Environment is a factor as well. People regularly exposed to environmental toxins require antioxidants such as vitamin C at higher levels than specified by the RDA guidelines. Athletes, or those with physically demanding jobs, are others who often require higher amounts of many vitamins and minerals.

It is also becoming better understood how certain pharmaceutical medications deplete vitamins and minerals from the body. For example, the birth-control pill and various types of antibiotics deplete vitamins B6 and B12 and folic acid. Cholesterol-lowering drugs such as Lipitor deplete CoQ10.

AND ONE TO GROW ON

All pregnant women should take prenatal vitamins; most obstetricians recommend them. They not only keep the pregnant woman healthier and prevent conditions such as anemia, but they could have lasting benefits for the baby as well. It is very important that women of childbearing age take a multivitamin before becoming pregnant as folic acid and B12 help prevent birth defects.

Most children should be on a full-spectrum multivitamin. A wide variety of vitamins and minerals are required for growth and development. It makes more sense to prevent a nutrition-related disease than to treat one. In one study, 60 children ages 12 to 13 were examined for the effect of a multivitamin on intelligence. Each child was given either a multivitamin or placebo for eight months. Only the group receiving a multivitamin showed improvement in non-verbal intelligence.

GOOD HEALTH INSURANCE

I like the analogy of comparing a multivitamin to an insurance policy. Seeing that vitamins and minerals are required for life, and that when used properly they do not pose toxic side effects, it makes sense to take one.

One of the problems with multivitamins is that people don't always feel a difference when taking them. In other words, some multivitamin users do not feel a tremendous surge in energy, or improvement in mood or concentration. This, of course, depends on the existing health of the person and the potency and quality of the multivitamin.

Remember that most chronic diseases take years to develop. Long-term nutritional deficiencies are often at the root of these chronic maladies.

The immune system requires many vitamins and minerals to function optimally. This is especially true in the elderly. One study examined the effect of a multivitamin on the immune function in the elderly. Those who received the multivitamin supplement had significantly fewer infections compared with those who received placebo.

Another study found that a multivitamin and trace element supplement resulted in stronger immune cell markers, compared with those who took placebos, who showed a reduction in immune-cell parameters. Also routinely taking a multivitamin has been shown to reduce inflammation; improve mood; prevent birth defects; reduce the risk for heart disease, cataracts, and cognitive decline; and slow age-related DNA damage.

Many of my patients who have no major illnesses often notice improvements such as healthier hair and nails, better skin health,

and fewer cravings for sweets and other junk foods. However, I do not find, nor do I expect, that multivitamins by themselves make a major noticeable impact on existing disease. For example, it is rare to see a patient with arthritis who starts taking a multivitamin and notices that his arthritic pain dramatically improves.

DOSAGE

The term "multivitamin" refers to a supplement that contains the essential vitamins and minerals. Look for a formula that contains a wide blend of vitamins and minerals. Ask your natural healthcare provider or pharmacist to recommend a high-quality product. There are a wide range of products on the market, varying in quality and potency. Following is an example of an adult full-spectrum multivitamin and mineral formula:

VITAMINS

Vitamin A: 1,000 to 5,000 IU

Beta carotene: 2,500 to 25,000 IU (mixed carotenoid complex is even better)

Vitamin D: 400 IU to 1000 IU

Vitamin E (d-alpha tocopherol): 200 to 400 IU (mixed tocopherols is better)

Vitamin K: 65 to 200 mcg

Vitamin C: 100 to 1,000 mg

Vitamin B1(thiamin): 10 to 100 mg

Vitamin B2 (riboflavin): 10 to 50 mg

Vitamin B3 (niacin): 10 to 100 mg

Niacinamide: 10 to 50 mg

Vitamin B5 (pantothenic acid): 25 to 100 mg

Vitamin B6 (pyridoxine): 25 to 100 mg

Folic acid: 400 to 800 mcg

Vitamin B12: 200 to 400 mcg

Choline: 10 to 100 mg

Inositol: 10 to 100 mg

MINERALS

Calcium: 250 to 1,000 mg

Magnesium: 250 to 500 mg

Chromium: 200 to 400 mcg

Copper: 1 to 2 mg

Manganese: 5 to 15 mg

Molybdenum: 10 to 25 mcg

Selenium: 200 mcg

Boron: 1 to 3 mg (not allowed in Canadian formulations)

Silica: 1 to 20 mg

Vanadium: 50 to 100 mcg

Zinc: 15 to 30 mg

I prefer capsules and powders to tablets for improved absorption, although some tablets are absorbed well (depending on the brand). Most high-potency multivitamins require 2 to 6 capsules or 2 to 4 tablets daily. Beyond obtaining a high-quality multivitamin, the most important consideration is consistency in taking it.

WHAT ARE THE SIDE EFFECTS?

Some people may experience digestive upset. This can be avoided by taking the supplement with meals and by using a high-quality product. Also, users can occasionally be sensitive to an ingredient in the multivitamin. This is more of a risk with cheap brands that use fillers, colorings, or other added chemicals. Choose a hypoallergenic multivitamin formula.

I recommend that you avoid a multivitamin that contains iron, unless your doctor has determined that you have iron-deficiency anemia. Iron supplements are suspect in causing oxidative damage when used by those who do not have an iron deficiency.

Pregnant women should not take vitamin A in dosages above 2,500 to 5,000 IU.

Occasionally, I have a patient who cannot tolerate multivitamins. For these patients I either recommend starting with a multivitamin that comes in lower dosages (for example, a formula where four capsules equals the daily dosage, and have the patient start with one capsule daily and slowly increase their dosage), or using whole food supplements.

Some people's livers cannot handle higher dosages of vitamins and minerals, and they may require a detoxification program first before using a multivitamin.

N-acetylcysteine

"I have had bronchitis for a week now and I nearly gag on all the mucus I cough up. Do you think I need antibiotics?" asked Dean, a computer technician.

"No, it's most likely a viral infection. What we will do is put you on some N-acetylcisteine (NAC) both as a supplement and as an inhalation treatment. That will clear you up," I replied. Sure enough over the next two days Dean began doing much better.

Over the years I have increasingly relied upon NAC to help my patients with a variety of health problems. NAC is an amino acid–like substance derived from the amino acid L-cysteine. NAC has many unique functions in the body. First it is a powerful antioxidant since it increases levels of glutathione. Glutathione is regarded by many as the master antioxidant in the body. Yet as a supplement glutathione does not appear to be very stable and may not have much benefit. Also, NAC supports kidney and liver detoxification. This mechanism com-

bined with its antioxidant benefit makes it useful in treating toxin exposure. It's even used in the intravenous form in hospitals to treat certain types of acute drug toxicities such as acetaminophen overdose. NAC also reduces excessive inflammatory responses by the immune system. Lastly, NAC is a mucus thinner and has long been used in conventional medicine for this benefit.

Dosage

For cold and flu prevention, I recommend 600 mg twice daily. For general health prevention take 300 to 600 mg daily. For the treatment of bronchitis, I typically prescribe 2,400 to 3,000 mg daily.

What Are the Side Effects?

I do not find side effects to be very common. Higher dosages may cause digestive upset. NAC contains the mineral sulphur, which causes a foul odor (rotten egg type smell) in the supplement form.

N-ACETYLCYSTEINE
RECOMMENDATIONS FROM THE NATURAL PHYSICIAN FOR . . .

ACETAMINOPHEN POISONING
NAC is used in hospital settings both orally and intravenously to treat acetaminophen overdose and reduces the

mortality rate. Since acetaminophen, a common over-the-counter nonsteroidal anti-inflammatory drug, depletes the body's glutathione level, it is prudent to supplement NAC when using acetamino-phen for an extended time period.

CHRONIC KIDNEY DISEASE

Oral NAC has been shown to reduce the risk of heart attack and stroke for those receiving dialysis for end-stage kidney disease, a result published in *Circulation*. The dose used in the study was 600 mg twice daily.

COLORECTAL CANCER

A study where participants taking 800 mg of NAC daily for 12 weeks showed reduced proliferation of colon polyps compared to those taking placebo.

CONTRAST DYE-INDUCED KIDNEY DAMAGE

Contrast dyes such as gadolinium are com-monly used with magnetic resonance imag-ing (MRI) and computerized tomography (CT) testing. At the University of Michigan researchers evaluated the available body of research on how best to shield kidneys from iodinated contrast agent–induced damage. They studied the results of 41 randomized controlled trials that involved data on the protective effects of agents administered to prevent kidney damage after coronary angiograms. They found that NAC was an inexpensive nutrient that in those with exist-ing compromised kidney function could help prevent kidney damage from contrast dyes. These results were published in the February 19, 2008, issue of *Annals of Internal Medicine*.

EPILEPSY

A small study found oral NAC to be help-ful with myoclonus epilepsy, the brief, involuntary twitching of muscles.

FLU PREVENTION

One cost-effective way to prevent the flu is supplementing NAC. Italian researchers found that people taking 600 mg twice daily developed few if any flu symptoms even though blood tests confirmed infec-tion. At the first sign of symptoms, increase your intake to 2,000 to 3,000 mg daily for two to three days. If you are fighting a full-fledged cold or flu, maintain this higher dose for a week.

HOMOCYSTEINE

NAC is one of the supplements that can reduce blood levels of homocysteine, an amino acid that increases the risk of heart disease, rheumatoid arthritis, and Alzheimer's disease. Other nutrients that reduce homocysteine include folic acid, vitamins B6 and B12, and trimethylglycine.

RESPIRATORY TRACT INFECTIONS

NAC is used by conventional physicians both orally and as an inhalation treat-ment to treat bronchitis, chronic obstruc-tive pulmonary disease (COPD), cystic fibrosis, and other respiratory conditions where mucus thinning is required. I have found it works well orally and as an inha-lation treatment. I have also had good results combining NAC with glutathione and licorice extract as an inhalation ther-apy for asthma, bronchitis, and emphy-sema. A study published in *Respiratory* demonstrated that in people with mod-erate to severe COPD, 600 mg daily of NAC combined with standard therapy reduced the number of flare-ups by 41%. Also, oral doses between 400 to 1,200 mg of NAC have been shown in studies to reduce exacerbations in those with chronic bronchitis.

Nettle

"Is there something you can recommend for my mother?" Todd asked. "She has terrible hay fever symptoms this spring."

Though Todd was a long-term patient of mine, I had never met his mother. Nevertheless, he couldn't go wrong with a remedy that used to be part of every home herb garden.

"Stinging nettles," I suggested.

Todd looked at me as if I'd just offered to poison his mother.

"Don't worry," I assured him. "When you take these nettles in the supplement form, they don't really sting. You can pick them up from the health-food store. Have her start with two capsules taken three times daily."

A few weeks later, when I saw Todd again, I asked how his mother was doing with her hay fever.

"She noticed an improvement in three days," Todd said. In fact, his mother had asked him to pick up another bottle of nettles, to make sure she didn't miss a single dose. "She doesn't want to run the risk of her allergies coming back," he told me.

"Great. At some point she can probably cut down the dose and still get the same benefit," I replied.

UNSTUNG HERO

Though stinging nettle (*Urtica dioica*) is a threatening-looking plant, the roots and leaves have the components of a remarkably effective herbal medicine. Curiously, each part of the plant has different medicinal uses. The leaf is used for allergies. A rich source of minerals, it also serves as a mild diuretic, and it's often recommended for arthritis. The root has become popular for the treatment of prostate enlargement.

The Latin name of *Urtica* means "to sting." The plant does, indeed, have small fibers or spines that sting the skin, and it can be seriously irritating. But as I explained to Todd, the herbal supplement has no such properties at all.

There are many different species of nettles, but most herbalists use *Urtica dioica*. (You should find the species name on the label of any supplement package you buy.) Though it's native to Europe, similar species grow in North America. When I was attending National College of Naturopathic Medicine in Portland, Oregon, students regularly plucked leaves from some of the nettles growing around the campus courtyard.

Nettle has been used as a medicinal food for many centuries. It's often taken in Europe for arthritis, kidney disease, anemia, and skin ailments. Native American women, when pregnant, boiled nettles to make a nutritive tonic that ensured the baby's health and was also reputed to ease labor. The tradition of giving nettle tonic during pregnancy continues to this day: Naturopathic obstetricians often recommend it to pregnant women to prevent anemia and fatigue.

Herbalists and naturopathic physicians often recommend nettle leaves as an essential part of any detoxification program. In fact, it was so often given to patients in springtime that it became known, literally, as a "spring tonic." Part of this "tonic" effect may be the natural diuretic action, which removes toxins through the kidneys.

GOOD GREENS

Herbalists recommend the young greens rather than mature plants. Naturopathic physician Sharol Tilgner has specified that nettle should never be harvested after the flowers appear as it may cause urinary tract irritation.

Young nettles can be prepared like a vegetable. When steamed or simmered in water, nettle looks like spinach, and the taste is similar. If you like the taste, you can use them in soups or salads.

Nettle has many active or beneficial constituents including lignans, sterols (including beta sitosterol), polysaccharides, histamine, acetylcholine, potassium, calcium, magnesium, carotenoids, iron, vitamin C, and silicic acid. The plant is also a good source of chlorophyll.

Most of the vitamins and minerals are located in the leaves, which also harbor the compounds that help prevent allergies. Lignans and sterols are found in the root. These are the compounds that seem to be so important in relieving the symptoms of an enlarged prostate.

DOSAGE

◦ *Nettle Leaf*

I recommend two capsules of 600 mg taken two or three times daily. The freeze-dried capsules are best.

Nettle-leaf tincture is also available. Take 30 drops or 0.5 mL two or three times daily.

Alternatively, you can drink two or three cups of nettle leaf tea.

◦ *Nettle Root*

For capsules, try to get a total of 320 to 1,200 mg daily.

(**NOTE:** Nettle root is often combined in formulas containing saw palmetto that are sold in capsule form.)

The recommended dose of nettle root tincture is 0.5 mL (30 drops) two to three times daily.

If you're taking nettle root tea, drink two to three cups daily.

WHAT ARE THE SIDE EFFECTS?

Nettle is very well tolerated. Occasionally, people may experience digestive upset, which may be resolved if the nettle is taken with a meal.

If you're on diuretic medications, however, you should avoid taking the leaf form of nettle. Excessively large dosages should be avoided during pregnancy. The maximum dosage recommended during pregnancy is 2 to 4 capsules daily or 20 drops of the tincture twice daily, taken with guidance from your doctor.

NETTLE

RECOMMENDATIONS FROM THE NATURAL PHYSICIAN FOR . . .

◦ ANEMIA

Nettle is one of the most widely used herbs for the treatment of anemia. It is often referred to as a "blood builder" as it contains iron and many other minerals.

It can be used safely by anyone who is susceptible to anemia, including women who have heavy menstrual flow. Pregnant women can safely take 600 to

1,200 mg daily of nettle leaf. It combines well with the herb yellow dock, which improves iron absorption.

◦ ARTHRITIS

Nettle leaf has often been used as an external and internal treatment for rheumatoid

(continued)

arthritis and osteoarthritis. It has also been popular for relieving tendonitis and sciatic pain. In one clinical study, researchers found that the combination of nettle leaf and a pharmaceutical anti-inflammatory (diclofenac) was as effective at relieving the pain of arthritis as a full dose of the drug. Though the drug diclofenac is considered ineffective at dosages below 75 mg per day, many participants in the study were getting good results with just 50 mg of diclofenac when the drug was combined with stewed nettles. This is a good indication that nettle has a significant effect on pain relief. Other studies have shown that nettle blocks the release of inflammatory chemicals.

I generally find that long-term use of nettle works well for chronic conditions such as arthritis. I also find it works best in formulas that contain other effective supplements for arthritis.

❧ EDEMA

Since the herb has a mild diuretic effect, it can be beneficial if you have water retention or swelling—such as edema from pregnancy or varicose veins. It should not, however, be combined with diuretic drugs.

❧ GOUT

Nettle leaf is one of the herbs that has been used by European doctors to reduce uric acid buildup associated with gout. It can be given every two hours to relieve acute gout attacks and works well when taken on a long-term basis to prevent uric acid buildup. Combined with this treatment, I also recommend a plant-based diet—and no alcoholic drinks—for anyone who is prone to gout.

Historically, a related species of nettles, *Urtica urens*, was commonly used for the treatment of gout. In the early part of the twentieth century, Dr. Burnett of London was so successful treating gout with nettle that he drew patients from the farthest reaches of the United Kingdom, eventually earning the nickname "Dr. Urtica."

❧ HAIR PROBLEMS

Nettle has been used historically for hair loss and to improve hair health. This has not been scientifically studied, but my guess is that the minerals, particularly silica, are responsible for this effect.

Hair loss can be a symptom of anemia, so those who are anemic and take nettle leaf may indirectly notice hair improvement.

❧ HAY FEVER

When someone asks what one herb I consider most effective for hay fever, my immediate response is nettles. I find about 50% of people who use freeze-dried nettles for hay fever notice a substantial improvement. Take 2 capsules three times daily until the symptoms are under control.

After a week or two you may be able to reduce the amount by half and continue taking it as a maintenance dosage. Again, side effects are not an issue—which makes nettle very attractive for people who suffer drowsiness and other side effects from prescription antihistamine medications.

In a randomized, double-blind study, scientists looked into the effects of freeze-dried nettles on people who had hay fever ("allergic rhinitis"). It was found that after one week of use, 58% of the participants were helped by this herbal extract.

❧ PREGNANCY

There are few herbs I recommend women use during pregnancy. Nettle leaf is one of them. It helps to prevent and treat anemia. In fact, midwives and naturopathic obstetricians routinely recommend nettle during pregnancy as a nutritive herb. It also helps some women with the overwhelming fatigue that can accompany pregnancy. It can also help to alleviate muscle cramps. (In all likelihood, this benefit comes from the many minerals in nettle, including calcium, magnesium, and potassium.) It can also help relieve constipation associated with pregnancy.

As mentioned earlier, very high dosages are not recommended during pregnancy—so don't exceed 2 to 4 capsules daily (600 to 1,200 mg) or 20 drops of the tincture twice daily, and only with the consent of your doctor.

❧ PROSTATE ENLARGEMENT

Based on published clinical studies, nettle root has become very popular for the treatment of benign prostatic hyperplasia (BPH). Approximately 50% of men over the age of 50—and close to 90% of men in their 80s—have BPH. Common symptoms of prostate enlargement include an increasing need to urinate frequently, especially at night, and reduced force of the urinary stream.

Researchers found that men with BPH could reduce the symptoms of urinary frequency and nighttime urination in the span of 10 weeks if they took nettle. In one study, for instance, more than three-quarters of the men who took nettle reported "good" or "very good" results.

Nettle root is often used in formulas that contain other effective herbs for the prostate such as saw palmetto and *Pygeum africanum.* I typically recommend that it be used this way to make the most of synergistic effects among these herbs.

There have been some positive studies that show the combination of saw palmetto and nettle root works well for the treatment of prostate enlargement. One randomized, double-blind study found the combination of nettle root and saw palmetto worked as effectively as the pharmaceutical drug finasteride, which is commonly used to reduce the symptoms of BPH. Participants either took the combination of 240 mg of nettle root with 320 mg of saw palmetto extract—or took 5 mg of finasteride daily for 48 weeks. (None of the men knew whether they were getting the herbs or the drug.) Researchers noted the herbal combination had fewer side effects than were experienced by men taking the pharmaceutical drug.

Another landmark study showed that the combination of saw palmetto and nettle root worked to shrink enlarged prostate tissue. This has been the first study to confirm that these two common herbs can have such an effect.

When men are using herbs like nettle root or saw palmetto, I always recommend that they continue on regular dosages for at least six to eight weeks. It takes at least that long to see whether these herbs are having a positive effect.

Nux Vomica

Nux vomica is a homeopathic remedy required by tens of thousands of people every day in the United States. This remarkable remedy is the diluted extract of poison-nut. While the nut is very toxic and causes a multitude of symptoms that range from vomiting, cramps, and nerve reactions, the homeopathic remedy is completely safe. It's an extremely diluted form of poison-nut extract—so diluted, that only the vibrational frequency of the plant remains. No material is left in it. In this form, the extract from the nut can treat numerous symptoms, especially those related to intestinal problems or insomnia.

Miles, a 41-year-old patient of mine, suffered both from chronic heartburn and from insomnia. Before coming to me he had been through the full gamut of conventional therapies—including heartburn medications and a whole range of sleep medicines. He had even been to a world-renowned sleep clinic where he was treated for insomnia, but with no improvement.

Miles fit the profile of what homeopathic physicians call a "nux vomica personality." Friendly and outgoing, he was also a hard-driving businessperson, who owned two successful businesses and liked to be very involved. He was also a beer drinker—another nux vomica trait. Emotionally, he tended to get irritable and impatient, and he could be easily angered.

For Miles, nux vomica provided an incredible response. When he started taking it, the incidents of heartburn greatly decreased in frequency and intensity. Insomnia ceased to become a problem. He told me he could finally get a sound night's sleep.

A QUESTION OF DIGESTION

Nux vomica has a specific action on the digestive system. It is one of the best remedies for heartburn, ulcers, cramps, hiccups, food poisoning, and constipation. It also has a detoxifying effect on the liver.

There are also beneficial effects on the nervous system. Nux vomica has a relaxing and calming effect, so it helps reduce the effects of stress, including muscle spasms and cramps.

In addition, nux vomica is commonly used to cure hangovers. Many years ago, after a friend's wedding, I recall giving nux vomica to quite a few members of the wedding party. Fifteen minutes after taking the remedy, people were coming to me with the question, "What *was* that remedy?" In that very short time, they were already feeling better.

In homeopathic circles, nux vomica simply means "no vomit."

DOSAGE

For acute relief of symptoms, I recommend a 30C potency to be taken every 15 to 30 minutes. (If 30C is not available, you can use other potencies at the same interval.) For chronic health problems, I recommend a dose twice daily for two weeks and then as needed.

WHAT ARE THE SIDE EFFECTS?

I have never seen side effects with this remedy.

NUX VOMICA

RECOMMENDATIONS FROM THE NATURAL PHYSICIAN FOR . . .

ALCOHOLISM

Nux vomica helps reduce the craving for alcohol and facilitate the recovery process. It also helps recovering addicts to detoxify more effectively.

ALLERGIES

This remedy is effective with hay fever and other inhalant allergies. If you sneeze frequently and have a runny nose when you wake in the morning, nux vomica is the remedy of choice.

BACK PAIN

Many practitioners are not aware that nux vomica helps to relieve back pain. While it is particularly effective if taken just before you go to bed, it can also help relieve back spasms and cramps during the day.

BLADDER INFECTION

Consider nux vomica for the relief of bladder symptoms when you have a constant urge to urinate. If you find that hot baths help relieve the pain, then nux vomica can probably provide further relief.

CHEMOTHERAPY

Nux vomica helps people undergoing chemotherapy to experience fewer symptoms of nausea, vomiting, and constipation. It is the second most-common remedy that I prescribe to prevent or treat chemotherapy side effects. (The other remedy I prescribe is cadmium sulph.)

COLIC

Nux vomica is an excellent remedy for colic symptoms. If you have a baby who is typically constipated, irritable, and arches the back during bouts of colic, the infant is a good candidate for nux vomica. It is not uncommon for the infant to improve within seconds or minutes after receiving the remedy.

COLITIS

This remedy provides relief for people suffering from digestive conditions such as ulcerative colitis, Crohn's disease, and irritable bowel syndrome (IBS). It helps prevent and relieve symptoms of abdominal cramps that may be brought on from feelings of anger, poor food choices, or stress. When tight clothes around the waist make the symptoms worse—and warm applications and warm drinks help provide relief—nux vomica is an excellent remedy as well.

CONSTIPATION

Nux vomica is the most common homeopathic remedy for constipation. Even if you're getting plenty of fiber and water in your diet, nux vomica can provide further relief. It's the remedy to use when constipation occurs while traveling.

FLU

Nux vomica leads to faster recovery from the flu, particularly if you're feeling very chilled, nauseated, and achy.

HANGOVER

For anyone who's had a few too many drinks, nux vomica can alleviate symptoms

(continued)

of nausea, vomiting, fatigue, headache, and cramps. (Of course, the surest prevention is to drink in moderation or not at all.)

INSOMNIA

Nux vomica actually treats the biochemical imbalances that lead to insomnia. If you've had trouble sleeping because you've been thinking about work, nux vomica is particularly effective. Another "nux vomica symptom" is waking between 3 a.m. and 4 a.m.

ULCER

I have had fantastic results in treating ulcers with this remedy. Patti, a 42-year-old patient of mine in Canada, exemplified the kind of success that someone can have with this remedy. She actually had to visit the emergency room because of extreme pain from stomach ulcers—and when she called me afterward, she was still in pain.

After she had described her symptoms, she tried one kind of homeopathic remedy, then I switched her to nux vomica, which brought her relief the same day. Over the next two weeks, the nux vomica completely healed her ulcer.

Onion

Often, practitioners of natural medicine focus on looking for the "new." It's exciting to discover a potent healing supplement that is being researched or developed for the first time—or the newly discovered healing power of some food.

However, sometimes old news is the best news. There are certain foods that have been around for centuries. Their potent medicinal effects are no secret; their story deserves to be told again.

Such is the case with the lowly onion (*Allium sativum*).

Most cultures around the world use onions as a seasoning that lends pungency to many dishes. It has also been a medicine for many centuries, particularly in Chinese and Ayurvedic medicines. But whether you consume onion for its flavor or value its medicinal properties, there's no question that you get hearty benefits from the allium every time you take a bite.

During the Civil War, General Ulysses S. Grant requested and received a shipment of onions to treat the soldiers who had dysentery.

Just a generation ago, it was common for people to make an onion poultice to help cure sore throats—a practice that proved its usefulness from the wild frontier to the urban landscapes of America.

Today, the scientists who have explored the components of the common onion have discovered that it does, indeed, possess medicinal properties that are very similar to those of garlic. It has antimicrobial qualities, reduces blood pressure and elevated cholesterol, and helps lower elevated blood-sugar levels.

Onions contain dozens of powerful medicinal ingredients, including:

- Sulfur compounds called thiosulfinates, which are thought to have strong anti-inflammatory effects and help with detoxification
- Flavonoids
- Phenolic acids, sterols, pectin, and volatile oils
- Vitamin C

You don't need to restrict your appetite to one particular type of onion, either. Other members of the allium family are beneficial, too. Scallions—often called spring or green onions—contain even more vitamin C than white or yellow onions. The green kind are also high in folate, which is one of the essential nutrients. The small onions called shallots are very rich in vitamin A as well.

Onions have been shown to have strong antioxidant effects. They are a good source of the flavonoid quercetin, which is valued as a potent antioxidant. It is estimated that a medium-size onion contains as much as 50 mg of quercetin. It is possible to get therapeutic amounts of this antioxidant if you eat onions every day.

DOSAGE

Choose firm, small-necked onions with brittle outer leaves. Avoid dark-spotted or sprouting bulbs. To maintain good health, try to eat the equivalent of ½ to 1 cup of chopped onions every day.

Raw onions contain higher amounts of the disease-fighting chemicals, but cooked onions are also healthful.

WHAT ARE THE SIDE EFFECTS?

Aside from getting burning, watering eyes when you chop them, some people experience digestive upset and heartburn from onions. If you have asthma, be wary of pickled onions, which may contain sulfites that can trigger asthma attacks.

Another side effect is "onion breath." Eating a sprig of parsley with your meal can help prevent bad breath that's associated with eating onions.

ONION

RECOMMENDATIONS FROM THE NATURAL PHYSICIAN FOR . . .

ᗯ ASTHMA

Onions have been traditionally used for the treatment of asthma. Animal studies have shown that phytochemicals within onions, such as thiosulfinates and cepaenes, inhibit inflammatory compounds associated with inducing asthma.

Nutrition-oriented doctors commonly prescribe high dosages of supplemental quercetin (1,500 to 3,000 mg) to help prevent asthma. As I've mentioned, onion is a natural source of quercetin. If you need a large dose, onions can't compete with a supplement (you'd have to eat too many), but for anyone with asthma, it's helpful to get as much quercetin as possible in your diet.

ᗯ CANCER

A French study of 345 women found that risk of breast cancer decreased as consumption of fiber, garlic, and onions increased.

A study examined the relationship between allium vegetable intake (includ-

ing onion), and cancer of the esophagus and stomach in Yangzhong City, one of the highest-risk areas for these cancers in Jiangsu Province, China. The researchers suggested that allium vegetables, like raw vegetables, may have an important protecting effect not only against stomach cancer, but also against esophageal cancer.

Quercetin, which appears to be one of the key active substances in onions, has been shown to protect against colon cancer in studies involving animals.

ᗯ CHOLESTEROL AND HIGH BLOOD PRESSURE

In clinical studies, researchers have found that onions decrease cholesterol and triglyceride levels. If you eat lots of onions, you can also help lower your blood pressure. In fact, if I see anyone with these conditions, I encourage the person to incorporate onions into his or her daily diet on a long-term basis. One medium onion a day—raw or cooked—can be helpful. You can't expect immediate improvements, of course, but over time, the ingredients in onions give you cumulative benefits.

❧ DIABETES

Studies have shown that onion reduces elevated blood-sugar levels. Along with garlic, onions are an excellent food for people with this condition to consume on a regular basis.

If you have diabetes, you should check with your doctor before introducing quantities of onion or making any changes in your diet.

❧ IMMUNITY

Onion is helpful in protecting against bacterial, fungal, and worm infections. It is excellent to include in a soup or broth for sore throats and upper respiratory tract infections.

Oregano

One of the great medicinal herbs is oregano (*Origanum vulgare*), a member of the mint family. It has a rich history in Mediterranean and French cuisine. It contains volatile oils that contribute to its great antimicrobial effect. Two of the well-researched oils are known as thymol and carvacrol. The essential oils of oregano have been shown to have a broad action against various bacterial and fungal organisms.

Oregano has also been shown by the US Department of Agriculture to have a very high antioxidant level. As does rosemary, oregano contains a phytochemical known as rosmarinic acid, which provides potent antioxidant power.

DOSAGE

As a food, sprinkling chopped oregano on salads and other foods is a healthy addition.

The concentration of oregano products varies greatly. A typical capsule dosage is 200 to 500 mg taken three times daily. The liquid form is commonly available, and 5 to 10 drops is an average dose. Follow the dosage recommendations on the label.

WHAT ARE THE SIDE EFFECTS?

Some oregano supplements are very concentrated, particularly the liquid form. Digestive distress may occur with too high a dose. This may be prevented by taking oregano supplements with a meal. People with ulcers or reflux may notice irritation from oregano supplements and when using oregano should choose the capsule form. Pregnant or nursing women should avoid supplements of oregano. Caution should be used when applying oregano liquid topically as it can be irritating. Keep oregano oil away from the eyes.

OREGANO
RECOMMENDATIONS FROM THE NATURAL PHYSICIAN FOR . . .

ATHLETE'S FOOT

Oregano oil can be diluted and applied topically to athlete's foot, which is a fungal infection. Taking oregano internally is also a good idea for those prone to this condition.

CANDIDA

The overgrowth of the fungal organism *Candida albicans*, as well as other fungal organisms, can often be treated very effectively by the internal use of oregano supplements. The repeated use of antibiotics, chlorine-rich tap water, stress, and high sugar diets make many people susceptible to fungal overgrowth in the digestive tract. Oregano oil and other antifungal antimicrobials are my first choice before using antifungal medications. Women prone to reoccurring vaginal yeast infections can benefit from taking oregano supplements internally as well.

RESPIRATORY TRACT INFECTIONS

I prescribe oregano oil to treat throat and lung infections since it has such a diverse antimicrobial effect. The liquid form is the preferred choice for these infections because it comes in touch with the mucus membranes that line the respiratory tract. Oregano nasal sprays are also available in health-food stores and are very effective for the treatment of acute and chronic sinusitis. It is interesting to note that studies by Mayo Clinic researchers have demonstrated that a high percent of chronic sinus infections are due to fungal infection.

PARASITES

Oregano oil is effective for treating a variety of parasite infections, including *Blastocystis hominis*, *Entamoeba hartmanni*, and *Endolimax nana*.

Passionflower

"I have had insomnia for a few months now. At least a couple nights a week, I can't even fall asleep."

Tammy was a 40-year-old mother of three. All of her children were beyond the "crying baby" stage, but even so, she often found herself lying awake at night. For a while, she had tried the natural sleep aid valerian—but she didn't like it. "I felt groggy in the morning, like I was hung over," she said. So, she had come to me to ask for something that wouldn't have any side effects. "Is there anything else you'd recommend?" she asked.

"Let's start with passionflower," I suggested. "It is a gentle herb that has been used for centuries to help relieve insomnia."

Four weeks later Tammy reported that the passionflower had worked like a charm. She said, "Those nights I can't fall asleep I take the passionflower as you told me to, and within 30 minutes I am fast asleep. I also feel perfectly fine when I wake up in the morning."

THE REST IS HISTORY

Passionflower (*Passiflora incarnata*) was used by Spanish explorers and missionaries who visited Peru in the early 17th century. They were intrigued by the plant's resemblance to a crown of thorns on top of a cross—suggesting volumes of religious meaning—and in 1605, one intrepid missionary sent samples of the symbolic flower to Pope Paul V. Along with a name that suggested "Christ's passion," the passionflower was also referred to as the Holy Trinity flower and passion-vine.

A climbing vine that can grow upward of 28 feet, passionflower grows wild in the southern United States as well as South America. It's also found in the East Indies and in parts of Europe. Historically, Native Americans ate the leaves and fruit of the passionflower and used various parts of the plant to cure ailments. Today, all parts of the plant—root, leaf, stem, and fruit—are used medicinally, although it's mainly the flower parts that are included in capsules, teas, and tinctures.

Researchers believe that certain flavonoids are responsible for the nerve-relaxing properties of passionflower, although other constituents are likely involved as well.

DOSAGE

I recommend 500 mg of the capsule form, or 20 to 30 drops (0.5 mL) of the tincture form, or one cup of the tea, taken two to three times daily.

WHAT ARE THE SIDE EFFECTS?

I have not read any reports of side effects to passionflower, nor have my patients shown any sign of them. As with any herb, I do not recommend large dosages for pregnant women.

PASSIONFLOWER
RECOMMENDATIONS FROM THE NATURAL PHYSICIAN FOR . . .

🐾 ANXIETY AND STRESS

Passionflower is an excellent herb for anxiety and general stress. It helps to relax the nerves and muscles without any kind of sedating effect, so it's particularly effective if you want to take something during daytime hours to reduce the effects of stress and anxiety. Passionflower also helps to relax tight muscles.

🐾 HEART PALPITATIONS

This herb is commonly included in European formulas for treatment of heart palpitations, particularly when there's an underlying component of anxiety. It is often combined with hawthorn berry extract, which is used as a heart tonic.

🐾 HIGH BLOOD PRESSURE

I like to use passionflower or valerian in herbal hypertension formulas when stress and anxiety are at the core of a high blood-pressure problem.

🐾 INSOMNIA

Passionflower is particularly good for insomnia related to anxiety. People who experience side effects from sleep medications and even from valerian—as Tammy did—have no such problems when they take passionflower.

Passionflower does not cause the drowsiness associated with over-the-counter or prescription sleep medications.

If you are taking it primarily as a sleep aid, I recommend 30 drops of the tincture or 500 to 1,000 mg of the capsule form be taken half an hour before bedtime. It is commonly found in formulas that contain nerve-relaxing herbs such as kava, hops, chamomile, and valerian.

🐾 PMS AND MENOPAUSE

Passionflower is sometimes used to help reduce the anxiety and irritability experienced by women who have premenstrual syndrome. We commonly recommend it for the relief of PMS symptoms in a formula that also contains hormone-balancing herbs such as vitex. It is also effective for relief of some menopause-related problems, such as relief from irritability, depression, and insomnia.

Peppermint

"I have been following those diet changes you recommended as well as the digestive enzymes and have been feeling a lot better. But I still get some gas and cramps in my lower abdomen."

At the age of 29, Kristina had all the symptoms of irritable bowel syndrome (IBS), a painful digestive problem that often requires long-term treatment. The fact that she had already improved was significant—and for her remaining symptoms, I recommended peppermint (*Mentha piperita*).

"If it works as it should, you'll be pretty much symptom-free. The peppermint oil capsules help to relax the digestive tract and reduce spasms and gas."

Over the next month, Kristina experienced the same results as many patients with IBS who take peppermint. She found that this simple natural remedy made a tremendous difference in how she felt. It was just what she needed on days when she felt some "uneasiness" in her lower abdomen.

MAKING A MINT

Mentha piperita has long been used to help digestive complaints such as digestive cramps and spasms, flatulence, colic, and gallstones. While it's one of the best herbs to use for irritable bowel syndrome, it also helps resolve problems with the upper respiratory tract. It can help relieve the symptoms of a cold and clear out sinusitis and bronchitis. Herbalists and holistic doctors have long used peppermint for the treatment of headaches, as well. When it's made into a cream, peppermint is an excellent topical ointment for relief of joint and muscle pain.

Other "mints"—and there are quite a number—share some of the healing powers of peppermint. They were used by ancient Greeks, Romans, and Egyptians as herbs for cooking and medicinal purposes. Peppermint has also been used for thousands of years by doctors who practiced traditional Chinese and Ayurvedic medicines. Introduced to western Europe in the 1800s, it remains popular among British and European herbalists to this day.

Peppermint is actually a hybrid of two other mints—spearmint (*Mentha spicata*) and watermint (*Mentha aquatica*). It's the leaves that are used for medicinal purposes.

The key constituents of peppermint are essential oils that include menthol and menthone. Menthol is particularly important for its antispasmodic, gas-relieving, bile-stimulating, and pain-relieving qualities. Peppermint also contains flavonoids, tannins, tocopherols, carotenes, and other nutrients.

Peppermint is an aromatic herb that has a cooling effect on the body. According to traditional Chinese medicine, it has an affinity for the lungs and liver.

DOSAGE

❧ Tea

I recommend an infusion of 1 to 2 teaspoons of the dried leaf per 8 ounces of water, one to three times daily.

❧ Tincture

I recommend 20 to 60 drops (approximately 0.5 to 1.0 mL) one to three times daily.

❧ Capsule

I recommend 1 to 2 enteric-coated capsules (0.2 mL per capsule) two to three times daily between meals. This is the form recommended for irritable bowel syndrome or digestive problems that occur in the lower half of the digestive tract (e.g., flatulence).

WHAT ARE THE SIDE EFFECTS?

Peppermint may aggravate esophageal reflux (heartburn). It should also be avoided if you have cholecystitis (inflammation of the gallbladder) or severe liver disease. Peppermint essential oil—the kind that's sold for aromatherapy—should be used with caution in people with asthma. Inhaling the fragrance of the essential oil could cause a flare-up of asthma.

Note that peppermint essential oil, the kind used for aromatherapy, is for scent only. Like other essential oils, it should never be taken internally.

Use caution if you're applying peppermint oil externally as it may cause skin irritation. Don't use the oil topically around the eyes, especially with children.

I have found that too strong a concentration or too high amount of peppermint oil taken internally can cause digestive upset in children.

PEPPERMINT
RECOMMENDATIONS FROM THE NATURAL PHYSICIAN FOR . . .

🌿 COLD AND COUGH

Peppermint has been used for thousands of years in traditional Chinese medicine for the treatment of the common cold when someone has symptoms of fever, slight chills, headache, cough, and eye redness. It is also commonly used as a topical or inhaled preparation (including menthol extract) to help ease breathing and open the respiratory passages.

Peppermint has been shown to possess antiviral qualities. In addition, it is a common ingredient in cough formulas.

🌿 GALLSTONES

Menthol has been shown to be helpful in dissolving gallstones when combined with ursodeoxycholic acid. It's used in a proprietary formulation known as rowachol.

🌿 HEADACHES

Peppermint is also used internally and as an oil externally to relieve headaches, particularly tension headaches.

🌿 IRRITABLE BOWEL SYNDROME

Enteric-coated peppermint oil capsules have become very popular to reduce and sometimes eradicate the symptoms of irritable bowel syndrome (IBS). This common condition is characterized by constipation or diarrhea—or an alterna-tion of these two symptoms—as well as flatulence and intestinal cramping.

Peppermint oil helps to relax the smooth muscle of the digestive tract. It has also been shown to have antimicrobial effects against yeast and other bacteria that are often involved with IBS.

Several studies have shown that peppermint oil is effective for IBS. One randomized, double-blind, placebo-controlled trial of 110 people with IBS found that peppermint oil improved symptoms of abdominal pain, distention, flatulence, and other symptoms. Peppermint oil was significantly more effective than placebo. In a recent Italian study of 57 people with IBS, participants were given two 225-mg capsules of peppermint oil twice daily, or a placebo. Their symptoms were evaluated before therapy, upon completion of the four-week therapy, and as a follow-up four weeks after therapy ended. Patients who took peppermint oil had significantly fewer and milder symptoms at the end of therapy and also at follow-up than patients given a placebo.

🌿 MUSCLE AND BONE PAIN

Both peppermint oil and menthol have been shown to reduce pain when applied topically. For this reason they are commonly used in creams and gels for muscle pain and spasm.

Phosphatidylserine

"Doctor, I am having terrible memory problems," said 57-year-old Melanie. "I have trouble remembering my friends' phone numbers, and I'm always forgetting where I put things."

I noticed memory problems during her visit. She had difficulty with both short-term concentration and long-term recall. She had difficulty remembering names of people she knew well.

After completing a medical history, I prescribed phosphatidylserine—a dosage of 300 mg daily. (Melanie had already been taking ginkgo with limited results.)

She forgot her purse and car keys when she left my office. I dashed out to the parking lot to give them to her.

"This is always happening to me," she said with tears in her eyes.

Eight weeks later, Melanie reported excitedly that her memory was coming back. After five months, her memory had improved even more. No more forgotten keys!

THE "NEW GINKGO"

Phosphatidylserine (also called PS) is being hailed as the "ginkgo for the millennium." Studies have shown that this phospholipid extract from soy is effective in improving mental alertness, and especially the memory, in people with age-related mental decline.

PS is an important phospholipid that is a building block for cell membranes. It is found in every human cell, but is a very specific brain nutrient, being most highly concentrated in brain cells.

It has the following functions: It normalizes brain chemistry, improves cell-to-cell communication, regulates nutrients that enter brain cells and waste products that exit brain cells, stimulates production and activity of neurotransmitters, and supports stress-hormone metabolism.

PS is found in foods such as rice, fish, soy, and green leafy vegetables. It is thought that the amount of PS people get from foods is not enough for many people as they age. It is estimated that the average person gets about 70 to 80 mg of PS daily from diet. Studies show that up to 300 mg is required for therapeutic effects. Using a PS supplement is a way to achieve required levels.

Dr. Paris Kidd, one of the world's leading experts on phosphatidylserine, has reviewed some 3,000 peer-reviewed research papers on PS. "It is the single best nutrient (really, the single best means of any kind) for safely conserving and restoring crucial higher functions of the brain," according to Dr. Kidd. "The remarkable benefits of PS and its safety in use are now established beyond doubt. What remains is to spread the message to the people who can benefit from PS."

DOSAGE

I recommend starting with 300 mg daily for the first month. Optimally, 100 mg should be taken three times daily with meals. This initial dosage helps to saturate the brain cells with PS. After one month, most people can use a maintenance dosage of 100 to 200 mg. If one is suspected of having Alzheimer's disease or severe memory loss, then I would recommend not using less than 300 mg, and perhaps even a higher dosage such as 500 mg.

Make sure to buy phosphatidylserine and not phosphorylated serine. The latter is not the same and will not have the same effect. (Typically, this means looking for brands that have the Leci-PS logo.)

PS is available in formulas that contain other beneficial brain nutrients such as DHA, ginkgo, acetyl-L-carnitine, B12, folic acid, and others.

It works even better when combined with the following holistic program for optimal brain health:

- Eat brain-fortifying foods (fish, nuts, seeds, fruits, vegetables, and whole grains).
- Take nutritional supplements, including acetyl-L-carnitine and ginkgo biloba.
- Practice stress-busting lifestyle habits (proper sleep, exercise, prayer, etc.).

WHAT ARE THE SIDE EFFECTS?

There are no side effects to speak of, except digestive upset for a small number of people. However, I would recommend not taking PS before bedtime, as it keeps some people awake.

PHOSPHATIDYLSERINE
RECOMMENDATIONS FROM THE NATURAL PHYSICIAN FOR . . .

❧ AGE-ASSOCIATED MEMORY IMPAIRMENT (AAMI)

Many people experience impaired memory as they age. Some researchers feel that AAMI is the beginning of a continuum of memory decline, with the worst case of deterioration ending in Alzheimer's disease. AAMI is the condition that brings many people to see me for their memory problems. Generally, I find people improve with PS. Many people try ginkgo first because it is less expensive than PS—and some patients are already taking ginkgo on their own before they see me. But I find PS especially helpful when patients do not respond to ginkgo.

In a 1991 study of phosphatidylserine among people ages 50 to 75, doctors found positive results when they used 100-mg doses of PS, three times daily. Participants were given objective assessments at the beginning of the study and at three-week intervals. Researchers found a 30% improvement

in cognitive function that included memory, learning, recalling names, faces, and numbers. They also found that some people with the worst memory impairment were more likely to respond positively to PS.

In evaluating this supplement, Dr. Thomas Crook, a leading researcher on the effects of drugs and supplements on memory, concluded that PS is "by far the best of all drugs and nutritional supplements we have ever tested for retarding Age-Associated Memory Impairment."

❧ ALZHEIMER'S DISEASE

Alzheimer's disease is one of the most feared of all diseases. When someone has Alzheimer's, the progressive deterioration of the brain has an obvious impact on behavior. One loses the ability to retrieve memory, learn, and reason. It is not well understood what causes this disease, although we do know that brain cells die.

Aside from ginkgo, PS is one of the few natural treatments that has been shown to delay the progression of the disease. Note that it delays the progression; it does not reverse or cure Alzheimer's. There is currently no treatment that does.

Several studies have shown that people who have Alzheimer's, especially in the earliest stages, experience an improvement in memory and cognitive function if they take PS.

ATTENTION DEFICIT/HYPERACTIVITY DISORDER (ADHD)

PS is being recommended by holistic doctors as an alternative to pharmaceutical medications such as Ritalin. In an article in the *Alternative Medicine Review*, Dr. Paris Kidd states, "In a physician in-office study of 21 consecutive ADHD cases aged 4 to 19, dietary supplementation with PS benefited greater than 90% of the cases. At intakes of 200 to 300 mg per day of PS for up to four months, attention and learning were most consistently improved. Oppositional conduct proved most resistant to PS."

BRAIN INJURY

Anecdotal reports from emergency room physicians confirm that PS helps quicken recovery from brain injuries. I had a patient who sustained a brain injury after falling off a tractor. PS helped improve his cognitive function after a month of use.

DEMENTIA

Alzheimer's disease is probably the best known of the brain-related diseases that fall under the category of dementia. All cases of dementia involve memory loss as well as loss of motor function, vocabulary, and judgment.

Dementia can result from various things—a stroke, Parkinson's disease, drugs, nutritional deficiencies such as B12 or folic acid, or even brain trauma. Several studies have shown PS to be effective in alleviating various symptoms.

DEPRESSION

PS has been shown to improve mood and alleviate depression. It has a balancing effect on the neurotransmitters of the brain, which are largely responsible for our moods.

STRESS AND FATIGUE

Cortisol, a hormone produced by the adrenal glands, plays a role in both stress and fatigue. When you have acute stress, cortisol is released in high amounts to help your body deal with it. With a rise in cortisol comes an increase in blood-sugar and heart rate. Other physiological effects also occur. This type of response is required for normal functioning. However, prolonged elevation of stress leads to chronically elevated cortisol levels, which causes serious problems.

Prolonged elevation of cortisol kills brain cells, suppresses the immune system, and leads to a breakdown of the body. Stress, whether it be physical or mental, causes elevated cortisol levels. PS has been shown to have a balancing effect on the adrenal glands, the ones that control cortisol. It is one of the supplements to consider taking if you are under chronic stress or are recovering from chronic fatigue.

PS is also effective in helping athletes adapt to stress caused by exhaustive training.

Phytonutrients

Phytonutrients, also known as phytochemicals, are naturally occurring substances that give plants their characteristic flavor, color, aroma, and resistance to disease.

We get our phytonutrients from plant foods such as vegetables, fruits, nuts, seeds, grains, and legumes. Thanks to a great deal of research that's been done over the last few decades, we know many of the health benefits of these substances—and there are more than we suspected. While hundreds have already been discovered, I suspect that thousands more will be identified in the future.

Some have been in the news. The phytonutrients known as isoflavones are found in soy, and seem to have a great number of health benefits. The carotenoids found in yellow-orange fruits and vegetables such as carrots and squash also have a great reputation, because they seem to help prevent cancer and heart disease.

Many phytonutrients have potent antioxidant activity, even exceeding the well-known antioxidant properties of such vitamins as E and C. In fact, the phytonutrients known as polyphenols, which are found in green and black teas, are some of the most potent antioxidants known.

DETOX PROGRAM

Many phytonutrients promote detoxification in the body, which is critical to overall health and the prevention of disease. A great example is d-glucarate, which has been shown to help the liver metabolize pesticides, hormones, carcinogens, and other toxins. Certain phytonutrients also help damaged cells to repair themselves, which is important in treating conditions like arthritis.

When we don't consume adequate amounts of fruits, vegetables, and other plant foods, we're not only missing out on the benefits of fiber, vitamins, minerals, and enzymes—we're also losing the opportunity to eat some vital, powerful phytonutrients. So the first thing I recommend, if you want to get more disease-fighting phytonutrients, is to increase your consumption of plant foods.

The second best way to increase your levels of phytonutrients is to use whole-food supplements. In some cases it makes sense to take high dosages of supplemental phytonutrients for the treatment of certain diseases. For example, I highly recommend the phytonutrient lycopene for men with prostate cancer and help them shape their diets so they're getting as much as possible in their meals. Then I recommend lycopene supplements.

We already know a number of other phytonutrients that seem to be effective for treatment of specific health problems. Flavonoid-rich supplements such as grape seed extract or Pycnogenol are excellent for varicose veins. Anthocyanosides as found in bilberry are excellent for eye conditions such as cataracts or poor night vision. Curcumin extracted from turmeric has potent anti-inflammatory properties. Indole 3 carbinol is helpful for women with abnormal pap smears, indicating cervical dysplasia.

Studies are ongoing with regard to isolated phytonutrients and their benefit in the treatment of specific diseases. Phytonutrients are important for cancer prevention as well. Previous studies have shown that flavonoids—plant phytonutrient pigments in fruits, vegetables, soybeans, legumes, and green and white tea—reduce risk for breast cancer, but their effect on survival rates was unknown. In one study, recently diagnosed breast cancer patients, ages 25 to 98, completed a food questionnaire covering the previous 12 months. Women with the highest intake of flavonoids were 36% to 48% more likely to have survived over the following six years, compared with those who had the lowest intake.

DOSAGE

The recommended dosage for the supplemental form really varies depending on the phytonutrient and what it is being used for. Consult the listing and description in this section.

WHAT ARE THE SIDE EFFECTS?

Whether you're getting phytonutrients in food or taking specific supplements, side effects are rarely a problem. Some people have to be wary of grapefruit and grapefruit juice, however, because it affects the way the liver metabolizes certain drug medications. The fruit and concentrated juice have been shown to alter the blood levels of some heart medications and antidepressants, sometimes causing the drugs to have a greater than anticipated effect.

PHYTONUTRIENTS

RECOMMENDATIONS FROM THE NATURAL PHYSICIAN FOR . . .

Some phytonutrients seem very effective in boosting general good health, while others are ones I'd recommend for specific conditions. The following list of recommendations is a summary of what we've learned about these nutrients so far:

CHLOROPHYLL

Source: green plants and other colored vegetables

Properties: antioxidant; contains vitamin K, which is needed for blood clotting and to build bone cells

Conditions: anemia; detoxification; burns and wounds; cancer prevention

CURCUMIN

Source: turmeric

Properties: anti-inflammatory; antioxidant

Conditions: arthritis; inflammatory bowel disease; cancer

For more about the benefits of this nutrient, see Turmeric, page 450.

ELLAGIC ACID

Source: berries; grapes; apples; tea

Properties: detoxifies

Condition: cancer prevention

FLAVOGLYCOSIDES

Source: ginkgo; black tea

Properties: antioxidant; improves blood flow

Conditions: heart disease; kidney disease; varicose veins; depression; poor memory

FRUCTOOLIGOSACCHARIDES (FOS)

Source: Jerusalem artichoke; chicory root; garlic; bananas

Properties: detoxifies; increases beneficial bacteria

Conditions: digestive conditions such as irritable bowel syndrome, Crohn's disease, ulcerative colitis; yeast overgrowth; cancer; vaginitis

GALLIC ACID

Source: green tea; red wine

Properties: antioxidant; enhances immunity

(continued)

Conditions: infections; heart disease

GLUCOSINOLATES

Source: cruciferous vegetables (broccoli, cauliflower, kale, Brussels sprouts)

Properties: detoxifies; helps balance hormones

Conditions: cancer prevention; general detoxification

HYPERICIN

Source: St. John's wort

Properties: antiviral; may improve mood

Conditions: depression; anxiety; viral infection

For more about the properties of hypericin, see St. John's Wort, page 433.

INDOLES

Source: cruciferous vegetables (broccoli, cauliflower, kale, Brussels sprouts)

Properties: detoxifies; helps balance hormones

Condition: cancer prevention (especially prevention of hormone-dependent cancers such as breast and prostate)

ISOFLAVONES

Source: soy; red clover

Properties: helps balance hormones; lowers cholesterol; antioxidants; cancer prevention

Conditions: menopause; PMS; cancer prevention; high cholesterol

ISOTHIOCYANATES

Source: broccoli; cabbage; cauliflower; horseradish

Properties: detoxifies

Condition: cancer prevention

LIGNANS

Source: flaxseed; walnuts

Properties: immune enhancement; helps balance hormones

Conditions: cancer and cardiovascular disease prevention

For more about lignans, see Flaxseed, page 187.

LIMONOIDS

Source: citrus fruits and peels

Properties: detoxifies

Conditions: cancer and cardiovascular disease prevention

LYCOPENE

Source: tomatoes; red grapefruit

Properties: antioxidant

Condition: cancer prevention and treatment (particularly prostate)

See also Carotenoids, page 87.

ORGANOSULFUR COMPOUNDS

Source: garlic; onions; chives

Properties: antioxidant; immune enhancing; detoxifies

Conditions: cancer and cardiovascular disease prevention; immune enhancement; general detoxification

PHENOLIC ACIDS

Source: broccoli; berries; tomatoes;

cabbage; whole grains

Properties: antioxidant

Condition: cancer prevention

SILYMARIN

Source: milk thistle

Properties: antioxidant; liver cell regeneration

Conditions: hepatitis; elevated liver enzymes; fat malabsorption

See also Milk Thistle, page 322.

SULFORAPHANE

Source: cruciferous vegetables, such as broccoli, cauliflower, kale, and Brussels sprouts

Properties: detoxifies; helps balance hormones

Condition: cancer prevention

Pine Bark Extract

Rarely does a nutritional supplement come along that has the diverse number of uses and amount of scientific research as does pine bark extract. As a matter of fact there have been more than 230 scientific articles and clinical trials demonstrating the safety and efficacy of this natural extract over the past 40 years. This extract comes from the bark of the maritime pine tree that grows in southwestern France. Pycnogenol (pronounced *pik-NOJ-en-all*) is the brand name of the extract used in published studies, which is available from several distributors of supplements.

The use of maritime pine bark medicinally goes back to 1534 when French explorer Jacques Cartier and his crew were said to recover from deadly scurvy by following the custom of local natives and drinking teas prepared from pine needles and tree bark. This plant contains various flavonoids (plant pigments) that are potent anti-inflammatories and antioxidants (chemical compounds that protect cells from harmful molecules called free radicals). Additionally, it supports collagen and elastin formation of the skin and connective tissues, and supports the production of endothelial nitric oxide, which helps to vasodilate blood vessels and improves circulation.

DOSAGE

I recommend 50 to 200 mg daily.

WHAT ARE THE SIDE EFFECTS?

In the United States, Pycnogenol has the designation of "generally regarded as safe" status, so that it can be used in foods and beverages. Check with your doctor before using Pycnogenol if you take blood-thinning medication, such as aspirin or warfarin, because it also thins the blood; if you take medication for diabetes, because Pycnogenol can lower blood-sugar levels; or if you are pregnant or nursing. Rare side effects that have been reported include hives and tightness in the chest or throat.

PINE BARK EXTRACT
RECOMMENDATIONS FROM THE NATURAL PHYSICIAN FOR . . .

◆ ARTHRITIS

There are many good supplements that can be used to alleviate the symptoms of arthritis and the most important ones are found in this book. Many people are surprised to find out that Pycnogenol is effective in this way also. In one three-month, double-blind, placebo-controlled study, participants were given Pycnogenol or placebo daily. Seventy-seven people were given 100 mg of Pycnogenol and 79 were given placebo. Symptoms, mobility, and medication use were then assessed. Researchers found that walking distance improved from 68 meters to 198 meters in the treatment group, compared to 65 meters to 88 meters in the placebo group. The use of anti-inflammatory drugs decreased by 58% in the treatment group versus 1% using placebo. Digestive complications decreased by 63% in the treatment group, but by only 3% under placebo. After three months, swelling of the feet decreased in 79% of the Pycnogenol patients versus 1% of the controls. Overall treatment costs were reduced significantly with Pycnogenol, as compared with placebo.

Another published study examined the effect on people with osteoarthritis of the knees who supplemented with 150 mg Pycnogenol or placebo per day over a period of three months. Joint pain decreased by 40.3% after completion of the three months of supplementation with Pycnogenol. Also, 38% of patients in the Pycnogenol group required fewer non-steroidal anti-inflammatory drugs or other analgesic medications for joint pain.

◆ ASTHMA

I have had great results with Pycnogenol for the natural treatment of asthma in both kids and adults. Many times I have been able to get patients off inhalers using Pycnogenol and other dietary supplements, such as fish oil, combined with an anti-inflammatory diet that is also free of anything that tends to trigger food sensitivities. A double-blind, placebo-controlled, crossover study investigated the effect of Pycnogenol in 22 patients (18 to 50 years of age) who had been suffering from asthma since age 1 to 16 years. Participants were randomly assigned for four weeks to either the Pycnogenol group, receiving 1 mg per pound per day (without exceeding 200 mg a day), or to the group receiving placebo. At the end of four weeks, those taking Pycnogenol had better breathing scores and significantly lowered asthma scores. Also, Pycnogenol appreciably reduced the inflammatory chemical leukotriene values in the patients' blood. Other studies have shown that Pycnogenol blocks histamine release, which is a chemical involved in allergy reactions.

A very interesting study was done with children, one doctors should take note of. This double-blind, placebo-controlled study included 60 children, ages 6 to 18, with mild to moderate asthma, over a period of three months. All children were depending on rescue inhalers (with albuterol) to control recurring asthma attacks. Thirty children were assigned for three months to treatment with Pycnogenol (1 mg per pound per day) and another 30 children to the control group receiving placebo. The study showed that easiness of breathing improved significantly after one month of treatment with Pycnogenol, as measured using spirometry testing. After one month, 8 out of 30 children taking Pycnogenol didn't require rescue inhalers at all anymore, and the number increased to 12 and 18 completely off the inhaler after two and three months' treatment, respectively.

ATTENTION DEFICIT/HYPERACTIVITY DISORDER (ADHD)

Current pharmaceutical medications for ADHD are grossly overprescribed and come with the potential risk of serious side effects such as stunted growth, heart disease, stomachaches, headaches, and others. Dietary changes and targeted nutritional supplements can be helpful for many children and adults with ADHD. In one randomized, placebo-controlled, double-blind study, 61 children were supplemented with 1 mg per kg per day of Pycnogenol or placebo over a period of four weeks. Patients were examined using standard questionnaires at the start of the trial, one month after treatment, and one month after the end of the treatment period. Results show that one month of Pycnogenol supplementation caused a significant reduction of hyperactivity and improved attention and visual-motoric coordination and concentration in children with ADHD. In the placebo group no positive effects were found. The supplementation needs to be continuous since researchers found that one month after stopping Pycnogenol, symptoms relapsed.

CHEMOTHERAPY

A 2008 study demonstrated that chemotherapy patients taking 50 mg Pycnogenol three times daily had drug side effects that were half as severe as those for patients taking placebos. Symptoms such as nausea, vomiting, diarrhea, and weight loss were reduced. Patients undergoing radiation had reduced ulceration and soreness of the mouth, nausea, vomiting, diarrhea, water retention, and weakness. As well the incidence of blood clots was significantly lower for Pycnogenol users compared to those taking placebo. Speak with your doctor about supplementing Pycnogenol if you are undergoing chemotherapy treatments.

CHOLESTEROL

Pycnogenol has been shown in three clinical trials to lower LDL cholesterol and increase HDL. A study of men with mildly elevated cholesterol levels found supplementation with Pycnogenol over a period of three months statistically significant in lowering both total cholesterol and LDL by 9.4% and 16%. (Pycnogenol supplementation lowered total cholesterol and LDL and increased HDL, resulting in a better atherosclerotic index.)

Another study with 200 perimenopausal women showed a significant decrease of LDL, and an increase of HDL cholesterol increased significantly by 4.6%, during the six-month treatment period. (Pycnogenol significantly lowered LDL and increased HDL in 155 of the menopausal women during that time.) Overall, Pycnogenol does not seem to have much effect on triglycerides.

(continued)

CIRCULATION

Venous insufficiency is a medical term referring to poor return of venous blood to the heart from the lower legs. This can result in swelling of the ankles, with fluid and enlargement of varicose veins. Pycnogenol has been demonstrated in studies to improve swelling associated with venous insufficiency. It does this by strengthening capillary walls where fluid leaks. One interesting double-blind, placebo-controlled study looked at 160 passengers on a long flight. They were given Pycnogenol prior to departure and again six hours later. After the flight, tissue swelling was significantly lower in the Pycnogenol group as compared to the placebo group.

In addition, Pycnogenol has been shown to protect against blood clots from developing on long flights due to its natural blood-thinning properties, similar to those of aspirin. Pycnogenol reduces platelet activity, the cells that are responsible for blood clotting. This mechanism has been demonstrated with smokers who tend to have elevated platelet activity.

DIABETES

Another study published in *Life Sciences* involved 77 people with type 2 diabetes. Participants who took 100 mg Pycnogenol daily for 12 weeks showed significantly lower blood-sugar levels than those who took a placebo. Pycnogenol has been shown to inhibit an enzyme that breaks complex carbohydrates down into sugar. This prevents a spiking of glucose levels. Pycnogenol stays in the intestinal tract for four to six hours so a dose in the morning will reduce glucose absorption from the lunch meal.

DIABETIC ULCERS

People with diabetes are more prone to compromised circulation which increases the risk of diabetic ulcers. These wounds can become infected easily and are a serious health threat. Pycnogenol acts as a blood thinner and promotes microcirculation to the legs and other extremities. Studies have shown that, in both topical and oral form, it can help heal diabetic ulcers.

ENDOMETRIOSIS

This is a painful condition where endometrial tissue grows outside the uterine cavity. In one study, 58 women who had previously had surgery for endometriosis but had a relapse of the condition and a rating of moderate to severe for their symptoms, were given Pycnogenol or Lupron (a drug used to treat the condition by shutting off hormonal stimulation of the endometrial tissue) treatment. Pycnogenol was effective for slowly but steadily decreasing pelvic pain from severe to moderate pain.

EYE HEALTH

Retinopathy is a serious disease caused most often by high blood pressure, atherosclerosis, and diabetes. Capillaries supporting the retina become brittle and leak blood into the retinal tissue causing vision loss. Five studies involving 1,200 people have shown benefit from Pycnogenol for this condition. For example, in a study of 1,169 diabetic retinopathy patients treated with Pycnogenol, all of whom showed retinal degeneration and 49% of whom had previously received other medication, researchers found that Pycnogenol did not only successfully stop further deterioration of visual acuity but also improved the eyesight to some extent. The trend toward improved visual acuity was already noticeable after three months of treatment. Treatment was generally well tolerated; only 1.45% of the patients experienced side effects.

FERTILITY

Pycnogenol has been shown to improve the morphology of sperm in men given 200 mg for 90 days. This supplement should be considered for men with sperm morphology abnormalities.

HIGH BLOOD PRESSURE

In a study published in the peer-reviewed international journal *Life Sciences*, 58 participants who were taking prescription hypertension medication took either placebo or 100 mg per day of Pycnogenol. After 12 weeks, 57% of Pycnogenol users were able to halve their drug dosage while continuing to take the extract.

Also, a double-blind, placebo-controlled, crossover study with people with borderline hypertension not yet prescribed blood pressure medication looked at the effects of Pycnogenol. Supplementation over a period of eight weeks significantly lowered systolic blood pressure as compared to placebo. There was also a lowering of diastolic pressure.

MENSTRUAL PAIN

Several studies have demonstrated that Pycnogenol supplementation reduces pain during menstruation known as dysmenorrhea. In one double-blind, placebo-controlled study involving four Japanese hospitals and a total number of 116 women suffering from menstrual pain, the number of painful days due to menses was significantly decreased, from an average of 2.1 days prior to treatment to 1.3 days after.

PERIMENOPAUSAL SYMPTOMS

In a Taiwanese study, 155 women in perimenopause (the years leading up to menopause) took either a placebo or 200 mg Pycnogenol daily, and also assigned scores for the severity of their symptoms, such as hot flashes, sleep problems, poor memory, and anxiety. After six months, symptom scores improved for everyone in the Pycnogenol group, while the placebo users' scores did not change significantly. Also, among Pycnogenol users, blood tests showed that LDL or "bad" cholesterol dropped by 10% and antioxidant levels increased.

PREGNANCY

One Japanese study found that women in their third trimester obtained benefit from supplementation of 30 mg daily of Pycnogenol, for symptoms of low back pain, hip joint pain, pelvic pain, and pain due to varicose veins or calf cramps.

SKIN PROTECTION AND REJUVENATION

Pycnogenol has many anti-aging benefits for the skin. As an oral supplement it has been shown to protect the skin from ultraviolet light exposure, such as that from the sun. It also increases microcirculation to the skin, so that the nutritional status of the skin is improved. For those with skin pigmentation from sun exposure, known

(continued)

as chloasma or melasma, one study showed benefit from Pycnogenol. In the one-month study, oral Pycnogenol at a dose of 75 mg daily reduced the size of skin affected by hyperpigmentation significantly, by 37%.

The topical application of Pycnogenol (available in topical cream and serums) has been shown to accelerate wound healing and lower scar formation, and to combat sunburn and reduce sun damage to the skin. Also, a study of 40 women with acne found 75% had improvement with topical Pycnogenol treatment.

🐟 SPORTS NUTRITION

Pycnogenol has many different applications for sports nutrition. It has been shown to improve the antioxidant status of the body, improve circulation, strengthen blood vessel walls, enhance recuperation, prevent cramping with intense exercise, and improve endurance in athletes. Pycnogenol increases human endurance during exercise by 21%.

Pomegranate

Superfood has become a catchy term in recent years. Although all foods have their own unique nutritional composition, one must pay close attention to the super ones like pomegranate. Research has demonstrated that it is a food to be admired and consumed for optimal health. Recent studies have shown benefit for the cardiovascular system and prostate.

Pomegranates grow on a small tree that reaches up to 5 meters in height. It is native to the Middle East, in countries such as Iran and Israel. I have spoken to patients from these countries who confirm that pomegranate is very commonly found growing and consumed by the local people. It also is native to the Himalayas and was naturalized over the whole Mediterranean region during ancient times. A majority of the studies on the medicinal properties of pomegranate have been done in Israel.

The tree was introduced into California by Spanish settlers in 1769. As a matter of fact, pomegranates grow locally where I live in San Diego. The tough skin or rind is typically yellow overlaid with light or deep pink or rich red. The interior has membranous walls and spongy white material that has a bitter taste. Further interior compartments are filled with sweetly acidic juice, pulp, and seeds.

Interestingly, theologians have considered pomegranate to be a viable candidate for what is referred to in the book of Genesis of the Bible as the "forbidden fruit" in the Garden of Eden. It has also been mentioned in other ancient texts, including Ayurvedic, Greek, and Egyptian texts. Various parts of the pomegranate have been used in traditional medicine in a variety of cultures for infections, heart disease, and other ailments.

Pomegranate and its juice are rich in a number of healthy phytochemicals. The juice contains a multitude of antioxidant-rich phytochemicals known as polyphenols. These include anthocyanidins delphinidin, cyanidin, pelargonidin, and hydrolyzable tannins, including punicalin, pedunculagin, punicalagin, gallagic, and ellagic acid. Studies have shown that ounce for ounce pomegranate juice contains more polyphenols and antioxidant activity than red wine, green tea, cranberry cocktail juice, or blue-berry juice. Vitamin C is also a nutrient found in pomegranates. Pomegranate seeds also contain antioxidants and small amounts of naturally occurring estrogens. The leaves have been shown in animal studies to have glucose-lowering effects while the flower portion has been used in Eastern traditional medicine to treat diabetes. Research suggests pomegranate juice can increase nitric oxide synthetase activity in the blood vessel endothelium, which increases the availability of nitric oxide, leading to artery dilation and better blood flow.

A majority of studies on the medicinal properties of pomegranate have been done in Israel.

DOSAGE

As a general dosage, I recommend 2 to 8 ounces (50 to 240 mL) pomegranate juice daily. Consuming the flesh and seeds of a pomegranate is very nutritious as well, and these should be added to the diet such as in salads as often as possible.

WHAT ARE THE SIDE EFFECTS?

Pomegranate juice is very well tolerated. I recommend those with diabetes or those prone to gaining weight to be aware that most pomegranate juices contain a high amount of naturally occurring sugar. Those with these conditions can consume a few ounces a day without worry.

POMEGRANATE
RECOMMENDATIONS FROM THE NATURAL PHYSICIAN FOR . . .

⮞ ATHEROSCLEROSIS

A small but interesting three-year study published in *Clinical Nutrition* demonstrated pomegranate juice effective in reducing plaque in the carotid arteries. The study included 19 men and women with severe carotid artery blockage (70% to 90% blockage). Carotid artery plaque was measured by Doppler ultrasound, several times during and at the end of the study. Ten participants consumed 1.7 ounces (50 mL) of pomegranate juice daily, while nine received a placebo. Participants consuming pomegranate juice had a reduced thickness of their carotid arteries of up to 35% after one year. Also, systolic blood pressure was significantly reduced, by 12%, after one year and markers of antioxidant status were appreciably improved. Those who consumed a placebo had a 9% increase in artery thickness after one year.

⮞ CORONARY ARTERY DISEASE

People with coronary artery disease have impaired blood flow through their heart arteries. Pomegranate juice appears to be of benefit for this condition, according to a study published in the *American Journal of Cardiology*. This randomized, placebo-controlled, double-blind study involved 45 participants with coronary artery disease. Those given 240 mL (8 ounces) of pomegranate juice daily for three months had improved blood flow in the coronary arteries. The average improvement in myocardial perfusion (blood flow through heart arteries) was approximately 17%, compared

(continued)

to those getting placebo, who had a 18% worsening of myocardial perfusion.

🐟 DIABETES

People with diabetes are prone to higher levels of oxidative damage due to higher glucose levels. In a study published in *Atherosclerosis*, 50 mL daily of pomegranate juice was shown to improve antioxidant status for people with type 2 diabetes.

🐟 HIGH BLOOD PRESSURE

Studies using pomegranate juice have demonstrated that it can significantly lower systolic blood pressure. One study found it reduced systolic blood pressure by an average of 12% after one year. It appears to naturally prevent the constriction of arteries with a mechanism similar to ACE (angiotensin converting enzyme)-inhibiting medications. Pomegranate juice should be considered as part of a comprehensive nutritional therapy for hypertension.

🐟 HIGH CHOLESTEROL

An Iranian study lasting eight weeks demonstrated that concentrated pomegranate juice at 40 g daily significantly reduced total and LDL cholesterol in patients with type 2 diabetes and elevated "good" cholesterol levels. Other studies have not found this benefit.

🐟 PROSTATE CANCER

A clinical trial for men with rising prostate specific antigen (PSA) after surgery or radiotherapy was conducted at UCLA and found that drinking eight ounces of pomegranate juice doubled the length of time it took for PSA to double. Although more research is needed, there is no risk in men with prostate cancer consuming this juice.

Potassium

Fred, a friend of mine, had just finished his daily jog when he arrived at my house. Actually, he had been experiencing cramps in his calves the last few times he went jogging, and wanted to talk to me about it.

"I don't understand why my legs are cramping," he said. "I've been drinking lots of water."

Considering that it was the middle of an unusually hot summer, and Fred usually jogged in the afternoon, I suspected he might have a potassium deficiency from all the sweating caused by the physical activity in the hot sun.

As a therapeutic experiment, I handed Fred a glass of water and three potassium tablets.

"Try these," I said.

"Sure, what are they?" Fred asked.

"Potassium," I replied. "I think you may be a little low because of this intense heat we are having."

After Fred took the tablets and drank the water, we sat down to talk.

About five minutes later, Fred said, "My cramps are gone! It usually takes hours for them to go away."

Our experiment had worked.

I told Fred to increase his intake of bananas and orange juice to prevent further cramping. I also recommended that he drink half a bottle of a sports drink (rich in potassium and other electrolytes) a half hour before jogging, and the other half immediately after. His cramps did not return for the rest of the summer.

A Vital Substance

Potassium is critical to life as it is required for the proper functioning of cells, including heart muscle cells. It interacts with sodium and other charged particles (magnesium, calcium, and others) known as electrolytes. Sodium and potassium are both positively charged, and compete with each other to get inside cells, which are negatively charged. This "ionic dance" creates the electricity that sustains life. So, think of potassium as an important part of your "cell's battery."

Adequate levels of potassium are required to prevent high blood pressure, muscle cramps, and for normal heart function. Potassium is also required for muscle contraction; nerve conduction; glucose, protein, and carbohydrate metabolism; kidney and adrenal function; and water balance.

A high amount of potassium can be lost through excessive sweating, frequent urination (caused by diuretic medications), and vomiting or diarrhea. Diseases such as untreated diabetes can also lead to excessive potassium loss.

Magnesium deficiency also contributes to potassium loss. To get the best use out of potassium, you need to make sure you get adequate amounts of magnesium from whole grains and green leafy vegetables.

A deficiency of potassium can lead to muscle cramps and weakness, irregular heartbeat, fatigue, mental confusion, irritability, and impaired growth.

Balancing Our Diets

The RDA for anyone over 10 years old is 2,000 mg daily. Potassium is found in many different foods, but particularly in fruits and vegetables. Good sources include carrots, avocados, tomatoes, apples, bananas, and oranges.

Dulse, a type of seaweed, is particularly high in potassium. Meat, fish, and milk are also good sources of potassium.

It is not only the total amount of potassium that is important, but also the balance with sodium. Many people are aware of the importance of reducing sodium (table salt) intake, but it is equally as important to increase potassium intake. Fruits and vegetables provide a high ratio of potassium to sodium.

According to nutritional researchers, most North Americans have a potassium-to-sodium ratio of less than 1:2. Experts recommend a potassium-to-sodium ratio of 5:1. Many fruits and vegetables have a potassium-to-sodium ratio of at least 50:1 and many times as high as 100:1. For example, bananas have a potassium to sodium ratio of 440:1, while oranges have a ratio of 260:1.

Dietary Reference Intake

0 to 6 months: 90 to 500 mg

6 to 12 months: 500 to 700 mg

1 to 10 years: 700 to 1,600 mg

11 to 18 years: 1,600 to 3,000 mg

18+ years: 2,000 to 5,000 mg

Pregnant/lactating: 2,000+ mg

It is best to increase potassium intake through foods, thus consuming other helpful vitamins and minerals as well. Another common way to increase potassium and reduce sodium is to use salt substitutes (such as Nu-Salt, No Salt, or Morton Salt Substitute), which are mainly composed of potassium chloride.

Most multivitamins contain potassium and help increase the daily intake. Potassium is also available as a supplement. Supplements are not allowed to contain more than 99 mg per dose. A dose of 500 to 3,000 mg is used by doctors for the therapeutic treatment of hypertension.

Remember, a diet rich in potassium and low in sodium will require a much lower dosage of potassium supplements. Consult a nutrition-oriented doctor to find the dosage of potassium that is correct for you.

WHAT ARE THE SIDE EFFECTS?

Some people should never take potassium unless they are advised to do so by their doctor. If you have kidney disease, you should not take potassium supplements without specific instructions from your doctor. Also, potassium supplements should not be used without a doctor's recommendation by people who are taking digoxin, ibuprofen, or naproxin, or potassium-depleting diuretics (such as lasix and thiazide diuretics), and cisplatin (chemotherapy drug).

Too high a dosage of potassium supplements can cause nausea, vomiting, diarrhea, and ulcers.

POTASSIUM

RECOMMENDATIONS FROM THE NATURAL PHYSICIAN FOR . . .

❧ HIGH BLOOD PRESSURE

Potassium is one of the most important minerals needed to prevent and treat high blood pressure. Studies have shown that taking potassium supplements significantly reduces systolic and diastolic blood pressure. Be aware that it is important to reduce sodium in the diet while increasing potassium. This is done by avoiding foods high in sodium, such as processed and packaged foods, canned foods, crackers, cheeses, and luncheon meats.

About 10% of people with high blood pressure have salt sensitivity. This means that even a small amount of sodium will drive up their blood pressure. (Other important vitamins and minerals to include for hypertension are calcium, magnesium, CoQ10, and vitamin C.)

❧ MUSCLE CRAMPS

As was shown earlier, muscle cramps and spasms, especially when caused by dehydration, are relieved by taking potassium. I recommend potassium if a patient has repeated muscle cramps that are not helped by increasing water intake, and taking calcium and magnesium.

❧ STROKE PREVENTION

Potassium helps to lower blood pressure, which is one of the leading risk factors for stroke. An eight-year study of 43,738 men, ages 40 to 75, found that those who consumed the highest amount of potassium (as well as calcium and cereal fiber) had a reduced risk of stroke.

Prayer

Shawn Mitchell, head pastor of New Venture Christian Fellowship in Oceanside, California, as well as chaplain for the San Diego Chargers, experienced the tragedy of his younger brother Andre succumbing to an aggressive form of kidney cancer in 1998.

Pastor Mitchell realized that he, too, should be tested to make sure he did not have cancer. At the time of his brother's death, the pastor realized that he had been experiencing fatigue for some time—and he wanted to make sure everything was okay. In 1999, Pastor Mitchell went through a battery of tests and scans.

Pastor Mitchell learned that the scans had detected a growth—what appeared to be a tumor—on one of his kidneys. His doctor recommended exploratory surgery to ascertain the extent of the growth and to remove it as soon as possible.

The news was stunning. Married, and the father of a young boy, Pastor Mitchell was gripped with the realization that he had the potential diagnosis of cancer.

Later, Pastor Mitchell would recall the moment when he broke down in tears, only moments before he was supposed to give a sermon. Even so, he found he was able to mount the pulpit, and once in front of the congregation, he began to preach his prepared sermon.

To his amazement, someone in the congregation requested to pray for his healing. One longtime member stood up and said he had heard that the pastor might have a serious cancer, and requested the opportunity for the congregation to pray for his healing. The service came to a halt as the congregation invited the preacher to come down from his pulpit and join them. Pastor Mitchell was surprised by the suggestion, but appreciative of the congregation's care.

As he walked into the middle of the congregation, many of the parishioners laid hands on him while praying for his recovery.

Pastor Mitchell had been scheduled for exploratory surgery within days—and the doctor did a follow-up scan to pinpoint the location of the tumor. Two days later, a call came from the doctor, reporting on the new scan. Since the pastor was not at home, his wife took the call. Her dread and fear quickly changed to relief when she heard the doctor's first words.

"Something has happened—your husband has a textbook-perfect kidney. We can't explain it, but the repeat scan shows that the growth is not there now."

The doctor admitted that neither he nor any of the other doctors at the hospital could explain the results of the scan. But the evidence was there for all to see—where once there had been a tumor, it was gone. The tumor that was previously so apparent had completely disappeared.

Tests and scans were repeated. A number of other doctors joined the team that examined the results with intense thoroughness. All agreed: There were no signs of cancer in Pastor Mitchell's body. Pastor Mitchell was shown the first scans, where the growth on the kidney was large and obvious—then, the subsequent scans, which were normal. Since no medical treatment had been attempted between the two scans, none of the doctors could conjure any explanation for the "miraculous cure." And 10 years later Pastor Mitchell suffered a hemorrhagic stroke and was told the bleeding in his brain was too great. After seeing his brain scans, the attending emergency room doctors stated sorrowfully that surgery could not be performed in the emergency room. He was told by the attending physicians it was unlikely he would live to see the next morning. Again, with many people praying,

Pastor Mitchell not only survived until the next morning but, although hard to believe, he made a full recovery.

On his final visit to the doctor, Pastor Mitchell stated, "I know how this happened. The Lord answered our prayers."

WHAT'S GOING ON?

As I write, Pastor Mitchell has been tested at regular intervals. There are no signs that the kidney growth has returned and his brain MRI scans have normalized.

Not so very long ago, a story like this would have been greeted by most rational, scientific medical doctors with incredulity or, at the very least, cynical disbelief. Now, even the most research-oriented doctor is much more likely to admit that there's good research and some very compelling arguments for the power of prayer. Many conventional and complementary practitioners have also accepted that prayer is a powerful weapon in the battle against disease and a tool that can be utilized more effectively than "great bedside manner" for the optimization of health.

There is no doubt in my own mind that prayer is good medicine. In fact, I recommend that patients pray, and I pray for them. Like other doctors and practitioners, I've discovered that I do indeed get a higher rate of response to treatment and healing if I make a conscious decision to pray for all my patients.

PRAYER WHEN YOU NEED IT

Perhaps the best thing about prayer is that you never need to wait for an appointment. Long before there were doctors—as we use that term today—people have used prayer for healing. Even today, whenever I see a new poll about religion in America, the results show that most Americans do use prayer in their daily lives.

Sometimes, we pray for others; often, it's for ourselves. Dr. Larry Dossey, author of *Healing Words: The Power of Prayer and the Practice of Medicine*, refers to these two types of prayers as petitionary and intercessory. Depending on the studies—and Dr. Dossey cites many of them—both types of prayer are effective.

But studying and measuring the health benefits of prayer is a challenging enterprise, as you can well imagine. How can you control the amount of belief that someone feels? Surely, if someone gives up control to a "higher being," that could be a great stress reliever, and we know that stress is an important factor in health.

What we do know, however, is that people need more than just physical healing. According to Dr. Dossey, who reviews the studies on prayer, "The evidence is simply overwhelming that prayer functions at a distance to change physical processes in a variety of organisms, from bacteria to humans. These data . . . are so impressive that I have come to regard them as among the best-kept secrets in medical science."

My recommendation is simple—a daily routine of prayer, offered in faith, to enhance health and wellness. Prayer can be used to prevent illness, maintain good health, and heal the most serious of diseases.

Prebiotics

Probiotics have become popular in health-food circles, and even mainstream medicine acknowledges the importance of these healthful bacteria. However, not as many people know about prebiotics. First, a primer on probiotics: Beneficial bacteria, such as *Lactobacillus acidophilus* and *Bifidobacterium*, are found in yogurt, miso, kefir, and other cultured foods (and in supplements, too). Called probiotics, these good bacteria populate the digestive tract as well as the respiratory and urinary tracts. Probiotics play an important role in digestion, detoxification, synthesis of various nutrients (such as B vitamins and vitamin K), and a healthy immune system.

Also vital to good health are "prebiotics." These nondigestible portions of foods contain unique sugar chains, which stimulate the growth and activity of certain probiotics (particularly *Bifidobacterium*) in the colon.

One important group of prebiotics is known as inulins. Great examples include wheat, all types of onions, leeks, bananas, garlic, Jerusalem artichokes, and chicory root (available as a coffee substitute).

Inulin-type prebiotics include inulin, oligofructose, and fructooligosaccharides (FOS). These inulin-type prebiotics are used as functional food ingredients in beverages, yogurts, biscuits, spreads, and also as dietary supplements, especially FOS.

It has been estimated that typical North American diets contain 1 to 4 g inulin-type prebiotic compounds daily, a relatively low daily intake compared to other regions of the world, such as Europe, with an estimated average daily intake of 3 to 11 g.

Another group of prebiotics, called soy oligosaccharides—found in soy, peas, and most beans—also stimulate the growth of *Bifidobacterium* so dominantly found in the large intestine.

DOSAGE

Incorporate at least three ½-cup servings of prebiotic foods into your diet every week. For the supplement form, I recommend a 2.5 to 5 g daily and as high as 10 g.

WHAT ARE THE SIDE EFFECTS?

Due to an alteration in gut flora, a small percentage of people may experience gas, bloating, and abdominal pain. These symptoms are often temporary or will go away when the dose is reduced.

PREBIOTICS

RECOMMENDATIONS FROM THE NATURAL PHYSICIAN FOR . . .

CANCER
Preliminary animal studies have demonstrated that FOS may prevent colon cancer in part by improving immune activity in the colon.

CONSTIPATION
Since healthy flora make up an important percentage of fecal weight, prebiotics such as FOS can help with constipation. A study with elderly men demonstrated that FOS benefits constipation.

FUNGAL OVERGROWTH
The body keeps the overgrowth of fungal organisms in check with friendly flora. By increasing the count and activity of friendly flora, FOS can be used to prevent fungal overgrowth in the digestive tract.

INFLAMMATORY BOWEL DISEASE
Infectious organisms can be at the root of inflammatory bowel disease and prebiotics support friendly flora levels that guard against infection. Also improved

digestion and detoxification from prebiotics are reasons that benefit this condition as well.

➤ **IRRITABLE BOWEL SYNDROME**
This condition can be caused by dysbiosis, an imbalance between friendly and harmful organisms in the digestive tract. Prebiotics improve the levels of friendly flora, so that harmful organisms like Candida do not wreak havoc in the digestive tract.

Probiotics

Every so often the evidence for the health benefits of certain nutritional therapies accumulates to such an overwhelming degree that mainstream medicine cannot ignore it. Such is the case with probiotics, also referred to as "friendly bacteria" or "good bacteria." The term *probiotic* actually means "for life," as these healthy live bacteria or yeasts are essential to the functioning of the human body. The World Health Organization and the Food and Agriculture Organization of the United Nations define probiotics as "live microorganisms, which, when administered in adequate amounts, confer a health benefit on the host." Probiotics are widely available in foods and supplements.

It was Dr. Eli Metchnikoff, a colleague of Louis Pasteur's, who did the first, groundbreaking work in the study of Lactobacilli and other "good" bacteria. Dr. Metchnikoff was awarded the Nobel Prize in 1908 for discovering that these bacteria played an important role in immunity. Most disease, he surmised, begins in the digestive tract. When the "good" bacteria were not successfully controlling the "bad" ones, Dr. Metchnikoff labeled the condition dysbiosis, which simply means that the bacteria were not living in mutual harmony. His research led to the understanding we have today of the numerous benefits of the good bacteria and the importance of their role in balancing the "bugs."

It is amazing to realize that *Acidophilus* and *Bifidobacterium*, as well as the other friendly flora, are part of the 100 trillion bacteria that live together in the human digestive system. All told, these bacteria comprise as much as four pounds of our body weight!

This fertile colonization of the human body begins even before birth. An infant enters the world with a measure of both good and potentially harmful bacteria. With the very first breath, a baby inhales bacteria from the environment, bringing those "bugs" into the mouth and mucous membranes. From there the bacteria go on to colonize the rest of the body.

From then on, the balance of bacteria is in a continuous state of adjustment. Breastmilk supplies beneficial bacteria, so as long as a child is nursing, he or she has the benefit of an extra boost. Aided by the friendly flora in mother's milk, *Acidophilus* and other beneficial bacteria set up their own territories where they act to prevent the potentially harmful accumulation of bugs that might attack the body.

In recent years, researchers have come to understand many of the chemical and biological reactions that characterize *Acidophilus* and other beneficial bacteria. *Acidophilus* produces an acidic environment, which inhibits the reproduction of many harmful bacteria. *Acidophilus* also produces substances called bacteriocins, which act as natural antibiotics to destroy harmful microorganisms. Along with other friendly flora, *Acidophilus* also activates the immune system by increasing antibody response in the mucous tissues.

As well, friendly bacteria help produce what are known as short-chain fatty acids. These fatty acids are important as they help the regeneration of colon cells. They also have anticancer effects.

Acidophilus and the friendly flora of the digestive system help break down foods in the colon, particularly undigested fiber from fruits and vegetables. They help to digest milk sugar and promote regular bowel movements. *Acidophilus* also works to prevent the growth of *H. pylori*, a bacteria implicated in many cases of stomach ulcers.

While most physicians know something about the benefits of friendly flora, other rewards are less well recognized. For instance, many physicians are unaware that *Acidophilus* and the other good flora help manufacture vitamins in the body. These include vitamins B2, B3, B5, B12, biotin, and vitamin K. Probiotics are also important for proper absorption of minerals in the small intestine.

Probiotics are named after the species of good bacteria they're part of, plus the subspecies (for example, *Lactobacillus ruteri*) and are commonly abbreviated (*L. ruteri*).

When it comes to probiotic foods, many people think only of yogurt. However, many societies throughout the world have recognized the health benefits of other cultured foods that are high in probiotics. Many interesting and tasty options abound. Kefir is a drink made from fermented milk and grains and available in health-food stores and some grocery stores. Japanese consume miso and tempeh, both of which include fermented soybeans and are widely available in North America. Other examples include a food consumed by the Koreans known as kimchi (a spicy vegetable dish), German sauerkraut, and Southeast Asian fermented fish sauces and pastes, common in Thai foods. Just about every cuisine includes some type of probiotic-rich food.

Your digestive tract is home to more than 500 species of bacteria. In fact, each of us has within us about 10 times more bacteria than we have human cells, with the bacteria accounting for several pounds of our weight. Our relationship with them is symbiotic: They feed on some of the nutrients we consume, and in turn, they help keep us healthy—as long as we give them some TLC.

Most of the bacteria in our digestive tract live in harmony with each other, even though their "neighborhood" is crowded and diverse. But our own poor eating habits, drinking chlorinated water, exposure to mercury from dental fillings and fish, stress, and some medications (particularly antibiotics) can disrupt this bacterial neighborhood, leading to a microbial imbalance called dysbiosis. Consequences may include flatulence, diarrhea, reduced immunity, hormone imbalances, eczema, vaginal infections, allergies—and possibly an increased cancer risk.

Consuming just one or two types of probiotics can strengthen your gut's entire bacterial environment, and taking even more can yield even greater health benefits. Different probiotics increase the body's production of many different immune compounds (such as immunoglobulin A and M) and release small amounts of chemicals (like lactic acid and hydrogen peroxide) that won't hurt you but will make life uncomfortable for disease-causing germs.

DOSAGE

Eat one probiotic food source at least every other day. Fortified beverages and yogurts are becoming popular, but many contain added sugars, and lactose intolerance and dairy sensitivity is common. I often recommend that patients take probiotic supplements, which are at least five times as potent as yogurt. For probiotic supplements, a wide range of choice exists. Look for products that use strains with benefit proven through human studies, such as *Lactobacillus acidophilus*, *rhamnosus*, and *plantarum*; *Bifidobacterium bifidus*; and *Saccharomyces boulardii*. For preventative purposes, take 1 to 5 billion organisms daily. For acute illness such as diarrhea take 10 billion or higher. Follow directions on the label. Buy the freshest product possible, indicated by the farthest-off expiration date on the bottle. I also recommend taking probiotics at the end of a meal or between meals, so food will buffer your stomach acid, which otherwise may destroy the probiotics.

WHAT ARE THE SIDE EFFECTS?

Side effects may include minor digestive upset, such as gas and bloating. This is often a positive sign that harmful bacteria are being destroyed. These symptoms usually reduce or go away in a few days. If not, you can take a lower dose of the probiotic supplement or try a nondairy food containing probiotics.

PROBIOTICS
RECOMMENDATIONS FROM THE NATURAL PHYSICIAN FOR . . .

ANTIBIOTIC-INDUCED DIARRHEA

Although oral antibiotics are sometimes necessary, they're like medical cluster bombs. They kill off disease-causing bacteria and wipe out beneficial bacteria at the same time. Opportunistic bacteria, such as *Clostridium difficile*, can quickly multiply, often leading to a secondary infection and diarrhea. It's important to use probiotics while taking antibiotics and for at least a month after you stop taking antibiotics. For the prevention of *Clostridium*, the most well-studied probiotics are *Saccharomyces boulardii* and *Lactobacillus rhamnosus*. These should be taken preventatively if one is hospitalized since infection is more common for those in hospitals.

CHEMOTHERAPY-INDUCED DIARRHEA

A study of people with colorectal cancer receiving chemotherapy with 5-fluorouracil who took a probiotic supplement containing *Lactobacillus rhamnosus* and *Lactobacillus GG* had significantly reduced severe diarrhea, less abdominal discomfort, reduced hospital care, and fewer chemotherapy dose reductions due to gastrointestinal side effects.

COLON AND BREAST CANCER

The studies have been with laboratory animals, not people, so they are preliminary—but they have been positive, demonstrating that *Lactobacillus* probiotics stimulated the activity of immune cells to fight these two types of cancer. The probiotics may also suppress bacteria that create cancer-causing compounds in the colon, and they may alter the inflammatory response so it does not stimulate breast cancer cells as well. Probiotics also help break down potentially harmful estrogens as they pass through the digestive tract.

❧ CONSTIPATION

Probiotics can be one of the key supplements to use in cases of chronic constipation for both children and adults. It normally takes a week or two for benefit to be achieved.

❧ ECZEMA

Studies have shown that probiotics can help alleviate eczema in children ages 1 to 13. Probiotics appear to reduce milk allergy and an overreactive immune system. There is some evidence that pregnant mothers taking probiotics can reduce food-allergy-related eczema, allergic rhinitis, and asthma in their children. The treatment was equally effective when taken by the breast-feeding mother or by the bottle-feeding infant.

❧ IMMUNITY

Some species of intestinal bacteria, such as *Lactobacillus*, play a fundamental role in the immune system, protecting us against infections and cancer. Researchers at the University of Cologne, Germany, discovered that destroying the intestinal bacteria of laboratory animals brought their immune system activity to a screeching halt—and with probiotics, immune function was restored. The scientists also found that these bacteria secreted protein-like compounds called peptides that kept the immune system running at a low idle, ready to respond to disease-causing infections. More research has found that probiotics activate a wide range of immune compounds that fight harmful bacteria and viruses.

❧ INFECTIOUS DIARRHEA

Probiotics can prevent or resolve infectious diarrhea, particularly in infants and children. After analyzing nine studies, scientists at the University of Washington, Seattle, concluded that treatments with *Lactobacillus* cultures could lead to a faster recovery. Probiotics secrete their own types of antibiotics, called bacteriocins and microcins, which fight pathogens. I recommend my patients take a probiotic supplement preventatively when traveling, especially to foreign countries.

❧ IRRITABLE BOWEL SYNDROME (IBS)

When disease-causing bacteria find a home in your gut, they can trigger inflammation, damage the intestinal wall, and set the stage for IBS. Studies have demonstrated that probiotics can play a major role in resolving IBS and inflammatory bowel disease.

❧ LACTOSE INTOLERANCE

Acidophilus also helps to produce the milk sugar enzyme lactase. It is well known that 75% of adults (except those of northwest European descent) have a deficiency of this enzyme, which means their digestive systems cannot break down milk sugar products effectively. This leads to lactose intolerance, indicated by symptoms that include diarrhea, gas, bloating, and bad breath.

❧ RESPIRATORY TRACT INFECTIONS

A study found that children, ages 1 to 6, attending day-care centers, who supplemented with a milk containing *Lactobacillus GG* had fewer and less severe respiratory infections.

(continued)

✦ ULCERATIVE COLITIS

A high-potency probiotic containing *Lactobacillus*, *Bifidobacteria*, and *Streptococcus* can prevent increases in harmful bacteria and relapse in ulcerative colitis patients. This probiotic has been shown to induce remission in up to 53% of patients with active mild-to-moderate ulcerative colitis who don't adequately respond to conventional treatment, and it produces at least a positive response in 24%.

✦ VAGINAL INFECTIONS

Probiotic bacteria and a type of probiotic yeast, *Sarrcharomyces boulardii*, can often resolve vaginitis, an inflammation of the vaginal tissues, as well as Candida infections. Live-culture yogurt, oral probiotic supplements, and even vaginal suppositories have been used successfully.

Progesterone

"Please tell me you have something else other than horse urine to help my hot flashes!" said Leanne, a 49-year-old artist.

"Oh, you know all about Premarin," I replied.

Leanne nodded. Her gynecologist had told her all about the synthetic forms of progesterone—with the trade names Premarin and Provera—and after asking a few questions, Leanne realized that Premarin is made from substances taken from horse urine. She was also alarmed by some reports that synthetic hormones could raise the risk of breast cancer.

"I asked my doctor if she thought I looked like a horse," said Leanne. "Plus, breast cancer is the last thing I want."

"I have never prescribed Premarin or Provera and likely never will. Tell me more about what you have been experiencing."

"It really isn't all that bad. I have three to four hot flashes during the day and then sometimes at night. Other than that, I can't complain."

"Have you had a bone density test lately?" I asked.

"Yes, and the doctor said it looked good," replied Leanne.

I also asked Leanne about her family history to determine whether there was any record of breast, uterine, or other types of cancer in the family. She told me that both her grandmother and aunt had died of breast cancer.

"Any problems with depression, anxiety, low libido, insomnia, vaginal dryness?" I asked.

"Not really," replied Leanne.

"Have you tried herbal or other natural supplements for your menopausal symptoms?"

"I saw an herbalist who recommended a few different herbal menopausal formulas, but they didn't seem to stop the hot flashes," Leanne said.

By the end of the examination, I had concluded that natural progesterone would be good for Leanne to try. I explained to her that the term "natural" was the best possible description of what it actually was. "This is exactly the same progesterone that your body produces."

Leanne had heard of it. She said that some of her friends had used it with positive results. She was ready to give it a try.

Two weeks after Leanne started using a natural progesterone cream, she reported a decrease in the number of hot flashes. Before long, they were only occurring at rare intervals.

HORMONAL WORKINGS

Progesterone is one of two main female hormones, the other being estrogen. (Actually, men have progesterone, too.) A cascade of biochemical events causes the production of progesterone by the corpus luteum in the ovary, by the placenta when a woman is pregnant, and by the adrenal glands during menopause. (In men, the production task goes to the adrenal glands and testes.) In the conversion process, cholesterol is turned into the hormone pregnenelone, which is then converted into progesterone.

The progesterone secreted by the adrenal glands also acts as a precursor for the formation of estrogen, testosterone, and corticosteroids.

Progesterone is secreted by the ovaries just prior to ovulation. It helps maintain normal function in the endometrium of the uterus. It also works to maintain a balance with estrogen to regulate the menstrual cycle and prevent side effects related to "estrogen dominance," a condition caused when estrogen levels are too high relative to the progesterone levels. Progesterone is an important precursor hormone for the synthesis of other hormones.

Progesterone has many important functions, including the following:

- It protects against fibrocystic breasts.
- It's a natural diuretic—that is, it helps the body rid itself of excess water.
- It helps turn fat (lipids) into energy.
- It acts as a natural antidepressant.
- It helps thyroid hormone action.
- It normalizes blood clotting.
- It can help restore the sex drive.
- It helps normalize blood-sugar levels.
- It normalizes zinc and copper levels.
- It restores proper cell oxygen levels.
- It has a thermogenic (temperature-raising) effect.

In addition, it has a number of protective effects, helping to guard against endometrial cancer and breast cancer. It may slow the advance of osteoporosis, and it also has anti-inflammatory effects.

THE QUEEN BEE OF HORMONES

All things considered, progesterone is an extremely important hormone, and not the least of its functions is its role in balancing estrogen. Imagine a scale, with estrogen on one side and progesterone on the other. The body produces these two hormones to maintain balance and for proper biochemical and hormonal activities.

Many women in our society have a progesterone deficiency, which tilts the balance with their estrogen levels. One reason that researchers have discovered is that many women have a problem with xenoestrogens. These are estrogenlike compounds found in such things as pesticides, herbicides, fungicides, cosmetics, and many materials derived from petroleum products such as plastics. Once in the body, xenoestrogens attach to estrogen receptors and mimic the action of estrogen.

Another reason for relatively low levels of progesterone in women is that many women do not ovulate regularly. Since most progesterone is released when ovulation occurs, there's a shortage of this hormone when ovulation is infrequent. This is a major problem related to conditions such as polycystic ovary syndrome (PCOS) and irregular menstrual cycles.

For women reaching the age of menopause, an imbalance of progesterone and estrogen levels is predictable. Progesterone levels drop more dramatically than estrogen levels during menopause.

Natural Versus Synthetic

More doctors are beginning to realize that there is a difference between synthetic and natural progesterone. Simply put, the term natural progesterone refers to progesterone that is identical to what you find in the human body (termed as bio-identical). Synthetic progesterone, which has been labeled progestin, refers to progesterone that is synthetically created and is not identical to the progesterone in the human body.

Progestins are the synthetic hormones found in most pharmaceutical products for menopause and for PMS. They're also in birth-control pills. They are known to cause many different side effects.

Most holistic doctors prefer to use natural progesterone as it appears to be much safer than the synthetic version. Potential side effects of Provera, for instance, include water retention, weight gain, and irritability. Some women also experience spotting or breakthrough bleeding between menstrual cycles. Others have breast tenderness, blood clots, headaches, nausea, and high blood pressure.

Dosage

Natural progesterone is available commercially as a transdermal cream that is applied to the skin in areas with high capillary density for absorption. The areas of the skin where it's best applied include the forearms (palm side), breasts, cheeks, and bottom of feet (as long as there are no calluses). It is a good idea to rotate sites with each application.

The advantage of this is that this direct absorption bypasses the liver. Conventional progesterone pills require more metabolism by the liver, which increases the risk of liver toxicity and degrades the progesterone into metabolites so the concentration is not so high. The disadvantage is that the absorption and utilization varies depending on the woman and it is not known whether it prevents the buildup of the endometrium in women taking estrogen therapy.

Through trial and error, and with the help of a doctor knowledgeable in natural hormone replacement, you can find the dose right for you and your condition. Saliva hormone testing is recommended to evaluate and monitor your hormone levels.

In considering natural progesterone products, you may become aware of the "wild yam cream" sold by a number of companies and promoted as having natural progesterone in them. In fact, however, many of these wild yam creams contain no progesterone at all. Your body cannot convert the diosgenin in wild yam cream into progesterone; it needs to be done in a lab. Thus, the term "wild yam scam" has been used to describe these types of products.

The dosage and scheduling of natural progesterone varies depending on what condition is being treated. When you buy natural progesterone cream commercially, make sure to purchase a product that contains actual progesterone. Look for natural progesterone creams that contain 960 mg per two ounces. Thus, ¼ teaspoon of natural progesterone cream is equivalent to 20 mg of progesterone.

This typically works out to ¼ teaspoon applied to the skin twice daily, or ½ teaspoon applied daily. See the recommendations for specific dosing schedules.

Another source of natural progesterone is oral microionized progesterone (OMP), which comes in capsule form. It has been shown to prevent endometrial hyperplasia when taken in conjunction with estrogen. OMP is available only with a doctor's prescription. The dosage varies depending on what condition is being treated, and needs to be adjusted depending on the woman.

There are other delivery mechanisms for progesterone as well. For example, sublingual progesterone comes in tablet and drop form, taken orally. You hold the tablet under your tongue until it dissolves.

Find a physician experienced in natural hormone replacement if you want to use natural progesterone. Every woman is different and requires a different dosage; there is no "typical dosage."

WHAT ARE THE SIDE EFFECTS?

Even though natural progesterone is "natural," it is still a hormone and must be used correctly to avoid side effects. Herbal, nutritional, and homeopathic therapies should be used as a first line of treatment for hormone balance as they are inherently safer. However, natural progesterone is needed in certain cases.

Overall, natural progesterone appears to be very safe when used properly. However, I have seen women experience symptoms such as increased breast tenderness and irritability when the dosage is too high.

Women who use natural progesterone to relieve menopausal symptoms can experience a period of spotting over the course of one to three months; this usually stops when the body adjusts to the progesterone. If the bleeding does not stop after three months, consult your doctor.

I recommend that women who are taking hormones (natural or synthetic) should also take supplemental phytonutrients such as calcium-d-glucarate and indole 3 carbinol to help the liver break down the metabolites of these hormones effectively.

PROGESTERONE

RECOMMENDATIONS FROM THE NATURAL PHYSICIAN FOR . . .

✒ AUTOIMMUNE CONDITIONS

A number of my female patients with autoimmune conditions, such as rheumatoid arthritis and lupus, showed improvement after being on a hormone-balancing program.

I have found natural progesterone quite effective for women who want to continue using Premarin. It has a balancing effect, reduces inflammation, and improves circulation for these women.

(continued)

Research has shown that synthetic estrogen replacement can worsen lupus.

🐦 ENDOMETRIOSIS

Natural progesterone has helped quite a few women manage this sometimes difficult-to-treat condition by acting as an estrogen balancer. (Estrogen stimulates endometrial tissue growth.) Apply ¼ teaspoon of the cream twice daily for three weeks and then discontinue during menses (one week). Some women require a different medication schedule prescribed by a knowledgeable doctor. It can take up to six months of use to notice improvements.

🐦 FIBROCYSTIC BREASTS

Natural progesterone helps most women with this condition. The dosage is ¼ teaspoon to ½ teaspoon applied twice daily from ovulation to the day before menses. It should be applied to the breast for direct benefits.

It works even better if you take a daily dosage of 800 IU of natural vitamin E and essential fatty acids such as flaxseed or fish oil and evening primrose oil.

🐦 MENOPAUSE

Many doctors tell their female patients who are going through perimenopause and menopause that their hot flashes and other symptoms are caused by a decrease in estrogen. Although estrogen does decline, progesterone drops much more dramatically (to almost zero), and is more likely responsible for a lot of the symptoms. Many women find that natural progesterone works extremely well to manage their perimenopausal and menopausal symptoms. It helps with hot flashes, mood swings, and low libido to name a few.

Menopausal women should apply ¼ teaspoon of natural progesterone twice daily for two to three weeks a month. Perimenopausal women who are still having a menses should discontinue using it during the five to seven days when they're having their period.

Postmenopausal women should apply ¼ teaspoon one to two times daily for three weeks a month.

Women who are taking a hormone replacement (e.g., Premarin) and wish to use natural progesterone can do so by applying ¼ teaspoon twice daily on the days they take Premarin. The dosage of Premarin often needs to be reduced by half or more when it is used with natural progesterone. Consult with your doctor about dosage issues.

🐦 MIGRAINE HEADACHES

I have had women use natural progesterone to prevent migraine headaches that are tied to their menstrual cycles. I have them apply ¼ teaspoon twice daily three to four days before their menses, or three to four days before the time they usually get the migraine headaches.

🐦 OSTEOPOROSIS

Natural progesterone may be helpful in the prevention and treatment of osteoporosis. One researcher has found that natural progesterone increases bone density in women.

The dosage for postmenopausal women is ¼ teaspoon of natural progesterone cream applied twice daily for three weeks of the month. For those women who are perimenopausal, the dosage is the same except that it is taken for two weeks before the menses (days 15 to 26).

◦❧ OVARIAN CYSTS

Natural progesterone can be effective for shrinking ovarian cysts. Have a knowledgeable doctor prescribe the correct dose specifically for you.

◦❧ PREGNANCY COMPLICATIONS

Natural progesterone vaginal suppositories are often used by obstetricians and fertility specialists for pregnant women who have a history of miscarriage. It is used during the first trimester.

◦❧ PMS

For women who do not respond to nutritional, herbal, and homeopathic treatments for PMS, I recommend applying ¼ teaspoon of natural progesterone twice daily beginning in the middle of the cycle (day 15). I usually advise continuing the applications twice daily until one day before the start of their period, then stop.

However, if the PMS symptoms begin near ovulation (near day 14), apply ¼ teaspoon daily from days 8 to 14 and then ¼ teaspoon twice daily until one day before the menses starts. Stop using it when your period begins.

It can also be helpful for acne associated with menses.

◦❧ UTERINE FIBROIDS

More than 50% of all women have uterine fibroids. The goal of natural treatment of uterine fibroids is to slow down, halt, or shrink their growth until menopause (when estrogen levels decrease). Natural progesterone can be quite helpful in managing this condition. Apply ¼ to ½ teaspoon twice daily for three weeks of the month. Discontinue during menses.

◦❧ VAGINITIS

Women who are prone to vaginal yeast infections may have an estrogen/progesterone imbalance. Some cases respond well to natural progesterone. Apply ¼ to ½ teaspoon of progesterone cream twice daily for one week before your period begins.

Propolis

Another miracle of nature, propolis is a very popular health product in Europe and is becoming better known in North America. Bees gather propolis from the buds and barks of certain trees and carry it to the hive, where they are met by other worker bees that help them unload this precious material. The worker bees add salivary secretions and wax flakes, then spread the finished product on the beehive walls, from the entrance all the way to the individual chambers. Hence, propolis is also referred to as "bee glue."

The propolis within the beehive actually does more than glue the walls together. Researchers have found that propolis actually prevents disease in the colony by inhibiting the growth of microbes such as bacteria, viruses, and fungi. As bees enter and exit the hive, they brush against the propolis, which acts like an instant decontaminant. Everything inside and outside the hive, including the interior cells where the queen lays her eggs, is covered with a thin coating of propolis.

Propolis is also used as an embalming agent for bugs or insects that have invaded the hive. The Greek translation of propolis is fitting as it means "for or in defense of the city."

Propolis is one of the most powerful topical antimicrobial agents humans can use.

THE PROPERTIES OF PROPOLIS

Although I was aware of propolis, I never understood all of its medicinal effects until I heard them described by Jan Slama, a Canadian herbal scientist and researcher. Citing all the European research that had been done with this product, he spoke passionately and enthusiastically about the almost-miraculous antiseptic properties of this bee-manufactured substance.

Knowing that Jan Slama is a reliable source, I immediately decided that it was time to start paying more attention to propolis and its potential benefits for my patients. I reviewed the medical literature to confirm Jan's findings and quickly discovered that hundreds of investigations had been conducted to probe the medicinal properties of propolis.

Hippocrates, the Greek widely regarded as the first "modern" physician, was one of the first to recommend propolis. He said it would heal ulcers of the skin and digestive tract. In *The History of Plants*, written by John Gerard in 1597, propolis was praised for its ability to provide quick and effective healing for several of the conditions mentioned by Hippocrates, as well as other conditions. Ancient Egyptians also used propolis for a variety of different ailments. Propolis has a history of use for cancer in Japan.

Until recently, most clinical information on propolis has come from Europe, though a few studies are now being conducted in the United States, sparked by rising interest in this natural product. Most of the research has focused on immune-stimulating and topical, antimicrobial qualities. However, researchers are also exploring the antioxidant properties of bee propolis, as well as considering its possible uses as a cancer treatment, anti-inflammatory, and dental product. It may also prove useful for surgical recovery and—in a throwback to Hippocrates's original recommendations—as a palliative for ulcers of the skin and digestive tract.

ACTIVE INGREDIENTS

There are more than 150 active components in propolis. Researchers now think that the substances called flavonoids—responsible for its bright yellow color—are responsible for most of its therapeutic activity. These are the same healing flavonoids that are found in such plants as ginkgo, grapes, as well as many other herbs and foods that have human health benefits.

But scientists have been interested to note that the flavonoids found in propolis are totally unlike those found in plants. Their unique biochemical makeup might account for the powerful therapeutic activity of propolis.

In addition, bee propolis contains a class of chemicals known as phenols that seem to be responsible for many of its antimicrobial effects. The bee product also has B vitamins and amino acids, more essential components of human health. Finally, it contains an essential oil that likely contributes to its medicinal effects.

DOSAGE

Propolis is available commercially in the following forms.

Capsules

I recommend capsules to enhance immunity. The typical adult dosage is 500 to 1,000 mg daily.

Tincture

This form can be taken internally to enhance immunity, especially if you have a sore throat or upper respiratory tract infection. The dose is 1 to 3 mL taken three times daily. It can also be diluted in water—10 parts water to 1 part propolis—and applied topically.

Throat Spray

A few companies offer propolis in a spray form. This is ideal for throat and mouth infections.

Cream

This form is ideal for preventing skin infections if you have a cut, scrape, or other type of small wound.

WHAT ARE THE SIDE EFFECTS?

Propolis is not known to have any toxicity to humans, but some people may have an allergic reaction. The most frequent reaction is dermatitis when propolis is applied topically. If you notice skin inflammation, sometimes accompanied by bumps and itchiness, it might be caused by the propolis. (Paradoxically, bee propolis is also used in Europe for the treatment of contact dermatitis.)

If you take an oral dose, you need to be cautious about the possibility of a severe allergic reaction, although only a few cases have been reported. To see if you are sensitive, apply a small amount on your skin or tongue. If no sensitivity or allergy is observed in four hours, you can take a regular dose.

It is recommended that individuals sensitive to balsam of Peru or poplar bud exudates (major source of propolis for bees in Europe) avoid the use of bee propolis.

PROPOLIS

RECOMMENDATIONS FROM THE NATURAL PHYSICIAN FOR . . .

DENTAL CONDITIONS

Propolis has demonstrated benefit for common dental conditions such as gingivitis, mouth ulcers, and periodontal disease. This has led to its inclusion in a number of European dental-care products such as toothpastes and mouthwashes. Russian and Bulgarian researchers have found that the alcohol extract (tincture) of propolis has weak local anesthetic activity, so it helps to numb the gums for pain relief.

DIGESTIVE CONDITIONS

Propolis is commonly used in Europe for the treatment of peptic ulcers and ulcerative colitis. Because the flavonoids have anti-inflammatory properties, they are thought to have a healing effect on internal digestive organs, including the stomach and intestines.

HERPES

Genital herpes is a prevalent, sexually transmitted disease that is carried by more than 45 million Americans. Antiviral drugs such as acyclovir are prescribed by conventional doctors to suppress the outbreak of herpes lesions.

I find natural therapies to be very effective for this condition, and they have the advantage of carrying few or no side effects. In one study involving 90 men and women, investigators compared an ointment made of Canadian propolis to the pharmaceutical acyclovir. (Both were compared with a group that got no treatment at all.) The participants were examined on the third, seventh, and tenth days of treatment by doctors at seven different medical centers.

When doctors accumulated their results, they found that improvement in the propolis group far outpaced the acyclovir group. (Those who got no treatment at all lagged even farther behind.) The authors concluded that propolis ointment appeared to be more effective than both acyclovir and placebo ointments in healing genital herpetic lesions, and in reducing local symptoms.

This study is important because it provides scientific proof of propolis in the treatment of genital herpes. People with this condition can dramatically benefit from propolis if they suffer an outbreak. It would be interesting to have a similar study where people with genital herpes not only used propolis to heal acute outbreaks, but also took propolis internally for long-term immune system support to prevent outbreaks.

🐝 INFECTIONS

One of the unique characteristics of propolis is its broad-spectrum antimicrobial effects. By this I mean the ways it can defend the body against bacteria, viruses, parasites, and fungus.

Propolis has been called "Russian penicillin," giving a nod of credit to research that Russian scientists have done on this substance. Though many of the antibacterial properties have only been demonstrated in test-tube studies, it's interesting that propolis has been shown to improve the effects of certain antibiotics. In some cases, antibiotics were 10 to 100 times more effective in destroying bacteria when propolis was added to the mix. Also, test-tube studies have shown that antibiotics such as erythromycin and tetracycline became more effective against disease-resistant bacteria if their power was enhanced with propolis. In fact, these antibiotics were unable to fight the disease-resistant bacteria strains until the medicines were combined with propolis. It's now been shown that propolis helps prevent bacteria cells from dividing and forming more of those disease-causing cells.

A similar effect has also been demonstrated with propolis and antifungal medications. The propolis actually boosts the power of the medications. Propolis has also been shown in animal studies to activate antibody formation and increase the activity of macrophages, immune cells that help protect our bodies by gobbling up invading microbes.

🐝 WOUND HEALING

Propolis has incredible healing effects when it's applied to topical wounds. Russian and European doctors use it routinely for the healing of surgical wounds. Compared with conventional therapies, topical use of propolis provides up to an 80% faster healing rate for burns, ulcers, and surgical wounds.

The bee product actually has two distinct properties important to wound healing. First, propolis accelerates tissue healing. Second, it prevents wound infection. In a remarkably revealing study of 42 hospitalized people who were suffering from burns, doctors found that topical application of napkins saturated with propolis were enormously helpful to the patients. In fact, the average length of hospital treatment was 11 days less among those who got the propolis applications, as compared with those who didn't.

Pulsatilla

Hundreds of my patients and family members have benefited from this remedy.

Pulsatilla is the homeopathic preparation from the pulsatilla plant, also known as the windflower. The leaves on pulsatilla are very soft, almost velvety. According to homeopathic physicians, that's a good description of the personality types who can benefit from this healing remedy—that is, people who have very gentle spirits and personalities, who are very sensitive to the feelings of others, and go the extra mile to avoid hurting anyone else's feelings. Their own feelings are hurt easily.

Being well-liked is extremely important to a pulsatilla type. Like the windflower, they can be easily swayed by more domineering types. Depending on what an influential person around them thinks or what the majority of a group feels, their decisions and opinions can be easily altered. This is analogous to the light-weighted flowers of pulsatilla that move in different directions depending on which way the wind is blowing.

Jolene is a good example of the constitutional type requiring pulsatilla. During our visit, she broke down in tears several times because her relationship with her boyfriend was not going smoothly. He would get mad at her when she wanted to go out with her friends and so she would cancel plans with her friends who she missed being with. At the same time, her friends would get upset with her for never going out with them and would criticize her boyfriend for being so controlling. Jolene felt like she was in a no-win situation. In conventional medicine, of course, the influence of personality and relationships are rarely taken into account when making a diagnosis. But as Jolene talked about her feelings, she also mentioned that her PMS was becoming increasingly worse over the past year. She would get very weepy and moody, she craved chocolate, and she suffered from intense menstrual cramps.

BALANCING ACT

Pulsatilla is one of the top hormone-balancing remedies, and given Jolene's personality, I decided that the remedy would probably be right for her. Over the next two months, Jolene took the pulsatilla as I recommended. She found that her PMS symptoms dramatically improved. Even after her menstrual cycle was over, she felt that her general mood had stabilized. (Interestingly enough, she also started to become more assertive with her boyfriend and months later I found out that she had broken off their relationship and was feeling in much more control of her life.)

Pulsatilla is also one of the important grief remedies. Death of a loved one, broken relationships, and other traumatic events that lead to grief are inevitable in life.

Pulsatilla helps those who have longstanding issues with grief move in the direction of emotional healing.

Pulsatilla is one of those homeopathic remedies that parents or caretakers of children should have in their "home remedy kit." It's easy to spot the children who can be helped with this remedy. Loving and cuddly, they always want to be held. Often, they are shy around strangers and take a lot of time to adapt to new kids or situations. In a group of children, the "pulsatilla type" tends to be timid—they're followers rather than leaders.

Even body temperature is distinctive among the adults and children who fit the pulsatilla picture. A pulsatilla type tends to be on the warm side. If you find that you get warm easily—compared to other people—and you feel uncomfortable in a warm room, you may be a pulsatilla type. Also, you probably prefer to have a window open and feel better when you can breathe in fresh air. (Another sign: You throw off the covers at night, or like to sleep with your feet exposed to the night air.)

Pulsatilla is also one of the most important acute remedies. It can be very effective in cases of respiratory ailments such as asthma, ear infections, bronchitis, sinus infections, and conjunctivitis.

DOSAGE

For acute treatment I recommend the 30C potency two to four times a day or as needed for relief of symptoms. For chronic use, take a 6C or 30C potency one to two times daily for a couple of weeks. If you see improvement, then just use the remedy whenever needed.

WHAT ARE THE SIDE EFFECTS?

Side effects are rare, though I have seen cases where the symptoms get worse when a patient takes the remedy too frequently. If that happens, just take the remedy less often until symptoms start to improve again.

PULSATILLA
RECOMMENDATIONS FROM THE NATURAL PHYSICIAN FOR . . .

⮞ ANXIETY

I find many women who have problems with anxiety benefit from this remedy. I believe there are two reasons why this is so. First, the constitutional types that resonate with this remedy are usually very concerned about other people's feelings toward them, and much of their anxiety is actually fear of the unknown. Do others *really* like and accept them?

Second, I have found that hormone imbalance, specifically estrogen and progesterone balance, can lead to increased feelings of anxiety. So pulsatilla simultaneously helps the anxiety that's associated with imbalances in hormone levels.

⮞ ARTHRITIS

Pulsatilla is a more common remedy for women than for men, and it seems to be especially effective with women who have arthritis. One of the reasons that pulsatilla helps certain cases of arthritis is that it is a hormone balancer. Recent research has shown that hormone imbalance and the use of synthetic hormones is associated with various types of arthritis in women.

I would prescribe pulsatilla if a woman has arthritic pains that move around to different parts of the body—what doctors call "wandering" or "migratory pains." Also, I prescribe it if the patient tells me her arthritis feels better with warm applications such as a hot shower, heating pad, or a hot tub.

ASTHMA

Asthma can be associated with a great many factors—stress, pollution, and nutritional deficiencies, to name a few. I have helped many patients cut down or get off their asthma inhalers or reduce the use of steroid medications by prescribing the homeopathic remedy pulsatilla. It is especially rewarding when this remedy helps young children who have asthma, because it gives them a chance to lead a more normal lifestyle.

Before you give pulsatilla to a child who has asthma, however, I recommend discussing the symptoms with a homeopathic doctor. No asthma medications should be stopped without the guidance of the doctor who prescribed them.

BLADDER INFECTION

I have found pulsatilla to be effective in curing chronic cases of bladder infections in women. It has a tonic effect on the urinary tract. Also, hormone imbalance can make a woman susceptible to bladder infections, and pulsatilla can correct this problem.

BRONCHITIS

You may have experienced a case of bronchitis where you felt feverish, coughing up yellow or green mucus, and had trouble falling asleep due to the cough. Pulsatilla helps to eradicate the infection and ease the cough.

When parents call in the evening and tell me their child has a bad cough that is preventing the child from sleeping, I always consider pulsatilla the remedy of first choice if a child fits the pulsatilla type. After a dose or two, the child goes to sleep and wakes up with a less severe cough.

CONJUNCTIVITIS

Many years back my sister called me when her family was on holidays. One of my nephews woke up with one eye "stuck closed" from a yellowish discharge. My sister wanted to know which remedy I'd recommend for his eye infection.

Pulsatilla did the job, clearing up the infection within 24 hours.

Nor was this an isolated incident. Recently, my wife, son, and I were taking a vacation together. The evening before our return, my son's eye was infected with yellow-green mucus that caused his eyelashes to stick closed. We knew we would be traveling for at least eight hours the next day, and it would be a miserable trip if my son was dealing with the discomfort of an eye infection the whole way. So I gave him a dose of pulsatilla before he went to bed that night. He awoke the next morning with a 90% improvement. After

(continued)

another dose that morning, the infection was completely cleared.

❧ DEPRESSION

I have seen many cases where pulsatilla helped both men and women recover from longstanding cases of depression. The "pulsatilla type" is someone who gets some relief of depression when comforted. The person tends to consume sweets, especially chocolate, during periods of emotional despair. Pulsatilla helps to correct the underlying biochemical causes of depression.

❧ ENDOMETRIOSIS

Since it is such a great hormone balancer, pulsatilla is one of the major remedies to consider for women who have endometriosis. The remedy can work at a deep level and in some cases totally alleviate this serious condition.

❧ HEADACHE

Cynthia, a quiet and shy 35-year-old, came to me for natural treatment of chronic migraine headaches. After taking her history, it became obvious to me that her headaches were hormone related. The migraine headaches occurred during the first three days of her menstrual period.

Cynthia's doctor had recommended that she take birth-control pills to prevent or cure the migraines—but before she went that route, Cynthia came to me for a holistic approach. Her symptom picture, and her personality, suggested that pulsatilla would be effective.

Her headaches were less intense after the first month of treatment with pulsatilla. She was free of the headaches by her second menstrual period. A few more

months on the remedy, and her chronic headaches were history.

❧ MENOPAUSE

Along with the remedies lachesis and sepia, pulsatilla is one of the three most prescribed remedies for menopause. Characteristic symptoms include hot flashes, general increase in body temperature (even the women who generally "felt chilly" before menopause may stick out their feet or throw off the covers at night). When the pulsatilla type is in menopause, she may also have a strong craving for sweets and chocolate, and probably feels an increase in mood swings, particularly feelings of weepiness and sadness.

❧ MENSTRUAL CRAMPS

Pulsatilla is a top homeopathic remedy to cure the excruciating menstrual cramps from which so many women suffer. Also known as dysmenorrhea, menstrual cramps occur in about 25% of the patients I see. But treatment is highly effective with many of these patients.

It all goes back to hormone imbalance. If the hormones are balanced, the cramps won't occur in the first place. Pulsatilla helps to alleviate acute menstrual cramps and cures the chronic susceptibility as well.

❧ ORCHITIS

Orchitis refers to inflammation of the testicles. This condition is typically a complication that occurs among young men after they've had the mumps, because the virus gets carried to the testicles. Pulsatilla is one of the most important remedies for clearing up this condition.

PSORIASIS

In cases where someone is a pulsatilla type, the remedy can greatly improve this aggravating skin disease. I have had a number of cases respond to pulsatilla.

SINUSITIS

You can take pulsatilla if you have a case of sinus infection or inflammation where yellow-green mucus forms.

VARICOSE VEINS

Pulsatilla can help your circulation and also help improve varicose veins. The remedy is particularly recommended if you have varicose veins that have a deep blue color or the kind that form during pregnancy.

Quercetin

"My asthma is acting up again, I think it's this darn pollen." As soon as Holly told me that, I asked what she had been taking. She named a number of pharmaceutical items as well as supplements. But quercetin was not among them.

I urged her to pick up some quercetin from her local health-food store. I knew that the quercetin would act as a natural antihistamine to alleviate the allergies, which were causing her asthma to flare up.

Two days later, I had another call from Holly.

"I'm taking the quercetin, but it doesn't seem to make a difference," she said.

"Let's double the dose to 3,000 milligrams a day," I said.

Sure enough, a day later, she called and reported that her symptoms started to subside. She now finds that 1,500 mg daily keeps her asthma symptoms at bay.

QUERCETIN QUESTIONS

Quercetin is one of the many types of flavonoids. Flavonoids are plant pigments that give fruits and flowers much of their color. They also have potent medicinal effects on the body. There are thousands of different flavonoids, each having a slightly different molecular makeup. (Many people are familiar with the citrus bioflavonoids, often found in vitamin C supplements.) Quercetin is found in many different plants and is the most common of all the flavonoids. Studies also show it to be the most active of all the flavonoids.

Common food items that contain quercetin include apples, onions, tea, berries, and brassica vegetables (such as kale, turnips, Chinese cabbage), as well as many seeds and nuts. It is also found in herbs such as ginkgo biloba and St. John's wort.

Quercetin is the major flavonoid in the human diet. The estimated average daily dietary intake of quercetin by an individual in the United States is 25 mg.

Quercetin has several different functions in the body. It acts as an antioxidant. This prevents oxidative damage of LDL cholesterol (a process that initiates atherosclerosis), skin, and nerve tissue. It acts as an anti-inflammatory. It has an inhibiting effect on enzymes related to inflammation (e.g., lipoxygenase and cyclooxygenase) and other inflammatory chemicals such as prostaglandins. It also prevents the release of histamine, thus having an anti-inflammatory and antiallergy effect. Quercetin also enhances the action of vitamin C.

Quercetin is also proving to be valuable for cardiovascular protection, cancer prevention, ulcers, allergies, cataracts, and antiviral activity.

DOSAGE

For acute inflammation I generally recommend a dosage of 500 to 1,000 mg taken three times daily. There is some information showing that quercetin is not well absorbed, so it is important to use this dosage to achieve therapeutic results. For general prevention one can take 500 mg daily.

WHAT ARE THE SIDE EFFECTS?

Quercetin is very safe. The only reactions I have seen are in people who are sensitive to

citrus, and use quercetin in a formula containing vitamin C or citrus bioflavonoids. Some have reported mouth sores, headaches, and digestive upset.

QUERCETIN
RECOMMENDATIONS FROM THE NATURAL PHYSICIAN FOR . . .

ALLERGIES

Quercetin is often recommended in high dosages for the relief of environmental allergies, particularly allergies to pollen. By inhibiting the release of the inflammatory chemical histamine, quercetin acts like a pharmaceutical antihistamine to prevent allergic symptoms. Some practitioners recommend it for people with food sensitivities as well.

Quercetin is helpful for conditions such as sinusitis, arthritis, and inflammatory bowel disease.

CANCER PREVENTION AND TREATMENT

Quercetin has been shown to have anticancer effects in test-tube and animal studies. Human studies are under way with quercetin to see how effective it is for human cancers. Most of the studies used very high dosages, and often given intravenously. Quercetin has been shown to increase the effectiveness of the chemotherapy drug cisplatin, as well as protect the kidney cells from the toxicity of this drug.

CARDIOVASCULAR PROTECTION

Quercetin is one of the many valuable antioxidants that helps to protect the heart and cardiovascular system.

It protects LDL cholesterol from being oxidized. This is important to prevent free-radical damage to the blood vessel walls and protect against plaque buildup. It also protects vitamin E that is incorporated into LDL to act as an antioxidant.

Quercetin prevents the aggregation of platelets so that circulation is improved and reduces the chances of blood-clot formation.

One study looked at the relationship of dietary flavonoid intake and risk of coronary heart disease in men between the ages of 65 and 85. Researchers found that the risk of heart disease mortality decreased significantly as flavonoid intake increased. It should be noted that the flavonoid-containing foods most commonly eaten in this study contained a high amount of quercetin—tea, onions, and apples.

DIABETES

Aldose reductase is an enzyme that plays a part in the formation of diabetic cataracts, neuropathy, and retinopathy. This enzyme converts glucose to sorbitol, which in the case of a diabetic cataract builds up in the lens of the eye. Quercetin

(continued)

has been shown to be a strong inhibitor of human lens aldose reductase.

DIGESTIVE DISORDERS

Since quercetin has anti-inflammatory effects, it is often incorporated into the treatment protocol of patients with inflammatory bowel disease such as Crohn's disease and ulcerative colitis. It is also thought to be helpful in repairing leaky gut syndrome, a situation where malabsorption takes place in the small intestine.

Quercetin is also used in the treatment of ulcers. It has been shown to inhibit the growth of *Heliobacter pylori*, a bacterium implicated in many cases of ulcers.

PROSTATITIS

This is a condition characterized by pain of the pelvic floor or abdomen, difficulty urinating or pain with urination, and a variety of other possible symptoms. It can be caused by a bacterial, viral, or fungal infection or sometimes the cause is unknown. Research shows that supplementing quercetin reduces pain and improves quality of life for men with prostatitis.

R

Red Yeast Rice

"My total and LDL cholesterol are way too high. My doctor insists that I take a statin drug to lower my levels but I know a lot of people get side effects from these medications. What can I do instead?" asked Melvin, a 55-year-old property manager who had genetic predisposition for high cholesterol. My solution was red yeast rice extract, which over the next two months helped to normalize his cholesterol levels.

Cholesterol is an essential substance found in every cell of your body. Patients are surprised to learn that approximately 85% of cholesterol in the body is manufactured by the liver and, to a lesser degree, the small intestine. The rest comes from your diet. Cholesterol circulates in the bloodstream in carrier packages called lipoproteins, which have fat (lipid) inside and protein outside.

I believe that elevated cholesterol levels, especially total cholesterol, is over-focused on. It is true that LDL and more specifically its subparticles, such as VLDL, should not be excessively high. This type of cholesterol when it becomes damaged from oxidation contributes to inflammation in the arteries and resulting plaque buildup. Also, it is beneficial to have high levels of HDL cholesterol, which transports cholesterol out of the arteries.

It seems the LDL cholesterol levels established in 2004 by the National Institutes of Health's National Cholesterol Education Program make most adults eligible for statin drugs. It was later revealed that eight of the nine authors of the new LDL recommendations had financial ties to manufacturers of statin drugs that were not disclosed. So much for objectivity!

For patients who really need cholesterol lowering due to genetics, I prefer diet changes, exercise, and supplements such as red yeast rice, fish oil, and niacin. Red yeast rice is certainly worth using before cholesterol-lowering pharmaceuticals that come with a host of risks, including liver damage, muscle breakdown, muscle and joint pain, memory loss, and potentially increased cancer risk.

Red yeast rice has been historically used as a food coloring and preservative agent for fish and meat in Chinese and Japanese cooking. It is formed from rice fermented with *Monascus purpureus* yeast.

Red yeast rice contains an ingredient called monacolin K, which inhibits the action of an enzyme in the liver (HMG-CoA reductase) involved in the synthesis of cholesterol. It is thought to have a similar effect to that of statin drugs such as lovastatin (Mevacor). Yet studies have not yet found elevated liver enzymes or muscle pain and weakness to be a problem with red yeast rice.

The amount of monacolin K in the red yeast rice is quite minute compared to what is found in lovastatin. Other ingredients in red yeast rice may also account for its powerful cholesterol-lowering properties, such as a family of eight other monacolins, sterols, and fatty acids.

DOSAGE

The amount used in published studies has been 1,200 to 2,400 mg daily. I normally start patients at 1,200 mg twice daily and retest after two to three months. Some patients are able to maintain lower cholesterol levels at 1,200 mg daily.

WHAT ARE THE SIDE EFFECTS?

Mild side effects such as heartburn, dizziness, and gas may occur, although my patients do not report these very often. Those with an existing liver disorder should use red yeast rice extract with caution although liver problems have not been found thus far in studies with the product. Since its safety during pregnancy and breast-feeding is unknown, the extract should be avoided by women at these times. I recommend those taking red yeast rice extract also supplement 50 mg to 100 mg coenzyme Q10 to prevent any possible deficiency.

RED YEAST RICE

RECOMMENDATIONS FROM THE NATURAL PHYSICIAN FOR . . .

❧ CANCER

A very interesting study published in the *American Journal of Cardiology* found that those given red yeast rice were 48% less likely to die from other causes such as cancer than were people in the placebo group. This may be due to an anti-inflammatory effect of the supplement.

❧ HEART DISEASE

The same *American Journal of Cardiology* study looked at the impact of red yeast rice extract on the risk of heart disease in Chinese people with a history of cardiovascular disease. The trial involved 1,445 people, ages 65 to 75. For four years, about half were given 600 mg Xuezhikang (a red yeast rice extract) two times per day, and the other half were given a placebo two times per day. The treatment group had a rate of new coronary events, including nonfatal heart attacks, sudden death from cardiac causes, and other heart-related deaths, reduced by almost 37%. Those taking red yeast rice extract were 48% less likely to die from stroke than were people in the placebo group.

❧ HIGH CHOLESTEROL

I often recommend red yeast rice extract for patients with genetically elevated cholesterol levels, particularly high LDL cholesterol. In my opinion it should be used before pharmaceutical cholesterol-lowering medications. Researchers at the UCLA School of Medicine found red yeast rice significantly reduced cholesterol levels. This 12-week double-blind study involved 83 healthy people (46 men and 37 women, ages 34 to 78) with high cholesterol levels. Red yeast rice at a dose of 2,400 mg a day or a placebo was given as well as instruction to consume a diet similar to the American Heart Association Step I diet. At weeks 8 and 12, total cholesterol, LDL cholesterol, and triglycerides were significantly reduced in the group supplementing red yeast rice extract compared to placebo. There were no differences in HDL levels between the two groups. Side effects were not a problem in the study. I commonly see a 30- to 40-point total cholesterol level drop, and have had a few patients with very high cholesterol see a 100-point drop. LDL levels can also be reduced by 30 to 40 points or more.

Reishi

Reishi (*Ganoderma lucidum*) is a spectacular healing remedy. Unfortunately, many people in the West are unaware of this prized mushroom, which has a 4,000-year history of use in traditional Chinese and Japanese medicine. In China it is known as ling zhi and given the descriptions of "Herb of Spiritual Potency" and the "Ten-Thousand-Year Mushroom."

It grows wild in the coastal areas of China and is cultivated commercially in North America, Taiwan, Japan, Korea, and China. There are six different colors of reishi but the red variety is the one most commonly used for medicinal purposes. The fruiting body is the component used for the making of reishi teas of supplements.

In Chinese and naturopathic medicine, reishi is regarded as an overall health tonic and adaptogen. Indeed, studies have demonstrated that this medicinal mushroom is beneficial for the health of the cardiovascular and immune systems, as well as liver function. It contains immune-enhancing polysaccharides. Also it contains compounds known as triterpenes, which have adaptogenic, blood-pressure-lowering, and antiallergy effects.

DOSAGE

Take two to five 400- to 500-mg capsules of standardized extract twice daily. Take 375 mL of the decoction form twice daily, or 1 mL daily of the tincture form.

WHAT ARE THE SIDE EFFECTS?

There is no reported toxicity. Some people experience digestive upset. Reishi has blood-thinning properties, so check with your doctor first if you take blood-thinning medication. If you take medication for diabetes, be aware that supplementing with reishi may require a lower dose of your medication. Caution should be used by those who have had organ transplants or who are using immunosuppressive agents, because reishi boosts immune function.

REISHI

RECOMMENDATIONS FROM THE NATURAL PHYSICIAN FOR . . .

↬ ALTITUDE SICKNESS

Reishi is used by mountain climbers to prevent altitude sickness. It is best used daily starting two weeks before mountain climbing and continuing during the climb.

↬ CANCER

Reishi is a good natural therapy for long-term immune support such as the

(continued)

complementary treatment of cancer. In one placebo-controlled study, 48 patients with advanced tumors were given reishi mushroom extract for 30 days. Researchers found a marked immune modulating effect as demonstrated by an increase in T lymphocytes and decrease CD8 counts. Patients also reported reduced side effects due to chemotherapy or radiation as well as post-operation recovery.

☙ CARDIOVASCULAR SUPPORT

Reishi has been shown in some studies to have a mild blood-thinning effect, which may benefit stroke prevention. It can also reduce blood pressure. In a study of 33 people with hypertension researchers found blood pressure was significantly reduced over two weeks' time with reishi supplementation. Chinese practitioners prescribe reishi for the treatment of high cholesterol.

☙ CHRONIC BRONCHITIS

Studies in China have demonstrated a substantial improvement for patients with chronic bronchitis. In a study of more than 2,000 patients with chronic bronchitis, there was a 60% to 90% improvement within two weeks of beginning a reishi syrup.

☙ DIABETES

Preliminary animal and test-tube studies show reishi has a blood-sugar-lowering effect. This is thought to be due to polysaccharides known as ganoderans A, B, and C. I don't use reishi as a primary natural treatment for those with diabetes, although it could be a supportive natural treatment.

☙ LIVER PROTECTOR

Reishi is commonly used for improving liver function. In one small study, people with hepatitis B and elevated liver enzymes (SGOT/SGPT) and bilirubin were given 6 g reishi for three months. Significant reduction in liver enzymes were observed within one month. After three months all values were within normal range.

Resperate

"Even with my changes in diet, exercise, and the many supplements I take, my blood pressure is still 10 points too high, and I don't want to go back on medication for it. The blood pressure medications make me tired," stated Joseph, a 58-year-old sales manager.

"How is your stress level?" I asked, already knowing it was a problem.

"Terrible as always," he replied. My solution was not another pill or diet change, but instead a well-studied machine that would help him relax his nervous system and bring his blood pressure down. My recommenda-tion—which worked to achieve his goal—was an interactive device called Resperate.

Resperate has three components—a small computer unit that looks like a portable CD player, a headphone set, and a sensor belt to wrap around the chest or upper abdomen. The first time you use the device, it detects your baseline (normal) breathing pattern. With this information, the computer develops a personalized melody—with high tones indicating inhalation and low tones indicating exhalation—that gradually guides you into a slower breathing pattern. You can follow this tailor-made breathing pattern effortlessly and almost unconsciously, the same way your toes automatically tap out the rhythm as you listen to music. Resperate is designed to slow your respiration rate from the average of 12 to 19 breaths per minute to the hypertension-lowering rate of 10 or fewer breaths per minute.

If you're like most people, you usually breathe shallowly, taking air only into the tops of the lungs. You also may unconsciously hold your breath many times throughout the day, especially when you feel anxious or are concentrating on a task. I think another contributing factor is the habit many people have of holding in the tummy all the time—a practice that slims the silhouette but interferes with the ability to take long, deep "belly breaths" that carry oxygen all the way down deep into the lungs. Breathing slowly and fully from the abdomen helps to reduce blood pressure. This type of breathing balances the messages from the nervous system that constrict or relax the arteries, in addition to helping control the "fight or flight" stress response. As the body relaxes and anxiety eases, constricted blood vessels dilate and blood flows more easily.

DOSAGE

It is recommended that you use Resperate for at least 40 minutes per week, typically in three or four 15-minute sessions. After you complete a session, your breathing will naturally return to its normal rate—but the lowered blood pressure achieved during your session usually remains throughout the day. And company studies have shown that the more you use Resperate to achieve a rate of 10 breaths per minute, the greater your blood pressure reduction is likely to be. After eight to ten weeks of regular use of Resperate, many patients are able to reduce their hypertension medication dosage, under their doctor's supervision. For sustained health benefits, you must continue to use Resperate for the rest of your life—just as it is necessary to exercise regularly and eat healthfully for life.

WHAT ARE THE SIDE EFFECTS?

This device is safe for everyone and has no side effects. It can be used in conjunction with blood pressure medication.

RESPERATE

RECOMMENDATIONS FROM THE NATURAL PHYSICIAN FOR . . .

ANXIETY AND STRESS REDUCTION

Although formal studies have not used Resperate for these conditions, I have found it is effective as a long-term natural treatment. Deep breathing helps to relax the nervous system and balance stress hormones, so it makes logical sense that this machine is helpful.

HIGH BLOOD PRESSURE

Research on hypertension has demonstrated that a reduction of 10 points for systolic pressure and 5 points for diastolic pressure yields measurable health benefits. Studies show that after three to

(continued)

four weeks of regular use, Resperate reduces blood pressure on average by 14 points for systolic pressure and 8 points for diastolic pressure. Some users have experienced significantly greater decreases in blood pressure after using Resperate—as much as 36 points systolic and 20 points diastolic. My patients routinely achieve significantly lower blood pressure with its use.

A study on the device appeared in the *Journal of Human Hypertension* in 2001. It involved 61 men and women whose blood pressure was around 155/95 mmHg on average. For 10 minutes each day, one group of participants used the Resperate device and the other group listened to a portable stereo playing quiet music. After eight weeks, the average decrease in the Resperate group was 15.2 points for systolic pressure (the top number) and 10 points for diastolic pressure (the bottom number) compared with the music group's average reduction of 11.3 points (systolic) and 5.6 points (diastolic). Furthermore, six months after treatment stopped, the Resperate group's average diastolic pressure remained lower than the music group's.

Resveratrol

You probably have heard about the "French paradox." The French have a relatively low risk of developing coronary heart disease even though they eat a lot of fatty foods. A possible explanation emerged about 10 years ago. While studying the natural constituents of red wine (also part of a typical French diet), scientists discovered trace amounts of an antioxidant called resveratrol.

Resveratrol (pronounced *res-VAIR-uh-traul*) is one of the thousands of antioxidant compounds found in blueberries, raspberries, apples, and other fruits. What makes resveratrol distinctive is its ability to increase the activity of Sirtl1, a gene that promotes longevity.

Will resveratrol enable you to extend your life? Although the research is tantalizing, so far nearly all of it has been done in test tubes, or on yeast, worms, fruit flies, fish, or mice—not people. But intensive research continues to be done on this fascinating substance. The pharmaceutical industry has been researching resveratrol and developing synthetic molecules that work in similar ways.

Sources of resveratrol include red wine, red grape skins, purple grape juice, mulberries, blueberries, bilberries, and peanuts. It is also found in other plants such eucalyptus (*Eucalyptus wandoo, Eucalyptus sideroxylon*), spruce (*Picea excelsa*), *Bauhinia racemosa*, and a root used in traditional Chinese and Japanese medicine known as *Polygonum cuspidatum* (hu zhang). Higher levels of resveratrol can be ingested via supplements. The main research focus of resveratrol is as a treatment for diabetes, weight loss, reduction of heart disease, and longevity.

DOSAGE

Consume a variety of food sources in your diet daily. The supplemental dose depends on the type of product, but a typical dosage is 200 mg daily.

WHAT ARE THE SIDE EFFECTS?

There has not been much research published on the side effects of the supplement form of resveratrol. I note that some patients feel overstimulated from the supplement form. Pregnant or nursing women and children should avoid the supplement form until more research is conducted.

RESVERATROL
RECOMMENDATIONS FROM THE NATURAL PHYSICIAN FOR . . .

❧ DIABETES

Researchers at the Harvard Medical School fed high-calorie diets to laboratory mice. Not surprisingly, all of the mice gained weight. But only those that received resveratrol did not also develop diabetes. They were given megadoses of the antioxidant—11 mg per pound of body weight per day, or the equivalent of the amount a human would get by drinking 1,000 bottles of red wine daily! Meanwhile, in a small study of men with type 2 diabetes, resveratrol reduced fasting blood-sugar and improved insulin sensitivity, changes that would protect against diabetes.

❧ HEART DISEASE

Cell and animal studies suggest that resveratrol may reduce the risk of coronary heart disease. Resveratrol has mild blood-thinning properties and appears to reduce inflammation, a factor in heart disease. It might also help prevent the oxidation of cholesterol, a change that makes the blood fat more likely to clog arteries.

❧ LONGEVITY

In the Harvard study, mice receiving resveratrol had higher activity in the Sirt1 gene, maintained normal liver function, and had low levels of growth factor-1, an insulin-like hormone that is a risk factor for cancer. Significantly, their average lifespan increased by about 15%—despite the bad diet—and the mice maintained physical activity and motor skill activity more characteristic of younger mice. Another recent study found that modest doses (the human equivalent of 340 mg daily) also slowed aging in mice.

Rhodiola

"Dr. Stengler, I have tried ginseng before for energy, but I don't feel well when I take it. Is there something else I can use instead to help me with stress and energy?" My advice: The herb rhodiola.

Rhodiola, also known as roseroot or goldenroot, has become a popular energy and antistress nutritional supplement. You can find a variety of different brands in health-food stores and several multilevel companies now promote it as a key ingredient in "energy tonics." It is claimed to help strength, mental capacity, athletic performance, depression, enhance immunity, enhance fertility, and help the body adapt to different types of stress.

There are many different species of rhodiola. The most well researched and commonly available is *Rhodiola rosea* (*R. rosea*). *R. rosea* grows at high altitudes in the arctic areas of Asia and Europe. It is also native to Alaska. It has been used as a medicinal plant in Russia for several hundred years. Since 1960 there have been more than 180 studies published on its chemistry and clinical use. Unfortunately, many of these studies are published in Slavic and Scandinavian languages. The second best researched species is *Rhodiola crenulata*. The crenulata species grows in the high altitudes of the Tibetan mountains. It has been used in Tibetan medicine for more than 2,000 years.

R. rosea has been used extensively in Siberian and Russian medicine as an adaptogen, a substance that improves the resistance of an organism to the effects of physical, mental, and emotional stress without causing a disruption in normal body functions. R. rosea has been shown to have strong antioxidant properties that may protect the brain and nervous system from the damaging effects of negatively charged molecules known as free radicals. It appears to stimulate the release of neurotransmitters in the brain which may explain why it can help cognitive function.

DOSAGE

For R. rosea the dosage is 200 to 300 mg daily of a product standardized to contain a minimum of 3% rosavins. Be wary of products that list rhodiola as "Rhodiola spp.," as this does not tell you what form of rhodiola you are getting. In my opinion, it is best to stay with the well-studied form of rosea, and second best is the Tibetan form known as crenulata.

WHAT ARE THE SIDE EFFECTS?

Side effects are uncommon with R. rosea and crenulata. Patients report increased energy, better mood, and sharper focus without an overstimulating effect. Patients that tend to be sensitive to the energizing effects of supplements should start with a lower dosage to see how they tolerate it. It is recommended that people with bipolar disorder avoid using this plant extract. It should also be avoided by pregnant and nursing women.

RHODIOLA

RECOMMENDATIONS FROM THE NATURAL PHYSICIAN FOR . . .

❧ ANXIETY

There is preliminary evidence that rhodiola extract may decrease anxiety in people with generalized anxiety disorder. This is likely due to its ability to improve functioning of the adrenal glands as an adaptogen, so people can respond to stress more effectively.

❧ ENERGY AND RECOVERY

A number of studies have shown that R. rosea increases physical work capacity and shortens recovery time between bouts of high-intensity exercise.

In a randomized, double-blind study of 60 people with stress-related fatigue, researchers found that rhodiola extract exerts an anti-fatigue effect that increases mental performance, particularly the ability to concentrate, and decreases cortisol response to awakening stress in burnout patients with fatigue syndrome.

❧ HYPOTHYROIDISM

Animal studies have shown that R. rosea enhanced thyroid function without causing hyperthyroidism. It was also shown to help the thymus (immune system) and adrenal glands (stress glands) function better.

❧ MEMORY AND CONCENTRATION

Several studies have shown benefit with R. rosea and cognitive function. In one study, 170 mg *R. rosea* extract was given to 56 young, healthy physicians on night call. A statistically significant improvement in mental performance tests was observed in the treatment group (*R. rosea*) during the first two-week period. No side effects were reported. Other similar studies have shown a sustained benefit on cognitive function.

Rhus Toxicodendron

Todd, a 60-year-old retired farmer, came to see me for his arthritis. He was very much into natural therapies. He pulled out a bag of supplements that he had tried for his osteoarthritis. They included glucosamine sulfate and about 12 other supplements as well.

"I hope you have something else that can help me," he said. "I'm taking all these supplements and even so, it's getting hard to walk."

He also complained of the expense of the supplements, which were costing him about $150 every month.

After asking Todd about all the symptoms he experienced, I recommended rhus toxicodendron (commonly called rhus tox).

He asked me two questions: "Is this going to work?" and, "How much is the medicine going to cost me?"

"It should help reduce the joint pain and stiffness," I replied, "even in the first couple of weeks. As far as cost goes, you can buy a month's supply at the health-food store for about seven dollars."

"Seven dollars, that's all it costs?" he questioned.

"That's it," I replied.

I suggested that Todd stop taking all the other supplements, as he had not noticed any improvement in his condition. I advised him to take only the rhus tox. When he came to my office for a follow-up visit six weeks later, Todd reported a 70% improvement in his arthritic symptoms.

PALLIATIVE FROM A POISON

Rhus tox is the homeopathic dilution of poison oak. We know this as a plant that causes a nasty, blistering rash. However, this homeopathic is one of the best skin remedies for relieving symptoms in people who have touched poison ivy. It is also effective in treating eczema, where the skin is very itchy and feels better after the application of very hot water.

I have also used this for people with shingles. The itching, burning pain of the shingles blisters can be relieved in a few days with rhus tox.

DOSAGE

The typical dosage for rhus tox is 30C potency taken two to three times daily for a day or two for conditions such as stiffness from overexertion. For long-term use for eczema or arthritis, I generally start with a lower dose such as 6C taken two to three times daily.

WHAT ARE THE SIDE EFFECTS?

While rhus tox has few side effects, some people may experience skin irritation. People with chronic eczema or arthritis may experience a flare-up of their condition at the beginning of treatment. This is usually a sign that the remedy is working (known as a healing aggravation).

If you do have a flare-up and you begin taking the rhus tox less frequently, you'll probably notice that the flare-up subsides. Soon after, you'll probably notice an improvement in your condition.

If you are not sure whether you should use rhus tox, consult a homeopathic practitioner.

RHUS TOXICODENDRON
RECOMMENDATIONS FROM THE NATURAL PHYSICIAN FOR . . .

🍂 ARTHRITIS

Rhus tox is commonly used for osteoarthritis and rheumatoid arthritis. This is probably the right remedy for you if you notice certain characteristics about your symptoms: they are worse in the morning, improve with motion and activity during the day, and then get worse again at night while in bed.

Rhus tox is also a good remedy if these arthritic symptoms flare up before a storm or in damp weather. It's probably the right remedy for you if hot baths and showers also provide joint pain relief.

🍂 FLU

Rhus tox is a good remedy for the type of flu that makes your joints and muscles stiff.

🍂 HERPES

Cold sores on the mouth or face, or genital herpes outbreaks can be helped greatly with rhus tox.

🍂 SHINGLES

This dormant chicken-pox virus erupts when the immune system is weakened. Many elderly people suffer from excruciating pain that is often not relieved with conventional medicines. Rhus tox has worked wonders in several cases I have treated.

🍂 STRAINS

Rhus tox should be used when ligaments and tendons are strained. It helps speed up the recovery process. Athletes should have a supply of rhus tox available at all times.

🍂 URTICARIA

Urticaria is a fancy way of saying hives. For hive breakouts that do not require emergency treatment (such as when the throat closes), rhus tox helps to relieve the itching and works to heal the lesions more quickly. It is also effective for relieving itching caused by mosquito bites.

Ribose

Ribose is a phenomenal supplement that every doctor should be recommending in his or her practice for common ailments such as heart disease, including coronary artery disease and congestive heart failure. It has been proven with my patients as well as in research to greatly benefit chronic fatigue and fibromyalgia.

Ribose, whose biochemical name is a-D-ribofuranose, is a simple sugar found in every cell in the human body as well as in small amounts in foods. Your body also synthesizes ribose from glucose. Ribose plays an important role in the body in the synthesis of compounds required for energy production. Your cells make ribose when there is a metabolic demand for it. No other naturally occurring sugar performs the functions that ribose does. Essentially, it helps your cells in energy recovery and is involved in the production of adenosine triphosphate (ATP), the energy fuel used by cells. Your body gets depleted of ribose from certain diseases, such as heart disease where there is often impaired blood flow. Other causes include aging and overexertion.

The main food source of ribose is red meat, especially veal. However, the amount is quite small relative to what is found in ribose nutritional supplements. For those with disease conditions, supplemental ribose is required for a therapeutic effect.

DOSAGE

For those who have one of the conditions described here a typical dose is 5 g taken two to three times daily. Otherwise 5 g daily is a preventative dose that can be used for those involved in athletic activity. Ribose is commonly available in powder form that can be blended into a drink.

WHAT ARE THE SIDE EFFECTS?

Side effects with ribose are not common. Some people may experience a reduction in blood-sugar for 60 to 90 minutes after ingestion causing hunger or light-headedness. To avoid this take ribose with a meal or a carbohydrate such as juice.

RIBOSE

RECOMMENDATIONS FROM THE NATURAL PHYSICIAN FOR . . .

ATHLETES

I have found personally and with those involved in strenuous exercise that ribose supports energy production and recovery after workouts. Taking 5 g ribose before and after physical activity may be beneficial.

CHRONIC FATIGUE SYNDROME

I find ribose supplementation helps many of my patients with chronic fatigue syndrome (CFS), in a nontoxic manner. A study published in the *Journal of Alternative and Complementary Medicine* found that ribose supplementation at 5 g three times daily improved energy, sleep, and sense of well-being in those with CFS.

CONGESTIVE HEART FAILURE

Surprising to many patients and their doctors is that several natural substances like ribose can improve and stabilize congestive heart failure. A study in the *European Journal of Heart Failure* demonstrated that ribose supplementation improved diastolic heart function as well as improved blood flow from the left atrium to the ventricle. In addition, patients had an enhanced quality of life.

CORONARY ARTERY BYPASS SURGERY RECOVERY

Supplementing ribose before and after cardiac surgery appears to be beneficial in improving heart function markers.

(continued)

✢ CORONARY ARTERY DISEASE (CAD)

One of the "must have" supplements for those with CAD is ribose. People with CAD are prone to having ischemia, where a lack of blood flow and oxygen to the heart causes angina (chest pain) or heart attack and heart damage. A study published in the *Lancet* demonstrated that oral administration of ribose improved the heart's tolerance to ischemia for people with CAD.

✢ FIBROMYALGIA

I routinely prescribe ribose to patients with fibromyalgia, a condition characterized by pain in the muscles, connective tissue, and sometimes joints. I find it helps the majority of patients I prescribe it to. One of the probable causative factors with fibromyalgia is poor energy production in muscle cells, resulting in pain signals. Research by conventional physicians has also shown ribose to benefit those with fibromyalgia.

S

SAMe

It was Sandy's first visit. A 40-year-old legal assistant, she had been suffering from on-and-off depression for more than 10 years.

"I've tried everything," she told me. Her list included St. John's wort, B vitamins, hypnosis, homeopathy, acupuncture, counseling. She refused to try antidepressant drugs—otherwise, those would have been on her list as well.

"What about SAMe?" I asked, pronouncing it *Sammy*.

"What is it?"

"It's the abbreviation for S-adenosyl-methionine, which is a substance naturally found in the cells of your body. There's some impressive research showing it helps depression and osteoarthritis. It is what we call a methyl donor."

The term methyl donor was obviously unfamiliar to her, so I went on to explain that SAMe could activate chemical reactions in the body. Among other things, it contributed to the way the brain used neurotransmitters to influence mood.

Sandy called me five days after starting SAMe and told me that she was doing better. I encouraged her to keep taking it, knowing that a positive response after five days of supplementation could well be a placebo effect, especially in someone who had a 10-year-old depression problem.

One month later, though, when Sandy returned to my clinic, she declared she had a new friend. "His name is Sammy."

She was thrilled to be feeling so much better. A year later, when she saw me again, Sandy continued to do very well on SAMe as her sole treatment for her depression.

FOR LOOSER LIMBS

I also recommend SAMe when patients have osteoarthritis, a common condition that affects almost everyone over the age of 50.

Troy, a 55-year-old carpenter, was a good example of what SAMe can do for this condition. When he came in the first time, the severe osteoarthritis in his knees and hips forced him to walk stiffly. He commented on how his joints "creaked" like an old wooden floorboard. Troy said his knees were always quite swollen and painful when he woke up in the morning.

Troy's chiropractor had him on some good supplements including glucosamine sulfate, vitamin C and other antioxidants, and MSM. For exercise, he swam five times a week. But after a year of taking these supplements and pursuing this regular exercise regimen, he still didn't feel much improvement.

Troy wondered whether it was just a matter of giving the supplements more time to work. But I told him that he should have noticed significant benefits within a few months. To speed up the process, I recommended that, for one thing, we work on his diet, since he might have digestive problems that were getting in the way of his improvement. I also had him stop taking his current supplements and start with SAMe.

The next time I saw Troy, three months later, he said that his joint pain had improved and the swelling had gone down. From observing his mobility, I judged that there had been a 70% improvement, at least.

WHAT MAKES SAMe RUN?

Needless to say, when something works, I stay with it—and I'm now a pretty strong advocate of SAMe for both depression and osteoarthritis. But how can one supplement address such different conditions?

Our bodies manufacture SAMe by combining the amino acid methionine with ATP (adenosine triphosphate, also known as the "energy molecule"). When this reaction occurs, the resulting compound becomes a "methyl donor," meaning that it can transfer a group of one carbon and three hydrogen atoms (CH3).

Numerous biochemical reactions require this "methylation" reaction—which helps to explain why it can be used for such different conditions. By taking SAMe as a supplement, you're essentially making sure that the "raw materials" are available for crucial chemical reactions to take place.

Some researchers have speculated that our bodies lose their ability to manufacture or utilize SAMe as we get older. Also, it appears that some people may have a genetic defect that prevents their bodies from utilizing the chemical very efficiently. (This could help explain why depression, in some cases, seems to be passed along genetically in families.) Vitamin B12 and folic acid deficiency can also interfere with the body's production of SAMe.

After SAMe donates its methyl group, it is converted to another substance called SAH (S-adenosyl-homocysteine). SAH then donates its sulfur group to other molecules, which is very important for a number of body processes, especially detoxification and cartilage formation.

THE LURE OF THE NEW

The popularity of SAMe has increased most sharply during the past decade or so, although it's been available commercially, at least in Europe, since 1975.

Before commercial introduction, SAMe was tested in 1973 as a treatment for people with schizophrenia. It didn't have a significant impact on the symptoms of schizophrenia, but during the treatments, doctors observed that schizophrenia patients became less depressed when given SAMe.

Thousands of studies have now been done with SAMe, mainly related to its use for osteoarthritis and depression. There is also research showing that it is effective for fibromyalgia and cirrhosis of the liver. It is an approved prescription drug in Italy, Spain, Russia, and Germany.

Interestingly, SAMe outsells Prozac in Italy, even though insurance companies only pay for Prozac. While its popularity may not be quite that high in the United States, SAMe can now be found in virtually every health-food store and pharmacy in North America. In all likelihood, SAMe's popularity will increase even more as its price steadily decreases.

DOSAGE

Most people will notice benefits when taking between 400 to 1,200 mg of SAMe on a daily basis. Many of my patients find that between 400 to 800 mg works well as a long-term dosage. The key is to find the dosage that works best for you.

SAMe is generally available in 200-mg tablets. Make sure it is enteric-coated, which is critical for maintaining stability. It should be taken a half hour before meals. I usually recommend that people take 800 mcg of folic acid and 1,000 mcg of B12 every day to help their bodies with the metabolism of SAMe—and some SAMe formulas already contain these two additional nutrients. If not, take a high potency 100-mg B-complex vitamin.

(The B-complex has other benefits as well. The B12, folic acid, and B6 included in a B-complex vitamin also help prevent depression and osteoporosis, so it's a perfect complement to SAMe.)

WHAT ARE THE SIDE EFFECTS?

SAMe is very safe. When extremely high dosages were given to animals, there were few signs of toxicity—and lower doses used in human studies have not shown any adverse reactions. As a matter of fact, in comparison tests, the people taking a placebo had more side effects than the people who were taking SAMe. (As in all scientific studies of this kind, neither group knew whether it was taking a real supplement or an inactive placebo.)

High dosages have sometimes been given intravenously without any harm. Oral dosages of 3,600 mg per day also produced no side effects in humans.

Rarely, some people find that taking SAMe on an empty stomach causes heartburn. If this happens, take it with meals or just try taking a different brand. If you get diarrhea or stomach upset at higher-than-recommended dosages, you can simply reduce the dosages; the symptoms will go away.

It is recommended that people with bipolar depression do not use SAMe or only do so under the guidance of a medical professional.

Pregnant or breast-feeding women should only use SAMe under a doctor's supervision. To date, there aren't any studies to indicate that SAMe can cause pregnancy problems or harm the unborn baby, but it is not known whether SAMe can be guaranteed safe for long-term use. My feeling is that it would be safer for the baby than pharmaceutical antidepressants, as SAMe is a normal constituent in the body.

SAMe has been used by psychiatrists in conjunction with pharmaceutical antidepressants. This approach helps the patient to feel better more quickly. Many antidepressant drugs take a full month to have an effect while SAMe can help in days. Also, people who continue on the pharmaceutical medication can usually reduce their dosage. European physicians commonly recommend a combination.

However, if you are on pharmaceutical medications, be sure to consult with your physician before starting SAMe. Your doctor will want to be able to monitor your progress and, of course, will need to decide whether your drug therapy may need to be reduced. It's also important to never stop taking a pharmaceutical antidepressant "cold turkey" when starting SAMe, as this could lead to worsening of symptoms.

Some researchers urge caution if you're taking MAO (monoamine oxidase) inhibitor antidepressants, as they suspect there may be some problem combining the MAOs with SAMe. This combination has not been well researched.

Some researchers feel that SAMe supplementation can lead to the buildup of homocysteine in the body, which is a substance associated with the risk of heart attack. Actually, the opposite may be true. SAMe increases the activity of an enzyme (cystathione-beta-synthetase) that converts homocysteine into the beneficial antioxidant glutathione. In any event, taking B vitamins as I recommended prevents the build up of homocysteine.

SAMe

RECOMMENDATIONS FROM THE NATURAL PHYSICIAN FOR . . .

◦❧ DEPRESSION

I recommend starting at 400 mg daily for two weeks. Stay at this dosage if you notice improvement. If there is little to no improvement, then increase the SAMe dosage to 800 mg daily for another two to four weeks. Some people may need to use up to 1,200 mg to notice an effect. This is fine as toxicity is not a concern.

There are different theories as to how SAMe works to alleviate depression. One is that it increases the cellular levels of phosphatidylserine, which is a substance found in very high concentration in brain cells. It improves cell-to-cell communication, allows the efficient passage of nutrients into cells, and helps remove waste products. Phosphatidylserine has been shown to help relieve depression.

The other thing SAMe accomplishes is the increase of concentration of the neurotransmitters responsible for controlling mood such as norepinephrine, dopamine, and serotonin. Researchers believe that, at the same time, SAMe improves the way your brain cells receive these important neurotransmitters. While the exact mechanism is unknown, the benefits are certainly related to the methyl-donor effect, which allows for biochemical reactions to occur more normally in the brain.

Several studies have shown that people with severe depression have markedly low levels of SAMe. When the published clinical studies on SAMe between the years of 1973 and 1992 were analyzed, researchers found a total of 38 studies that showed the effectiveness of the supplement. When SAMe was compared with a placebo and with pharmaceutical antidepressants, it was found to be more effective than the placebo and just as effective as the class of drugs known as tricyclic antidepressants.

A 1994 study at the University of California Irvine Medical Center compared the effectiveness of SAMe with the pharmaceutical antidepressant desipramine. This double-blind study found that 62% of the people taking SAMe and 52% of those taking desipramine improved significantly.

Given all the potential side effects of traditional antidepressants, it makes sense that natural compounds such as SAMe and St. John's wort be used as a first line of treatment. If you are currently taking pharmaceutical antidepressants, I recommend working with a doctor to add SAMe to your protocol. Medications always have side effects, and if you can reduce the dosage, you're likely to reduce or eliminate at least some of the effects.

SAMe works at a much deeper level than drug therapy. With the methyl-donor mechanism, it opens the door to more biochemical reactions. Drug antidepressants, by contrast, force a chemical change to take place.

◦❧ FIBROMYALGIA

SAMe does seem to have some benefit for fibromyalgia, though the results aren't likely to be so dramatic as they are for the treatment of depression and osteoarthritis. In one double-blind fibromyalgia study, 44 patients received either 800 mg of SAMe or a placebo. The SAMe group showed significant improvement, with less pain, relief from fatigue, less morning stiffness, and improved mood. However, there was no difference between the groups in respect to tender points and muscle strength.

Another double-blind study found that SAMe improved trigger-point pain and depression. It appears that SAMe has some effect on fibromyalgia symptoms and significantly relieves depression associated with fibromyalgia.

I recommend 800 mg daily as the average dosage for this condition. Some people may need to use higher amounts and some may only need 400 mg.

LIVER PROBLEMS

The highest concentration of SAMe is found in the liver. It is involved in various detoxification pathways, including the proper metabolism of estrogen. It also is involved in the production of bile salts that help to digest fats.

When people get cirrhosis of the liver (most commonly from alcoholism), they have depleted levels of SAMe, which is necessary for bile production and detoxification. With more SAMe, there's an increased level of glutathione—a beneficial substance that becomes depleted when liver function is impaired. (Glutathione is one of the most important antioxidants for detoxification.)

Since SAMe can be helpful in preventing liver degeneration, it's also a treatment for hepatitis.

For conditions like cirrhosis and hepatitis, it's important to consult an experienced doctor or practitioner before taking SAMe at any dosage. If you don't have these conditions, you can take SAMe as a general aid in detoxification, since it helps your liver remove impurities.

For cirrhosis, I recommend 800 to 1,200 mg daily. This can be taken indefinitely, with the consent of your doctor. For general liver and detoxification support, the dosage is 200 to 400 mg daily.

OSTEOARTHRITIS

Osteoarthritis is the most common type of arthritis, where symptoms include stiffness, pain, and swelling of the joints. SAMe is known as a "chondroprotective agent," meaning that it prevents damage and degeneration of cartilage. Specifically, SAMe prevents the breakdown of substances called proteoglycans.

Proteoglycans hold water in the cartilage, which helps keep it flexible. These substances also help to keep the joints lubricated, thus preventing friction, and reducing wear and tear. Similar to glucosamine sulfate, SAMe has been shown in animal and human studies to increase cartilage production, which is critical in counteracting the effects of osteoarthritis.

In the largest study on SAMe and osteoarthritis, researchers followed the progress of 20,641 people who took SAMe for eight weeks. Patients took 400 mg three times daily for the first week, 400 mg twice daily for the second week, and 200 mg twice daily during the third to eighth weeks. Seventy-one percent of SAMe users reported "good" or "very good" benefits, while only 9% reported poor outcomes.

Several studies have compared SAMe with popular NSAIDs (nonsteroidal anti-inflammatory medications such as Advil or ibuprofen). In general, SAMe was as

(continued)

effective in relieving pain, stiffness, and other symptoms common to osteoarthritis. One of the major advantages of SAMe as compared with standard drug treatment is that it does not carry the risk of side effects. With NSAIDs you can get internal bleeding, liver damage, and kidney problems—but SAMe produces none of these side effects.

There's another benefit to taking SAMe. If you have conventional treatment with an NSAID, aspirin, or steroids, there's a good chance you actually speed up the destruction of cartilage even though you may be relieving some of the pain. All the conventional drugs have that effect—but SAMe does the opposite, actually helping to build healthier, more flexible cartilage. Along with a good diet and exercise, therefore, SAMe is a primary treatment for reducing osteoarthritis symptoms and regenerating cartilage.

Start at 800 mg daily for the first month and then cut back to 400 mg as a maintenance dose. Since SAMe is one of the more expensive supplements, many patients start at 400 mg. If you can get a good response at that level, there's no reason to go higher.

Saw Palmetto

The old adage is "a dog is a man's best friend." If you were to talk to men over age 50, that saying may be changed to "saw palmetto is a man's best friend."

Saw palmetto (*Serenoa repens*) is an incredible herb for treatment of prostate enlargement, also known as benign prostatic hypertrophy (BPH). This common condition affects 50% of men over the age of 50—and close to 90% of men in their 80s have a problem with BPH. Youth is no guarantee of immunity, however. Nearly one out of every 10 men between the ages of 25 and 30 have BPH. Common symptoms of prostate enlargement include:

- Need to urinate more frequently, especially at night
- Delay in urination
- Slow stream of urine flow
- Incomplete emptying of the bladder
- Increased incidence of prostatitis (prostate infection)
- Increased incidence of bladder infections

The prostate is a walnut-shaped gland located beneath the bladder. It surrounds the neck of the bladder and encircles the urethra (the passageway from the bladder through the penis). If the prostate gland starts to enlarge, it puts pressure on the bladder wall, urethra, and the sphincter muscles that control the flow of urine out of the bladder—hence, the increased difficulty with urination. Since urine flow is impeded, there's a greater likelihood of infections.

A FLUID ROLE

The function of the prostate is to secrete prostatic fluid that creates a favorable environment for sperm to live. As a man ages and his hormones fluctuate, testosterone levels decline while other hormones, such as estrogen, increase. Specialists surmise that the prostate enlarges because, as men get older, a lot of testosterone is converted to a substance known as dihydrotestosterone

(DHT). The enzyme responsible for this conversion of testosterone to DHT is 5-alpha reductase. It is believed the activity of this enzyme increases as men age, so that DHT levels increase. DHT is implicated in the stimulation of the growth of prostate cells.

Recently, researchers have also given attention to the role of estrogen and its role in prostate enlargement. Some researchers feel that prostate cell growth is largely a result of the balance among estrogen, testosterone, and DHT.

It is interesting to note that the enzyme aromatase converts testosterone to a potent form of estrogen known as estradiol, which causes cells to grow and multiply. It is believed that this enzyme activity increases as men get older. As estrogen levels increase, hormones such as progesterone and prolactin may play roles as well.

One study showed that the combination of saw palmetto and the herb nettles helps shrink enlarged prostate tissue. While no definitive explanation has been agreed upon, hormone balance seems to play a role.

My patient Michael, a 54-year-old real estate entrepreneur, would agree that saw palmetto can work wonders for a man's prostate. Though he originally came to see me for a problem with insomnia, I quickly determined that he wasn't sleeping well because he had to get up three or four times every night to urinate. Once awake, he then had trouble getting back to sleep. On further questioning, I found out that he also had dribbling after urination—another symptom of BPH. In other words, Michael's waking up at night was actually a symptom of prostate enlargement.

Blood work and a prostate exam helped to confirm the diagnosis of BPH. Within four weeks of taking saw palmetto extract, Michael was just getting up twice a night, as opposed to the three or four wakenings he'd had previously. Three months later, after continued use of saw palmetto, he was getting up no more than once a night.

A BERRY TONIC

The credit for medicinal use of saw palmetto goes to Native Americans who (as far as we know) were the first to make a tonic for the prostate and urinary system out of saw palmetto berries. American settlers adopted saw palmetto for their own uses, and before long it was also being used in Europe, where it is still a very popular treatment for prostate enlargement and urinary tract infections. (Some European doctors also recommend it as an aphrodisiac.) Saw palmetto is native to Florida, Georgia, Louisiana, and South Carolina.

Saw palmetto berry contains about 1.5% oil that is high in fat-soluble fatty acids and sterols. It also contains flavonoids, carotene, essential oil, enzymes, and phytosterols. Saw palmetto berry extracts with a standardized fatty-acid content are approved by both the German and French governments for the treatment of BPH.

Research has shown that saw palmetto helps the prostate in a number of ways. Among its many activities in the body, saw palmetto:

- Inhibits the activity of the enzyme 5-alpha reductase, thus reducing the conversion of testosterone to DHT
- Blocks DHT from binding to prostate cells
- Reduces the effects of estrogen and progesterone on the prostate cells
- Causes smooth muscle relaxation (theoretically allowing the urethra

to open more effectively and prevent the backup of urine)

- Reduces inflammation and edema by inhibiting the effects of inflammatory-producing chemicals called prostaglandins
- Alters cholesterol metabolism in the prostate
- Modifies the levels of sex hormone binding globulin (SHBG)

Although saw palmetto is mainly used to benefit the prostate, it is also used by herbalists for:

- Acne, which is highly influenced by hormones
- Prevention of bladder infections related to BPH
- Premature balding, which is related to the conversion of testosterone to DHT
- Polycystic ovary syndrome, which typically is characterized by DHEA and testosterone excess

- Prostatitis-inflammation and infection of the prostate
- Prostate cancer, which is influenced by hormonal factors

DOSAGE

The saw palmetto extracts that I recommend contain 85% to 95% fatty acids and sterols. The total dosage should be 320 mg daily.

I tell my patients to give saw palmetto extract a "trial run" of at least four weeks, but that's a minimum. In some men it can take up to two months before improvements begin.

WHAT ARE THE SIDE EFFECTS?

The only reported side effect is stomach upset in a small percentage of users. If you have that problem, try taking the herb with meals.

SAW PALMETTO
RECOMMENDATIONS FROM THE NATURAL PHYSICIAN FOR . . .

◈ ACNE

While I don't know of any studies on saw palmetto as a treatment for acne, some herbalists have seen positive results. I include saw palmetto in acne formulas that contain other herbs such as vitex, burdock root, and milk thistle. The combination has helped some teenagers who have serious cases of acne. In theory, saw palmetto reduces hormonal stimulation of the sebum glands, so fewer pustules form.

◈ BALDNESS

Recently, some advertisers have been touting products that help balding men regrow their hair, and the ads mention a "special herb" that prevents high levels of DHT from building up in the scalp. That herb could only be saw palmetto. I haven't seen reports of studies on saw palmetto and baldness, and I would not expect dramatic effects—but on the other hand, I have not seen any evidence to refute the claims.

BENIGN PROSTATIC HYPERTROPHY (BPH)

I find that saw palmetto helps more than 80% of men with BPH who take the full dosage for four to six weeks. Saw palmetto also combines well with the herb *Pygeum africanum* for an effective treatment. To be even more aggressive with treatment, I ask men to take some extra zinc (50 to 100 mg with a few milligrams of copper), and the supplements calcium d-glucarate plus indole 3 carbinol (for their hormone-metabolism properties). In addition, essential fatty acid sources such as flaxseed/flaxseed oil, and pumpkinseed/pumpkinseed oil are effective for BPH.

Alternatively, you may be able to find a ready-made formulation that includes saw palmetto blended with herbs such as *Pygeum africanum* and nettle root. Another helpful supplement included in some formulations is cernilton, a rye pollen extract, which has also been shown in studies to be effective for BPH as well as prostatitis.

In one study involving 1,098 men over the age of 50, researchers compared the results of taking saw palmetto extract (320 mg) with a prescription dosage of the drug Proscar (5 mg daily). After a 6-month trial, researchers were able to report that the treatments were equally effective in reducing the symptoms of BPH. However, the men taking the prescription pharmaceutical Proscar had far more problems with sexual dysfunction, complaining of lowered libido, impotence, and ejaculatory disorders.

Based on studies like this, saw palmetto clearly shows the same benefits without the drawback of negative side effects.

The prestigious *Journal of the American Medical Association*—the bible of conventional medicine—summed up the findings in a number of reports on the healing effects and the safety of saw palmetto extract in men with prostate enlargement. When the authors reviewed 18 scientifically controlled trials involving 2,939 men with BPH, they concluded that, indeed, saw palmetto was just as effective as Proscar, and the side effects were fewer.

You may have heard about a study published in the *New England Journal of Medicine* that reported that saw palmetto was not effective for symptoms of BPH. The double-blind trial randomly assigned 225 men over the age of 49 years who had moderate-to-severe symptoms of benign prostatic hyperplasia to one year of treatment with saw palmetto extract (160 mg twice a day) or placebo. The headlines about this study ignored the more than 20 other well-designed studies showing the efficacy of saw palmetto. The media also failed to report that the men with BPH in the study had moderate to severe symptoms. Saw palmetto has shown unquestionably it is effective for mild to moderate symptoms of BPH.

BLADDER INFECTION

Bladder infections and urinary tract infections are much more likely to occur in men who have BPH. As urine flow is impeded and slowed down, bacteria are more likely to thrive and cause infection in the bladder and urinary tract. By reducing the prostate congestion and improving urination, saw palmetto treats

(continued)

the underlying condition that often leads to bacterial infection.

🐚 POLYCYSTIC OVARIAN SYNDROME

This condition involves hormone imbalance. Women who have this syndrome may begin to grow facial hair, gain weight, experience menstrual irregularities, and have ovulation problems. Higher-than-normal levels of the hormones DHEA and testosterone are found in some women with this condition. Herbalists theorize that saw palmetto may be helpful because it blocks the effects of these hormones. I doubt it would be effective by itself, but it's worth trying in herbal hormone-balancing formulas.

🐚 PROSTATE CANCER

There are no studies looking at saw palmetto's effect on prostate cancer. My view is that it would not hurt and may have some benefit as part of a comprehensive approach. After all, saw palmetto may prevent excess hormone stimulation of the prostate cells, so perhaps it reduces the stimulus for cell growth. Fortunately, saw palmetto does not appear to affect the PSA marker (test marker for prostate cancer), so there is no conflict in using it.

🐚 PROSTATITIS

Congestion and inflammation of the prostate leads to a condition known as prostatitis. This can cause serious pain in the prostate gland—pain that can be felt in other areas of the body such as the low back, abdomen, and testis. (Doctors call this "referred pain," since it affects body areas that are separate from the actual pain site.) Saw palmetto helps to reduce the congestion and alleviate prostatitis when used on a long-term basis. (The rye pollen extract cernilton has been shown in studies to treat prostatitis even more effectively than saw palmetto.)

Schussler Cell Salts

"Dr. Mark, I picked up the kali phos 6x that you recommended for my nerves. On the bottle it said 'Schussler Cell Salt.' What does that mean?" asked Florence, a patient of mine.

"Schussler cell salts refer to a group of homeopathic remedies that was developed by Dr. Schussler of Germany in the late 1800s. His research led him to believe that 12 inorganic minerals were the key constituents of cells. He referred to these 12 minerals as tissue builders and said that healthy cells contain normal amounts of these minerals. He theorized that disease occurs when there is a deficiency or imbalance of these cell salts. By taking the indicated cell salt or combination of salts, the proper structure and function of the cells could be restored. Healthy cells make for a healthy person. In your case, you are stimulating your cells to use potassium more effectively, which benefits your nervous system."

SIMPLE, BUT EFFECTIVE

There are more than a thousand homeopathic remedies. Each one has its own set of symptoms on which it is used. The Schussler cell salts are a simplified system that complements the other homeopathic remedies. As you will see, they are easy for the public and homeopaths to use. What is more important, they work!

Have you ever taken a mineral like magnesium to help reduce or prevent muscle cramps, and find that it does not help?

You may not be getting the benefit from the magnesium at the cellular level, no matter how much you are taking. In a case like this, I find that taking the cell salt, or the homeopathic form of the deficient mineral, works quickly to alleviate the condition. The cell salt stimulates a biochemical change at the cellular level, which then gives the desired result.

DOSAGE

Cell salts are used like other homeopathic remedies—and as with other homeopathics, they come in pellet, tablet, or liquid form. The most common potency available commercially is 6x.

Cell salts are best taken 10 to 20 minutes before or after you have any drink or meal. For an infant, you can crush a cell salt tablet and place it on the child's tongue. Or you can mix the tablet with an ounce of purified water and place a few drops in the child's mouth using a dropper or teaspoon. Children like the sweet taste of the pellets and tablets.

When you do take cell salts, however, you'll probably want to avoid strong odors, such as the fragrance of eucalyptus or essential oils.

For acute conditions, cell salts should be taken every 15 minutes or two hours, depending on the severity of the condition. For chronic conditions, cell salts are usually taken one to three times daily. Since they are of a low potency, they can be used on a long-term basis.

As described below, one type of cell salts—or a combination of them—can be taken to treat a particular symptom or condition. For example, mag phos helps to relieve muscle spasms. If a person is also experiencing nerve pain, then kali phos could be used as well. These different types of cell salts can either be taken at the same time

or in alternating doses throughout the day.

There are also some formulas that combine all the cell salts together in one formula. These are commonly known as bioplasma. They may be used preventatively or to recover from various chronic illnesses.

WHAT ARE THE SIDE EFFECTS?

Side effects are not an issue with cell salts. They either help or do nothing at all.

SELECTING THE APPROPRIATE CELL SALT

A list of various cell salts follows, with the conditions for which each is used.

⁓ *Calcarea Fluorica (Calc Fluor)*

This cell salt is involved in the formation of connective tissue, making it important for the skin, ligaments, and tendons. It is also found in bones. I recommend it for the following conditions:

Abnormal spine curvature

Brittle teeth and sore gums

Hard nodules of the breast or other tissues

Hemorrhoids

Spine that "goes out" easily (including during pregnancy)

Sprains and strains

Varicose veins, weak ligaments, tendons, and joints

⁓ *Calcarea Phosphorica (Calc Phos)*

This is the main cell salt for bone health. Interestingly, calcium phosphate is an important enzyme required for bone formation. Calc phos helps in bone formation. I recommend it for the following conditions:

Arthritis

Fractures

Growing pains

Osteoporosis

Teething

🐦 *Calcarea Sulphurica (Calc Sulph)*

This cell salt is a wound and skin healer. (It is especially recommended when there is a yellow discharge from the skin.) I recommend it for the following conditions:

Abscess

Acne

Boils

Bronchitis

Post-nasal drip

🐦 *Ferrum Phosphoricum (Ferrum Phos)*

This cell salt is homeopathic iron bound to phosphate. It is required for red blood cell formation and function. I recommend it for the following conditions:

Anemia treatment and prevention (iron deficiency)

Bleeding (acute and chronic)

Fever and infection

Heavy menstruation

🐦 *Kali Muriaticum (Kali Mur)*

This cell salt helps to dissolve mucus. I recommend it for the following conditions:

Fluid in the ears

Sore throat (with white mucus being produced)

🐦 *Kali Phosphoricum (Kali Phos)*

This is the primary cell salt for nervous tissue, including the brain. I recommend it for:

Anxiety and nervousness

Depression

Fatigue

Nerve injury

Poor memory and lack of concentration

🐦 *Kali Sulphuricum (Kali Sulph)*

This is another remedy for skin and mucous membrane discharges (especially where there is a yellow discharge). I recommend it for:

Bronchitis

Eczema

Psoriasis

🐦 *Magnesia Phosphorica (Mag Phos)*

This is the primary cell salt for the muscles—both internal and external. It also has a tonic effect on the nervous system as well. It can help with:

Anxiety and nervousness

Hyperactivity

Menstrual cramps

Muscle spasms and cramps

Seizures

Stomach cramps

Toothache

🐦 *Natrum Muriaticum (Nat Mur)*

This cell salt regulates water balance within the cells and tissues. I recommend it for the following conditions:

Cold sores

Depression

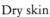

Dry skin

Edema

Grief

Hay fever

Skin rash from sun exposure

❧ *Natrum Phosphoricum (Nat Phos)*

This is the cell salt that is an acid-base balancer of the cells. I recommend it for the following conditions:

Bladder infections

Heartburn

Muscle soreness

Vaginitis

❧ *Natrum Sulphuricum (Nat Sulph)*

This remedy has a balancing effect on the fluids of the body. In addition, it tonifies the liver and digestive tract. I recommend it for:

Asthma

Head injury

Hepatitis

Newborn jaundice

Swelling

❧ *Silica*

This cell salt is found in the connective tissue, skin, glands, and bones. It acts as a tissue cleanser. I recommend it for the following conditions:

Acne

Asthma

Boils

Brittle hair and nails

Sinusitis

Selenium

Humans require very small amounts of the trace mineral selenium, yet it is involved in some very important functions in the body. Specifically, selenium is necessary for the production of antioxidant enzymes that remove toxic waste products formed from oxidative reactions.

Selenium works synergistically with vitamin E to prevent oxidative damage of cell membranes. Vitamin E works more effectively in the presence of selenium.

Selenium is also important for preventing heart disease, cancer, inflammatory conditions such as rheumatoid arthritis, and cataracts. It plays a role in the production of thyroid hormone, and it's needed during pregnancy for the growing baby.

Selenium binds to heavy metals such as mercury and may reduce their toxicity.

The dietary reference intake (DRI) for men and women is 70 mcg. Foods containing selenium include wheat germ, Brazil nuts, oats, liver, whole wheat bread, broccoli, red grapes, onions, and egg yolks.

Unfortunately, though these foods contain the nutrient, the actual concentrations are unpredictable. That's because the level of selenium in food depends on levels of selenium in the soil where the food was grown. Since soil's selenium levels vary from region to region, the broccoli raised in California is very likely to have a different concentration from the broccoli raised in New Jersey.

But there are also selenium supplements, and they are generally well absorbed. Selenomethionine and selenium-enriched yeast are good forms.

The greatest risks for those with selenium deficiency appear to be heart disease, cancer, and lowered immune function. Possibly the best evidence of this comes from a study of the residents of Nianning

County, China. There, the soil is deficient in selenium, and most of the food that's consumed in that area comes from the same region. Children and women of childbearing age who lived in this area had an abnormally high rate of a rare form of heart disease called Keshan disease. It was later discovered that the selenium deficiency made the children and women susceptible to a viral infection that caused the heart disease. Selenium supplementation significantly reduced the prevalence of this disease in these people.

DIETARY REFERENCE INTAKE

0 to 6 months: 10 mcg

6 to 12 months: 15 mcg

1 to 10 years: 20 to 30 mcg

11 to 18 years: 40 to 60 mcg

18+ years: 70 mcg

Pregnant/lactating: +5 mcg

I recommend a dosage of 200 mcg as an adult supplement. For those with viral infections, I recommend a dosage of 400 to 600 mcg daily.

Selenium is found in most multivitamin/multimineral supplements. If you're in gen-erally good health, strive for 200 to 300 mcg daily (most multivitamins contain 200 mcg). Don't take more, though, unless your physician recommends it, because high doses are potentially toxic. Alternatively, you could eat a handful of Brazil nuts (about six) each day—they're the richest natural source of selenium.

WHAT ARE THE SIDE EFFECTS?

Toxicity can occur with dosages above 900 mcg. A toxic dosage may interfere with sulfur metabolism, preventing you from absorbing sulfur in ways that are necessary for your health. Side effects of toxicity can include depression, nausea, vomiting, and nervousness. If you notice a garlic odor on your breath (even though you haven't been eating garlic) or if you perspire excessively, these symptoms might be a sign of toxicity. Also, you should be aware of any signs of hair loss or changes in the appearance of your fingernails.

Children and infants should not take separate selenium supplements unless instructed to do so by a physician. Some selenium may be included in multivitamin supplements for children, but this is acceptable since the controlled doses are very small.

SELENIUM

RECOMMENDATIONS FROM THE NATURAL PHYSICIAN FOR . . .

🐦 AIDS

People with AIDS tend to have low levels of selenium. That shortage puts a stress on the immune system, because selenium is needed to avoid oxidative stress. Selenium should be taken with other major antioxidants to optimize immune function.

🐦 CANCER

Several studies have shown that low levels of selenium are associated with an increased risk of cancer. This is especially true for stomach, esophageal, colon, rectal, and prostate cancers. Interestingly, garlic, onions, broccoli, and whole grains are recommended to prevent cancer, and all of them are good sources of selenium. As I've mentioned, selenium concentrations vary in these foods, but of course they also have other nutrients and phytochemicals that seem to help prevent cancer.

Smokers may benefit from increased selenium intake.

Some interesting research has been done on breast cancer and selenium. It is a component of glutathione peroxidase and thioredoxin reductase, which are powerful antioxidants made by the body.

Mutations in the BRCA1 genes are an established risk factor for breast cancer. Women of Jewish European heritage have a high risk of inheriting this gene, but it is also common in women of Mexican heritage. Men with BRCA1 gene mutations also have a higher-than-average risk of breast cancer. (**NOTE:** 1,600 men are diagnosed annually in the United States, compared to 200,000 women.) But once again, your genes don't have to be your fate.

The BRCA family of genes is involved in repairing damaged genes. Mutations can keep the BRCA genes from functioning properly. If they can't do a good job at repair, cell damage accumulates, increasing the risk of breast cancer. The good news is that a study in *Cancer Epidemiology, Biomarkers and Prevention* found that 690 mg of supplemental selenium, taken twice daily, normalized the rate of gene damage in women with BRCA1 mutations. Although the study was too short (only three months) to determine whether there would be a reduction in cancer risk, the findings are encouraging.

CATARACTS

Cataracts are the result of free-radical damage to the lens of the eye. Studies have shown that people with cataracts generally have low levels of selenium, so I recommend supplementation—both for prevention and treatment—to help provide antioxidant support.

HEART DISEASE

In his book *The Antioxidant Miracle*, Lester Packer states that research by Dr. Raymond Shamberger of the Cleveland Clinic has shown "that people who live in states with the lowest selenium content were three times more likely to die of heart disease than those who lived in states that were more selenium rich." The states that were found to have selenium-deficient soil include Connecticut, Illinois, Ohio, Oregon, Massachusetts, Rhode Island, New York, Pennsylvania, Indiana, Delaware, and District of Columbia. For people living in those areas, I would recommend 200 mcg of supplementation.

HEPATITIS C

I recommend selenium supplementation for those with hepatitis C to help keep this viral infection of the liver under control.

IMMUNITY

Selenium is important for the immune system, particularly the function of lymphocytes and macrophages. One study found that 200 mcg of selenium given to people with normal blood selenium levels resulted in a significant increase in immunity. It increases the ability of immune cells to kill cancer cells and various pathogens.

(continued)

PRENATAL INFANT GROWTH

Selenium appears to be important for proper fetal growth and is included in prenatal multivitamins.

RHEUMATOID ARTHRITIS

Selenium helps to reduce the production of inflammatory chemicals and supports the function of vitamin E in preventing joint inflammation and destruction.

SKIN

Selenium helps to prevent oxidative damage to the skin. It appears to help prevent skin cancer, but does not help once the cancer has already developed.

SUDDEN INFANT DEATH SYNDROME (SIDS)

Selenium deficiency may be a factor in sudden infant death syndrome. Breast-feeding mothers can provide adequate selenium for their infants by taking a multivitamin that contains this nutrient.

Sepia

Tiffany, a 25-year-old homemaker and mother of three, came to my office with a problem that seemed to be turning her life into an unrelenting torment: severe premenstrual syndrome. In fact, she was so upset by what was happening that she began crying as we talked.

She explained that she had always suffered from PMS, but the symptoms had become much more extreme since the birth of her last child. Her husband concurred. From his perspective, her PMS seemed to last the entire month.

Through her tears, she went on to confess that she had been struggling with depression and constantly felt tense and irritable, especially during the week before her menstrual cycle. What bothered her most was how short-tempered she had become with her kids, snapping at them for "normal" childhood mischief. She could not understand why she was acting this way, and her feelings of guilt were now beginning to overwhelm her.

Physically, Tiffany felt burned out. Her energy was at an all-time low. She experienced some improvement emotionally and physically after exercise, but the relief was temporary. She was constantly chilly, and some recent blood tests revealed that her thyroid function was close to being underactive. She also experienced extreme bloating just before the start of her menstrual flow.

All of this turmoil was putting a strain on her relationship with her husband. Not only was the communication between them breaking down, but Tiffany's libido had dwindled to almost nothing. She confessed that she actually felt repulsed by the thought of having sexual relations.

THE CRITICAL BALANCING ACT

As extreme and general as her condition sounded, however, when Tiffany mentioned one particular symptom—a craving for pickles—I realized immediately that her solution would be simple and specific: a homeopathic remedy, made from the ink of the cuttlefish, called sepia.

Very early in my clinical practice, I learned how valuable sepia can be for women. In fact, it has turned out to be one of the most effective natural therapies I've ever come across for treating hormone-related conditions. PMS, menopause, irregular menstrual cycles, ovarian cysts, fibrocystic breast syndrome, hormonal headaches, and many other conditions related to hormonal imbalance all respond wonderfully to sepia.

I explained to Tiffany that the underlying cause of her problem was most likely a hormonal imbalance. It's common for a woman's hormones to "get out of whack" after a pregnancy, and hormones are such powerful chemicals that when they fall out of balance, they can negatively affect the neurotransmitters of the brain, causing mental and emotional difficulties. Many women also find that the thyroid becomes sluggish after pregnancy, which can also cause problems with thinking, weight gain, chilliness, and constipation.

RELIEF AT LAST

The terrible feelings of guilt that had plagued Tiffany disappeared like vapor when she learned that she wasn't to blame for the way she had been feeling and behaving. Her problems clearly had a physical basis. We started her on sepia, and week-

---

DO YOU NEED SEPIA?

In homeopathy, the following signs often indicate that a person can be helped by taking sepia. If you have a few or more of these signs, it may be helpful.

Mental
- irritability
- sarcastic demeanor
- feeling better when alone, worse with company
- episodes of crying without knowing why they occur
- poor memory and concentration
- low libido

Head
- left-sided headaches
- cracking of lips

Digestive
- constipation
- hemorrhoids
- gas and bloating
- empty sensation in stomach not relieved by eating

- craving for sour foods (pickles, vinegar)

Urinary
- urine leak while laughing, sneezing, or exercising

Genital
- chronic vaginitis
- uterine prolapse
- genital warts
- scanty or irregular menses

Chest
- Loss of fullness and flatness in breasts

Skin
- dryness
- psoriasis

General
- chills
- symptoms grow worse between 2 p.m. and 5 p.m.
- problems ever since using the birth-control pill, pregnancy, miscarriage

by-week she saw improvement. First, her energy began to increase. After three weeks, her husband noticed that she was growing calmer. Her body temperature also slowly increased over time, indicating that her thyroid function was improving.

Last of all, her libido began to reassert itself. The last time I met with her, she had resumed sexual relations with her husband. She had not yet returned completely to normal in this part of her life, but she was headed in the right direction, and she described her marital relationship as "much better."

What pleased and relieved Tiffany most, however, was that she felt so much more patient with her children.

DOSAGE

I recommend starting with a lower potency of sepia, usually 6C taken two times daily, but many health-food stores and pharmacies carry the 30C potency—which is generally safe—that can be used as well. Try the remedy for one week. If you notice improvements in your mood, energy, or physical symptoms, continue daily use for another two weeks. Then use it only as needed.

WHAT ARE THE SIDE EFFECTS?

Occasionally, I see women who experience an initial aggravation of symptoms with this remedy if they take too high of a dosage or take it too frequently. If this happens, simply cut back to one dose every two or three days, or switch to a lower potency.

SEPIA

RECOMMENDATIONS FROM THE NATURAL PHYSICIAN FOR . . .

❧ BIRTH-CONTROL PILL SIDE EFFECTS

Sepia is an excellent medicine to use when a woman has stopped taking birth-control pills and begins to experience hormonal imbalances such as an irregular menstrual cycle, water retention, tender breasts, headaches, and irritability.

❧ BLADDER INFECTION

Sepia is one of the better remedies to use for women who are susceptible to chronic bladder infections. Hormonal changes, such as seen in menopause, lead to changes to the tissues of the bladder wall that can make a woman more susceptible to a bladder infection.

❧ DEPRESSION

Hormonal imbalance can lead to depression. Sepia can help improve depression that often accompanies irritability.

❧ FERTILITY

Hormone imbalance is one of the major causes of infertility, and sepia can be of benefit to women who have this problem. A history of miscarriages is an indication for using sepia.

❧ FIBROCYSTIC BREAST SYNDROME

Breast cysts that enlarge or become more tender on a cyclical basis can be helped by using sepia. I have seen this remedy clear up many cases within three to five months.

∼ GENITAL WARTS AND HERPES

Sepia is one of the more common remedies for the natural treatment of genital warts and genital herpes.

∼ HYPOTHYROID

I have found sepia to help a number of women with low thyroid function. Imbalances with estrogen and progesterone can suppress normal thyroid function. Sepia appears to balance estrogen and progesterone and thus free up thyroid activity.

∼ IRREGULAR MENSTRUAL CYCLES

Along with pulsatilla, sepia is one of the most common remedies for women who experience irregular menstrual cycles. It is also one of the most effective remedies for amenorrhea (no menstrual cycle).

∼ LIBIDO

One of the classic symptoms that can be helped by sepia is an unexplained dwindling of libido. Women requiring this remedy state they have developed a sexual aversion to their husband or partner but are not sure why. Taking the remedy does not increase libido immediately but usually helps after a few months of treatment.

∼ MENOPAUSE

Sepia is very effective in helping to reduce the symptoms of menopause, including hot flashes, irritability, depression, vaginal dryness, and low libido.

∼ MIGRAINE HEADACHES

Headaches that occur at about the same time each month, especially in relationship to the menstrual cycle, can show great improvement, or disappear altogether, after balancing the hormones by using sepia.

∼ NAUSEA DURING PREGNANCY

Sepia is an excellent remedy for ailments that occur during pregnancy, including nausea, which usually worsen during the time from 3 p.m. to 5 p.m. Craving for pickles or vinegar are indications for sepia, too.

∼ OVARIAN CYSTS

Many women needlessly suffer from ovarian cysts, which really is a condition of hormonal imbalance. Sepia is one of the main remedies for this condition (along with pulsatilla, lachesis, lycopodium, and folliculinum).

∼ PMS

Symptoms of extreme irritability, increased craving for chocolate or sweets, breast tenderness, and water retention can all be helped by sepia.

∼ PROSTATE ENLARGEMENT

This is one of the few male conditions that sepia can relieve. Symptoms include dribbling after urination and the sensation that "a ball is in the rectum."

∼ PSORIASIS

Sepia is one of the more common remedies to use for psoriasis. It has greatly helped several of my female patients.

∼ RAYNAUD'S SYNDROME

Hormones also influence blood circulation. Sepia is a good remedy for this condition (hands and feet that turn pale white or blue after brief exposure to cold), especially

(continued)

when other signs of hormonal imbalance are present. Raynaud's syndrome sometimes starts after taking birth-control pills or hormone replacement therapy (HRT).

🐦 SINUSITIS

Chronic sinusitis is another condition that sepia can alleviate.

🐦 URINARY INCONTINENCE

Women requiring sepia can sometimes leak urine while laughing, sneezing, or exercising. I have found this remedy works especially well for women who develop incontinence during menopause.

🐦 UTERINE PROLAPSE

Sagging of the uterus occurs when the ligaments that hold it in place become too lax, usually as a result of hormonal changes that occur after pregnancy or during menopause. Sepia can help prevent this problem.

🐦 VAGINITIS

Vaginitis, characterized by a white, offensively odorous discharge, can be helped by sepia, especially when the condition is chronic. Vaginal dryness during or after menopause is another indication for sepia.

🐦 VARICOSE VEINS

I have seen sepia help cases of varicose veins that became a problem during menopause.

Silicon

"I can't believe it, my hair and nails have been brittle for years, and now after just a month on this silicon supplement you recommended I can notice a huge improvement," were the words of Tracy, a 47-year-old homemaker.

Silicon, also referred to as silica or silicon dioxide, is a trace mineral that is somewhat of a nutritional secret in the medical world. It plays a role in the formation of hair, bones, skin, cartilage, tendons, nails, and healthy artery walls. Once silicon is consumed, it is converted in the digestive tract to orthosilicic acid, which increases its absorption. It is found in several foods, including whole grains, vegetables, fruits (such as bananas and raisins), lentils, beans, coffee, beer, and unfiltered drinking water. The average intake of silicon in adults is 14 to 21 mg per day. Do note that silicon is different than silicone, a chemical mixture used to make breast implants and other medical devices.

Studies show silicon improves bone formation and hair quality.

DOSAGE

A preventative dose for good health maintenance is 300 to 500 mcg silicon daily. For brittle hair, take 10 mg silicon a day in the form of choline-stabilized orthosilicic acid. Those with osteoporosis should take 6 to 12 mg daily.

WHAT ARE THE SIDE EFFECTS?

Silicon appears quite safe. Silicon supplements should be avoided by those with a history of silicon-containing kidney stones and people with chronic kidney disease. Supplementation has not been studied in pregnant or nursing women.

SILICON

RECOMMENDATIONS FROM THE NATURAL PHYSICIAN FOR . . .

❧ HAIR QUALITY

I have found silicon helps many men and women with brittle hair as well as hair thinning. In a study reported in *Archives of Dermatological Research*, for nine months 48 women with fine hair were given 10 mg silicon a day orally in the form of choline-stabilized orthosilicic acid beadlets, or they were given a placebo. Hair quality and tensile (strength) properties were evaluated before and after treatment. The supplementation of silicon had a positive effect on hair thickness, and tensile strength, including elasticity as well as break load.

❧ OSTEOPOROSIS

A study in the *Journal of Bone and Mineral Research* demonstrated that the intake of silicon in the diet correlated positively and significantly with bone density at all hip sites in men and premenopausal women, but not in postmenopausal women.

Also, research has demonstrated that supplementing with silicon improved several markers that reflect bone and connective tissue breakdown. The study investigated the effect over 12 months of a low dose of supplemental silicon on markers of bone turnover and bone mineral density in 114 women with osteopenia (mild bone loss) or osteoporosis. The women were divided into four groups. All received 1,000 mg calcium and 800 IU vitamin D3 (cholecalciferol) each day. Three of the groups also took supplements of 3 mg, 6 mg, or 12 mg of a usable form of silicon, sold as Biosil. Researchers found the silicon supplement enhanced the benefits of the calcium and vitamin D supplementation. Although bone-mineral density of the spine did not change significantly, a subgroup of 81 women who took 6 mg Biosil per day and whose thighbone density score was lower than average at the start of the study showed significant thighbone density improvements. For people with low bone mineral density and those at risk for osteoporosis—which includes people who have a strong family history of osteoporosis, thin bones, or a history of eating disorders, as well as those who have used steroids (prednisone) for long periods or who smoke—I recommend a supplement of 6 to 12 mg silicon daily in addition to calcium, magnesium, vitamin D, B vitamins, strontium, vitamin K, and essential fatty acids, all of which support bone metabolism.

Sitz Bath

"I'll get started on the diet and medicines you prescribed right away. Is there anything else I should do?" asked Bill, a 54-year-old high school teacher, who came to see me for his hemorrhoids.

"Yes, there is," I said, "and it will help give you some immediate relief. I want you to take a sitz bath."

"A sitz bath? I haven't heard that term since I was a teenager," replied Bill.

"Some of these old therapies are the most effective," I responded. "Plus, it doesn't cost you anything."

"I like that part. How do I do this sitz bath?" asked Bill.

"It's pretty simple."

I explained that I was actually recommending a hot sitz bath alternated with a cold one—so he would need two plastic or metal tubs, both large enough to sit in comfortably.

"Fill one tub with hot water—between 100 and 106 degrees Fahrenheit—but make sure it's not too hot—just tolerable. Fill the second tub with cold water—as cold as you can stand."

I recommended that he sit in the hot tub for three to five minutes, then sit in the cold bath for about thirty seconds. "Do this three or four times. Make sure the last tub you are in is the cold one. Then get out and dry off."

I had an additional recommendation as well. "Add an ounce of witch hazel to the water in each tub."

"I'm not looking forward to that cold tub," said Bill.

"I hear you; but it's the cold that really helps improve the circulation to the hemorrhoids and relieves a lot of the congestion and pain. So it is the more important part of the treatment."

"How many times should I do this?" asked Bill.

"Take the sitz bath every day for the next week, and then you should take two to three a week for a month after that."

Bill called, three days later, to tell me that the burning pain from his hemorrhoids had improved. He also mentioned that the bleeding had stopped after the second treatment.

SOOTHING WATER

The alternating sitz bath is a form of hydrotherapy. Using water as a medium to carry heat or cold, one can manipulate circulation to the pelvis and organs of the lower abdomen. With increased blood flow to this area, you're also bringing in the immune cells and nutrients that are carried in the blood—all of which helps to promote healing. Pain and inflammation are reduced as circulation improves.

Of course, you can try a single-temperature sitz bath, using either hot or cold water.

DOSAGE

For acute conditions, take a sitz bath one to two times daily. For chronic conditions, sitz baths can be taken two to seven times a week. I recommend resting after the sitz bath. You'll probably want to avoid physical activity for an hour or two afterward, until blood flow returns to normal. Purchase a plastic sitz bathtub that is placed on the toilet (available at drugstores). These are contoured to focus circulation on the buttocks. Next best thing: the bathtub. Fill the tub with water high enough to reach just under the navel while you are seated.

How to do it: Use a thermometer to determine water temperature. To alternate between warm and cold water, have two buckets of water ready or use both the purchased sitz bath and the bathtub. See the chart below for the best type of sitz bath for your condition.

WHAT ARE THE SIDE EFFECTS?

Sitz baths are as safe as regular baths. Of course, you need to be careful getting in and out of the tubs—and anyone who needs assistance should have a partner or helper nearby.

If you have diabetes, heart disease, or high blood pressure, speak to your doctor before taking a sitz bath because it can cause changes in blood pressure, pulse, or glucose levels.

SITZ BATH

RECOMMENDATIONS FROM THE NATURAL PHYSICIAN FOR . . .

Abdominal or Uterine Pain, Low Back Pain, Insomnia, Hemorrhoids, Muscle Spasms

Add 2 cups of Epsom salt.

Warm treatment: Water 106°F to 110°F, 5 to 8 minutes, one to two times daily.

Acute Bladder Infections, Itchy Rectum, Acute Urinary Tract Infection

Lukewarm treatment: Water 92°F to 97°F, 15 minutes to one hour (depending on your comfort level), one to two times daily.

Constipation, Prostate Enlargement, Uterus or Rectum Prolapse

Cold treatment: Water 55°F to 75°F, 5 to 8 minutes, one to two times daily.

Vaginal Infections, Prostatitis, Headache, Postpartum Recovery, Chronic Urinary Tract Infection

Alternating treatment: Warm water for 3 to 5 minutes followed by 30 to 60 seconds in cold. Repeat three times daily.

Soy

Soy (*Glycine max*) is a prime example of good eating that's good medicine. It's a staple of many diets throughout Southeast Asia, and as its many health properties are being uncovered and cooks are using it in more recipes, I find more soy sneaking into supermarkets as well as health-food stores. It comes in many forms—from the newly popular soy burgers in many varieties and flavors to the traditional soybean product, tofu, which has been part of Asian diets for thousands of years.

I recommend soy to my patients to prevent heart disease, because there's no question that it lowers LDLs, the "bad" kind of cholesterol. But I also recommend it because soy can help prevent some kinds of cancer and the onset of osteoporosis or delay its progress. Soy also reduces menopausal hot flashes and relieves PMS. It can help increase levels of the good bacteria *Bifidobacteria*, too.

PEAS IN A POD

A member of the pea family—and, therefore, a legume—the soybean is native to Southeastern Asia. More than 2,500 different varieties are cultivated.

Soybeans are rich in calcium, iron, zinc, B vitamins, and fiber. They are a great source of protein. Commercial soy foods such as tofu, as well as most of the soy-based products sold in supermarkets, are highly digestible.

Soy is a staple of the Chinese diet and has been used in that culture as a food and medicine for thousands of years. The Chinese discovered how to ferment soy to make it digestible, and it became a staple throughout Korea, Japan, and Southeast Asia.

Soy arrived in Europe in the 1700s; it was in the United States by the 1800s, brought by Chinese immigrants. It was also popular among Seventh-Day Adventists, who were largely vegetarian. Dr. Harvey Kellogg (founder of Kellogg's cereals) became an advocate of soy foods and recommended that people eat soy in place of meat products.

FRESH FROM THE FERMENT

Soy foods come in many different forms. Among the traditional fermented soy foods are tempeh and miso, as well as the now-common tofu. These represent the forms of soy that are used in population studies where researchers try to pinpoint the dietary benefits of soybeans.

Another popular food product—though not in the "fermented" category—is soy milk. If you have a problem with the lactose in cow's milk, you can safely drink soy milk without any side effects, so it's particularly appealing to people who are lactose intolerant. With calcium-enriched soy milk avail-able, soy milk has nearly all the benefits with none of the lactose problems that come with "regular" milk.

Soy protein powders (isolates) are used by people looking for nonanimal protein sources. Soy protein powder is also a popular supplement for athletes and for anyone who's active. It helps aid muscle recovery and acts as an energy source.

Roasted soy nuts and toasted soy flour are also popular.

ALL ABOUT ISOFLAVONES

Soy isoflavones are unique components that have caught the attention of researchers and the media. Chemically, isoflavones resemble the hormone estrogen. Thus, they are referred to as phytoestrogens (plant estrogens). But even though they resemble powerful hormones, the plant forms are much weaker, carrying about one-thousandth the potency of estrogen.

This is thought to be a good thing. Soy isoflavones may block strong or toxic estrogens from binding to receptor sites on hormone-dependent tissues such as the breast, uterus, and prostate. By occupying these sites and effectively taking the place of the more powerful forms, the phytoestrogens help prevent cancer growth.

Isoflavones, which are available in supplement form as well as in foods, are key compounds in decreasing cholesterol levels.

DOSAGE

Fermented soy foods should be eaten liberally for their health-protective qualities. Next best? Take fermented soy protein powders that have standardized isoflavone content and drink plenty of soy milk.

You also have a third option, which is getting isoflavone capsule supplements.

Though the supplements aren't as good a source as food, this may be the most practical way to increase intake of soy isoflavones (although the least-studied). Supplements are available in 50-mg capsules, and the usual dosage is 50 to 150 mg daily.

Look for foods and supplements that are non-gmo (meaning they are not genetically engineered). Also, look for soy products that list the isoflavone content. Not all of them do. (For example, some soy protein isolates have had the isoflavones removed by alcohol extraction.) There are other healthful components in soy, but we know that isoflavones are important active substances, so you want to make sure they're included in whatever soy product you're buying.

WHAT ARE THE SIDE EFFECTS?

Some people have a sensitivity reaction to soy, which can cause digestive upset. For some people, the side effect is preventable, as long as they take digestive enzymes before eating a meal that has soy in it—or even during the meal.

I have found that some children's eczema and recurring ear infections are brought on or worsened by soy products.

Raw soy beans (soy flour, or protein powders made from raw or unfermented or unroasted soybeans) may inhibit thyroid function, although this has not been proven in human studies.

There is speculation that the isoflavones in soy formula for infants and children may be a problem, but the American Academy of Pediatrics still endorses the use of the formula. More research will be needed to determine what problems, if any, the formula may cause. Thus far the published studies have not shown any problems. Moderate intake appears to be fine. For women with a history of breast cancer or family history of breast cancer, soy foods or supplements have not been shown to be a problem. Consult with your oncologist about optimal intake in your situation.

SOY

RECOMMENDATIONS FROM THE NATURAL PHYSICIAN FOR . . .

❧ CANCER

Many researchers feel that soy as a food works wonders to prevent many different forms of cancer. The death rate among women in China who have breast cancer is one-fifth what it is in the United States. The mortality from cancer in Japan is one quarter of the United States', and it's just one-tenth in Korea.

People in these countries eat many other plant foods that also account for the decreased susceptibility. But when researchers have focused on soy, they've found that it seems to be a key ingredient in preventing death from breast cancer in those countries.

People in Japan often consume an average of 200 mg of isoflavones daily as compared with the 1 to 3 mg Americans consume. Interestingly, in the populations of people who have moved from Japan to the United States, rates of cancer and prostate cancer have soared toward the same levels as Americans who have been raised on the classic Western diet comprised of many high-fat foods and fewer

(continued)

plant foods. Clearly, there is a strong dietary connection.

Many epidemiological studies suggest that soy as a food has a cancer-prevention effect. Soy consumption is associated with a decreased risk of breast, colon, rectum, lung, prostate, and stomach cancers.

Isoflavones seem to be the important cancer-preventing compounds. They have been shown to possess potent antioxidant activity and hormone-balancing qualities, both of which are believed to be important in preventing cancer.

Soybeans also contain protease inhibitors, and although most are lost through cooking, the small amount left appears to protect cell DNA from damage.

In addition, soy contains other potential anticancer compounds such as phytosterols, saponins, and phenolic acids.

While the significance of diet is clearly evident, however, we don't know much about the effectiveness of soy isoflavone supplements. I haven't seen any conclusive information about whether soy isoflavone supplements will prevent cancer, and we still haven't determined whether they're helpful in treating the disease.

✒ CHOLESTEROL AND HEART DISEASE

Soy has been shown to lower total cholesterol and LDL cholesterol, whether eaten as a food or taken in the form of isolated isoflavone supplements. As a matter of fact, the FDA approved the claim by manufacturers that a food containing 6.25 g of soy protein had cardiovascular benefits. It was found that 25 to 50 g of soy protein consumed on a daily basis can reduce cholesterol levels.

An analysis of 29 studies found that just 31 to 47 g of isolated soy protein or texturized soy protein decreased total cholesterol by 9% and LDL cholesterol by 13%.

✒ DIABETES

A study of postmenopausal women with type 2 diabetes found that taking 30 g of soy protein and 132 mg of isoflavones daily for 12 weeks lowered fasting insulin levels and hemoglobin A1c levels.

✒ KIDNEY DISEASE

Soy protein has been shown to reduce the amount of protein in the urine of those with kidney disease.

✒ MENOPAUSE

Soy is helpful for some women in reducing hot flashes and vaginal dryness. In one study, women were given 160 mg of isoflavones daily for three months. They experienced a significant reduction in their menopausal hot flashes and other menopausal symptoms.

✒ OSTEOPOROSIS

One study of postmenopausal women found that soy protein with high isoflavone content improved bone mineral density in the lumbar spine. In another study Chinese researchers analyzed nine studies involving 432 menopausal women, looking at the effect of *soy isoflavones* (soy-derived compounds that have estrogen-like effects) on bone breakdown and bone formation, as measured by markers in urine and blood. Women (especially Asians) who consumed as little as 90 mg daily of soy isoflavones in supplement form showed decreases in bone breakdown and increases in new bone formation.

Also, soy is a protein source that does not lead to urinary calcium excretion, as does protein from animal foods.

Spirulina

The longer I practice natural medicine, the more I am impressed with the visible benefits of some specific nutritional supplements. From my experience with patients, and based on nutritional studies, there is no doubt that most people benefit from taking vitamins and minerals. Not only can a vitamin or mineral supplement help prevent deficiencies, it can also help to therapeutically treat existing conditions.

However, we still have a lot to learn about the bioavailability and absorption of the active components in these supplements. How much of the active or beneficial components are actually taken into the body? How quickly can we experience the benefits? We don't have much information about nutrient interactions. That is, we still have to determine what are the positive and negative interactions when certain vitamins and minerals are combined together.

But we do have some limited knowledge. For example, we know that vitamin C enhances iron absorption. We also know that iron hinders calcium absorption. So if you're taking a supplement that's high in iron, it makes sense that you'd also try to get more vitamin C to make sure you absorb as much iron as possible.

But while we're continuing to learn more about the vitamins and minerals we need—and how best to get them—we also know that many of the processes of absorption are almost infinitely complex. Rather than trying to "create" the perfect supplement, or the exact mix of vitamins, minerals, enzymes, and phytonutrients, we also need to consider whole foods for their healing powers.

One potent whole food actually comes in supplement form—and it's called spirulina. This is called a whole food supplement because the actual plant itself, rather than its chemical or nutrient components, are contained in the supplement pill, capsule, powder, or other form. In the case of spirulina, nature seems to have provided a particular combination of nutrients and disease-fighting substances that is greater than the sum of its parts. That is, we don't know the most active or effective ingredients in this whole-food supplement, but we do know that it carries health benefits that are definitely worth enjoying.

SINK AND SWIM

Spirulina (rhymes with "ballerina"), is a blue-green algae that grows wild in warm-water alkaline volcanic lakes. It has long been a staple food for Mexicans going back to Aztec civilization. The two most common species used for human consumption include *Spirulina maxima* and *Spirulina platensis.*

Spirulina is also an important food for people in Eastern and Central Africa. For example, the people in the nation of Chad in Africa consume 9 to 13 g of spirulina in each meal.

Today, commercial algae farms cultivate spirulina that is exported to millions of people in more than 70 countries. The United States is the world's largest producer of spirulina followed by Thailand, India, and China.

Spirulina has great nutritional value. Between 62% and 71% of the plant is comprised of amino acids, and all are the essential amino acids. It is also a remarkable source of protein, and the protein is highly bioavailable, meaning it can be readily absorbed in the body with no harmful effects.

Spirulina contains beta carotene and a blend of the other carotenoids, as well as chlorophyll and the essential fatty acid GLA. It's also said to be the world's richest source of vitamin B12.

MOODY BLUE

One important component is phycocyanin, a phytonutrient that gives spirulina its dark blue-green color. Phycocyanin has been shown in animal studies to stimulate the production of red blood cells.

The probable reason why the bioabsorption is so great is that spirulina contains a soft cell wall composed of proteins and complex sugars that can be easily digested.

More than 100 published scientific references help support the case for the health benefits of spirulina. Some studies demonstrate that spirulina seems to possess anticancer effects and antiviral properties. Also, animal studies show that it is a powerful tonic for the immune system.

Spirulina activates many of the different immune cells, including macrophages, T-cells, B-cells, and natural killer cells. It also activates the organs involved with immune function such as the spleen, liver, bone marrow, lymph nodes, tonsils, and thymus gland. Naturopathic physicians often recommend it to treat high cholesterol, hypertension, and diabetes. It's also a popular product for detoxification.

Like other blue-green algae, spirulina is thought to help bind heavy metals, which is necessary before they can be excreted out of the body. In addition, it has been shown to increase the presence of beneficial bacteria such as *Lactobacillus* and *Bifidus* by acting as a "food" for these friendly flora.

Spirulina is also an important food supplement for children. It is used to prevent blindness in malnourished children. A recognized treatment for radiation sickness, it was given to children in the area of Chernobyl after the nuclear reactor.

DOSAGE

Spirulina comes in many different forms: capsules, tablets, flakes, and powders. The average intake for adults is 2,000 to 3,000 mg per day. The typical children's dosage is 500 to 1,500 mg daily. I often recommend spirulina in a formula with other "green superfoods" such as wheatgrass and chlorella.

WHAT ARE THE SIDE EFFECTS?

The safety of spirulina has been well researched. There have been extensive safety studies with animals and humans since the 1970s. It was found to have no toxic side effects.

Spirulina is well tolerated with only occasional reports of allergies or sensitivity reactions. Reputable companies make sure the spirulina has not been taken from water where they might have absorbed heavy metals such as lead, mercury, aluminum, and arsenic. Good quality products are also tested to make sure the spirulina has not been contaminated by algal toxins from other blue-green algae.

Since raw material suppliers cultivate their own spirulina, they can control and test for heavy metals and algal toxins.

Spirulina does not increase the flare-ups of gout in people who are susceptible. That's surprising, because spirulina is high in nucleic acids and protein—which, theoretically, increase the flow of uric acid, one of the contributing factors in gout attacks. But even when spirulina is consumed in high dosages (such as 50 g a day), it doesn't cause problems for people who have gout.

SPIRULINA

RECOMMENDATIONS FROM THE NATURAL PHYSICIAN FOR . . .

ANEMIA

Anemia is the deficiency of red blood cells. It can have various causes such as blood loss; insufficient bone-marrow production; or deficiencies of B12, folic acid, or iron. Phycocyanin, a phytonutrient found in spirulina, has been shown in animal studies to stimulate production of stem cells by the bone marrow. Stem cells are immature cells, which later mature into red and white blood cells.

Spirulina also contains B12. If absorption is sufficient, supplementing with spirulina may help prevent B12-deficiency anemia, which is a concern for strict vegetarians.

CANCER

Spirulina and its extracts have been shown to have anticancer activity in animal studies. Spirulina stimulates natural killer cells and similar anti-immune components of the immune system that can help fight cancer cells. Laboratory studies also show that spirulina polysaccharides can work to repair genetic material that has been damaged from toxins or from radiation.

It may also help people who have mouth cancer. In one study, tobacco chewers who had a type of mouth disease called oral leukoplakia were given 1 g a day of spirulina for one year.

Nearly half of those who took the supplement showed marked improvement, while only three out of 43 in the non-supplement group had any reversal of symptoms.

CHOLESTEROL

Animal and human studies have shown spirulina to reduce high cholesterol. A study looked at the effect of spirulina supplementation on 30 healthy men with high levels of cholesterol, triglyceride, and LDL. One group of men consumed 4.2 g daily for eight weeks and researchers found a 4.5% decrease in cholesterol levels. For such a short period of time, that is considered to be a significant decrease in cholesterol.

DETOXIFICATION

I have found spirulina to be a great supplement for helping patients with detoxification. The protein content also helps to stabilize blood-sugar.

IMMUNITY

As mentioned, spirulina stimulates many components of the immune system. Special extracts of spirulina have also shown potent antiviral activity. One type of spirulina, known as *Spirulina platensis*, was shown to inhibit the HIV virus (HIV-1) in a test-tube study. Another study found a spirulina extract known as Calcium Spirulan inhibited the replication of several viruses. Among the viruses that it helped control were herpes simplex type 1, cytomegalovirus, measles, mumps, influenza A, and HIV-1.

(continued)

🐟 MALNOURISHMENT AND VITAMIN A DEFICIENCY

Many authorities have recommended that spirulina be used on a large scale to combat world hunger because of its good nutritional value and cost effectiveness. Spirulina supplementation with children has been studied since the early 1970s with impressive results.

In a one-year program, 5,000 preschool children who lived in a rural area near Madras, India, were fed spirulina regularly. At the start of the program, all the children had the symptom of advanced vitamin A deficiency known as Bitot's spots. (This is a superficial foamy patch on the eye conjunctiva that mainly occurs in advanced vitamin A deficiency). During the program, the children consumed 1 g of spirulina daily for at least 150 days. In many of the children, the Bitot's spots went away, indicating the vitamin A deficiency had been corrected. Whereas 80% of the children had the spots at the beginning of the program, only 10% showed any sign of Bitot's spots by the time the program was ended.

This is an important finding, as vitamin A deficiency is the leading cause of blindness, and among children who have severe vitamin A deficiency, the death rate can be as high as 50%.

In another study of 400 school children, researchers found that spirulina increased their vitamin A status to the same level as those who were administered pure vitamin A. Beta carotene (and perhaps some of the other carotenoids) from spirulina have a high bioavailability and are converted to vitamin A very effectively. Because spirulina contains essential amino acids—which few plant foods do—you get the vitamin A as well as the amino acids, all in one.

🐟 RADIATION POISONING

As I've mentioned, spirulina was used to treat the children of Chernobyl who were suffering from radiation sickness as the result of eating food grown on radioactive soil. Since radiation sickness can produce bone-marrow damage, children with the sickness cannot produce enough red blood cells. They have a deficient immune system because the white blood cells are depleted, but along with that, they also become anemic because of the underproduction of red blood cells. This causes a susceptibility to allergies, infections, and cancer.

Remarkably, spirulina stimulates the production of both red and white blood cells. Children fed 5 g of spirulina tablets daily have been shown to make dramatic recoveries, a striking contrast to the children who did not have access to spirulina.

Stevia

Stevia rebaudiana (stevia) has been a popular natural sweetener in the US health-food industry for a long time. It is up to 300 times sweeter than sugar and has almost no calories. This plant grows in the rain forests of Brazil and Paraguay, as well as in Japan, Korea, Thailand, and China. The Guarani Indians of Paraguay have used stevia leaves for centuries to sweeten teas and medicinal potions, in addition to chewing it simply for pleasure. In the mid-1970s, stevia became popular in Japan as a tabletop sweetener, as well as an ingredient in a variety of food products. Stevia is available as a dietary supplement in the United States and Canada, and it sells very well in health-food stores. Interestingly, the world's largest soda pop companies are now using stevia as a "natural sweetener" in their products.

Dosage

Stevia is available in liquid, powder, and tablet form. To sweeten an eight-ounce beverage, such as coffee, tea, or lemonade, you need to use only one tablet, or a pinch of the powder, or 3 to 5 drops of the liquid. However, follow directions on the label, as the concentration and potency varies depending on the product. Stevia can also be used in cooking. Some bakers find that it works best when mixed with other natural sweeteners, such as honey, barley malt, lo han, and xylitol.

What Are the Side Effects?

Stevia contains sweetening substances known as steviol glycosides. The main constituent of these glycosides responsible for the sweet taste is rebaudioside A. Rebaudioside A has "generally recognized as safe" status in the United States for use as a sweetener for foods. No significant adverse effects have been found with stevia.

STEVIA
Recommendations from the Natural Physician for . . .

ᔋᐁ CAVITY PREVENTION

In my opinion, stevia is a better substance to use for sweetening products, instead of sugar, if you wish to prevent cavities.

ᔋᐁ DIABETES

My patients with diabetes report that stevia has no detrimental effects on their blood-sugar readings. In fact, some evidence suggests that stevia can reduce blood-sugar levels in people with type 2 diabetes.

ᔋᐁ HIGH BLOOD PRESSURE

Preliminary research demonstrates that stevia may reduce blood pressure in people with hypertension.

ᔋᐁ WEIGHT LOSS AND OBESITY

The most obvious benefit of stevia is that it has few calories compared to sugar. This makes it a popular product for those working to lose weight.

St. John's Wort

"I've been on Prozac for over a year now. I seem to be doing fine. I have my moments where I feel depressed, but don't we all?" said Tony, a 49-year-old money manager.

"Yes, that's part of life," I replied.

"My wife and I are concerned about side effects from Prozac. She feels it's the reason why my libido is so low. I'm worried about that as well as what I have read in the papers. I've heard it can sometimes cause suicidal depression!"

"Do you feel suicidal at times?" I asked.

"No, that was never a problem," replied Tony.

Then I asked, "Have you talked to your other doctor about getting off the Prozac?"

"Sort of. I brought it up and he kind of brushed me off, saying if I'm feeling good why go off it."

"Interesting. So you want to get off the Prozac?" I asked.

"Yes, I feel like this is a good time. Have you gotten other patients off Prozac?" asked Tony.

"I sure have." I went on to tell him how some patients were able to "wean themselves" off Prozac by using St. John's wort (*Hypericum perforatum*).

"I was going to ask you about that," said Tony. "My friend Tim says that St. John's wort works better than drugs to prevent depression."

"For some people it does. The other bonus is that it doesn't have the side effects like reduced libido," I replied.

"My wife will be happy when she hears that," said Tony with a smile.

I then explained that it is very important that he be monitored closely while switching over from the Prozac. Stopping the Prozac too rapidly could cause a rebound effect, sending him into very severe depression as his brain is deprived of the accustomed medication.

Tony was weaned off the Prozac over the next two months. It turned out to be a smooth transition for him. To prevent a recurrence of his depression, I also recommended he see a counselor to address underlying emotional problems. I felt these were at the root of his history of depression.

AN ANCIENT HERBAL HEALER

North Americans have been using St. John's wort for the treatment of mild to moderate depression for the past 15 years. This trend began when clinical research from Germany was publicized. Supplement companies helped to broadcast the information, which was readily picked up in the media. Today, St. John's wort is one of the top 10 bestselling herbs in the United States. In Germany, St. John's wort outsells pharmaceutical antidepressants.

More than 30 clinical studies have been done on St. John's wort, and several more are still underway, including some under the auspices of the National Institutes of Health.

St. John's wort is grown in many different areas, including North Africa, Europe, western Asia, Canada, Australia, China, and the United States (especially northern California and southern Oregon). The characteristic bright yellow flowers contain a red pigment, known as hypericin, which is one of the active constituents. When you get a "standardized" preparation of St. John's wort, it is standardized to hypericin. (That is, the preparation contains the percentage of hypericin that's stated on the label.)

The Latin translation of hypericum means "over an apparition." This refers to the belief that the scent of the herb would drive away evil spirits. Ancient Europeans believed that St. John's wort protected one against evil and disease.

Physicians in ancient times, such as Hippocrates and Dioscorides, used St. John's wort for depression as well as for burns, wounds, sciatica, ulcers, and poisonous reptile bites.

BACK TO THE ORIGINS

The name "St. John's wort" is believed to come from Christian tradition. There are different theories as to how the name came about. One is that the plant blooms around St. John's Day, which is June 24. Another is that red spots appeared on the leaves during the anniversary of St. John's beheading. These were thought to symbolize his blood. Yet another is that if you put the herb under your pillow, St. John would appear in a dream and bless you, and prevent a loved one from dying the following year.

As with many herbs, St. John's wort appears to have many different active constituents. Early research focused on the standardization of products to hypericin. In recent years there has been a movement toward the standardization to another active substance, hyperforin.

It is also believed that flavonoids play an important role in the antidepressant action of this herb. Other important constituents include essential oils and pseudohypericin.

At least one study has shown that a combination of constituents is responsible for the potent antidepressive effect. It is interesting to note that isolated extracts of hypericin and hyperforin are not effective antidepressants by themselves. Both need to be present, as they are in St. John's wort.

St. John's wort appears to act like SSRI (selective serotonin reuptake inhibitors) antidepressants such as Prozac and Zoloft, as well as tricyclic antidepressants, such as amitryptiline and imipramine. It causes an increase in the neurotransmitter serotonin, a powerful chemical that is responsible for good moods. It has also been shown that St. John's wort increases the neurotransmitters dopamine and norepinephrine, which are also responsible for moods.

There are studies that have suggested that St. John's wort affects GABA receptor sites (a neurotransmitter known for its calming effect) and lowers the stress hormone cortisol.

DOSAGE

For the treatment of depression, I recommend 300 mg of an extract to be taken three times daily. I recommend a product containing 3% to 5% hyperforin and 0.3%

hypericin. People usually notice improvement within two to six weeks.

The tincture can also be used. I recommend taking 30 drops (approximately 0.5 mL) three times daily.

The oil is used topically for skin conditions.

WHAT ARE THE SIDE EFFECTS?

St. John's wort has a good safety rating. However, one study reported that some people experienced digestive upset, fatigue, restlessness, and allergic reactions using St. John's wort extract.

A number of researchers have reported that St. John's wort may cause the skin to be sensitive to light. There have been a few reports of people's skin burning more easily, or of their eyes becoming more sensitive to light. I don't think it is a side effect to be overly worried about. If you have light skin, be more cautious in the sun; cover up with light clothing, and wear a hat as well as sunglasses.

I do not recommend St. John's wort for children unless it is used with the guidance of a doctor. There have been no studies done on children. However, if a child does need additional therapy beyond counseling, then St. John's wort seems like a better choice to me than a pharmaceutical antidepressant.

It is best to avoid this herb during pregnancy and while breast-feeding.

Do not combine St. John's wort with your pharmaceutical antidepressant as it could potentially lead to serious side effects. You need to be gradually weaned off your medication under a doctor's care.

Also, this herb should not be used if you are using the following medications: digoxin, cyclosporine, theophylline, warfarin, or the AIDS drug Indinavir.

ST. JOHN'S WORT

RECOMMENDATIONS FROM THE NATURAL PHYSICIAN FOR . . .

ANXIETY

St. John's wort has been found to be as effective as pharmaceuticals in treating anxiety.

BRUISES, BURNS, AND WOUNDS

St. John's wort has a long history of use for the treatment of bruises, burns, and wounds. The oil is applied topically and provides soothing relief as well as prevents secondary bacterial infections. It also helps to relieve nerve injuries and nerve pain. European herbalists also use the oil for the treatment of eczema.

DEPRESSION

St. John's wort has been the subject of some of the best and most intensive clinical and scientific research among all the herbs in the world. I find that it is helpful in about 70% of people who take it for depression. This is quite a high response rate, whether a pharmaceutical or natural therapy is used. In a review of 23 European clinical studies involving 1,700 patients, researchers found that St. John's wort was significantly more effective than placebo and equally as effective as standard drug therapy for mild to moderate depression.

You may have read in the past a headline stating that St. John's wort is ineffective for depression. This is not true. The study published in the *Journal of the American Medical Association* looked at the effect of this herb in a population of people with severe depression. This is a condition that's hard to treat with any therapy. The fact is that most studies with

St. John's wort have involved people afflicted with mild to moderate depression for which it comes out highly effective. Interestingly, a 2009 review involving a summary of studies including 18 placebo-controlled studies and more than 5,000 people found St. John's wort safe and effective for cases of severe depression.

Several studies have shown comparable effects when St. John's wort has gone head-to-head with pharmaceutical antidepressants. This includes two studies with the antidepressant imipramine. In the first study people took either 900 mg of St. John's wort or 75 mg of imipramine per day for six weeks. The St. John's wort users had a slightly better improvement and experienced fewer and milder side effects as compared with the imipramine group.

A similar study compared the two therapies but used double the amount of dosages. This study also looked at people with moderate to severe depression. People took either 1,800 mg of St. John's wort or 150 mg of imipramine for six weeks. Improvements in depression were about equal. Again, side effects were more common in those taking imipramine. This study was important because it examined people with moderate to severe depression. Most studies have been done on people with mild to moderate depression. Further studies will clarify the value of St. John's wort for severe depression.

Overall, I would recommend that doctors start antidepressant therapy with St. John's wort instead of with pharmaceutical antidepressants. My reasoning for this is that St. John's wort has proven to have less risk of side effects. For people who do not respond to adequate trials and dosages of St. John's wort, pharmaceutical treatment can be considered.

Like pharmaceutical medications, St. John's wort works most effectively when combined with counseling, hormone balancing, nutritional therapy, exercise, and other holistic therapies that treat the underlying cause of the depression.

Some people have been diagnosed with "genetic depression" and told they must take pharmaceutical antidepressants, that natural therapies would not be strong enough. I have found that St. John's wort and other natural therapies are strong enough for "genetic depression."

❧ PMS

One study found that St. John's wort improved symptoms of PMS by apprioximately 50% in some women.

❧ MENOPAUSE

The combination of black cohosh and St. John's wort has been shown in one study to help menopausal symptoms.

❧ SEASONAL AFFECTIVE DISORDER (SAD)

This is a condition where people experience depression and mood changes as the result of reduced light exposure during the winter. One small study showed that people who took St. John's wort in combination with either bright light or dim light therapy experienced significant improvement in SAD.

❧ VIRAL INFECTIONS

The constituents hypericin and pseudo-hypericin have shown in test-tube studies to have strong antiviral activity against herpes simplex virus—both type 1 (mouth) and type 2 (genital)—as well as influenza virus A and B, and Epstein–Barr virus.

Sulforaphane

Researchers from Johns Hopkins University and many other prestigious institutions have published a tremendous number of studies on a compound called sulforaphane, which is found in broccoli and similar vegetables. Sulforaphane helps prevent cancers of the breast, ovary, prostate, bone, brain, bladder, liver, lung, and stomach, and combats other conditions associated with aging and cell death.

It is no secret that the average American fails to consume the seven to nine daily servings of fruits and vegetables recommended to provide dietary protection against cancer. And for many people, the produce they do eat seldom includes the recommended one

to two daily servings of cruciferous vegetables (so called because the plants' flowers have four petals arranged like a crucifix or cross), such as cauliflower, kale, bok choy, rutabaga, radishes, turnips, Brussels sprouts, and of course broccoli. For instance, an analysis published in the *Journal of Nutrition*, which looked at dietary data on 4,806 men and women ages 25 to 75, revealed that just 3% of the group consumed broccoli during the two-year study period, and that consumption of dark green vegetables averaged just one-fifth of a serving per day.

Cruciferous vegetables contain cancer-fighting phytonutrients including thiols (such as the sulfur-containing glucosinolates) and indoles (which bind chemical carcinogens and activate detoxifying enzymes).

Scientists at Johns Hopkins University School of Medicine identified the compound sulforaphane glucosinolate (SGS)—a naturally occurring precursor to sulforaphane—in 1992 and began to research its cancer-fighting potential. The strategy was to support the body's natural detoxification capacity to fight cancer-causing chemicals and free radicals (negatively charged molecules that cause damage to cell DNA). It is well accepted that cell DNA controls cell replication, and that damage to cell DNA is an important factor in the development of cancer.

In 1994, these scientists looked at the impact of SGS on mammary (breast) tumors in rats exposed to a potent carcinogen. The results were astounding. The number of rats that developed tumors was reduced by as much as 60%, the number of tumors in each animal was reduced by 80%, and the size of the tumors that did develop was reduced by 75%. Subsequently, hundreds of other test-tube and animal studies have confirmed the anticancer properties of sulforaphane.

Toxins (both natural and man-made) go through phases of breakdown in the cells of the body, particularly the liver. Sulforaphane promotes the natural detoxification of harmful substances in the cells of the body by:

- Supporting the enzyme systems that eliminate carcinogens
- Stimulating longer-lasting protective enzymatic actions than other antioxidants (such as vitamins C and E) do
- Raising and replenishing the cells' levels of the amino acid glutathione, a powerful antioxidant that supercharges the immune system
- Inhibiting activation of COX-2, an inflammatory enzyme that contributes to cancerous changes in cells

- Decreasing the amount of DNA damage and uncontrolled cell proliferation

The Johns Hopkins team discovered that various types of fresh and frozen broccoli differed significantly in the amounts of SGS they contained—and that the older the broccoli was, the lower its SGS. Painstaking research uncovered certain varieties of three-day-old broccoli sprouts—which look like a cross between alfalfa sprouts and bean sprouts—that contained up to 50 times more SGS than mature, cooked broccoli. In other words, a single ounce of these special sprouts could provide as much SGS as three pounds of cooked broccoli.

This set the stage for a fascinating study, published in *Cancer Epidemiology Biomarkers & Prevention* in November 2005. It was led by the Johns Hopkins University School of Medicine and the Bloomberg School of Public Health, working with the Qidong Liver Cancer Institute, Jiao Tong University in Shanghai, and the University of Minnesota Cancer Center. The study was conducted in a rural area near Shanghai where the incidence of liver cancer is extremely high because the local grain is contaminated with aflatoxin, a powerful carcinogen produced by mold.

In the study, broccoli sprouts with known levels of SGS were grown at the site in China. Three days after the shoots emerged from the soil, the sprouts were picked and used to prepare a liquid extract to ensure standard dosages. One hundred local residents drank five ounces of diluted extract in tea form (equivalent to eating about two ounces of broccoli sprouts) daily for two weeks. A control group of 100 drank a tea that was indistinguishable in taste and appearance but contained no SGS. Analysis of the participants' urine showed that, in people who drank the SGS extract, carcinogens were being removed from the body—providing the first direct evidence that a particular food can enhance the human body's detoxifying system, reducing the risk of cancer.

DOSAGE

For optimal health benefits, eat ½ cup (1 ounce) of BroccoSprouts every other day. Each serving contains 73 mg SGS. They are most beneficial when eaten raw, so sprinkle them on salads or sandwiches. If you haven't yet sampled broccoli sprouts, you're in for a treat. The taste is similar to a radish, with a spicy flavor that results from the release of the sulforaphane as you chew. Even people who hate broccoli usually enjoy the tangy taste of broccoli sprouts. Also, the supplemental form is available, which contains 30 mg SGS per capsule. The dosage is one to four capsules daily.

WHAT ARE THE SIDE EFFECTS?

Broccoli sprouts and SGS are safe for everyone. Johns Hopkins researchers conducted a formal safety study on SGS, published in *Nutrition and Cancer*, which involved 12 healthy volunteers who were given varying doses of SGS extract. Thirty-two laboratory tests, including blood tests, were performed on subjects before, during, and after the treatment period. No toxicities were found.

SULFORAPHANE

RECOMMENDATIONS FROM THE NATURAL PHYSICIAN FOR . . .

✋ CANCER

Sulforaphane in the sprout or supplement form can be used as part of a comprehensive cancer prevention program. I also recommend it for people with existing cancers. If you have ever had cancer or are currently undergoing cancer treatment, increase to two to four capsules daily, under the supervision of your doctor.

✋ DETOXIFICATION

Sulforaphane is also an important phytonutrient that aids detoxification. It can be helpful for those requiring detoxification support, especially those who are or have been exposed to toxic and cancerous chemicals.

Sulphur

"I've had this rash all over my back and arms. One doctor calls it eczema and the next one calls it dermatitis."

There was confusion in Jeff's voice—but also a fair degree of outrage. A 40-year-old construction worker who had been trying to beat this problem for five years, he was obviously in search of some reliable answers.

"I've used creams and lotions," he recalled. "They usually help for a week or so, but after that, the rash comes back. It itches like mad.

Sometimes I think it'll drive me crazy. I have problems getting to sleep as it is—and the itching always gets worse at night."

After we had discussed his dilemma for a few minutes, I inquired whether he was the type of person who often felt too warm.

"Oh yeah, it can be freezing outside and I won't need a coat. I sweat like a pig when it's warm out."

"Well, I'm going to prescribe homeopathic sulphur for you. It should help to clear up that rash for good."

"I'm ready to try anything," said Jeff.

When I saw Jeff six weeks later, his rash was completely gone. We were both impressed. He was sleeping better, too.

"It's hard to believe those little white pellets could make such a difference," Jeff commented.

"Welcome to the world of homeopathy!" I replied.

MINERAL MAGIC

Sulphur is a mineral that's present in the foods we eat and the water we drink. It appears to be important for detoxification and for joint health. Historically, sulphur baths have been used as a means of detoxification and for healing. Homeopathic sulphur, a highly diluted preparation of this mineral, is one of the most important medicines used by homeopaths today.

Homeopathic sulphur affects many of the organs of the body. Specifically, it improves liver function and detoxification. It also has a profound effect on the entire digestive tract, stimulating healing. More important, sulphur works at the cellular level to stimulate cellular detoxification.

Homeopathic sulphur is used most commonly for skin ailments. This includes rashes, eczema, psoriasis, boils, cradle cap, and many other dermatological conditions. It is also an excellent remedy for digestive conditions such as ulcers, diarrhea, flatulence, and inflammatory bowel disorders. Sulphur is also a common homeopathic remedy for insomnia and headaches.

WHAT CHARACTER

Each homeopathic remedy has its own set of characteristics, and seems to work best with people who fit a particular description. The sulphur "constitutional" picture is unique. There are generally two types of people

requiring this remedy. First is the philosophical type. Described as a deep thinker who likes to let people know how smart he or she is, this philosophical type tends to be unkempt—since outward appearance is not important to him or her—and a loner.

The other sulphur "type" is more outgoing and social. This person loves to be around other people and is extroverted. Women who fit the constitutional type tend to be quick witted, leaders in their field, and, quite often, the leaders of their group or business. Children requiring sulphur are usually outgoing and are very curious, wanting to know how everything works and always asking "why?"

People requiring sulphur are almost always on the warm side. They sweat easily, prefer cool rooms, and often sleep with no blankets on (especially children).

They also tend to be thirsty, especially for ice-cold drinks.

There's also a profile for appetite. The sulphur type will have food cravings for sweets, spicy foods, fats, and alcohol, especially beer. I often see the strong craving for spicy foods with people who fit the sulphur constitutional type.

People requiring this remedy often are night people. They like to stay up late at night and prefer to sleep in when the morning comes.

DOSAGE

If you need to clear up a rash that you've had only recently, I recommend taking two pellets of 30C potency twice daily for two to three days.

When taking sulphur as a constitutional remedy to strengthen the body as a whole, you can take two pellets of a 6C or 12C potency twice daily for two weeks and then stop. If you notice improvement, take the remedy as needed in the future for a few days as a "tune up."

WHAT ARE THE SIDE EFFECTS?

Homeopathic sulphur is extremely safe. Side effects are uncommon. Some people with longstanding rashes or skin eruptions who take the remedy too frequently or in too high a potency may see their skin prob-lems worsen. This occurs because the body is detoxifying too quickly. When they stop taking the sulphur, this reaction will stop. They may not even need to take it anymore as the detoxification process will have been initiated. From then on, they can take the sulphur less frequently (e.g., once every two days instead of daily) or use a lower potency (e.g., 6C instead of 30C).

SULPHUR

RECOMMENDATIONS FROM THE NATURAL PHYSICIAN FOR . . .

❧ ATTENTION DEFICIT DISORDER (ADD)

One 12-year-old boy I treated for this con-dition was completely cured by this rem-edy without other types of therapies.

I sometimes recommend sulphur for the related condition attention deficit/hyperactivity disorder (ADHD).

❧ DIGESTIVE AILMENTS

Sulphur is indicated for many digestive disorders. Homeopathic doctors have found that it's especially likely to be effective if a person is prone to flatulence that has an odor like "rotten eggs."

Sulphur is commonly used for acute or chronic bouts of diarrhea, especially where there is burning. The diarrhea often occurs first thing in the morning. It is a common homeopathic for colitis, ulcers, and Crohn's disease.

❧ FATIGUE

Sulphur can be an excellent remedy to bring the energy levels back up if the person fits the "constitutional type." It improves energy production through improved cellular detoxification.

❧ HEADACHE

Sulphur is effective for headaches that occur only on the weekend and feel bet-ter after cold applications.

❧ INSOMNIA

Sulphur can be helpful for those who fall asleep for a few hours, then wake up and cannot fall asleep again. Peculiarly, those who are helped by sulphur prefer to sleep on their left side.

❧ LOW BACK PAIN

Sulphur may help relieve a weak low back that is going out all the time, and also reduce the frequency of episodes.

❧ MENOPAUSE

Sulphur helps to cool down a person. It will bring relief from hot flashes associ-ated with menopause.

❧ SKIN ERUPTIONS

The most common use of sulphur is for the various types of skin eruptions that people experience. These can range from

(continued)

a simple rash to a severe case of eczema, acne, or boils.

You'll know that there's a good chance of being helped with sulphur if the skin eruption is very red, inflamed, and extremely itchy. In fact, the itch can be so bad that you want to scratch it until it bleeds. The skin condition is worse from heat, bathing, touching wool, and at nighttime.

For nearly anyone with these condi-tions, sulphur soothes the skin and relieves the itching and sensitivity.

⊷ SORE THROAT

Sulphur can relieve a burning sore throat or chest infection. It's most likely to be helpful if you have the kind of burning sore throat or chest infection that feels better when you have ice-cold drinks, especially if you're very feverish.

Symphytum

Symphytum is the homeopathic prepara-tion of the herb comfrey, which has the interesting common name "bone-knit." That's precisely what the remedy and the herb can do—help heal broken bones.

Of course, if you've broken a bone, the first thing you do is go directly to the emer-gency room for evaluation and treatment. (On the way to the emergency room, how-ever, I'd advise taking some arnica to help with the pain.) Once there, the bone will be set and put into a cast—and you might have surgery, if that's necessary. Homeopathic care comes later.

I encourage patients to come and see me after a fracture has been evaluated and set in a cast—but not before. Homeopaths in the past have reported that symphytum heals the bone so quickly that it should not be given until the fracture is set. (If the bone heals in the wrong position, then it would need to be rebroken and reset again!)

While helping to stimulate healing of the fracture, symphytum also reduces the pain. Other painkillers might still be needed, but at least the homeopathic remedy helps to take the edge off the pain. (At the same time, I often recom-mend other complementary treatments for fractures, including acupuncture and magnet therapy.)

Many people who take symphytum are surprised at how quickly their fractures begin healing—and so are their doctors. Some doctors have observed that fractures heal 50% faster among people who take symphytum during the healing process.

DOSAGE

The typical dosage is a 30C potency taken twice daily for one week. Practitioners of homeopathy may give a single dose of a high potency such as 200C, 1M, or higher.

WHAT ARE THE SIDE EFFECTS?

I have not read about or seen any side effects with symphytum.

SYMPHYTUM

RECOMMENDATIONS FROM THE NATURAL PHYSICIAN FOR . . .

❧ EYE INJURY

Symphytum is a remedy to consider when there is blunt trauma to the eye or to the orbit (the bone that surrounds the eye). Typically, I'll try arnica first; if that doesn't give relief, I recommend symphytum instead.

❧ FRACTURE

While symphytum is the most common homeopathic remedy for healing fractures, homeopathic calc phos should be considered in the small percentages of cases where the bones do not unite together even after using symphytum. Not only does symphytum speed bone healing, it also helps to heal the soft tissue that covers the bone (the periosteum). It also helps treat pain, whether or not a fracture has occurred, such as when a soccer player has been kicked in the front of the lower leg.

In the case of fractures, however, it's important to note that symphytum should be accompanied by other natural remedies that encourage bone healing. I encourage patients to make sure they are on a proper diet and getting the nutrients that are required for bone healing, with special emphasis on calcium-rich foods such as broccoli, orange juice, and almonds. At the same time, it's important to avoid food products that cause the loss of calcium and other bone minerals. These culprits include caffeinated beverages such as soda and coffee.

I encourage people to avoid eating large amounts of red meat and to stop smoking. (For quicker bone healing, some of the most beneficial vitamins and minerals include calcium, magnesium, vitamin C, vitamin K, B vitamins, silica, and boron. I usually recommend a comprehensive bone formula or a high-potency multivitamin and a separate calcium/magnesium supplement, supplying at least 1,000 mg of calcium and at least 500 mg of magnesium.)

T

Tea Tree Oil

"This toe fungus just won't go away," said Marlene, a 33-year-old patient of mine. "I tried a couple of antifungal creams for it and there was no improvement. One doctor recommended a prescription for an antifungal medication that you take internally, but after reading that it could damage my liver, I said forget it."

"Let me take a look." It didn't take long to ascertain that she had a very mild case. "Tea tree oil should clear that up," I suggested.

"Is that something I need a prescription to get?"

"Oh no, you can get it at any health-food store as well as many pharmacies."

We discussed some of its properties, and then I described how to use it.

"First you need to cut your nails really short so that the tea tree oil can come in contact with the fungus. Then each morning and evening wash your feet with tea tree soap. Dry your feet, and then apply a few drops of tea tree oil to those three toes that have the fungus. You can use a cotton swab to apply it. Over the next four weeks the fungus should be killed by this treatment. The area of skin where you apply it will become dry and slough off."

"That's all I have to do?" asked Marlene.

"Pretty much. But I also want you to stay away from sugar products."

"So you think that will clear this up?"

"It should."

Another possibility was to use a bleach solution, but I would reserve that for a more serious case of the fungus. I suspected it wouldn't be necessary as long as she followed my initial recommendations.

Two months later Marlene was back for a return visit.

"Take a look," she said as she showed me her feet. "The tea tree oil really did work. I've been recommending it to my friends who have the same problem."

A TREASURE FROM DOWN UNDER

Tea tree oil (*Melaleuca alternifolia*), also referred to as ti tree oil, or cajeput oil, has become very popular for its antiseptic and healing properties to the skin. This oil comes from the leaves of the Australian *Melaleuca alternifolia* tree, and early settlers in Australia made tea from these leaves—which explains the origin of its most common name. But even before the arrival of Europeans, Aborigines of the area were well aware of the medicinal benefits of the oils from this tree.

Most of the research on the medicinal effects of tea tree oil has focused on *Melaleuca alternifolia* in the New South Wales area of Australia.

The first scientific investigations of tea tree oil began in Sydney in 1922 when a government chemist noticed the antiseptic effects of tea tree oil. Though the oils were potent, he observed, they were nontoxic and nonirritating. His initial investigations were followed up by numerous studies, especially in the years between 1922 and 1930. The benefits of this oil became so well established that it was included as standard medical issue in the Australian Army during World War II.

ALL STEAMED UP

Melaleuca alternifolia oil is extracted from the leaves using a steam-distillation process that extracts only the essential oils. There are approximately 100 chemicals in tea tree oil. Two of the key active constituents are terpinen-4-ol and cineole.

A standard for tea tree oil was established in 1985. It requires a minimum content of 30% terpinen-4-ol and less than 15% cineole. Higher quality oils contain 40% to 47% terpinen-4-ol and 2.5% cineole. The balance between these two constituents is important, with a high-quality product having oils high in terpinen-4-ol and low in cineole. The oil has natural anti-inflammatory, analgesic, and antiseptic properties. It destroys bacteria, fungus, and viruses.

Tea tree oil can be used topically for almost any skin condition. Examples include acne, athlete's foot and fungal infections of the skin, boils, bruises, burns, cold sores, cuts, dandruff, insect bites, rashes, lice, and warts. It can also be used for gingivitis and vaginitis.

DOSAGE

Make sure to get a product that is 100% *Melaleuca alternifolia* oil. An organic product is best. Tea tree oil is generally used in one of three ways: topically, oral rinse, or inhaled.

ᵔᵕ *Topically*
When used topically, the oil is placed on the skin. The oil itself can be used, or you can use a cream or gel formula. It can also be used in baths.

Do not apply tea tree oil on infants' skin. Do not use tea tree oil near the eyes.

ᵔᵕ *Oral Rinse*
When using it as an oral rinse, dilute a few drops in water, gargle, and spit out. It can be used for conditions like gingivitis, toothaches or tooth infections, and sore throat.

ᵔᵕ *Inhaler*
To inhale it, add a few drops of tea tree oil to a mister or steamer. You can also put a few drops on a tissue and smell it.

(**NOTE:** Tea tree oil also makes a good disinfectant for washing clothes. Look for laundry detergents made with tea tree oil or add 5 to 10 drops in your washing machine with each load of laundry.)

WHAT ARE THE SIDE EFFECTS?

Tea tree oil is very safe for topical use. It is generally nonirritating and nontoxic. It has a pH balance that is almost neutral, so it is not caustic. As with any substance, however, some people could be sensitive to tea tree oil; it is not common but it has been reported in the literature. You can test your sensitivity by putting a couple of drops on your skin before going to bed and seeing if an irritation occurs by morning.

Pure undiluted tea tree oil should not be applied to the skin of children or pregnant or lactating women. These people should use a commercial cream or gel.

TEA TREE OIL
RECOMMENDATIONS FROM THE NATURAL PHYSICIAN FOR . . .

ACNE

Tea tree oil has become popular as a treatment for acne. It is applied most commonly as a gel or cream. One study showed that a 5% tea tree oil gel extract was comparable to benzoyl peroxide in the treatment of mild to moderate acne. Tea tree oil users experienced fewer side effects (dryness, burning, redness, and itching). Another technique is to dab the oil on the pimples with a cotton swab before bedtime.

ATHLETE'S FOOT AND TOE FUNGUS

Fungal infections of the feet (athlete's foot), toes, and toenails (onychomycosis) are very common and can be stubborn to treat. Tea tree oil has become a popular treatment for this problem.

One study compared 100% tea tree oil to the antifungal topical drug clotrimazole for the treatment of toenail fungus for a period of six months. Results indicated very similar results with the two treatments.

I usually have patients trim their toenails, wash feet with soap or tea tree soap, and then apply tea tree oil to the infected area. This needs to be repeated on a daily basis for weeks and sometimes months to eradicate the infection. Another technique is to add 10 drops of tea tree oil to 1 quart of warm water. Soak the feet for 10 minutes and then dry the feet thoroughly with a towel and hair dryer. Continue the treatment for at least six weeks.

Tea tree oil can also be used to combat foot odor (bromhidrosis).

COLD SORES

Tea tree oil can be dabbed onto the sores at the first signs of an outbreak. This will keep the lesions under control and prevent the infection from spreading.

LICE

Approximately 12 million cases of head lice infestation are discovered each year, mostly in preschool- and elementary school–age children. Lice are extremely small parasites that live and feed on skin. For those seeking a natural, nontoxic approach to this irritating condition, try the following:

Mix 1½ teaspoons of tea tree oil and 1½ teaspoons of lavender oil into 4 ounces of olive oil or 4 ounces of your child's shampoo. Massage this mixture into the hair and scalp. Do not rinse. Cover the head with a shower cap until morning and then comb the hair with a fine-tooth comb. Add 5 drops of tea tree oil to the comb before using it to get out the eggs. Rinse hair and then blow dry for 5 to 10 minutes. (This helps to destroy the eggs.) Repeat this procedure for seven days.

Tea tree oil can also be used in a shampoo to help treat dandruff.

MOUTH AND GUM INFECTIONS

Tea tree oil is used for mouth and gum infections, including gingivitis and tooth abscess. Use it as a gargle by adding 3 drops of tea tree oil to 1 ounce of warm water. It can also be purchased commercially as a mouthwash. This treatment can also be used daily for bad breath.

❧ SKIN INFECTIONS AND ERUPTIONS

Tea tree oil is excellent for the topical treatment of skin infections. It has been shown to be effective against many different types of bacteria and fungus, including *Staphylococcus aureus, Candida albicans,* and many others. It can be used in cream or gel form to treat skin infections such as acne, impetigo, and boils. It also helps to alleviate the infection and inflammation caused by insect bites. Its soothing and anti-inflammatory properties make it helpful for burns and rashes such as eczema.

❧ VAGINITIS

Tea tree oil solutions have been shown to be effective for vaginitis caused by *Candida albicans* and trichomonas. This treatment should be done only under a doctor's care.

❧ WARTS

Tea tree oil can be applied topically to warts as it has antiviral properties. It is especially useful for plantar warts.

Tocotrienols

What natural nutrient both improves cholesterol levels and reduces plaque in the arteries? Many people are surprised to hear that one answer to this question is tocotrienols. Vitamin E is not just one vitamin, but rather a family of eight slightly different molecular structures that function differently in the body. There are two principal categories of vitamin E—tocopherols and tocotrienols. Each of these has four subcategories—alpha, beta, gamma, and delta. The vitamin E chapter in this book (page 474) mainly focuses on the tocopherol family, while this chapter discusses the equally important tocotrienols.

There are several food sources of tocotrienols. One rich source that the supplemental form is often extracted from is palm oil, taken from the fruits of the oil palm. Other food sources include rice bran, barley, wheat germ, and rye.

As a supplement, tocotrienols have been shown to have several benefits for the cardiovascular system such as reducing cholesterol levels, decreasing plaque in the arteries, and preventing excessive blood clotting. In addition, studies have demonstrated anticancer effects and skin protection against UV radiation. Like their relatives the tocopherol family, the tocotrienols also have super antioxidant properties. The delta fraction has the highest antioxidant activity compared to alpha, beta, and gamma tocotrienols.

DOSAGE

There is currently no government-recommended intake for tocotrienols. For healthy individuals the optimal dose is 30 to 50 mg daily. For those with existing disease such as atherosclerosis or high cholesterol the recommended dosage is 240 to 300 mg daily. Tocotrienols are fat-soluble and are best taken with food for optimum absorption.

WHAT ARE THE SIDE EFFECTS?

Toxicity studies have shown tocotrienols to be very safe. They do have a cholesterol-lowering and blood-thinning effect. Consult with your doctor before combining tocotrienols supplements with blood-thinning and cholesterol-lowering medications or if you are scheduled for surgery.

TOCOTRIENOLS

RECOMMENDATIONS FROM THE NATURAL PHYSICIAN FOR . . .

ATHEROSCLEROSIS

One of the most phenomenal effects of tocotrienols is their ability to reduce existing plaque in the arteries. This was demonstrated in a four-year study at Elmhurst Medical Center in Queens, New York. The study included 50 participants with plaque in the carotid arteries (arteries that carry blood flow to the brain). Among the patients who took 240 mg tocotrienols and 60 mg alpha-tocopherol daily, 88% experienced stabilization or actual reduction of plaque. Among participants taking a placebo, 60% experienced a worsening of their condition and only 8% stabilized or improved! In addition to lowering cholesterol and protecting against the oxidative damage that initiates plaque formation, tocotrienols also protect the arteries and heart by reducing triglycerides; promote dilation and flexibility of arteries; reduce platelet clumping, which improves blood flow; and lower blood pressure.

CANCER

Animal and in vitro studies have demonstrated that tocotrienols have anticancer properties. This includes inhibiting human breast cancer cells regardless of estrogen status. In the studies, delta tocotrienols had the strongest effect in inducing cancer cell death. A study in human prostate cancer cells also demonstrated benefit. As well, alpha tocotrienol and gamma tocotrienol have been shown to prolong the life span of cancer-infected mice. Delta tocotrienols have been shown to reduce blood supply to tumors. While more human studies are needed, it appears that tocotrienols have beneficial anticancer properties.

HIGH CHOLESTEROL

Tocotrienols also reduce high cholesterol levels by decreasing the liver's production of cholesterol. A study review published in the *Journal of the American Nutraceutical Association* reported that supplementation with gamma and delta tocotrienols at 75 to 100 mg per day for two months reduced total cholesterol levels by 13% to 22% and cut LDL "bad" cholesterol by 9% to 20%. In addition, tocotrienols change LDL cholesterol into a form that does not promote plaque formation.

Tryptophan and 5-HTP

"There is no doubt I am depressed, and I am having trouble sleeping, which just compounds my problem," explained a 40-year-old construction worker who was requesting natural therapy for his depression.

"Let's start you on 5-HTP. It is an amino acid that will increase the level of serotonin in the neurotransmitters in your brain. As a result, you will feel less depressed and more relaxed, and you will sleep better. In the meantime, we will work on your diet, exercise, and stress-reduction techniques so that you are not so susceptible to depression."

Tryptophan and its metabolite 5-HTP (5-hydroxytryptophan) are both amino acids that play an important role. Tryptophan, more formally known as L-tryptophan, is an essential amino acid and must be consumed in the diet. Tryptophan is one of the many amino acids used to manufacture protein. It also is a precursor in the formation of the neurotransmitter serotonin and the B vitamin niacin. Eggs are one of the highest sources of tryptophan. Other sources include oats, mangos, milk, fish, chickpeas, cottage cheese, spirulina, sunflower seeds, chocolate, and poultry such as chicken. Many people believe that high amounts of turkey from a celebratory meal such as Thanksgiving or Christmas results in drowsiness as the result of high tryptophan levels. This is not likely to be true since turkey has a tryptophan amount comparable to other meats. It likely has more to do with all the carbohydrates consumed, including alcohol!

5-HTP is converted by the liver into serotonin. 5-HTP crosses the blood-brain barrier. My experience is that 5-HTP has a quicker onset of action than tryptophan. Both are available over the counter as supplements.

DOSAGE

For depression and anxiety, take 500 to 1,000 mg L-tryptophan three times daily on an empty stomach or 100 mg 5-HTP three times daily on an empty stomach. For insomnia, take 1,000 mg L-tryptophan before bedtime, on an empty stomach, or 100 to 200 mg 5-HTP before bedtime, on an empty stomach.

WHAT ARE THE SIDE EFFECTS?

In 1991, tryptophan was banned for sale as a dietary supplement in the United States due to illnesses that appear to have been related to a contaminated batch from a Japanese supplier. It came available again over the counter in 2002. I have not found side effects to be common for L-tryptophan or 5-HTP. For both supplements side effects may include digestive upset and drowsiness. Since both supplements increase serotonin levels they should not be combined with psychiatric medications such as antidepressant, antianxiety, or seizure medications unless you are instructed to do so under the guidance of a doctor. Patients with Down syndrome are advised to avoid the use of 5-HTP.

TRYPTOPHAN AND 5-HTP
RECOMMENDATIONS FROM THE NATURAL PHYSICIAN FOR . . .

ANXIETY

5-HTP is effective in my clinical practice in helping patients control anxiety. Along with stress reduction techniques, and treating low blood-sugar and hormone imbalances, the use of 5-HTP is quite useful. A small study in the *Journal of Affective Disorders* found 5-HTP indeed helpful for alleviating anxiety.

DEPRESSION

5-HTP has been shown to be very effective in treating depression as demonstrated by several studies. I use supple-

ments like 5-HTP while also addressing underlying issues related to depression such as grief, trauma, and hormone imbalance. Some people have a genetic inability to produce enough serotonin; 5-HTP supports the brain in manufacturing more of this important neurotransmitter. 5-HTP has even been shown to help people with treatment-resistant depression.

(continued)

FIBROMYALGIA

A low serotonin level is considered to be one possible cause of fibromyalgia. Serotonin works to relax the muscles. Studies show that 5-HTP reduces pain severity, morning stiffness, and sleeplessness in these patients.

INSOMNIA

I have not seen any studies researching 5-HTP and sleep problems, although I have found it helps many patients to fall asleep. L-tryptophan seems to be a better choice for those who can fall asleep but wake up several hours later. 1,000 mg L-tryptophan before bedtime is helpful for some who wake up the middle of the night and have trouble returning to sleep.

PREMENSTRUAL DYSPHORIC DISORDER (PMDD)

PMDD is a condition characterized by severe depression, irritability, and tension before menstruation. These are similar symptoms to PMS but more intense. My experience is that these women can have their problem resolved by balancing their hormones, usually increasing their progesterone level. Also, L-tryptophan at a dose of 6,000 mg daily was shown in a study to decrease mood swings, tension, and irritability in women with PMDD.

RESTLESS LEG SYNDROME

Low serotonin is thought to be one of the possible causes of restless leg syndrome. Several of my patients have found help for this condition by supplementing with 100 to 200 mg 5-HTP before bedtime.

SEASONAL AFFECTIVE DISORDER (SAD)

Interestingly, a study in the *Journal of Affective Disorders* found that tryptophan was equally as effective as light therapy for the treatment of SAD.

SMOKING CESSATION

L-tryptophan has been shown in the *Journal of Behavioral Medicine* to reduce withdrawal symptoms for those quitting smoking.

WEIGHT CONTROL

5-HTP is one of the supplements I prescribe for those I am treating for obesity and overweight. A double-blind study in the *American Journal of Clinical Nutrition* examined the effect of 5-HTP on 20 obese people. They were randomly assigned to receive either 5-HTP 900 mg a day of 5-HTP or a placebo. Significant weight loss was observed in the 5-HTP-treated patients. Also, a reduction in carbohydrate intake and a consistent presence of early satiety were also found.

Turmeric

In India the smell of turmeric, a bright yellow spice used in curries, fills almost every restaurant and home. Indians eat turmeric because they like it, but rapidly growing evidence indicates that the spice is giving them much more than flavor. Thousands of years ago, Ayurvedic and traditional Chinese medicine recognized turmeric as a healing agent for everything from flatulence to liver disease, and now modern research demonstrates that properties in this zesty spice may be useful for lowering rates of breast, prostate, lung, and colon cancers and for treating breast cancer, inflammatory bowel disease, Crohn's disease, and possibly cystic fibrosis and Alzheimer's disease.

Turmeric is a powder made from the root of the plant *Curcuma longa*, which grows in southern Asia. The part of the plant that is responsible for healing is the yellow pigment, called *curcumin*. And when it comes to health-giving properties, curcumin gives twice. It is a potent anti-inflammatory agent, but without the potential side effects of anti-inflammatory drugs. Next, curcumin is a powerful antioxidant—it tracks down and reduces free radicals, disease-causing molecules that otherwise would cause damage in the body.

Turmeric is a member of the ginger family. The rhizome is the part that is used and is cured (boiled, cleaned, sun-dried, and polished). It has long been cultivated in India, China, and other tropical countries. India is the major producer of turmeric, responsible for 94% of the world's production.

Turmeric has been used in Asian culture throughout the ages for many different purposes including as a spice, dye, food preservative, and medicine. Many of the medicinal uses have come out of Ayurvedic and Chinese medicines—treating liver disease, digestive problems, painful menstruation, and as a poultice for sprains and arthritis. In the West, it has become a major ingredient in curry powder, and it's also a coloring agent for prepared yellow mustard.

MELLOW YELLOW

Turmeric has many different active constituents. One group of these constituents that

is thought to be important for its antioxidant and anti-inflammatory properties is curcuminoids. Curcuminoids give turmeric its bright yellow-orange color (which makes for a good dye).

Curcumin is one of the curcuminoids that has been the focus of a lot of research. Its antioxidant activity is comparable to that of vitamins C and E. Similar to capsaicin in cayenne, curcumin depletes substance P so that pain messages are not sent through the nerves.

Turmeric also contains volatile oils, which contribute to its medicinal effects.

NATURAL BENEFITS

It is not fully understood how turmeric reduces inflammation in the body. Researchers feel that curcumin and the volatile oils play a major role in this. Studies confirm that these turmeric extracts have potent anti-inflammatory effects.

For example, one study examined 40 men with swelling and tenderness of the spermatic cord following surgery for a hernia or hydrocele. At the end of the six-day study, it was found that curcumin was nearly identical to the anti-inflammatory medication phenylbutazone in reducing inflammation.

Turmeric and its constituent curcumin also reduce cholesterol levels and increase the good HDL cholesterol. It reduces the levels of lipid peroxides (oxidants that can initiate atherosclerosis). The turmeric inhibits platelet aggregation, which is thought to prevent the risk of stroke.

DOSAGE

Turmeric is excellent to use in the diet. As a supplement, the typical adult dosage is 450 to 600 mg of curcumin, but you can take up to 2 g a day. Use it liberally as a spice in food. I encourage all my patients, especially those over 50, to consume 1 or 2 teaspoons a day of turmeric. You can sprinkle it into egg salad or over vegetables while sautéing; add it to soups or broths; put it on fish or meat or in lentil curries; and use it to flavor rice or a creamy vegetable dip. It is important to purchase turmeric as a separate spice. Lab tests show that many curry powders in this country have almost no turmeric.

Those who don't love turmeric—or who want to get even more of its protective effects—can take curcumin in supplement form. I prescribe supplements of 2,000 mg a day for people who have a strong family history of Alzheimer's disease or who show signs of dementia, and those with inflammatory conditions like arthritis or colitis.

WHAT ARE THE SIDE EFFECTS?

Turmeric is quite safe as a spice and supplement. However, pregnant women should not use it in supplement form. Also, people with gallstones should check with their doctors before using it, as it stimulates bile production. People taking blood-thinning medications should check with their doctors before using turmeric as a supplement.

TURMERIC

RECOMMENDATIONS FROM THE NATURAL PHYSICIAN FOR . . .

🍃 ALZHEIMER'S DISEASE PREVENTION

In healthy people, immune cells attack and destroy *amyloid-beta plaques*—a build-up of proteins between neurons in the brain. But in people with Alzheimer's, this immune response is less efficient and allows plaques to form. Plaque triggers inflammation and free radicals, both of which cause cell damage in the brain. Curcumin slows this harmful process in a number of ways: It forms a powerful bond with the amyloid protein that prevents the protein from clumping; preliminary research demonstrates that it may break down plaques as well; and finally, as I noted before, curcumin reduces the oxidative damage and brain inflammation that are believed to contribute to Alzheimer's.

🍃 ARTHRITIS

Turmeric extract is commonly found in arthritis supplements to reduce pain and inflammation. A study of people with rheumatoid arthritis found that taking 1,200 mg of curcumin per day for two weeks significantly improved morning stiffness, joint swelling, and walking ability.

This is important because natural anti-inflammatories like curcumin do not have the toxicity that standard conventional anti-inflammatory drugs have. I like to use nutritional formulas containing curcumin to reduce pain and inflammation while treating the underlying cause of the disease—such as poor digestion, nutritional deficiencies, diet, hormone imbalance, stress, and lack of exercise.

🍃 CANCER

Turmeric and curcumin suppress the cancer-causing effects of mutagens and carcinogens such as tobacco smoke and other chemicals. A study of smokers who took a supplement of 1.5 g of turmeric a day had reduced urinary excretion of mutagens (substances that cause damage to cell DNA, which can lead to cancer formation).

❧ CHOLESTEROL

Studies demonstrate that curcumin reduces cholesterol. In one study, healthy volunteers took 500 mg of curcumin supplements every day for one week. The result was reduced levels of total cholesterol and lipid peroxides (markers of free radical damage to fats).

❧ DIGESTIVE AND LIVER PROBLEMS

Turmeric has a long history of use for digestive problems. It stimulates bile pro-

duction and reduces intestinal gas. Also, curcumin protects the liver cells from toxins as a result of its antioxidant properties. It is also used to lower elevated liver enzymes. For these reasons, it is often included in digestive formulas that target the liver and gallbladder.

❧ INFECTION

Studies have shown that turmeric inhibits the growth of several bacteria as well as fungi. I especially recommend it for respiratory tract infections and for hepatitis.

Uva Ursi

"I think I have a urinary tract infection. I feel burning when I go to the bathroom and feel feverish today."

Karen, my 25-year-old patient, also looked feverish—and a quick check with the thermometer confirmed that she had a low-grade fever. My suspicions were confirmed when the nurse came by a few minutes later with the results of the urinalysis. The report indicated that there were bacteria in her urine—a moderate amount, but still, they were there.

I let Karen know that I'd send out for a culture just in case she needed antibiotics. "But I really want to avoid antibiotics if possible," I went on.

Karen agreed with me. She'd had yeast infections in the past, and if she took antibiotics there was a good chance the drug would lead to a new flare-up. (Antibiotics knock out the "good" bacteria that help control yeast as well as the "bad" bacteria that cause infection—and yeast can begin to thrive if they aren't naturally controlled by your body's healthy supply of bacteria.)

"I know antibiotics could bring back that yeast problem," Karen acknowledged. Clearly, neither of us thought antibiotics were a good idea.

"The trick is to get the infection under control in the first 48 hours," I told her. "We especially want to make sure that this infection doesn't spread to your kidneys."

"Should I drink cranberry juice?" asked Karen.

"Unsweetened cranberry juice would be fine to take, but I find it works better for the prevention of urinary tract infections rather than actually treating them."

I had other recommendations. "I want you to drink lots of water, at least eight tall glasses a day. And I don't want you eating any sugar products while we're treating you for this. Sugar can suppress the immune system. Also, I want you to take some herbs that help to eradicate the infection."

At that point, I told her about uva ursi. I also told her my experience with it—that I had seen evidence that it could help eradicate bacteria in the urinary tract very quickly.

During the next two days, Karen reported that the burning she experienced during urination was dramatically reduced. A week later, she had a repeat urinalysis, and the test didn't turn up any signs of infection.

I kept Karen on uva ursi—as well as a number of other bacteria-fighting herbs—for another week. I just wanted to make sure the infection was completely gone. Only when the urinalysis continued to be negative did we decide to stop the treatment.

BERRY USEFUL

Uva ursi (*Arctostaphylos uva ursi*), also known as bearberry, is one of the best herbs for treatment of urinary tract infections. The leaves, long used by practitioners of herbal medicine, have antiseptic effects. The leaf extract is also a diuretic, helping to remove excess liquids from the body. As a popular home remedy, uva ursi was traditionally used for treatment of bladder and kidney infections, and kidney stones. It was also recommended for treatment of bronchitis.

In my own practice, I most often recommend it for treatment of urinary tract infections, bladder infections, and even kidney infections. Uva ursi is considered to be an astringent. It is slightly sweet tasting and has cooling and drying properties.

Uva ursi leaves contain a substance known as arbutin, which is converted to hydroquinone. This acts as an effective antimicrobial agent.

Uva ursi also works to make the urine more alkaline, which improves the effectiveness of hydroquinone. But there are many other active substances as well—including flavonoids, tannins, phenolic acids, volatile oil, resin, and gallic and egallic acid.

DOSAGE

For acute urinary tract infections, the dosage is 500 mg of the capsule (10% to 20% arbu-

tin) or 60 drops (1 mL) of the tincture taken four times daily. It should not be taken with anything that will acidify the urine.

WHAT ARE THE SIDE EFFECTS?

Because the effects of uva ursi have not been thoroughly researched as yet, I do not recommend that pregnant or breast-feeding women take it without the advice of a doctor. It should also not to be given to children under age 12.

Digestive upset, such as nausea and vomiting, can occur in some people. Those with kidney disorders should not use it. Very high dosages may cause tinnitus (ringing in the ears), vomiting, delirium, difficulty breathing, convulsions, and loss of consciousness. Do not take more than the recommended dosage as given in this section unless you are seeing a practitioner who is familiar with the herb.

UVA URSI

RECOMMENDATIONS FROM THE NATURAL PHYSICIAN FOR . . .

❧ KIDNEY STONES
A number of physicians and researchers have reported that uva ursi can be helpful for the prevention of kidney stones.

❧ URINARY TRACT INFECTIONS
I recommend uva ursi for any infection of the urinary tract. I usually combine it in

formulas with herbs such as echinacea, goldenseal, buchu, marshmallow, and usnea. A number of companies produce variations on this formula for people who have urinary tract infections.

V

Valerian

There were lots of reasons why Steve couldn't sleep. A 40-year-old lawyer who worked long, grueling hours under intense pressure, he'd always had trouble winding down after work. He'd also recently been through a divorce. This was a man with a lot on his mind—and it all conspired to throw a monkey wrench into his sleep patterns.

Wisely enough, he had talked to a doctor. But he was reluctant to accept the doctor's advice.

"My sister said Valium could be dangerous," he admitted.

I was not at all surprised to hear him mention one of the most often prescribed drugs for anxiety. But I was quick to reassure him that there were many other options.

"There are a lot of natural approaches we could use to help with the anxiety and insomnia. Are you seeing a counselor?" I asked.

"Yes, just started last week," replied Steve.

"Good, that will be very helpful. While you are working on the emotional issues, I'd like to recommend a natural medicine to help you cope better. My first choice is the herb valerian for a situation like yours. It does not have significant side effects."

I also observed that it wasn't "dangerous" in the way that Valium could be. No one, in my experience, had ever become addicted to valerian—while new cases of Valium addiction were cropping up every day.

Several days after he left the clinic, Steve reported that the valerian was working for him. He was taking it nightly to help him sleep, and he'd found that it also helped to reduce anxiety during the day.

FROM SEIZURES TO SHELL SHOCK

Valerian (*Valeriana officinalis*) was used by the ancient Greeks and Romans to treat menstrual cramps, seizures, digestive problems, and other common health conditions. Europeans used it during the 16th century for anxiety and insomnia, and it was also prescribed to ease digestion.

After World War I, physicians favored it for treatment of shell shock. Then during World War II, when England endured the bombings, Londoners would take valerian to help them sleep.

Valerian is used in Ayurvedic medicine for the treatment of hysteria, neurosis, and epilepsy. It's considered a "warming herb" in Chinese and Ayurvedic medicines. Early American physicians, known as the Eclectics, learned of the use of valerian from English colonists. Today, valerian is approved for over-the-counter distribution in pharmacies throughout Germany, France, Belgium, Italy, and Switzerland—countries where doctors regularly prescribe the herbal remedy.

TRAVELS WITH VALERIAN

Though it was first found in northern Asia and Europe, today *Valeriana officinalis* is cultivated in many parts of the world, including North America. The roots and rhizomes are collected for medicinal use.

More than 200 species of valerian are used to treat a very wide range of ailments that include not only insomnia, anxiety, and stress, but also pain, hypertension, menstrual cramps, muscle spasms, and stress-related digestive disorders.

It is not clear how valerian works to promote relaxation. According to one theory, valerian has an effect that's similar to Valium's, but without the side effects of Valium such as impaired mental function. Another theory holds that valerian contains the neurotransmitter GABA, which has a calming effect on the brain, or that it somehow influences GABA concentrations in the brain.

Also, some researchers believe that valerian has an effect on serotonin levels similar to antidepressant drugs such as Prozac. Volatile oils, valepotriates, valeric acid, and velerenic acid are all constituents of valerian that may contribute to its sedative effects. In the most recent experiments, however, scientists have focused on the effects of valeric acid.

DOSAGE

If you're using valerian to treat insomnia, take the herb 30 to 60 minutes before you go to bed. You can take it two to four times throughout the day for treatment of stress and anxiety.

The recommended dose of tincture is 30 to 60 drops (0.5 to 1.0 mL). If you prefer the capsule or tablet, I recommend between 300 and 500 mg. Valerian also makes a tea, though some people strenuously object to its flavor.

Valerian combines well with the herbs scutellaria, kava, lemon balm, and passionflower for relaxation.

WHAT ARE THE SIDE EFFECTS?

While valerian does not, generally, produce the "hangover effect" that people usually get from Valium, some people seem to be very sensitive to it and may feel very groggy after taking valerian. I've also noticed that a small number of people find it stimulating, actually causing them insomnia and bad dreams.

These reactions would be considered completely understandable in traditional Chinese medicine. Valerian is a warming herb, so if you take it by itself, the herb may cause too much "heat." This would explain why it overstimulates those who already—again, in Chinese medicine terms—are constitutionally warm.

A small number of people may experience stomach upset. If you take a dose that's too high, you may have symptoms that include blurred vision, change in heartbeat, headache, nausea, and uneasiness. Lowering the dose will probably alleviate these side effects, but by all means, avoid taking high doses if you intend to drive or operate machinery.

Valerian should never be combined with tranquilizers or antidepressant medications—and you should never discontinue these prescription medications without consulting your doctor. If you're taking medications, be sure to talk to your doctor before you take any dose of valerian.

VALERIAN

RECOMMENDATIONS FROM THE NATURAL PHYSICIAN FOR . . .

🌿 ANXIETY AND DEPRESSION

One study found the combination of valerian and St. John's wort to be equivalent to the antidepressant drug amitryptiline, but without the side effects such as dry mouth and lethargy.

🌿 DIGESTIVE PROBLEMS

Valerian can be helpful for digestive conditions associated with stress, such as irritable bowel syndrome (IBS).

🌿 HYPERTENSION

I like to add valerian to herbal hypertension formulas to help relax the nervous system. Stress and anxiety can play major roles in high blood pressure for some people.

🌿 INSOMNIA

I find that valerian works well for many people to help alleviate insomnia. Those who have sleep disturbance due to anxiety and stress seem to be particularly well served by this herb, and several clinical studies confirm that valerian is effective for insomnia.

In a scientifically controlled study that involved 121 people who had insomnia, researchers studied the effects of 600 mg of valerian that was administered in tablet form. Not knowing whether they were getting the herbal treatment or an inactive placebo, all participants took tablets one hour before bedtime for 28 days. When the results were analyzed, researchers saw that people who took valerian reported significant improvement in their feelings of being rested after sleep. They also reported better sleep quality than those taking the placebos, with better dream recall and less daytime fatigue.

Reported side effects in the study were rare.

🌿 MENSTRUAL CRAMPS

Valerian has been historically used to help relieve the pain of menstrual cramps. It is commonly included in menstrual cramp formulas.

🌿 MUSCLE SPASMS

I readily recommend valerian in combination formulas for relief from muscle spasms.

🌿 STRESS

While valerian does not treat the cause of someone's stress, it can be used to help calm the nervous system so that one can cope more effectively and deal with the underlying cause.

Vanadium

Paul, a new patient of mine, had just been diagnosed with type 2 diabetes.

"What's the deal with vanadium?" he asked me bluntly.

I wasn't surprised. It had been in the news. One of Paul's relatives had mentioned it to him—but he wasn't about to try it without doing his homework first. So he had come to me.

Quickly, I gave him a rundown of this trace mineral and what it was said to do. "Trace mineral simply means that you require it in very tiny amounts," I explained. "There have been a few studies in recent years showing that it helps to lower elevated blood-sugar and cholesterol levels."

"Should I use it instead of chromium?" asked Paul.

"I wouldn't advise it. But if someone has diabetes, it makes sense to take chromium *along with* vanadium. Both help to normalize blood-sugar levels. In fact," I added, "many blood-sugar-related nutritional formulas already contain vanadium."

Understandably enough, vanadium started to gain attention as the evidence mounted that this substance could help with blood-sugar and cholesterol metabolism. Animal studies show that high dosages improve the mineralization of bones and teeth, adding calcium and other minerals that improve bone density.

There is still a lot more to learn about the role of vanadium in the human body. For instance, though we know it helps lower blood-sugar levels, the mechanism that makes that happen is still under investigation.

There's some speculation about vanadium, too. One theory holds that vanadium helps insulin transport glucose more effectively in the cells.

But whatever the exact role of vanadium, researchers feel that this trace mineral is probably an essential nutrient for humans.

Food sources of vanadium include shellfish, mushrooms, dill, black pepper, soy, corn, and cereals.

DOSAGE

Studies have used a form of vanadium that's combined with another substance to create vanadyl sulfate, which is an excellent form for absorption. The usual dose used in studies is 300 mg per day of vanadyl sulfate. With regard to elemental vanadium, up to 100 mcg daily is thought to be safe.

WHAT ARE THE SIDE EFFECTS?

There is not a lot known about the side effects of vanadium and there have not been any long-term human studies to investigate adverse effects. Digestive upset was the main side effect in one human study where vanadyl sulfate was used. If you're taking a diabetes medication, it's essential to consult with your doctor before you start taking vanadium.

VANADIUM
RECOMMENDATIONS FROM THE NATURAL PHYSICIAN FOR . . .

☙ TYPE 2 DIABETES

This is the only condition for which vanadium seems to be a particularly effective treatment. Small human studies involving vanadium have all been done with people who have noninsulin-dependent diabetes (type 2). The most recent study involved 16 people with type 2 diabetes, who were studied before and after they had been treated for six weeks with vanadyl sulfate at three different dosages (75, 150, and 300 mg). The signs of blood-sugar problems decreased significantly in those taking 150 and 300 mg of vanadyl sulfate.

Vitamin A

"Is there anything else I can take for this bronchitis? The herbs I've been using just don't seem to be working," said Simon, a 29-year-old patient of mine.

"Yes, let's get you on some vitamin A. Take 50,000 IU for the next two days and let's see how you do."

A few days later, Simon called to report that he was doing much better. "The vitamin A seems to be working."

I have so often seen marked improvement using vitamin A—particularly for respiratory tract infection—that I agree that this deserves the name of "anti-infective vitamin."

Vitamin A, which is also called retinol, is important for normal growth and development. It can improve vision, and it also provides benefits for the immune system. I've recommended this vitamin to improve health of epithelial tissue, which includes mucus membranes, lining of the digestive system, lungs, urinary tract, vagina, and skin. In addition, it has antioxidant activity.

Vitamin A also benefits the brain and nervous system. Researchers have also discovered that children need vitamin A in order to learn properly. That's an important fact, with global implications, since an estimated 190 million children worldwide have a vitamin A deficiency.

GETTING ALL A'S

Food sources of vitamin A include beef liver, chili peppers, carrots, sweet potatoes, parsley, kale, spinach, mangoes, broccoli, and squash. Milk and butter are commonly fortified with vitamin A, as well.

Carotenoids, such as beta carotene, found in foods or taken as a supplement, are converted into vitamin A—so any orange or yellow-colored fruit or vegetable, or any dark green type of lettuce—is potentially a good source of vitamin A because it's a source of carotenoids.

DIETARY REFERENCE INTAKE

0 to 6 months: 2,000 IU or 400 mcg

6 to 12 months: 2,000 IU or 400 mcg

1 to 3 years: 2,000 IU or 400 mcg

4 to 6 years: 2,500 IU or 500 mcg

7 to 10 years: 3,500 IU or 700 mcg

11 to 18 years: 4,000 IU or 800 mcg

18+ years (male): 5,000 IU or 1,000 mcg

18+ years (female): 4,000 IU or 800 mcg

Pregnant/lactating: 4,000 IU or 800 mcg

Severe vitamin A deficiency can cause a wide range of health problems, from eye inflammation and blindness to impaired growth, weight loss, improper tooth and bone formation, and reduced resistance to infection. While most people in the United States have access to plenty of foods that can provide vitamin A, some people do suffer from deficiencies because their bodies don't absorb the nutrient properly or because they're on very low-fat diets.

Vitamin A is especially important for growth and development and proper immune function in children. Vitamin A supplements are associated with a significant reduction in mortality. When given to impoverished children who had been deprived of the nutrient, vitamin A literally saves lives.

DOSAGE

Multivitamin supplements often contain vitamin A or beta carotene in the amount of

1,500 to 5,000 IU. (If it's in the form of beta carotene, it's converted into vitamin A once you take the supplement.) This is adequate to take as a preventative dosage.

Higher amounts may be needed for therapeutic levels to treat specific diseases. For example, 50,000 IU is usually recommended for the short-term treatment of a respiratory tract infection.

I wouldn't advise any higher dosages unless you're under the guidance of a nutrition-oriented doctor. It's especially important to not take high dosages for long periods of time.

Vitamin A is best taken with meals for better absorption.

WHAT ARE THE SIDE EFFECTS?

Vitamin A is a fat-soluble vitamin and gets stored in the tissues. High amounts taken over prolonged periods of time can result in toxicity.

An overdose of vitamin A can produce symptoms of vomiting; joint pain; abdominal pain; bone abnormalities; dry, cracking skin; headache; gingivitis; irritability; and fatigue. Symptoms disappear after you stop taking the supplement.

Tolerance to high vitamin A dosages varies. For example, 50,000 IU taken by an adult for several months or years may result in toxicity. If you're taking any amount higher than the RDA, I recommend consulting with a doctor.

Pregnant women should be extremely cautious. Vitamin A can cause birth defects if you take a very high dose. It is advised that pregnant women take vitamin A supplements below a dosage of 5,000 IU.

People with liver diseases such as cirrhosis or hepatitis should use vitamin A with caution as it can build up to toxic levels more easily.

Children can safely handle the amounts found in a children's multivitamin. They should not use vitamin A supplements on a long-term basis, however, unless under the supervision of a doctor.

VITAMIN A

RECOMMENDATIONS FROM THE NATURAL PHYSICIAN FOR . . .

ACNE

High dosages of vitamin A can be helpful for acne but should be used only under the direction of a nutrition-oriented doctor, as side effects can become a problem. When other supplements—such as vitamin E, zinc, and selenium—are used, a much lower dosage of vitamin A can be taken so that side effects are not an issue.

The common acne drug Accutane is actually a synthetic version of vitamin A.

AIDS

Anyone with AIDS may benefit from vitamin A supplementation. One study found that vitamin A deficiency is associated with many people who are HIV positive. Researchers have found that vitamin A can improve the immune function—in particular, raising the concentration of CD4 T-cells.

DRY EYES

Practitioners of natural medicine find that vitamin A eyedrops can help alleviate dry eyes. Check with your local pharmacist.

(continued)

📚 NIGHT BLINDNESS

If you have trouble with night blindness, the condition could be related to a vitamin A deficiency. For people who are having this problem, I usually recommend zinc in combination with vitamin A. An ideal combination is 5,000 to 10,000 IU daily of vitamin A along with 50 mg of zinc.

📚 RESPIRATORY TRACT INFECTIONS

I have found that vitamin A works well for respiratory tract infections such as bronchitis and pneumonia. It is particularly good to help improve immune function against viral infections.

Vitamin C

"It's wintertime again. I wonder how many colds and infections Jeremy and Tim will get?" pondered Samantha, the mother of two boys in grade school.

"Do they get sick a lot in the winter?" I asked.

"Yes, it seems like they come down with something every other week," replied Samantha.

"Why don't you give them each some extra vitamin C? I know they already take a children's multivitamin, but I have found that a little extra vitamin C—100 to 200 mg—can make a big difference in reducing the amount of colds and infections for kids in the winter. They'll love the chewable vitamin C. Just make sure they rinse their mouths with water afterward because the acidity can be hard on their gums and tooth enamel."

I went on to recommend vitamin C for Samantha and her husband as well. "You two can take an extra 500 mg each day," I noted. "It won't hurt and it will probably be helpful."

Five months later, Samantha reported that her boys had considerably fewer colds and sick days as compared with other winters. She also noted that she had fewer episodes of sinusitis since taking the vitamin C.

C CHANGE

Vitamin C (ascorbic acid) is one of the most widely used supplements in the world. Interestingly, while most animals can manufacture their own vitamin C, humans need to get it from their diet or as a supplement.

Many animals have an enzyme that converts glucose to vitamin C. Goats, for example, can produce up to 13,000 mg of vitamin C a day. Unfortunately, a number of animals lack this ability, including humans, guinea pigs, a type of fruit-eating bat from India, and a songbird called the red vented bulbul.

Historically, humans experienced great suffering before learning about vitamin C. Severe vitamin C deficiency caused scurvy, a condition that devastated people who didn't have access to fresh fruits or vegetables (the best natural sources of vitamin C). Sailors on long voyages, who went months without eating fresh food, often had all the symptoms—bleeding gums, skin hemorrhage and easy bruising, weakened bones, poor wound healing, susceptibility to infection, and depression. Numerous shipboard deaths were attributed to scurvy, even before the cause was known.

As far back as 1227, an explorer by the name of Gilbertus de Aguilla began advising sailors to carry fruits and vegetables on trips to avoid scurvy. But this was considered off-the-cuff advice until, in the mid 1700s, a British physician by the name of James Lind conducted an experiment and found that sailors who ate lemons and oranges were able to reduce the effects of scurvy.

GETTING YOUR VITAMIN C

Vitamin C is found mainly in plant foods, particularly in fruits and vegetables. Citrus fruits, tomatoes, peppers, dark green leafy vegetables, broccoli, kale, strawberries, and potatoes are all rich in vitamin C.

Dietary Reference Intake

0 to 12 months: 40 to 50 mg

1 to 10 years: 20 to 25 mg

11 to 18 years: 45 to 75 mg

18+ years: 75 to 90+ mg

Pregnant/lactating: 45+ mg

NOTE: Smokers should add an additional 35 mg to their DRI.

While you'll never be deficient in vitamin C if you meet these minimum levels, your needs for optimum health may actually be higher. For example, if you're exposed to environmental pollutants or already have a disease that requires extra vitamin C—such as heart disease, arthritis, cataracts, or cancer—you should take more. Vitamin C is nontoxic and very safe for people who can benefit greatly from higher dosages.

Vitamin C was first isolated from the red pepper in 1928 by Albert Szent-Gyorgi. For this he was awarded the 1937 Nobel Prize for Medicine.

Today, new attributes of vitamin C are still being discovered.

HOW IT WORKS

Vitamin C is an important antioxidant. A water-soluble antioxidant, it protects cells and cholesterol from oxidative damage. It helps to regenerate vitamin E in the body and is one of the few supplements that can elevate red blood cell levels of glutathione, another one of the body's potent antioxidants. It also prevents premature aging of the skin, cataract formation, and many other conditions related to free-radical damage.

It is also critical for the liver's ability to detoxify substances that get into the body. It does this by acting as an antioxidant and increasing the levels of glutathione.

As is true of many antioxidants, vitamin C is important for reducing the risk of heart disease. Vitamin C prevents oxidation of cholesterol, which is a major factor in the formation of atherosclerosis.

Vitamin C is required for the production of collagen. This is a type of protein that forms the connective tissue that holds our skin together. Collagen is also an important component of cartilage, tendons, ligaments, bone, and blood vessels.

Also, vitamin C strengthens the capillaries and may be helpful for those who bruise easily. It generally helps people to recover from bruises more quickly.

The immune system requires vitamin C to work properly. The late Dr. Linus Pauling touted vitamin C as a cure for the common cold, and a number of studies have since shown that it does help prevent and reduce the severity and length of the common cold.

Vitamin C is very concentrated in white blood cells, the most critical components of the immune system. This vitamin increases the activity of those cells and improves antibody response—that is, the way those cells fight against invading microbes. Vitamin C also increases interferon—an antiviral chemical produced by the body that is required to manufacture protective hormones and is also needed to help fight cancer.

DOSAGE

The dosage for vitamin C depends on the individual. People who regularly consume fruits and vegetables generally do not require vitamin C supplements. A general recommendation for adults requiring supplements is 500 mg daily.

For those with conditions such as cancer, weakened immunity, diabetes, and cataracts, a much higher dosage is recommended. For acute infections such as the common cold, you can take 500 to 1,000 mg every two to three hours. Most people can take 2,000 mg daily without side effects. Doctors can use intravenous vitamin C for the treatment of serious conditions such as cancer or hepatitis.

It is best to take vitamin C in divided doses during the day.

Vitamin C works synergistically with other antioxidants such as vitamin E. Therefore, it makes sense to take it as part of antioxidant or multivitamin formulas.

Vitamin C is available in capsule, crystal, powder, and tablet forms. Most people do fine with regular ascorbic acid. However, the combination of vitamin C with bioflavonoid mixtures is more effective, providing that there is an adequate amount of bioflavonoids. For example, 250 to 500 mg of bioflavonoid complex per 500 mg of vitamin C will improve the effects of vitamin C.

Some people are sensitive to regular vitamin C. The acidity upsets their stomach or causes heartburn. This is a problem for people who have general citrus fruit sensitivity. If you have this problem, I recommend taking buffered vitamin C, where the acidity is reduced by combining calcium, potassium, sodium, or magnesium with ascorbate. The calcium ascorbate form is probably the best. (Another option that works well is to use Ester-C, although this is more expensive.)

Skin creams and topical liquid serums that contain vitamin C are now available. These products fight wrinkling of the skin. Look for a product that contains 5% vitamin C stated on the label.

WHAT ARE THE SIDE EFFECTS?

Vitamin C is nontoxic. However, if people ingest too much, they suffer diarrhea and digestive upset. This is reversible when the dosage is reduced.

If you need to take high dosages of vitamin C, you can try increasingly larger doses every day. You'll know you've reached the maximum level of toleration if you start to have diarrhea. If that occurs, just cut back the dose to a more comfortable level. The diarrhea stops immediately. This is known as "bowel tolerance."

There has been concern about high dosages of vitamin C causing kidney stones. This appears to be unwarranted. In fact, one study showed that men who consumed 1,500 mg daily were less likely to get kidney stones than those who consumed less than 250 mg. Urinary oxalate—the mineral that goes into the makeup of kidney stones—doesn't increase unless you're taking more than 4,000 mg daily, which would be a very high dose.

VITAMIN C

RECOMMENDATIONS FROM THE NATURAL PHYSICIAN FOR . . .

AGE-RELATED MACULAR DEGENERATION (AMD)

Taking 500 mg of vitamin C in combination with 80 mg of zinc, 400 IU of vitamin E, and 15 mg of beta carotene daily was shown to provide a risk reduction of 27% for visual acuity loss and a risk reduction of 25% for progression of AMD in patients with advanced AMD.

ALLERGIES AND ASTHMA

If you're allergic to environmental pollutants, you may also be more prone to getting asthma. Vitamin C works to reduce the allergenic response, though I usually find it works best in combination with other antioxidants. Anyone with asthma is more susceptible to respiratory tract infections, but you can reduce the risk by supporting the immune system with vitamin C. Anyone with asthma, including children, should take vitamin C and antioxidant supplements.

In one study, people with asthma received 1,000 mg of vitamin C for 14 weeks, and their health was compared with others with asthma who were taking a placebo. Those receiving vitamin C had 73% fewer asthma attacks than those receiving placebo. Also, the asthma attacks the vitamin C users had were less severe than the ones experienced by people taking the placebo.

Another study, done in Italy, analyzed the diets and respiratory health of 19,000 children ages six to seven. Children who consumed the most vitamin C–rich fruit were 36% less likely to experience wheezing.

ARTHRITIS

Vitamin C has natural anti-inflammatory properties that make it effective for all different types of arthritis. It is required for the production of cartilage and prevents joint destruction due to its antioxidant properties. I find it most helpful when used as part of an antioxidant formula or nutritional arthritis formula.

ATHEROSCLEROSIS

Vitamin C supplementation has been shown to reduce the risk of atherosclerosis and peripheral artery disease.

CANCER

Many studies show that a diet rich in vitamin C is protective against many different types of cancer. Vitamin C protects the genetic material in cells—their DNA—from damage. This is significant because researchers think DNA damage is one of the leading reasons why people have cancer.

Vitamin C also supports proper functioning of the white blood cells and immune cells, which help keep cancer cells in check. In addition, it is an important component of general detoxification. To the extent that you can detoxify your liver and other body organs, you help to metabolize or "burn up" some of the cancer-causing chemicals and excrete them from your body.

Many nutrition-oriented doctors like me recommend vitamin C–rich foods, supplementation, and even intravenous treatments.

(continued)

CATARACTS

Vitamin C is important in preventing cataract formation. It prevents oxidation in the lens of the eye, and the oxidation process is what contributes to formation of cataracts.

COMMON COLD

Many studies have confirmed that vitamin C reduces the length and severity of the common cold. Australian and Finnish scientists analyzed data from 30 studies involving 11,350 participants to determine the effects of taking 200 mg or more daily of vitamin C for the prevention and treatment of colds. In the general population, vitamin C did not reduce the risk for catching a cold. However, people who were taking vitamin C when they contracted a cold experienced slight reductions in duration and severity of their illness, compared to those taking a placebo. Among marathoners, skiers, and soldiers exposed to significant physical stress or frigid weather, participants who took vitamin C contracted 50% fewer colds.

A previous review of 21 controlled trials using 1 to 8 g of vitamin C found that vitamin C reduced the duration of episodes and the severity of the symptoms of the common cold by an average of 23%.

I find it works best when people load up on it at the first signs of symptoms and take it consistently for the next 48 hours.

DIABETES

Vitamin C and glucose compete to get into the cells, and glucose usually wins. Thus, people with diabetes often have a vitamin C deficiency. If you have diabetes, you need to eat foods that are rich in vitamin C, and you may need to take supplements as well to help prevent such complications as poor wound healing, bruising, and high cholesterol. For anyone with diabetes, I'd recommend a minimum dose of 500 mg of vitamin C, taken twice daily.

GALLSTONES

An increasing amount of research is showing that vitamin C reduces the risk of developing gallstones. It activates an enzyme that breaks down cholesterol into bile acids—which is significant because gallstones occur when your blood is too highly saturated with cholesterol. In one study that included more than 13,000 women, researchers found that those who consumed the greatest amount of vitamin C had a 39% lower risk of developing gallstones.

GINGIVITIS

If you have gum inflammation and your gums seem to bleed easily, it's an indication that you might be suffering marginal vitamin C deficiency. Extra supplements can help improve this condition.

GLAUCOMA

This disease is characterized by increased pressure within the eyeball. Vitamin C is one of the supplements that has been shown to help decrease the pressure.

HEART DISEASE

Numerous studies have demonstrated that vitamin C reduces the risk of cardiovascular disease. It prevents the oxidation of LDL cholesterol and lipoproteins, which are often the precursors of atherosclerosis or "hardening of the arteries." Vitamin C also raises the good HDL cholesterol.

A higher level of vitamin C is also associated with lower blood pressure. Since elevated blood pressure is one of the greatest risk factors for heart disease, the more you can bring it down, the better.

Third, vitamin C strengthens the collagen in the artery walls, which means that the walls become sturdier and less susceptible to scarring. (Cholesterol buildup seems to be worst—and the danger of blockage the greatest—in areas where the artery walls have been scarred.)

In a UCLA study, researchers discovered that men who took 300 mg of vitamin C each day had a 45% lower risk of heart disease than men who took less than 49 mg daily. This well-publicized study, published in the *Journal of the American Medical Association* in 1997, first looked at the short-term effect of a high-fat meal on the arteries. Researchers found that healthy people who were given a high-fat meal and supplementation of 1,000 mg of vitamin C and 800 IU of vitamin E had no negative effects in blood flow through the arteries. By comparison, those who ate a high-fat meal *without* taking these two supplements had blood flow that was negatively affected for up to four hours after eating the fatty meal.

HEPATITIS

Vitamin C is commonly recommended by nutrition-oriented doctors for people with hepatitis, especially the B and C types. It activates the immune system's white blood cells, which helps keep the hepatitis virus under control.

INFECTIONS

Vitamin C can be used as an adjunctive therapy for pretty much any type of infection as it supports normal functioning of the white blood cells.

MALE INFERTILITY

Vitamin C protects against DNA sperm damage and prevents sperm cells from clumping together. One study examined a group of men with infertility due to sperm agglutination (clumping). Some were given 500 mg of vitamin C twice daily. Within three weeks, researchers found that the sperm clumping was reduced, and thus the number of normal cells increased.

There was another interesting result. Pregnancy occurred in the wives of all the men who took the vitamin C for two months. No pregnancies occurred in the wives of the men who were not given vitamin C.

OSTEOPOROSIS

Vitamin C is necessary for proper bone health. It is one of the many vitamins required to prevent and treat osteoporosis, as well as to heal fractures.

PREGNANCY COMPLICATIONS

Vitamin C appears to be one of the important nutrients for preventing preeclampsia, a condition that can be potentially fatal to the mother and infant.

STRESS

Vitamin C is one of the more important nutrients to help your body cope with stress. It not only acts as an antioxidant and improves immune status, it is also involved in the production of stress hormones by your adrenal (stress) glands.

(continued)

🐚 SUNBURN

As an antioxidant, vitamin C helps to retard some of the harmful effects of the sun's ultraviolet rays. This makes it useful when taken internally and used topically.

🐚 WOUNDS

I find that skin wounds such as cuts, burns, and even bedsores heal more quickly if you take extra vitamin C supplements.

🐚 WRINKLES

New research is showing that vitamin C creams may be helpful in reducing wrinkles.

Also, researchers from England conducted the first study to examine the association between nutrient intake and skin-aging appearance in more than 4,000 women, ages 40 to 74. Researchers found that women who ate a diet high in vitamin C were 11% less likely to have wrinkles and 7% less likely to have dry skin due to aging compared to those whose diets were low in vitamin C. Higher linoleic acid (a polyunsaturated fatty acid found in many vegetable oils) intakes were also associated with a lower likelihood of dryness and skin thinning (25% and 22%, respectively).

Vitamin D

Vitamin D used to be known as a nutrient that helped calcium absorption for supporting bone formation. It now has become a superstar nutrient even in the conventional medical field. Why is there now such widespread acceptance that vitamin D supplementation is required? The simple answer is that a ton of studies published in major medical journals have shown that vitamin D deficiency is a major health risk in many different categories that range from osteoporosis, heart disease, arthritis, and mental health to diabetes and cancer (at least 17 different varieties). For example, a study in the *Archives of Internal Medicine* found that three out of every four Americans don't get adequate amounts of vitamin D. This was particularly problematic among non-Hispanic blacks (97%) and Mexican Americans (90%) in the researchers' analysis of National Health and Nutrition Examination Survey (NHANES) data.

Where I practice, in sunny San Diego, it is amazing to see how many of my patients have low vitamin D levels. Genetics comes into play when it comes to the amount of sun people need in order to make their own vitamin D. Common gene mutations interfere with how people use this vitamin. According to a study in the journal *Metabolism*, 35% of Americans have a genetic variation (known as VDR bb) that reduces their ability to use vitamin D. And more impressively, vitamin D targets more than 2,000 genes in the human body.

Low levels of vitamin D occur not just in northern states that are sun-starved during the winter. A new study found that one quarter of adults in sunny southern Arizona were deficient in vitamin D.

People who are obese are also more prone to vitamin D deficiency as are infants not exposed to sunlight.

TYPES OF VITAMIN D

There are three different forms of vitamin D. They include:

🐚 *Cholecalciferol (Vitamin D3)*

Cholecalciferol is the naturally occurring form of vitamin D. It is made from sunlight that hits the skin. It is commonly available as a supplement.

✒ *Calcidiol (25(OH)D3 or 25D3)*

Calcidiol (25-hydroxyvitamin D) is known as a prehormone in your blood. It is made from cholecalciferol (vitamin D3) in the liver. When being tested for vitamin D deficiency, they measure the calcidiol in your blood, known as the 25-hydroxyvitamin D level.

✒ *Calcitriol (1,25(OH)2D3 or 1,25D3)*

Calcitriol (1,25-dihydroxyvitamin D) is made from calcidiol in both the kidneys and other tissues. It is also derived from cholecalciferol (vitamin D3) and known as the active form of vitamin D3. Calcitriol has potent anticancer properties. It is sometimes referred to as the active form of vitamin D.

SUNLIGHT

We need sunlight. As I mentioned, sunlight is key to manufacturing vitamin D in the body. When you are out in the sun and your skin turns pink, you make between 10,000 and 50,000 units of cholecalciferol in your skin. What about vitamin D overdose from sunlight? Our bodies have been designed so that, at about 20,000 units of vitamin D production, ultraviolet light from the sun begins to degrade cholecalciferol. This maintains a steady state and prevents toxicity of vitamin D from the sun.

Thanks to UV-blocking car windows, sunscreens, and clothing to cover up all body parts due to the fear of skin cancer, vitamin D deficiency is a problem. It is also a problem for the elderly who often do not get outside and those living in northern climates who are indoors during the winter months.

Want to absorb your calcium? No one disputes that vitamin D is necessary for calcium absorption. However, since so many people

---

GETTING YOUR D'S

People can become deficient in vitamin D from poor dietary intake. Strict vegetarians may be more prone to such deficiency.

A number of different kinds of fish are particularly good food sources of vitamin D, including salmon, herring, mackerel, and sardines. Other sources are butter, egg yolks, and vitamin D-fortified milk. Most plant sources are low in vitamin D, but you can glean some from mushrooms and dark green leafy vegetables.

Fifteen minutes of direct sunlight daily is recommended. Be aware that sunscreen blocks the UV rays from activating vitamin D synthesis.

There is broad consensus that the dietary reference intake (DRI) for children and adults is woefully inadequate to prevent vitamin D deficiency. Most children should be supplementing 1,000 IU of vitamin D daily and teenagers and adults closer to 2,000 IU. Of course, sunlight exposure plays a factor in the amount one requires. However, these supplement dosage recommendations are generally safe and effective. A simple blood test can show how deficient one may be or if their vitamin D supplementation is adequate.

Dietary Reference Intake

0 to 6 months: 400 IU or 10 mcg
6 to 12 months: 400 IU or 10 mcg
1 to 3 years: 400 IU or 10 mcg
4 to 6 years: 400 IU or 10 mcg
7 to 10 years: 400 IU or 10 mcg
11 to 18 years: 400 IU or 10 mcg
18+ years (male): 400 IU or 10 mcg
50+ years: 400 IU or 10 mcg
Pregnant/lactating: 200+ IU or 5+ mcg

are deficient in vitamin D, their calcium absorption is impaired. Instead of popping megadoses of vitamin D people well need to find out if their vitamin D levels are low and then optimize them along with a regular intake of calcium. For example, a study in the *Journal of American College of Nutrition* showed that people with higher levels of vitamin D3 (86 nmol) absorbed 65% more *calcium* than those with levels of 50 nmol/L.

There are two main forms of vitamin D: vitamin D2 (ergocalciferol) and vitamin D3 (cholecalciferol). Vitamin D2 is the type added to milk and other foods. Vitamin D3 is found in animal foods such as fish, oils, and eggs. This is also the kind that's produced by human skin when you are exposed to sunlight. Most supplements contain vitamin D3.

IN HIGH DEMAND

Vitamin D has several functions. Most important, it promotes calcium absorption and enhances bone mineralization. But it also performs a kind of "blood rescue" function. If blood levels of calcium are too low, a form of vitamin D, synthesized in the kidneys, helps draw some calcium and phosphorous from the bones and deliver these crucial minerals to the blood, bringing blood-calcium levels up to snuff.

Since the liver and kidneys are involved in the activation of vitamin D, diseases of these organs can cause vitamin D deficiency-related diseases.

The symptoms of severe vitamin D deficiency are quite extreme. Children can get a condition called rickets, evidenced by bowed legs, knock-knees, softening of the skull bones, spinal curvature, and increased joint size. In adults, a deficiency can result in osteomalacia, which means softening of the bone. This is more common in people who are not exposed to sunlight or women who have had a number of closely spaced pregnancies—which can deplete a mother's reserves of vitamin D.

It also appears that people lose some of their ability to produce vitamin D from sunlight as they get older. Studies show that people over the age of 61 produce only one-fourth the amount of vitamin D from ultra-violet rays as do people who are under 31 years of age.

Children, especially, need to get enough vitamin D, as good bone density in childhood is associated with a reduced likelihood of developing osteoporosis when they grow into adulthood.

It has also been shown that breast-fed infants who received vitamin D supplements during the first year of life had increased bone density in later childhood.

DOSAGE

Those with fair skin can get enough by spending 10 to 15 minutes outdoors daily in the summer sun, while people with darker complexions likely need 30 to 40 minutes. Unfortunately, most people don't get nearly enough sun.

People in nursing homes and people who are hospitalized are particularly susceptible to a deficiency and must take vitamin D supplements. An average dose is 1,000 to 2,000 IU daily. My experience is that most people need close to 2,000 IU daily for supplementation. I recommend people have a vitamin D3 level of 50 to 80 ng/mL (or 125 to 200 nM/L) year-round. Many people in northern climates need to increase their vitamin D dosage during the winter months.

Certain drugs are known to cause vitamin D deficiency, including anticonvulsants, cimetidine (Tagamet), corticosteroids, heparin, and diuretics.

Children should also be on vitamin D supplements with 1,000 IU the average dose.

WHAT ARE THE SIDE EFFECTS?

Very high doses of prolonged supplementation of vitamin D above dosages of 1,200 IU may result in side effects such as calcification of internal organs, soft tissue damage, kidney damage, kidney stones, digestive upset, and headaches. However, this is uncommon and unneccesary seeing as blood vitamin D levels can be easily monitored. Researchers have learned in recent years that vitamin D toxicity is quite rare. I commonly have patients supplement 2,000 to 5,000 IU daily while monitoring their levels.

If you have hyperparathyroidism or sarcoidosis, you should not take vitamin D supplements unless your doctor instructs you to do so.

A few cautions should be observed if you are taking certain drugs. If you're taking cholesterol-lowering drugs—such as cholestyramine and colestipol—that prevent bile acid reabsorption, then you shouldn't take vitamin D within an hour *before* you take the medications, nor within six hours *after* taking the medication. Also, don't take mineral oil within two hours of taking vitamin D—*either* before or after. You should also not take any vitamin D supplements at any time if you're taking the drug verapramil.

VITAMIN D
RECOMMENDATIONS FROM THE NATURAL PHYSICIAN FOR . . .

◌ AUTISM

One possible theory for the cause of autism may be vitamin D deficiency in the pregnant mother and/or the developing child. There is some research demonstrating that autism is more common in areas of impaired ultraviolet B penetration such as northern latitudes, urban areas, areas with high air pollution, and areas of high precipitation. Also, autism is more common in dark-skinned persons and severe maternal vitamin D deficiency. Genetic defects in the ability to utilize vitamin D may be an issue as well. The reduction in vitamin D levels in the past 20 years may be an issue, too. Vitamin D is involved in proper brain development and neurotransmitter balance.

◌ AUTOIMMUNITY

An increasing amount of information is demonstrating that vitamin D deficiency is a risk factor for a variety of autoimmune diseases such as rheumatoid arthritis, lupus, and multiple sclerosis. Activated vitamin D in the body has a balancing effect on the immune system.

◌ CANCER

Vitamin D has many anticancer effects such as inhibiting improper cell division and metastasis, reducing blood vessel formation around tumors, and regulating proteins that affect tumor growth.

Vitamin D levels are emerging as an important factor in the prevention of cancer. A study in the *Journal of the National Cancer Instutite* found that low levels of vitamin D may be associated with increased cancer incidence and mortality in men, particularly for digestive-system cancers. Men with higher

(continued)

blood vitamin D levels had a 17% reduction in overall cancer incidence, 29% reduction in cancer-related mortality, 43% reduction in gastrointestinal cancer incidence, and 45% reduction in gastrointestinal cancer-related mortality.

Also, men and women with higher blood levels of vitamin D had a decreased risk of colorectal cancer–related mortality.

Another study, this one a 16-year study of more than 88,000 women, found that higher intakes of vitamin D were associated with significantly lower breast cancer risk during premenopause.

There are also studies demonstrating a link between low vitamin D levels and risk of prostate and several other cancers. Adequate vitamin D levels appear to be very important in the holistic approach to preventing a variety of different cancers.

⛭ CHRONIC PAIN

A variety of studies have found a correlation between different forms of chronic pain and low vitamin D levels. Vitamin D supplementation may help some people with the recovery from chronic pain such as low back pain or arthritis of the knees.

⛭ DEPRESSION

Researchers are finding a correlation between low vitamin D levels and risk of depression. Vitamin D supplementation should be considered for those with a history of depression.

⛭ COGNITIVE FUNCTION

Vitamin D has many physiologic effects on the brain. A deficiency has been shown to be associated with reduced cognitive function in older adults and possibly dementia.

⛭ DIABETES

Vitamin D plays a role in the secretion of insulin and glucose balance. Population studies show that those with lower vitamin D levels have a significantly higher risk of type 2 diabetes compared to people with higher vitamin D levels.

Vitamin D supplementation has not been shown to treat type 2 diabetes, although it may help in a multifactorial approach. However, vitamin D supplementation with infants during the first year of life reduces the risk of type 1 diabetes later in life.

⛭ FALL PREVENTION

Studies suggest that increased vitamin D levels can help prevent falls in the elderly.

⛭ FIBROMYALGIA

Low vitamin D levels may be one causative or associated factor with fibromyalgia. I recommend all patients with fibromyalgia get adequate vitamin D levels through sun exposure and supplementation.

⛭ HEART DISEASE

Population studies suggests that people with low vitamin D levels have a significantly increased risk of developing cardiovascular disease. This includes heart attack, stroke, heart failure, cardiovascular mortality, and all-cause mortality compared to those with higher vitamin D levels. In a large study, researchers from Drew University of Medicine and Science in Los Angeles analyzed data collected by the National Center for Health Statistics to evaluate the association between vitamin D and cardiovascular disease. They examined blood levels of vitamin D in 7,186 men and 7,902 women and found that, compared to those with the highest levels of vitamin D, those with the lowest levels were significantly more likely to suffer from heart disease risk factors, including obesity, diabetes, and high blood pressure. The study authors noted that further research is needed to assess the effect of vitamin D supplementation on cardiovascular risk factors.

HIGH BLOOD PRESSURE

Lower vitamin D levels are a risk factor for high blood pressure, which in turn is a risk for heart disease.

HIGH CHOLESTEROL LEVELS

Research demonstrates that a low vitamin D level is associated with higher cholesterol and triglyceride levels. If your lipid levels are elevated, have your vitamin D level checked as a root cause.

HYPERPARATHYROIDISM-RELATED BONE LOSS

Vitamin D should be supplemented in those with high levels of the hormone parathyroid, which takes calcium from the bones. Vitamin D supplementation can help improve bone turnover.

MULTIPLE SCLEROSIS

Vitamin D levels appear to be very important in the prevention of this disease. Population studies suggest that long-term vitamin D supplementation decreases the risk of MS in women by up to 40%.

OSTEOPOROSIS

Though vitamin D is always necessary for good health, it's particularly critical for prevention and treatment of osteoporosis.

Several studies have shown that the combination of calcium and vitamin D is more effective in slowing bone loss or increasing bone density than calcium alone. One study examined 249 healthy postmenopausal women with an average age of 61. All the women received a calcium supplement, bringing their total combined dietary intake to 800 mg a day. Half the women received 400 IU of vitamin D and the other half a placebo. Bone density was measured three times over the course of one year. The group receiving the calcium only (calcium citrate malate) had no bone loss over the course of the year. The women who received additional vitamin D supplementation along with the calcium had a significant gain in bone density of the spine. Another study found that 700 to 800 IU daily of vitamin D3 supplementation with or without calcium seems to reduce fracture risk in ambulatory and institutionalized elderly people. For my patients with osteoporosis, it is not uncommon for me to prescribe 3,000 to 5,000 IU daily, depending on their blood levels.

Vitamin D is very important in preventing hip fractures (as are magnesium, vitamin K, and calcium). Researchers from across the United States examined previously collected data on 93,676 postmenopausal women. Vitamin D status in 400 women who had suffered a hip fracture was compared to 400 age- and ethnicity-similar women who had not suffered a hip fracture. They found women with the lowest vitamin D blood concentrations were 71% more susceptible to fracture.

TOOTH LOSS IN THE ELDERLY

Vitamin D along with calcium supplements

(continued)

have been shown to help prevent tooth loss in the elderly.

🐚 UPPER RESPIRATORY TRACT INFECTION

Data analyzed from approximately 19,000 adolescent and adult participants found that those who had the lowest blood levels of vitamin D were about 40% more likely to have had a recent respiratory infection than subjects who had vitamin D levels of 30 ng/mL or greater.

🐚 WEIGHT LOSS

Recent studies show that it is harder to lose weight when one is deficient in vitamin D.

Vitamin E

"I read in the newspaper that vitamin E should not be supplemented to prevent heart disease, and that it can actually increase your risk of heart disease. I have been taking vitamin E for years. Was that a mistake?" questioned Fred, a 58-year-old electrician.

"No, you have been taking the natural form of vitamin E. Many of those studies used synthetic vitamin E and populations of people that were unhealthy to begin with," I replied.

Like many supplements, vitamin E has been under attack in recent years. However, when the supposed negative studies are scrutinized more closely along with the positive studies, vitamin E stands strong in terms of its scientific support.

Vitamin E has been shown to be important as a supplement for people with specific diseases such as Alzheimer's and diabetes or those with a high susceptibility to certain diseases, such as bladder cancer and eye disease. Vitamin E prevents LDL "bad" cholesterol from becoming oxidized (damaged), thereby helping to guard against plaque formation in the arteries, known as atherosclerosis. Also, low vitamin E levels are associated with an increased risk of major depression, rheumatoid arthritis, and preeclampsia (a condition during pregnancy characterized by swelling of the hands and face and high blood pressure). In addition, those with the genetic condition cystic fibrosis have trouble absorbing vitamin E.

Vitamin E really refers to a family of compounds. There are more than 12 vitamin E compounds found in nature (currently eight forms are available in supplement form). There are two main groups of compounds—tocopherols (found in foods such as corn, soy, and peanuts) and tocotrienols (found in rice, barley, rye, and wheat). Many foods contain a blend of these two groups. Both have subgroups called alpha, beta, gamma, and delta.

The most commonly used supplement form is alpha tocopherol, and most studies (positive and negative) have researched this form. But taking just alpha tocopherol can reduce the blood levels of beneficial gamma and delta tocopherols. Epidemiological studies indicate that higher blood gamma tocopherol levels correspond to the reduction of prostate cancer and coronary heart disease. Also, delta and gamma tocotrienols reduce the liver's production of cholesterol. One of the positive aspects of the negative vitamin E studies I mentioned above is that they have pushed researchers to look deeper into what vitamin E supplements should really contain.

According to Barrie Tan, PhD, adjunct

professor of food science at the University of Massachusetts, Amherst, believes that vitamin E supplements used for disease prevention should be a blend of both tocopherols and tocotrienols. I agree with this view because these forms are more similar to what we find in food.

THE E IN GREENS

Vitamin E was first discovered in 1922 when researchers found that an unknown substance in green lettuce prevented rats from miscarrying. It was later isolated in wheat germ oil in 1936. Vitamin E is often referred to as alpha-tocopherol, which is the most biologically active form of the tocopherols.

The term tocopherol translated from Greek means "to bear children." Therefore, vitamin E has been referred to as the "fertility" or "antisterility" vitamin.

Vitamin E is very important as the body's most significant fat-soluble antioxidant. It prevents cell membranes and cholesterol from becoming damaged by the process of oxidation, which is similar to the chemical process that leads to rusting in metal and rotting in fruit and vegetables. Vitamin E is important for a healthy immune system, cardiovascular disease protection, and cancer prevention.

People with certain diseases, such as diabetes and Parkinson's disease, should always have extra vitamin E supplementation—and there's ample research to support this view. But there are, in addition, many other conditions for which vitamin E can be helpful, ranging from arthritis to skin wounds.

Athletes require additional antioxidant support from the free radicals generated by exercise. Vitamin E is important for reducing muscle inflammation and soreness from strenuous exercise.

A severe vitamin E deficiency is rare in North America, except in infants who are born prematurely and in adults who require kidney dialysis. But people who have cystic fibrosis may lack vitamin E because they can't absorb it properly, and vitamin E deficiencies have also shown up in some people who have genetic disorders such as sickle cell disease.

Symptoms of a vitamin E deficiency can include nerve problems, muscle weakness, anemia, and poor coordination. More commonly, people in our society experience less overt symptoms of vitamin E deficiency—the kinds of slow-developing problems that tend to lead to health problems over prolonged periods of time. These include heart disease, skin problems, and a weakened immune system.

GETTING YOUR VITAMIN E

Vitamin E is found in the fats of vegetables. Polyunsaturated vegetable oils such as wheat germ oil contain high amounts of the tocopherols. Interestingly, vitamin E is found in nature in foods that contain high amounts of polyunsaturated fatty acids (such as safflower oil, corn oil, and soybean oil), which help protect the foods against rapid oxidation. Theoretically, then, we would get vitamin E from commercial vegetable oils—but unfortunately, they're so altered in processing that they have little vitamin E left by the time they reach the store shelves, and they don't have a good blend of tocopherols and tocotrienols. The same holds true for most grains, which start out with vitamin E, but are depleted as they're processed into the flours that are used in most breads and other baked goods.

Vitamin E is found naturally in wheat germ, nuts, seeds, whole grains, egg yolks, and leafy green vegetables. Animal products are a poor source of vitamin E. Serious vitamin E deficiency is rare, although many Americans don't get enough vitamin E, especially those on low-fat diets because fat is needed for absorption of vitamin E.

Tocotrienols are also a part of the vitamin E family. More information can be found in the tocotrienols chapter.

DIETARY REFERENCE INTAKE

0 to 12 months: 4 to 5 mg

1 to 10 years: 6 to 10 mg

11 to 18 years: 11 to 15 mg

18+ years: 15+ mg

Pregnant/lactating: 4+ mg

THE MEDIA HAS IT WRONG

As I mentioned there has been a lot of media hype on the safety and efficacy of vitamin E in the press. For example, two well-publicized studies raised questions about vitamin E. The first is a meta-analysis (a study of other studies) led by researchers from the Johns Hopkins School of Medicine. The researchers reviewed 19 vitamin E studies that followed almost 136,000 patients. Most of these studies targeted populations at high risk for a chronic disease, usually coronary heart disease. Nine of the 19 studies focused on vitamin E alone, while the other 10 studies combined vitamin E with other vitamins or minerals. These studies ranged from 1.4 to 8.2 years in length. Vitamin E dosage varied from 16.5 IU to 2,000 IU per day, with a median dosage of 400 IU per day. The meta-analysis found that those taking 400 IU or more of vitamin E daily for at least one year were 10% more likely to die from all causes than those who did not.

There were several problems with this analysis. First, researchers combined data

that used both natural (the same as found in food) and synthetic forms of vitamin E. Previous research has shown that natural forms of vitamin E are better utilized by the body than cheaper, synthetic forms. The 1996 Cambridge Heart Antioxidant Study used only a natural form of vitamin E and found that a dose of at least 400 IU daily substantially reduced the rate of nonfatal heart attacks after one year of treatment.

However, the biggest criticism of the meta-analysis was that most of the studies included elderly people who had existing diseases such as cancer, Alzheimer's disease, heart disease, and other potentially fatal illnesses. Even the authors of the study stated, "The generalizability of the findings to healthy adults is uncertain. Precise estimation of the threshold at which risk increases is difficult."

Another study, which was published in the March 16, 2005, issue of the *Journal of the American Medical Association*, focused on patients who were 55 or older with vascular disease or diabetes. The study's conclusion was that for people with vascular disease or diabetes, long-term vitamin E supplementation does not prevent cancer or cardiovascular events and may increase risk for heart failure. This study provides no evidence that vitamin E is unsafe for people who are healthy.

This chapter describes the many studies that demonstrate both the safety and effectiveness of vitamin E.

DOSAGE

I recommend that adults get an average of 200 to 400 IU of natural vitamin E daily, preferably the mixed vitamin E form that contains a blend of tocopherols and toctorienols. Higher doses are required for those with a history of deep vein thrombosis or Alzheimer's disease and up to 2,000 IU may be required. Some people (those with a history of heart disease or cancer) may require a higher dosage, such as 800 IU daily. Vitamin E works synergistically with vitamin C, lipoic acid, and coenzyme Q10.

Always choose the natural form, which is d-alpha tocopherol, as opposed to the synthetic version, which is d,l-alpha tocopherol. So, if it has an "l" in it, then "leave" it alone. Although it costs more, the natural form is two to three times more absorbable to your body tissues than synthetic vitamin E. It would be rare to find synthetic vitamin E products in a health-food store.

There are several medications that can deplete vitamin E levels and supplementation should be considered. These include bile acid sequestrants such as cholestyramine (Questran) and colestipol (Colestid); epiliptic drugs such as carbamazepine (Tegretol), phenobarbitol, and dilantin; and weight medication such as orlistat (Xenical, Alli).

WHAT ARE THE SIDE EFFECTS?

Vitamin E is quite safe when used at a dosage of 1,200 IU and lower, although studies have shown it to be safe even at 2,000 IU. Consult with your doctor if you plan to take more than 400 IU of vitamin E if you are on a blood-thinning medication. Also, vitamin E supplements are usually stopped seven to ten days before and after surgery.

VITAMIN E
RECOMMENDATIONS FROM THE NATURAL PHYSICIAN FOR . . .

ACNE
I have found that vitamin E helps teenagers and adults with mild to moderate acne, especially when combined with vitamin A supplementation.

AIDS
Vitamin E is an extremely important antioxidant for people with AIDS. Studies have shown that those with this disease are often deficient in vitamin E and that taking vitamin E helps to slow down the progression of the disease.

ALZHEIMER'S DISEASE
Although the cause of Alzheimer's disease is unknown, research is showing that free-radical damage in brain cells accelerates progression of this disease. Vitamin E protects against cell oxidation.

In a study done in the late 1990s, researchers found that vitamin E sup-plementation reduced the risk of reaching the most severe stages of Alzheimer's disease as compared with those taking standard drug therapy or placebo. I recommend vitamin E and the other major antioxidants for those who have or are suspected of having this disease.

ANGINA
Vitamin E is recommended by nutrition-oriented doctors to help prevent and treat angina. I always combine it with other heart-healthy nutrients such as CoQ10 and magnesium, and herbs such as hawthorn, ginkgo, and cactus.

ARTHRITIS
Vitamin E appears to have a natural anti-inflammatory effect and can be helpful for

(continued)

persons suffering from different types of arthritis, particularly rheumatoid arthritis.

✤ BURNS, WOUNDS, AND SCARS

Vitamin E promotes the healing of burns and wounds to the skin. It is excellent to take internally and to apply externally to prevent scarring or reduce newly formed scars. You can open up a capsule of the mixed form of vitamin E gel capsules to apply to scars or purchase creams that are rich in vitamin E.

✤ CANCER

Studies have shown that people with low vitamin E levels are more susceptible to different types of cancers. Vitamin E appears to be especially important for the prevention of prostate and lung cancer. One study found that supplementing 200 IU of vitamin E evreyday for greater than 10 years was associated with a reduced risk of bladder cancer mortality.

Tocotrienols have been shown to be important for the prevention and treatment of cancer, especially breast cancer. Gamma tocopherol has been shown to be important for the prevention of lung cancer for those who smoke.

✤ CAROTID STENOSIS

Tocotrienols appear to be one of the few effective alternatives to surgery for carotid stenosis, the buildup of plaque that narrows the carotid artery blood flow to the brain. The surgery for carotid stenosis (carotid endarterectomy) is quite dangerous, with a 1 in 10 risk of stroke and death. So it's much preferable to try to avoid the necessity of such surgery by taking tocotrienols. See the Tocotrienols (page 447) for more information.

✤ CATARACTS

Cataracts occur as the result of oxidation of the lens in the eye. Vitamin E is one of the important antioxidants that can help to prevent this condition.

✤ DIABETES

Vitamin E has been shown to improve glucose tolerance in people who have diabetes. In addition, it helps to protect against nerve damage associated with free radical damage caused by the disease.

✤ ECZEMA

Vitamin E taken both internally and applied externally can be helpful to reduce eczema.

✤ FERTILITY

Vitamin E has been shown to help male fertility in several studies. For example, in one study, men with low sperm counts and motility demonstrated that vitamin E supplementation achieved impregnation at a rate of 21% compared to none for similar patients receiving placebo.

✤ FIBROCYSTIC BREAST SYNDROME

I have found that women with this condition respond very well to a dosage of 800 IU of vitamin E.

✤ HEART DISEASE

The most popular use of supplemental vitamin E is for the prevention of heart disease. Vitamin E prevents the oxidation of cholesterol, which is a leading culprit in the buildup of atherosclerotic plaque in the arteries.

Polls of cardiologists have shown that nearly 50% take vitamin E themselves.

The Cambridge Heart study of 2,000 patients with heart disease found that those who took between 400 to 800 IU of vitamin E had a 77% decrease in cardiovascular disease over a year's time. In a Nurses Health study involving 87,000 women, doctors learned that women who took vitamin E for two years or more had a 41% reduction in the risk of heart disease. Women taking 200 IU had more protection than those taking 100 IU.

A further study was conducted with 11,000 seniors, ages 67 to 105, over a nine-year period. Doctors found that those who took a vitamin E supplement of 400 IU daily had a 41% reduction in heart disease. Results were even better when people took vitamin C in addition to vitamin E.

Vitamin E also helps to reduce another important marker of cardiovascular disease. C-reactive protein is an inflammatory marker—and inflammation of the blood vessels sets the stage for artery disease. Elevated C-reactive protein levels are associated with a 4.5 times increased risk of having a heart attack. Vitamin E also reduced another marker of inflammation known as interleukin-6 by 50%.

Vitamin E has natural blood-thinning properties; this is thought to be why it helps to improve circulation as well as prevent strokes. In one study, where people took 600 IU of vitamin E daily for two weeks, researchers found immediate evidence that the vitamin delayed blood clotting—a good indication that it was acting as a blood thinner.

HIGH CHOLESTEROL

Vitamin E prevents the oxidation of cholesterol, particularly the "bad" LDL cholesterol. It also increases the "good" HDL cholesterol in young adults who have abnormally low HDL levels.

Rice bran tocotrienols are proving to be powerful in their ability to lower cholesterol (especially LDL) and increase the protective HDL cholesterol.

INFECTIONS

Vitamin E is one of the many nutrients required for a healthy immune system. People with chronic infections such as hepatitis or those with susceptible immune systems may benefit from taking vitamin E supplements.

MACULAR DEGENERATION

Studies have shown that vitamin E can help prevent and improve this eye disease, which is a leading cause of blindness. Combining 400 IU vitamin E with 80 mg zinc, 500 mg vitamin C, and 15 mg beta carotene daily showed a risk reduction of 27% for visual acuity loss and a risk reduction of 25% for progression of age-related macular degeneration in patients with advanced cases of this condition.

MENOPAUSE

Vitamin E helps to reduce hot flashes as well as vaginal dryness in menopausal women. Studies have shown that vitamin E in dosages of 400 to 800 IU reduces the frequency of hot flashes.

Also, taking a vitamin E supplement during this transitional time is important as the risk of heart disease increases greatly with the hormonal changes.

(continued)

🐚 MUSCLE STRENGTH WITH ELDERLY

Vitamin E was shown in a study to improve muscle strength and physical performance in the elderly.

🐚 MULTIPLE SCLEROSIS

I recommend that people suffering from this autoimmune disease take a vitamin E supplement to help prevent relapses. Vitamin E helps to protect against oxidative damage to the myelin sheath.

🐚 PARKINSON'S DISEASE

Researchers speculate that free radicals—the electrically charged molecules that speed up oxidation—play an important role in Parkinson's disease. Since vitamin E is one of the antioxidants that helps control free-radical activity, it should be included in a comprehensive treatment program.

🐚 PERIPHERAL VASCULAR DISEASE

As a natural blood thinner, vitamin E helps to improve blood flow to the hands and feet. For example, researchers from Harvard analyzed data from nearly 40,000 women, ages 45 and older, who took 600 IU of vitamin E or a placebo every other day for about 10 years. Compared to placebo users, vitamin E users were 21% less likely to develop venous thromboembolism (VTE), a potentially fatal clot in a lung artery or deep vein. In the vitamin E group, risk fell by 18% for women with no history of VTE, by 44% for those with a history of VTE, and by almost 50% for women with a genetic mutation that increases VTE risk.

🐚 PMS

Vitamin E supplementation of 400 IU daily for three months can reduce symptoms of depression, anxiety, and cravings in women with PMS.

Vitamin K

"I think I am taking all the vitamins and minerals needed for bone health and to improve my bone density," stated Bonnie, a new patient of mine with mild osteoporosis.

"Let me take a look at your list," I replied as I scanned through her list and the dosages of the many supplements she was taking. It turned out that Bonnie was missing one critical vitamin, which recent research has shown to play a key factor in bone health, as well as the cardiovascular system—vitamin K.

Vitamin K has long been known for its role in blood clot formation. It is essential for the functioning of several proteins involved in blood clotting because of the role it plays in transporting calcium. Vitamin K is was named based on the German word *koagulation*. Coagulation is the process by which blood clots are formed. This vitamin is also important for bone calcification, whereby calcium is transported from the blood into the bones to keep them strong. To accomplish this, the body requires the assistance of the protein osteocalcin, and osteocalcin cannot do its job without vitamin K. So both major roles of vitamin K in blood clotting and bone calcification revolve around its key role in calcium transportation.

There are two main forms of vitamin K: phylloquinone (K1) and menaquinone (K2).

Vitamin K1 is abundant in the diet in dark green leafy vegetables such as lettuce, spinach, and broccoli. Vegetable oils are also sources of vitamin K; soybean, cottonseed, canola, and olive oils all contain vitamin K, with olive oil being the healthiest choice. However, vitamin K2 is better absorbed and remains active in the body longer than vitamin K1. The best food source of vitamin K2 is natto (fermented soybeans) and, to a lesser degree, fermented cheeses (the type with holes, such as Swiss and Jarlsberg), butter, beef liver, chicken, and egg yolks. Also, friendly flora in the large intestine synthesize vitamin K2.

Studies by the USDA demonstrate that vitamin K deficiency in the American diet is more common than was once thought. This is particularly true of Americans ages 18 to 44, who tend not to consume vitamin K–rich foods.

DIETARY REFERENCE INTAKE

0 to 12 months: 10 to 20 mcg

1 to 10 years: 15 to 60 mcg

11 to 18 years: 50 to 100 mcg

18+ years: 100+ mcg

Vitamin K deficiency can result in impaired blood clotting. This can manifest as easy bruising or bleeding. A deficiency can also contribute to impaired bone metabolism and calcification of the arteries. Vitamin K deficiency is more common in those on blood-thinning medications such as Coumadin (warfarin) because users are advised to abstain from vitamin K–rich foods or vitamin K–containing supplements. Also, those with liver disease and people with digestive disorders that have impaired fat absorption are at increased risk of vitamin K deficiency. Exclusively breast-fed newborn babies are said to be at an increased risk of vitamin K deficiency, although I have not observed this in practice. There are several medications that can cause vitamin K deficiency, including broad-spectrum antibiotics; diet medications that block fat absorption (orlistat); mineral oil; cholesterol-lowering medications known as bile acid sequestrants, such as cholestyramine (Questran) and colestipol (Colestid); salicylates; anticonvulsant medications; and anticoagulants, such as Coumadin (warfarin). Vitamin K supplementation should be considered when long-term use of these medications is required.

DOSAGE

Vitamin K is available in supplement form. I find higher-quality multivitamins often include vitamin K, as do several bone formulas. Most adults can benefit from 25 to 200 mcg vitamin K depending on their dietary intake and their health status. Dosages of oral vitamin K up to 45 mg per day have been used in studies to treat osteoporosis. Vitamin K is fat-soluble so it is best taken with food.

WHAT ARE THE SIDE EFFECTS?

Vitamin K appears to be quite safe except for those who require lower intakes, such as those on blood-thinning medications such as Coumadin (warfarin). However, vitamin K supplementation and vitamin K–rich foods may still be consumed when kept at a steady level. This requires a doctor's supervision. Those receiving dialysis treatments for chronic kidney disease should avoid excessive vitamin K supplementation.

VITAMIN K

RECOMMENDATIONS FROM THE NATURAL PHYSICIAN FOR . . .

ATHEROSCLEROSIS

When vitamin K is deficient, calcium that is free in the blood goes looking for a place to land—and heads for the arteries, which in turn become stiffer and more prone to allowing formation of dangerous blood clots. In other words, vitamin K promotes beneficial bone calcification but also protects against harmful arterial calcification.

Recent research indicates that vitamin K2 is especially protective against artery calcification. The Rotterdam Study, an ongoing European clinical trial started in 1990, evaluated (among many other things) how vitamin K intake affected 4,807 subjects over a period of 7 to 10 years. Results published in the *Journal of Nutrition* showed that a diet providing 45 mcg per day of vitamin K2 was associated with 50% less arterial calcification, a 50% decrease in cardiovascular mortality risk, and a 25% reduction in risk of dying from any cause. Clinical trials also have demonstrated that vitamin K2 improves elasticity of the carotid arteries, thereby promoting better blood flow.

People taking Coumadin (warfarin) are at higher risk for atherosclerosis and osteoporosis (brittle bones) because the drug increases arterial calcification and decreases bone calcification. A study in the journal *Pharmacotherapy* demonstrated the safety and benefit of low-dose vitamin K supplementation in patients taking warfarin. However, it is imperative that a person who takes blood thinners use vitamin K2 only under the close supervision of a doctor so that blood clotting times are monitored.

HEMORRHAGIC DISEASE OF THE NEWBORN

Vitamin K deficiency can result in bleeding in a newborn infant. However, this is uncommon since vitamin K is routinely given after birth in the United States.

OSTEOPOROSIS

Vitamin K should be utilized more by physicians in the prevention and treatment of osteoporosis, a disease that is epidemic in the United States. As mentioned in this chapter, vitamin K is intricately involved with the bone-forming protein osteocalcin. Adequate vitamin K intake reduces bone loss and fracture rates. Studies on the benefit for people with osteoporosis are conflicting. However, a meta-analysis in *Archives of Internal Medicine* that reviewed previous randomized controlled trials that gave adult participants oral vitamin K supplements for longer than six months, which included 20 trials, and found that all studies except one showed benefit of vitamin K in reducing bone loss.

Vitex

"My menstrual cycle is out of control! It's been irregular for the last five years."

When I asked Sherry, a 24-year-old nurse, to explain what she meant, she described a menstrual cycle that did, indeed, seem out of control. One month her menstrual flow might last 20 days; the next month, only seven.

"Sometimes I go a month or two without a period," she continued. "It's so frustrating! My gynecologist wants to put me on the birth-control pill and that's the last thing I want to take. I want to get pregnant in the near future. Anyway, a friend of mine told me that you helped her out with a similar problem. She said that you could balance hormones naturally."

"Yes, usually. Are there any other hormone-related symptoms or conditions you have?" I suspected that she might also have PMS, ovarian cysts, or other problems.

"I have mood changes and breast tenderness for three or four days each month. My husband calls me the PMS monster during this time. I have had cysts show up on my pelvic ultrasounds in the past. Do you have different treatments for all these things?" Sherry asked.

"It's all pretty much the same treatment," I said. "Once we balance your hormones, most of these problems should clear up."

I wanted Sherry to appreciate that hormones are very powerful chemicals. If they were out of balance, some major problems could occur, exactly like the ones she was having.

"Based on what you've told me about your menstrual pattern, it appears that you are not ovulating regularly," I observed.

"That's what my gynecologist said, too," replied Sherry.

I explained that while the birth-control pill often helps to regulate the menstrual cycle—because of the estrogen and progesterone it contains—it does not help ovaries to ovulate. In fact, it actually prevents ovulation.

"So we need to regulate your cycle and make sure you're ovulating regularly," I concluded. "I have had good results in cases like this with the herbal extract vitex, commonly called chasteberry. It helps to increase the pituitary gland's release of luteinizing hormone, which then stimulates the ovaries to ovulate. You get a release of progesterone once this happens, so that ultimately you have a balance between estrogen and progesterone, and the menstrual cycle balances out."

"And it will also help my fertility because I will be ovulating," Sherry added.

"Yes. In fact, I have found it helps some cases of infertility related to anovulation (no ovulation)."

Sherry began taking vitex extract every day.

By the second month, her period was lighter than usual and she was less irritable than she had been during previous cycles. After five months of continuous use, Sherry began having regular menstrual cycles. Each period occurred once a month and lasted about five days. Also, she no longer had a problem with breast tenderness.

I asked Sherry to continue taking vitex for another five months.

Soon after, she reported that she was pregnant. I cannot say she became pregnant because of vitex—as there is no way to prove that—but I do know that vitex has definitely helped other women who wanted to become pregnant.

A History of Helping

Vitex agnus-castus, also known as chasteberry or chaste tree, is the most important herb for women in western and European herbal therapy. If I were limited to one herb for women's health, vitex would be the one I would pick, as it is so versatile. It can help acne, fibrocystic breast syndrome, infertility, lactation, menopausal hot flashes, menstrual disorders, ovarian cysts, and PMS. In other words, it is a woman's best herbal friend.

The long history of medicinal use dates back to the fourth century BC, when Hippocrates wrote about the capabilities of this remarkable herb. In fact, the terms "chasteberry or chaste tree" were originally applied to this plant because people believed that it somehow made chastity easier. To Ancient Greeks, vitex was an appropriate symbol of chastity to display during festivals that honored the goddess Demeter.

Later, the Christian Church adopted a similar type of symbolism. Vitex was the plant of choice for the pathway to the monastery that monks would follow during their initiation. The herb was thought to restrain the libido of monks who might go astray. (Whatever its effect on men, however, vitex has no reported dampening effect on women's libido.) The practice of planting vitex along the monastery pathways continues to this day in Italy.

Another common name for vitex is "monk's pepper." The vitex fruit smells like pepper and was used as a spice on monastery meals.

Vitex does not contain hormones. Rather, it acts on a part of the brain known as the hypothalamus and the pituitary gland (located in the brain) to increase the production of luteinizing hormone (LH). LH is responsible for stimulating the ovaries to ovulate.

When ovulation occurs, there is a release of progesterone during the second half of the cycle. This is important to maintain a balance with estrogen. Many women do not ovulate on a regular basis, and therefore have a relative higher elevation of estrogen to progesterone, referred to as "estrogen dominance." By helping to normalize progesterone levels, vitex promotes hormone balance. This is why it is effective for so many female conditions, which are in large part caused by an estrogen–progesterone imbalance.

Also, vitex has been shown to lower levels of prolactin. This hormone, which is also secreted by the pituitary gland, is associated with PMS, irregular menstrual cycles, and infertility.

DOSAGE

I most often use the capsule form of vitex. I have had good results with a dosage of 80 to 240 mg (usually one to three capsules) of a 0.6% aucubin extract. Products containing 0.5% agnuside are also frequently used. There is no agreed-upon standardization for vitex. It is generally recommended that the product contain 30 to 40 mg of the dried fruit, and that it be taken daily.

Clinical studies have used 40 drops of a standardized tincture extract taken once a day in the morning, so that's probably the minimum dose for effectiveness. However, I sometimes recommend 40 drops of the tincture form to be taken three times daily.

Vitex is best used on a long-term basis. Women may notice improvements within two menstrual cycles; however, it often needs to be taken for a minimum of four to six months. Long-standing conditions such as infertility, amenorrhea, irregular menstrual cycles, or endometriosis may require vitex supplementation for a year or longer.

WHAT ARE THE SIDE EFFECTS?

Vitex is quite safe. In rare cases, there may be mild digestive upset, nausea, headaches, and skin rash. Vitex should not be taken by women who are also taking birth-control pills. Also, you should not take vitex if you're also taking drugs that block dopamine receptors, such as haloperidol.

So far, we don't know whether vitex interferes with hormone replacement that is given for menopause, so caution should be used. I have, at times, had women use vitex who were on hormone replacement, and none of them reported problems.

As with most herbs, it is best avoided during pregnancy, although some herbal practitioners recommend it for the first trimester for women who have a history of miscarriage due to progesterone deficiency.

Some women experience an "adjustment phase" with vitex during the first few months of use. During this phase, the cycle shortens or lengthens. Menstrual flow can become lighter or heavier than what it was previously. This "adjustment phase" almost always normalizes after three to four months of use.

VITEX
RECOMMENDATIONS FROM THE NATURAL PHYSICIAN FOR . . .

ACNE

Acne is a hormone-dependent condition. As a hormone balancer, vitex is especially effective in reducing menstruation-related acne.

I have also found it to work well for teenage acne, for both boys and girls. They can usually see improvement in a few months.

AMENORRHEA

Vitex is one of the most specific herbs to use for amenorrhea. It has been used mainly in cases of secondary amenorrhea (where there has been menstrual flow in the past but it has stopped).

There can be different causes of amenorrhea—lack of ovulation being one of them. This is the type that vitex is indicated for, since vitex increases the production of LH by the pituitary gland to stimulate ovulation and progesterone production.

Vitex also reduces elevated levels of the hormone prolactin by binding to dopamine receptors of the pituitary gland, where prolactin is secreted. A study of 52 women who did not ovulate due to high prolactin levels found that vitex extract taken for three months reduced prolactin levels. As a result, the progesterone levels were normalized as well as the cycle itself.

FIBROCYSTIC BREASTS AND BREAST PAIN

Benign breast cysts are very common, and women frequently turn to their gynecologists when they have cysts. Often, the first sign is an increase in sensitivity or pain right before menstruation. This is thought to be a result of estrogen dominance.

I have found vitex to eliminate or improve benign breast cysts and cyclical breast pain. Again, this usually takes up to three months to be effective and up to six months for some women.

A study of 104 women who suffered from premenstrual breast pain found that vitex extract significantly reduced breast pain. Improvements were noticed within

(continued)

two cycles. (Vitamin E and essential fatty acid, such as evening primrose oil, are very helpful as well.)

🐚 INFERTILITY

Vitex is indicated for cases of infertility resulting from insufficient progesterone production (which means there's no ovulation) and due to high prolactin levels. I have seen it help women begin to ovulate when they were previously unable to do so. Work with your doctor to incorporate vitex into a treatment protocol for infertility.

One study of women with menstrual disorders found that vitex improved cases of polymenorrhea (too frequent) as well as cases of women with menorrhagia (excessive bleeding).

🐚 LACTATION

Vitex has long been used to increase milk supply during lactation. Recently, I had a female patient who stopped breast-feeding a few days after the birth of her child because she was put on medication. A week later, she had problems resuming breast-feeding because her milk production had greatly diminished. I recommended vitex. Over the next 10 days, it helped to reestablish her milk flow.

A study of 353 breast-feeding mothers with poor milk production found that vitex supplementation for seven days resulted in significant improvement.

🐚 MENOPAUSAL HOT FLASHES

Vitex has been used by European doctors to help relieve hot flashes for women going through the transition of menopause. I normally prescribe it in a menopausal formula that contains herbs such as black cohosh.

🐚 MENSTRUAL DISORDERS

The hormone-balancing effects of vitex make it a superior herb for a wide variety of menstrual disorders. This includes painful periods, medically known as dysmenorrhea. It does not work well for the acute relief of dysmenorrhea, but is excellent for long-term treatment to correct the hormone imbalance that is causing the problem.

Also, it helps with irregular menstrual cycles that are too long or too short. I particularly like vitex for young teenage girls who suffer from abnormal menstrual cycles or dysmenorrhea. It seems like a much better option than the birth-control pill.

Speaking of the birth-control pill, vitex is commonly used by herbalists to normalize the menstrual cycle after a woman has discontinued using the pill and then suffers from menstrual irregularity.

🐚 OVARIAN CYSTS

Ovarian cysts, another condition related to hormone imbalance, can often be eliminated with vitex. A separate condition known as polycystic ovary syndrome can also be helped with regular vitex supplementation.

🐚 PMS

Balancing hormones is the key to treating the underlying cause of PMS. Most of the research on vitex has been done with regard to PMS. Again, it helps to reduce high levels of prolactin and to lower the levels of progesterone—both of which are associated with PMS.

One survey involved more than 1,500 women with PMS who supplemented with vitex extract. The women took 40 drops of vitex for an average of 166 days. Fifty-seven percent of the patients reported improvement, and another 33% reported complete relief of symptoms. The physicians reported positive results in 92% of the cases.

In another study, 127 women were given 200 mg of vitamin B6 or vitex extract for three menstrual cycles. While both groups had good responses, the women using vitex had a greater overall decrease of symptoms, especially breast tenderness, bloating, and depression. Overall, 77% of the vitex group had improvement compared with improvement of these symptoms in 61% of those taking vitamin B6.

As you can see from these studies, natural and nontoxic therapies such as vitex and vitamin B are quite effective. I consider them nature's "PMS busters." I certainly favor their use over conventional therapies for PMS, which include the birth-control pill, diuretics, antidepressants such as Prozac, and tranquilizers such as Xanax.

Vitex works well for PMS if you take the herb by itself, and I consider it essential in any PMS formula. As a matter of fact, if a PMS formula does not contain vitex, then I would advise you don't bother purchasing it.

UTERINE FIBROIDS

Vitex is one of the better herbs to use for uterine fibroids. It helps to keep the fibroids from enlarging in mild to moderate cases. If a woman can keep the symptoms at bay until she is past menopause, the fibroids will shrink on their own, due to the decrease of estrogen. While I don't recommend vitex as a general preventative, I will recommend it in some cases.

Fortunately, most fibroids do not cause symptoms. For severe cases, we recommend natural progesterone. In a small number of cases, surgery is required.

W

Water

I remember a span of about three weeks during medical school when I experienced dull headaches, dizziness, and lethargy. It seemed like my thinking was cloudy. While I couldn't explain all these symptoms, I assumed that the mounting stress of my classes, plus all the hours I'd been working in the clinic, were beginning to take their toll.

Then, one day, when I decided I was tired of feeling this way, I sat down and analyzed everything I had been doing. I was eating pretty well and exercising a reasonable amount. It seemed very unlikely that I was suffering any kind of nutritional deficiency.

But even while I contemplated possible explanations, I happened to notice someone getting a glass of water at a nearby watercooler. Then it occurred to me. Many of my symptoms suggested dehydration. It was just possible that I was experiencing these symptoms because I wasn't consuming enough water.

As I reviewed my actions of the last few days, I realized I'd really had very little water—possibly two tall glasses a day, total. That wasn't nearly enough, considering that I was exercising regularly, under stress, and mentally active. I decided that was a good time to start doing exactly what I was recommending to many patients—drinking more water.

With the phrase "physician heal thyself" dancing in my head, I immediately resolved to triple the amount of water I was consuming. After that small revelation, I started drinking approximately six 8-ounce glasses a day.

My symptoms disappeared over the next three days. It was a long, roundabout route, but I'd been forced to the simple rediscovery that water is one of the fundamental necessities of good health. Few of us are regularly in danger of dying of thirst—but I suspect that many of us are seriously slowed down by unrecognized thirstiness.

WAITER, MORE WATER!

As we all probably learned in school, water is composed of two hydrogen molecules and one oxygen molecule. More than half of our total body weight is water, and a newborn is about three-quarters fluids and one-quarter solid, living human matter.

The brain, surprisingly, is the most concentrated reservoir. There, the concentration of water is almost 85%.

About two-thirds of the water in our systems comes from those glasses of fluids that we drink. The rest comes from food and from the leftover "disposables" of cellular metabolism.

Our bodies are really the middle of a streambed. While the water is coming in through various pathways, it's exiting in the urine (60%), evaporating from skin (20%), hissing out through the respiratory tract (15%), and departing in stool (5%).

Water is involved in every single biochemical activity in the body and is required as a solvent for many processes. It is an important component of blood (plasma) and fluids inside and outside the cells. All the tissues of the body—including cartilage and skin—are unquenchable water drinkers. The medium of water is a traveling road show, where electrolytes move around, enabling the cells to perform their duty as they generate electrical activity. You need water for detoxification, because waste products course their way out of the body through the multitude of aqueducts—veins, arteries, glands, and organs—that pump, feed, and carry fluids from place to place. Throwing in some thermostatic responsibilities, water also provides a means for temperature regulation.

BODY LUBE

Humans have a thirst mechanism that is activated when our body is becoming low in reserves of water. Researchers have noted that there is often a long delay between the time when your body actually becomes dehydrated and the moment when you experience the sensation of thirst. In other words, by the time you feel thirsty, you're *already* somewhat dehydrated.

I've already mentioned the symptoms of dehydration that I experienced myself, but there are others. Thirst, naturally, is one— and any time your mouth feels dry or "sticky," you probably need fluids. Dark urine is another sign.

Many people are in a constant, low-grade state of dehydration. They won't faint, nor do they need to be hospitalized. But that low-grade dehydration can sap vitality and contribute to many of the symptoms I've noted.

Of course, there are situations that lead, almost automatically, to dehydration. If you're in a hot climate, exercising heavily, and not drinking very much, your water reserves drop fast. But excessive sodium intake—eating a lot of salty foods, including heavily processed food products—will draw water out of the tissues. (I am always reminded of the effects of sodium a couple hours after eating sushi with soy sauce, or foods containing lots of sodium.)

THE DEHYDRATORS

If you drink a lot of beverages containing caffeine—coffee and soda, for instance— you're sure to have some dehydration unless you also drink lots of water. Alcoholic beverages also have a dehydrating effect.

Any medication that's described as a diuretic, or drugs that have diuretic side effects, will require you to compensate for water loss by getting more fluids every day.

Conditions I see that are related to insufficient water intake include headaches, dizziness, heart palpitations, high blood pressure, irritability, cloudy thinking, skin rashes, kidney pain, and fatigue. Other physicians have noted even more conditions associated with dehydration, ranging from colitis and rheumatoid arthritis to obesity, asthma, and allergies.

Of course, while I'm recommending that people drink sufficient water, I'm acutely aware that many are concerned with the quality of their drinking water. Thousands of people suffer from parasites and other infections related to contaminated water each year. Industrial pollutants and chemicals are traceable in many sources of drinking water. Even the chemicals used to purify water— such as chlorine—have in some cases been linked to cancers such as bladder cancer and, possibly, aggravating asthma. Heavy metal contamination such as lead, mercury, and aluminum are problems as well.

I advise people to invest in a high-quality filtration system or drink tested bottled water. I also recommend having your local water tested.

DOSAGE

Drink at least six to eight 8-ounce glasses of water daily. If you drink coffee, consume one 8-ounce glass of water for every cup of coffee you drink.

If the weather is hot, drink a glass or two before exercising, and have more than eight glasses during the day.

People on detoxification programs often need to increase their water intake to help flush toxins out of the body.

WHAT ARE THE SIDE EFFECTS?

In rare cases, too much water consumption may place stress on your heart or kidneys. If you have kidney or heart disease, consult with your doctor before drinking larger-than-normal amounts of water.

You may feel bloated if you haven't been drinking very much water and then abruptly increase your water intake. The bloating comes from swallowing extra air—but it won't take long for your body to adjust to increased water intake.

WATER

RECOMMENDATIONS FROM THE NATURAL PHYSICIAN FOR . . .

🐟 CLOUDY THINKING

I call this symptom "brain fog," and most people know instantly what I mean. The mind is not clear, and you find it hard to concentrate. I have seen these symptoms improved with increased water consumption.

🐟 DIZZINESS

Unexplained dizziness may be related to dehydration. Water is required for normal blood pressure. When you're dehydrated, your circulation may be poor, which deprives cells of needed nutrients. Dizziness is one outcome.

🐟 FATIGUE

Unexplained fatigue can be a result of dehydration. Many people notice increased energy when they drink more water.

🐟 HEADACHES

Patients with chronic, low-grade headaches are often dehydrated. It is often described as a fuzzy sensation in the head.

🐟 HEART PALPITATIONS

Occasionally a patient reports a history of heart palpitations. These episodes may improve or cease completely when water intake increases.

🐟 HIGH BLOOD PRESSURE

You'd think that anyone consuming lots of water would be raising their own blood pressure, but the opposite is true. When you're dehydrated, your body tries to compensate by increasing blood pressure. For anyone with high blood pressure (hypertension), it's especially important to increase water intake.

🐟 IRRITABILITY

There are many reasons for irritability, of course, but if you think dehydration might be one possible cause, there's a quick way to find out—just start drinking a lot more water, and see if your mood improves.

(continued)

❧ KIDNEY PAIN

A number of patients experience kidney pain when they are not drinking enough water. Any kind of kidney pain should be taken seriously. But while you should see the doctor and explain your symptoms, it's also advisable to increase your intake of water. It can't do any harm—and that just might turn out to be the explanation of the problem.

❧ SKIN RASHES

The skin is a major organ of detoxification. If you're not getting enough water in your system to aid detoxification, you can begin to develop skin rashes of many sorts. Increase water consumption, and you'll help expel some of the accumulated toxins in the body. This is the quickest "first aid" I can think of for treatment of skin rashes.

❧ WEIGHT GAIN AND EDEMA

Your body will retain water if you are chronically dehydrated. This condition, called edema, contributes to weight gain as well. Thus, increased water consumption is an important therapy for helping these conditions.

Wheatgrass

Juice bars around the country offer wheatgrass as a natural way to detoxify and bolster one's nutritional status. Indeed I have spoken to many people who feel that regular consumption of wheatgrass has made a noticeable difference in their health, including better energy, healthier-looking skin, improved bowel regularity, and better immunity.

Wheatgrass is rich in chlorophyll, a phytonutrient that has potent antioxidant properties. It also contains vitamins A, C, E, K, and B-complex; iron; calcium; magnesium; selenium; and amino acids.

DOSAGE

One ounce daily of fresh wheatgrass is a common dosage. For the treatment of ulcerative colitis the recommended dose is 100 mL. Wheatgrass is also available in capsule or powder form from health-food stores. Take as directed.

WHAT ARE THE SIDE EFFECTS?

Nausea from straight wheatgrass juice can occur. Use with caution if on blood-thinning medications as wheatgrass contains vitamin K.

WHEATGRASS

RECOMMENDATIONS FROM THE NATURAL PHYSICIAN FOR . . .

❧ BAD BREATH

Wheatgrass and its rich chlorophyll content are helpful for some people with bad breath. However, I am unaware of any studies researching this effect.

❧ DETOXIFICATION

Wheatgrass is used by natural practitioners to aid detoxification. The naturally

(continued)

occurring nutrients and antioxidants in wheatgrass likely support the detoxification pathways.

🐦 ULCERATIVE COLITIS

A study of 21 patients with active ulcerative colitis was randomized so they received either 100 mL wheatgrass juice or placebo daily for one month. Researchers and physicians monitored rectal bleeding and number of bowel movements, and performed a sigmoidoscopic evaluation to determine the efficacy of treatment. They found that patients who received wheatgrass juice had a significantly lowered overall disease activity index and rectal bleeding compared to those on placebo.

Wormwood

The herb wormwood (*Artemisia absinthium* and other species) has a long history of use in for a variety of conditions in China and Europe (and more recently America). It is also known by the common name mugwort. Traditional uses include treatment of fever, inflammation, digestive ailments, headache, bleeding, and parasitic and other infections, such as malaria.

Wormwood has been the subject of controversy because it is a flavoring and color agent in absinthe, an alcoholic beverage that was banned in the United States and Europe in the early 1900s because it was thought to cause hallucinations and even insanity. A component of wormwood—the chemical thujone—was believed to have these mind-altering properties. But some experts have since questioned the science behind this belief, and in the 1990s Europe lifted the ban on the manufacture and consumption of absinthe without any related increase in mental illness. In 2007, the US government began allowing thujone-free absinthe to be imported into the country (wormwood as an herbal supplement has long been available in the United States, both in health-food stores and as part of professional supplement lines). Wormwood products that are thujone-free have "generally recognized as safe" status for use in foods in the United States.

Newer research shows that this herb is helpful in fighting some insidious health conditions. My experience with wormwood has been positive. I have mainly used it to treat digestive ailments, such as infections of the digestive tract, and more recently Crohn's disease.

DOSAGE

The dosage for wormwood varies greatly depending on the product being used. It is commonly used in Chinese and Western herbal formulas that contain many other ingredients. For the treatment of Crohn's disease, 750 mg of a specific type of extract has been used.

WHAT ARE THE SIDE EFFECTS?

I have not commonly seen problems with herbal products containing wormwood. The most commonly reported reaction is digestive upset. If you are using antacid or seizure medication, check with your doctor first, since negative interactions have been reported. Pregnant and nursing mothers should avoid using wormwood.

WORMWOOD

RECOMMENDATIONS FROM THE NATURAL PHYSICIAN FOR . . .

CANCER

Some research suggests that extracts of wormwood might have anticancer benefits. However, the research has been limited to small-scale cell and mouse studies so there is not enough information yet to evaluate it properly for this use.

CROHN'S DISEASE

A study published last year by doctors at the Yale University School of Medicine found that wormwood significantly reduced symptoms of Crohn's disease, a form of inflammatory bowel disease. Forty patients were given either 750 mg wormwood extract (brand name SedaCrohn) or a placebo twice daily for 10 weeks. After eight weeks, 13 of the 20 patients (65%) taking wormwood had experienced almost a full remission of symptoms. As a result, they were able to reduce their use of corticosteroid drugs. For most of the patients taking placebos, symptoms worsened.

MALARIA

A very close relative of wormwood called sweet wormwood (*Artemisia annua*) has been found beneficial in treating malaria, which is caused by a mosquito-borne parasite. *Artemisia annua* contains artemisinin, an interesting compound that has the known antimalarial effect of suppressing the ability of Plasmodium (the parasite species that causes malaria) to replicate in red blood cells. A 2008 study found cure rates with wormwood extract artemisinin comparable to drug therapy for a seven-day treatment. Another study found that cure rates were 74% with artemisinin compared with 91% for quinine, a commonly used malaria drug. However, symptoms reappeared at much faster rates in the artemisia groups.

Although most Americans are not likely to contract malaria, the disease is still a major problem in Africa and throughout the developing world. The World Health Organization has approved the use of wormwood-based compounds in the treatment of malaria—a sign of the herb's efficacy and safety.

PARASITIC INFECTIONS

Wormwood has a long history of use in traditional Chinese medicine and in Western naturopathic medicine for treating a variety of parasitic infections. I have also found it to be effective in treating many of these conditions.

Xylitol

Xylitol is a white crystalline substance that looks and tastes like sugar. It is found naturally in fruits, vegetables, and the bark of some trees. Birch trees and corncobs are the commercial sources of xylitol. The human body also produces xylitol naturally from other food sources. Used in foods since the 1960s, it is approved as a food additive by both the World Health Organization and the FDA. Xylitol has 40% to 50% fewer calories than sugar. It has no detrimental effects on blood-sugar levels and is safe for people with diabetes.

This natural sweetener works very well for beverages. However, because yeast cannot metabolize xylitol, the product should not be used for baking breads or other foods that contain yeast.

DOSAGE

Varying doses are found in natural products or in sweetening formulas. For dental cavity prevention, a minimum of 1 g daily is required. For ear infection prevention approximately 8.5 g daily is used in children in the form of chewing gum, syrup, or lozenges.

WHAT ARE THE SIDE EFFECTS?

In some people, xylitol can trigger diarrhea. To avoid this, start with a small amount and let your digestive tract adjust to it gradually. Xylitol has "generally recognized as safe" status in the United States.

XYLITOL
RECOMMENDATIONS FROM THE NATURAL PHYSICIAN FOR . . .

CAVITIES

Unlike table sugar, which is notoriously bad for the teeth, xylitol actually reduces formation of cavity-causing plaque such as of *Streptococcus mutans*, prevents bacteria from adhering to the mucous membranes of the mouth and sinuses, improves saliva flow rates, stimulates activity of the antimicrobial enzyme lactoperoxidase in saliva, and helps to build tooth enamel. More than a dozen studies have shown that xylitol reduces tooth decay by up to 80%, which is why it has the support of six national dental associations. Xylitol is used in sugar-free chewing gums, mouthwashes and toothpastes—which I buy for my own family.

EAR INFECTION PREVENTION

A double-blind, randomized study published in the *British Medical Journal* found xylitol effective for treating children with a history of reoccurring ear infections (otitis media).

❧ WEIGHT LOSS AND OBESITY

Like the natural sweeteners stevia and lo han, xylitol is an excellent low-calorie sweetener.

Z

Zinc

Jim was concerned about his son's acne.

"Is there anything you can give him?" Jim asked me. "Randy is 17 years old now, and we actually thought his acne would start to get better. But it's not."

"There are lots of good natural treatments," I answered. "But I'd start by giving him zinc."

I explained that I'd seen zinc help in many cases of teenage and adult acne, and I recommended that Randy start at a high dosage.

"Have him take 30 milligrams three times daily, with meals, for a month. Then cut back to 50 milligrams a day as a maintenance dosage. You should also make sure he gets a few milligrams of copper to maintain a balance with zinc."

"That high dosage won't harm him in any way, will it?" asked Jim.

"No. We prescribe dosages like that all the time. The studies show that long-term usage of dosages of 150 to 200 milligrams daily can cause toxicity problems, and I'm not recommending a dosage near that high," I replied.

After taking the zinc supplement for two months, Randy noticed a marked improvement in his skin. Although his acne still broke out at times, it was much less noticeable and the daily blemishes were greatly improved.

THE QUALITIES OF ZINC

Zinc is a mineral with many important functions. Found in all the cells of the body,

it's known as a cofactor—that is, a substance required for numerous enzymatic reactions, including detoxification.

It is important for the synthesis and activity of many hormones such as thymic hormone, growth hormone, and insulin, as well as testosterone and other sex hormones. It is necessary for proper immune function and wound healing. It is also needed for protein and DNA synthesis.

Zinc is needed for proper vitamin A metabolism. It is involved in bone formation and in taste.

There are several reasons why people may develop zinc deficiencies. Poor dietary intake is one reason. For example, vegetarians may be more prone to zinc deficiency, as zinc in plant foods is not as bioavailable as in animal products.

Other factors come into play such as genetic susceptibility and some problems with absorption. We also know that certain medications, such as ACE inhibitors like captopril, enalapril, and lisinopril that are commonly used to lower blood pressure, can cause zinc deficiency. Other problematic drugs are aspirin and the birth-control pill.

The elderly are more prone to a deficiency because digestive powers decrease as we age, and our bodies don't absorb zinc as well. Alcoholics are at risk for zinc deficiency, as is anyone with a metabolic disease such as diabetes. When people have diseases of the digestive tract such as Crohn's or celiac disease, or just have general malabsorption—caused by leaky gut syndrome, for instance—they may have impaired mineral absorption.

WHEN ZINC IS MISSING

Severe nutritional deficiencies are not that common—but I often see people who have marginal or subclinical deficiencies. Symptoms and conditions associated with zinc deficiency include the following:

- Poor wound healing
- Lowered immunity; susceptibility to infections
- Poor skin and nail health (nails may have white spots)
- Fatigue
- Loss of taste and smell
- Poor growth and development
- Blood-sugar imbalance
- Anorexia; reduced appetite
- Delayed sexual development and maturation
- Night blindness (due to involvement with vitamin A metabolism)
- Infertility
- Skin abnormalities
- Dandruff
- Impaired nerve conduction
- Hair loss
- Prostate enlargement
- Birth malformations
- Psychiatric illness

GETTING YOUR ZINC

Good food sources include fish and seafood such as oysters and other shellfish. Red meat is also high in zinc.

Eggs and milk also contain ample amounts of zinc. Plant foods such as whole grains and cereals, legumes, nuts, and seeds (particularly pumpkin seeds) contain good amounts of zinc, but the mineral isn't as bioavailable as the zinc that comes from animal products.

Breast milk contains a good supply of zinc, so infants are well protected.

DIETARY REFERENCE INTAKE

0 to 6 months: 3 mg

6 to 12 months: 5 mg

1 to 10 years: 10 mg

11 to 18 years: 15 mg

18+ years: 15 mg

Pregnant/lactating: 7+ mg

DOSAGE

Adults can benefit from supplementing with an extra 15 to 30 mg daily of zinc. Most high-potency multivitamins contain this amount.

Children under one year of age can use a pediatric multivitamin that contains up to 5 mg. Children over the age of 1 can take a children's multivitamin that contains 5 to 15 mg in each daily dose.

For specific conditions, such as wound healing or acne, higher dosages of up to 100 mg daily may be required for a limited amount of time.

Avoid the use of zinc sulfate, which is not readily absorbed. I recommend other formulas such as zinc picolinate, zinc monomethionine, zinc citrate, and zinc chelate.

(**NOTE:** If you are taking a calcium supplement, take it at a different time from when you take your zinc supplement. The calcium may hinder zinc absorption.)

WHAT ARE THE SIDE EFFECTS?

Zinc is actually quite a safe supplement, though some people may experience digestive upset if they take zinc on an empty stomach.

High dosages of 150 to 200 mg or more, taken over a long period of time, might cause depressed immunity. But I don't recommend taking such high doses anyway, even if you're treating a condition such as severe acne.

One concern is the possibility of developing copper anemia if you are taking high dosages of zinc without taking copper. In the absence of copper, red blood cells change shape; when that happens, they don't carry oxygen as efficiently.

ZINC

RECOMMENDATIONS FROM THE NATURAL PHYSICIAN FOR . . .

✎ ACNE

Zinc is involved in the metabolism of testosterone. As that "male hormone" is metabolized, it is converted to a metabolite hormone known as DHT (dihydrotestosterone). High levels of DHT are associated with the development of acne, because it increases sebum production. Zinc works to reduce the conversion and also promotes skin healing. Many studies have shown that zinc is beneficial for acne treatment, and at least one indicated that zinc is as effective as tetracycline.

✎ AIDS

People with AIDS are prone to several nutritional deficiencies. Zinc is one of the critical minerals for the immune system, therefore an essential supplement if you have AIDS.

✎ ALZHEIMER'S DISEASE

Zinc may be helpful in slowing the progression of Alzheimer's disease. In a study that included 10 people who had Alzheimer's, researchers found that supplementation with zinc helped 8 of the people improve memory and communication.

✎ ATHEROSLCEROSIS

Zinc appears to be one of the many nutrients that helps to prevent atherosclerosis.

✎ ATTENTION DEFICIT/HYPERACTIVITY DISORDER

Children with a zinc deficiency can have symptoms of this condition improved with an increased intake of zinc.

✎ BIRTH COMPLICATIONS

Zinc is important during pregnancy because it is required for cell division. A deficiency of zinc is linked to conditions such as premature birth, low birth weight, growth retardation, and preeclampsia. A good prenatal multivitamin should help prevent a zinc deficiency when used in combination with a balanced diet.

✎ BURNS, CUTS, AND WOUNDS

Zinc is needed for cell division and protein synthesis, both of which are required for skin and wound healing. Burns, cuts, and other skin traumas can be relieved with zinc supplements. By taking supplements, you can also speed healing.

✎ COMMON COLD

Several studies have shown that zinc lozenges reduce the severity and duration of the common cold, and also help to relieve sore throats that accompany a cold. It is helpful to take zinc lozenges

(continued)

containing 15 to 25 mg of elemental zinc gluconate or acetate at the first signs of a cold every 2 hours for two days. I find they are particularly good for healing a sore throat.

EATING DISORDERS

Zinc is involved in producing stomach acid as well as stimulating a normal appetite. Studies have shown that people with anorexia and bulimia have deficient zinc levels and may benefit from zinc supplements. Holistic practitioners recommend zinc as part of a comprehensive protocol for people with these eating disorders.

MACULAR DEGENERATION

Zinc is important in maintaining normal vision. One study of 155 people with macular degeneration found that 45 mg of zinc per day significantly slowed the rate of visual loss.

The macula is the portion of the eye that is responsible for fine vision, and when there's degeneration in that area, the sight begins to go. In fact, macular degeneration is the leading cause of blindness in the aged. There are two main types—"dry" and "wet." Nutritional therapy is mainly used for the dry type.

I usually recommend combining zinc supplementation with other important supplements including vitamin C, selenium, carotenoids, taurine, lutein, and the herbs ginkgo and bilberry.

MALE INFERTILITY

Men who are deficient in zinc may have decreased testosterone and sperm production. Studies have shown that zinc supplements increase sperm counts and testosterone in men who previously had deficiencies that prevented conception.

In one study, 11 men who were infertile were treated with 55 mg of zinc daily for six to 12 months. They showed an increase in sperm count and motility—and three of the men's wives became pregnant during the study.

PROSTATE ENLARGEMENT

Zinc is an effective treatment for prostate enlargement. The mineral inhibits the enzyme 5-alpha reductase, which converts testosterone to dihydrotestosterone (DHT). Since high levels of DHT are believed to promote prostate enlargement, I generally prescribe 90 to 100 mg daily for men with this condition. After two months, I recommend reducing the zinc dosage to a maintenance level of 50 mg.

WILSON'S DISEASE

Zinc is one of the primary treatments for this genetic disease in which copper accumulates in the liver and body, causing brain damage. High doses of zinc help to hinder copper absorption.

REFERENCES

For a complete list of references used for this book, please go to www.lajollawhole health.com.

QUICK CURE FINDER
An A-to-Z Guide to Health Conditions and Therapies

THE FOLLOWING LIST is a reference guide to help you quickly find solutions to your health problems. Just look up a health condition in the list below, then turn to the specific healing-therapy chapters for complete information about recommendations and dosages.

(**NOTE:** This section is solely intended to guide you to healing therapies in the book. For the complete index, please see page 515.)

A

ABSCESSES: cell salts

ACNE: B-complex vitamins; burdock; cell salts; flaxseed; goldenseal; guggul; saw palmetto; tea tree oil; vitamin A; vitamin E; vitex; zinc

ADRENAL FATIGUE: adrenal glandular; ashwagandha; *Cordyceps sinensis*; DHEA; ginseng; pantothenic acid; rhodiola; vitamin B5; vitamin B12; vitamin C

AGE-ASSOCIATED MEMORY IMPAIRMENT (AAMI): acetyl-L-carnitine; fish oil; ginkgo biloba; phosphatidylserine; turmeric; vitamin B12

AGING: antioxidants; ashwagandha; chlorella; ginseng; melatonin; multivitamins; prayer

AIDS: aloe; selenium; vitamin A; vitamin E; zinc

ALCOHOLISM: B-complex vitamins; lachesis; milk thistle; nux vomica; thiamin

ALLERGIES: acupressure; adrenal glandulars; apis; *Arsenicum album*; bee pollen; butterbur; DHEA; eyebright; food-sensitivity therapy; milk thistle; MSM; nux vomica; quercetin; vitamin C

ALTITUDE SICKNESS: reishi

ALZHEIMER'S DISEASE: alpha GPC; acetyl-L-carnitine; ginkgo biloba; huperzine; L-carnitine; phosphatidyl-serine; vitamin B12; vitamin E; zinc

AMENORRHEA: acetyl-L-carnitine; vitex

ANEMIA, IRON-DEFICIENCY: ashwagandha; cell salts; ferrum phosphoricum; gentian root; iron; nettle; phytonutrients; spirulina

ANESTHESIA SIDE EFFECTS: ginger root

ANGINA: amino acids; arginine; bromelain; coenzyme Q10; hawthorn; L-carnitine; magnesium; vitamin E

ANOREXIA: ignatia; L-carnitine

ANTIBIOTIC-ASSOCIATED COLITIS: acidophilus; probiotics

ANXIETY: aconite; acupressure; amino acids; *Arsenicum album*; Bach flower remedies; black cohosh; carbo vegetabilis; cell salts; chamomile; exercise; gelsemium; ignatia; kava; mental imagery; passionflower; phytonutrients; pulsatilla; Resperate; rhodiola; St. John's wort; tryptophan and 5-HTP; valerian

AORTA ELASTICITY PROBLEMS: garlic

APPETITE, LOSS OF: dandelion; gentian root; ginger root

ARRHYTHMIAS: coenzyme Q1O; hawthorn; L-carnitine; magnesium

ARTHRITIS: antioxidants; apis; ashwagandha; bee pollen; black cohosh; boswellia; bromelain; cayenne; cell salts; enzymes; evening primrose oil; exercise; feverfew; fish oil; flaxseed; food-sensitivity therapy; ginger root; glucosamine sulfate; hyaluronic acid; hydrotherapy; ledum; lycopodium; MSM; nettle; phytonutrients; pine bark extract; pulsatilla; rhus toxicodendron; turmeric; vitamin C; vitamin E

ASTHMA: adrenal glandulars; aloe; American ginseng; *Arsenicum album*; boswellia; butterbur; carbo vegetabilis; cell salts; fish oil; ipecacuanha; lachesis; magnesium; MSM; onions; pine bark extract; pulsatilla; quercetin; vitamin C

ATHEROSCLEROSIS: antioxidants; artichoke; bromelain; cayenne; coenzyme Q1O; fiber; fish oil; garlic; green tea; guggul; L-carnitine; pomegranate; tocotrienols; vitamin B12; vitamin C; vitamin D; vitamin E; vitamin K; zinc

ATHLETE'S FOOT: oregano; tea tree oil

ATTENTION DEFICIT DISORDER (ADD)/ATTENTION DEFICIT-HYPERACTIVITY DISORDER (ADHD): evening primrose oil; fish oil; food-sensitivity therapy; ginkgo biloba; sulphur

AUTISM: food-sensitivity therapy; vitamin D

AUTOIMMUNE CONDITIONS: DHEA; enzymes; food-sensitivity therapy; MSM; progesterone; vitamin D

B

BACK PAIN: fish oil; glucosamine; horse chestnut; hyaluronic acid; MSM; nux vomica; sitz bath

BACTERIAL INFECTIONS: echinacea; goldenseal

BAD BREATH: chlorella; peppermint; wheatgrass

BALDNESS: saw palmetto

BEE STINGS: apis

BIRTH-CONTROLL PILL SIDE EFFECTS: sepia; vitex

BLADDER INFECTIONS: cell salts; cranberry; echinacea; goldenseal; nux vomica; pulsatilla; saw palmetto; sepia; sitz bath

BLEEDING: cell salts; ferrum phosphoricum

BLOATING: enzymes; food-sensitivity therapy; gentian root; ginger root; lycopodium

BLOOD THINNING: bromelain; enzymes; green tea; vitamin E

BOILS: cell salts; tea tree oil

BONE DENSITY: calcium; DHEA; ipriflavone; magnesium; silicon; vitamin D

BONE PAIN: MSM; peppermint; symphytum

BRAIN INJURY: arnica; phosphatidylserine

BREAST CANCER: astragalus; coenzyme Q10; D-glucarate; fermented wheat germ extract; green tea; maitake; probiotics

BREAST CANCER PREVENTION: black cohosh; fermented wheat germ extract; flaxseed; ginseng; green tea; maitake; phytonutrients; vitamin D

BREAST PAIN: evening primrose oil; progesterone; vitex; vitamin E

BREAST TENDERNESS: evening primrose oil; progesterone; vitamin E; vitex

BREAST-FEEDING: chlorella; vitex

BREASTS, HARD NODULES OF: cell salts

BRONCHITIS: astragalus; bromelain; butterbur; carbo vegetabilis; cell salts; echinacea; elderberry; food-sensitivity therapy; goldenseal; hydrotherapy; ipecacuanha; pulsatilla; reishi; vitamin C

BRUISES: arnica; bromelain; hyaluronic acid; ledum; St. John's wort

BURNS: aloe; bromelain; calendula; cantharis; phytonutrients; St. John's wort; vitamin E; zinc

C

CANCER: *Agaricus blazei*; *Arsenicum album*; astragalus; bromelain; burdock; cat's claw; coenzyme Q10; coriolus; enzymes; fermented wheat germ extract; fiber; fish oil; green tea; hydrotherapy; maitake; melatonin; mental imagery; phytonutrients; prebiotics; probiotics; quercetin; red yeast rice; reishi; spirulina; sulforaphone; tocotrienols; vitamin D; wormwood

CANCER PREVENTION: acidophilus; antioxidants; B-complex vitamins; bromelain; carotenoids; coriolus; D-glucarate; fish oil; flaxseed; garlic; ginseng; green tea; hydrotherapy; maitake; onions; phytonutrients; prebiotics; probiotics; quercetin; red yeast rice; selenium; soy; sulforaphane; turmeric; vitamin C; vitamin D; vitamin E

CANDIDA: echinacea; food-sensitivity therapy; garlic; gentian root; oregano; phytonutrients; prebiotics; probiotics

CANKER SORES: aloe; B-complex vitamins; licorice root; probiotics

CARDIOMYOPATHY: arginine; coenzyme QlO; hawthorn; L-carnitine; magnesium; ribose

CARDIOVASCULAR DISEASE: antioxidants; arginine; B-complex vitamins; bromelain; calcium; carotenoids; cayenne; coenzyme Q10; DHEA; enzymes; exercise; fish oil; flaxseed; folic acid; garlic; ginger root; green tea; hawthorn; L-carnitine; magnesium; phytonutrients; pine bark extract; pomegranate; pyridoxine; quercetin; reishi; Resperate; ribose; selenium; soy; tocotrienols; vitamin B12; vitamin C; vitamin D; vitamin E

CARDIOVASCULAR DISEASE PREVENTION: *see* Cardiovascular Disease

CAROTID STENOSIS: bromelain; garlic; pomegranate; tocotrienols; vitamin E

CARPAL TUNNEL SYNDROME: bromelain; hypericum; pyridoxine; St. John's wort; vitamin B6

CARTILAGE DEGENERATION: glucosamine sulfate; hyaluronic acid

CATARACTS: bilberry; ginkgo biloba; multivitamins; selenium; vitamin C; vitamin E

CAVITIES: probiotics; stevia; xylitol

CELLULITIS: aloe; calendula; echinacea; goldenseal

CHEMOTHERAPY: antioxidants; chlorella; *Cordyceps sinensis*; coriolus; fermented wheat germ extract; ginseng; milk thistle; maitake; nux vomica; pine bark extract

CHEMOTHERAPY SIDE EFFECTS: *see* Chemotherapy

CHOLESTEROL: *Agaricus blazei*; amino acids; antioxidants; artichoke; calcium; cayenne; chromium; cinnamon; fiber; fish oil; flaxseed; garlic; ginger root; glucomannan; green tea; guggul; niacin; onions; pantothenic acid; phytonutrients; pine bark extract; pomegranate; red yeast rice; soy; spirulina; tocotrienols; vitamin D; vitamin E

CHRONIC FATIGUE SYNDROME: adrenal glandulars; Ashwagandha; B-complex vitamins; chlorella; coenzyme Q10; *Cordyceps sinensis*; DHEA; gelsemium; L-carnitine; magnesium; rhodiola; ribose; vitamin B12

CHRONIC OBSTRUCTIVE PULMONARY DISEASE: *Cordyceps sinensis*; fish oil; N-acetylcysteine

CHRONIC PAIN: *see* Pain

CIRCULATION: bilberry; cayenne; cinnamon; DHEA; enzymes; fish oils; garlic; ginger root; ginkgo biloba; hawthorn; horse chestnut; lachesis; milk thistle; pine bark extract; vitamin E

CIRRHOSIS: artichoke; liver glandulars; milk thistle; SAMe; turmeric

CLOUDY THINKING: fish oil; ginkgo; phosphatidylserine ; vitamin B12; water

COGNITIVE FUNCTION: fish oil; ginkgo biloba; huperzine; multivitamins; phosphatidylserine; vitamin D

COLD FEET: cayenne; ginger root; ginkgo biloba; hawthorn; thyroid glandular

COLD SORES: aloe; B-complex vitamins; cell salts; food-sensitivity therapy; lysine; tea tree oil

COLIC: chamomile; enzymes; nux vomica; peppermint

COLITIS: boswellia; bromelain; chamomile; fish oil; food-sensitivity therapy; lycopodium; nux vomica; peppermint; prebiotics; probiotics; wormwood

COLON CANCER: calcium; coriolous; fermented wheat germ extract; garlic; lutein; N-acetylcysteine; onions; prebiotics; probiotics; vitamin D

COLON CANCER PREVENTION: *see* Colon Cancer

COMMON COLD: aconite; acupressure; andrographis; astragalus; cinnamon; colloidal silver; echinacea; essential oils; garlic; gelsemium; ginger root; goldenseal; lomatium; peppermint; vitamin C; zinc

COMPLEMENTARY CANCER TREATMENT: *see* Cancer

CONCUSSION: arnica

CONGESTIVE HEART FAILURE: amino acids; arginine; carbo vegetabilis; coenzyme QlO; ginseng; hawthorn; L-carnitine; magnesium; ribose

CONJUNCTIVITIS: calendula; eyebright; pulsatilla

CONSTIPATION: acupressure; artichoke; bitter aloe latex; burdock; cascara sagrada; chlorella; dandelion; eyebright; fiber; flaxseed; food-sensitivity therapy; gentian root; glucomannan; hydrotherapy; juicing; milk thistle; nux vomica; prebiotics; probiotics; reishi; sitz bath

COUGHS: acupressure; colloidal silver; echinacea; elderberry; goldenseal; licorice root; peppermint

CORONARY ARTERY DISEASE: *see* Atherosclerosis

CRADLE CAP: biotin; fish oil; flaxseed

CROHN'S DISEASE: *see* Colitis

CUTS: calendula; colloidal silver; vitamin C; zinc

CYCLICAL BREAST TENDERNESS: evening primrose oil; progesterone; vitamin E; vitex

D

DANDRUFF: fish oil; flaxseed; tea tree oil

DEMENTIA: *see* Cognitive Function

DENTAL CONDITIONS: *see* Cavities

DEPRESSION: acetyl-L-carnitine; amino acids; black cohosh; cell salts; chromium; essential oils; exercise; fish oil; food-sensitivity therapy; ginkgo biloba; ignatia; kava; multivitamins; phosphatidylserine; phytonutrients; pulsatilla; SAMe; sepia; St. John's wort; tryptophan and 5-HTP; valerian; vitamin D

DETOXIFICATION: antioxidants; artichoke; burdock; chlorella; D-glucarate; dandelion; exercise; fiber; garlic; green tea; hydrotherapy; juicing; licorice root; milk thistle; onion; phytonutrients; reishi; spirulina; sulforaphane; sulphur; turmeric; wheatgrass

DIABETES: *Agaricus blazei*; aloe; antioxidants; B-complex vitamins; biotin; burdock; chromium; cinnamon; coenzyme QlO; dandelion; DHEA; evening primrose oil; exercise; fiber; ginseng; glucomannan; gymnema sylvestre; L-carnitine; magnesium; maitake; milk thistle; onions; pine bark extract; pomegranate; quercetin; reishi; resveratrol; soy; stevia; vanadium; vitamin C; vitamin D; vitamin E

DIABETIC NEUROPATHY: acetyl-L-carnitine; alpha lipoic acid; cayenne

DIABETIC RETINOPATHY: bilberry; ginkgo biloba; pine bark extract

DIARRHEA: *Arsenicum album*; bilberry; fiber; food-sensitivity therapy; gelsemium; ginger root; goldenseal; probiotics

DIGESTION: aloe; artichoke; astragalus; carbo vegetabilis; chamomile; cinnamon; enzymes; essential oils; flaxseed; ginger root; green tea; hydrotherapy; licorice root; nux vomica; peppermint; propolis; reishi; sulphur; turmeric

DIGESTIVE DISORDERS: *see* Digestion

DIZZINESS: ginkgo biloba; water

DOWN'S SYNDROME: L-carnitine

DRUG-ADDICTION RECOVERY: B-complex vitamins; lachesis; milk thistle; nux vomica

DRY EYES: bilberry; fish oil; vitamin A

DRY SKIN: cell salts; evening primrose oil; fish oil; flaxseed

DYSBIOSIS: prebiotics; probiotics; wormwood

E

E. COLI: colloidal silver; goldenseal; probiotics

EAR INFECTIONS: aconite; colloidal silver; echinacea; food-sensitivity therapy; goldenseal; lachesis; pulsatilla; xylitol

EARACHES: *see* Ear Infections

EARS, FLUID IN: cell salts; nettle; quercetin

EATING DISORDERS: ignatia; zinc

ECZEMA: calendula; cell salts; evening primrose oil; fish oil; flaxseed; food-sensitivity therapy; licorice root; prebiotics; probiotics; pulsatilla; sulphur; vitamin E

EDEMA: arginine; cell salts; dandelion; enzymes; hawthorn; horse chestnut; nettle; water

EMOTIONAL BLOCKAGES: Bach flower remedies; ignatia; prayer; pulsatilla

ENDOMETRIOSIS: lachesis; pine bark extract; progesterone; pulsatilla; sepia

ENERGY: *see* Chronic Fatigue Syndrome

EPILEPSY: calcium; fish oil; magnesium; N-acetylcysteine

EPSTEIN-BARR SYNDROME: astragalus; echinacea; gelsemium; lomatium

ERECTILE DYSFUNCTION: arginine; ginkgo biloba; ginseng; maca

ESOPHAGEAL CANCER: beta-carotene; coriolus; fermented wheat germ extract

EXHAUSTION: *see* Chronic Fatigue Syndrome

EYE INFECTIONS: colloidal silver; eyebright; goldenseal; pine bark extract

EYES, DRY: *see* Dry Eyes

EYES, INJURY TO: symphytum

EYESTRAIN: acupressure; bilberry; eyebright

F

FALL PREVENTION: vitamin D

FAT MALABSORPTION: artichoke; dandelion; enzymes; milk thistle; phytonutrients

FATIGUE: *see* Chronic Fatigue Syndrome

FEARS: Bach flower remedies

FELINE LEUKEMIA VIRUS: aloe; astragalus; colloidal silver; echinacea; lomatium

FEVER: aconite; burdock; cell salts; cinnamon; colloidal silver; echinacea; ferrum phosphoricum; goldenseal; hydrotherapy; pulsatilla; sulphur

FIBROCYSTIC BREAST SYNDROME: evening primrose oil; progesterone; pulsatilla; sepia; vitamin E; vitex

FIBROMYALGIA: black cohosh; calcium; chlorella; ignatia; magnesium; MSM; ribose; SAMe; tryptophan and 5-HTP; vitamin D

FISSURES: cell salts; sitz bath

FLATULENCE: chamomile; dandelion; enzymes; ginger root; lycopodium; peppermint; prebiotics; probiotics; sulphur

FLU: aconite; acupressure; andrographis; *Arsenicum album*; colloidal silver; echinacea; elderberry; gelsemium; lomatium; N-acetylcysteine; nux vomica; rhus toxicodendron; vitamin C

FOOD ALLERGIES: enzymes; gentian root; MSM; probiotics

FOOD POISONING: *Arsenicum album*; ginger root; nux vomica

FOOD SENSITIVITIES: enzymes; gentian root

FOOT PAIN: ginkgo biloba; MSM

FRACTURES: calcium; cell salts; ipriflavone; magnesium; silicon; symphytum; vitamin D

FREE RADICALS: antioxidants; carotenoids; green tea

FUNGAL INFECTIONS: echinacea; prebiotics; tea tree oil

G

GALLBLADDER CONDITIONS: artichoke; dandelion root; enzymes; food-sensitivity therapy; milk thistle

GALLSTONES: artichoke; dandelion; food-sensitivity therapy; milk thistle; peppermint; turmeric; vitamin C

GENITAL WARTS: lomatium; sepia

GINGIVITIS: coenzyme Q1O; tea tree oil; vitamin C

GLAUCOMA: bilberry; magnesium; vitamin C

GOUT: dandelion; nettle

GRIEF: Bach flower remedies; cell salts; ignatia; pulsatilla

GROWING PAINS: calcium; cell salts; magnesium; vitamin D

GUM INFECTIONS: calendula; colloidal silver; goldenseal; tea tree oil

GUMS, SORE: *see* Gum Infections

H

HAIR HEALTH: B-complex vitamins; fish oil; flaxseed; MSM; silicon

HAIR PROBLEMS: B-complex vitamins; cell salts; coenzyme Q10; essential oils; fish oil; flaxseed; nettle; silicon; tea tree oil

HANGOVERS: ipecacuanha; nux vomica

HAY FEVER: bee pollen; butterbur; cell salts; nettle; nux vomica

HEAD INJURY: cell salts

HEADACHES: acupressure; amino acids; food-sensitivity therapy; gelsemium; gentian root; hydrotherapy; ipecacuanha; lycopodium; melatonin; peppermint; pulsatilla; sitz bath; sulphur; water

HEART: coenzyme Q10; *Cordyceps sinensis*

HEART ATTACK RECOVERY: *see* Cardiovascular Disease

HEART DISEASE: *see* Cardiovascular Disease

HEARTBURN: aloe; calcium; cell salts; chamomile; enzymes; food-sensitivity therapy; licorice root; nux vomica

HEART PALPITATIONS: coenzyme Q10; hawthorn; L-carnitine; magnesium; passionflower; ribose; water

HEMORRHAGE: ipecacuanha; lachesis

HEMORRHAGIC DISEASE OF THE NEWBORN: vitamin K

HEMORRHOIDS: bilberry; butcher's broom; cell salts; food sensitivity therapy; horse chestnut; sitz bath

HEPATITIS: artichoke; cell salts; *Cordyceps sinensis*; coriolus; dandelion; hydrotherapy; liver glandulars; lycopodium; milk thistle; phytohutrients; selenium; vitamin C

HERPES: amino acids; apis; licorice; lomatium; lysine; propolis; rhus toxicodendron; selenium; sepia

HIGH BLOOD PRESSURE: *Agaricus blazei*; arginine; chlorella; coenzyme Q10; fish oil; garlic; glucomannan; hawthorn; pine bark extract; magnesium; pomegranate; red yeast rice; Resperate; stevia; valerian; vitamin D

HIV: DHEA; L-carnitine

HIVES: apis; quercetin; rhus toxicodendron

HORMONE IMBALANCE: black cohosh; D-glucarate; dandelion; glandulars; lachesis; licorice root; milk thistle; progesterone; maca; N-acetylcysteine; sepia; vitex

HYPERACTIVITY: amino acids; cell salts; essential oils; fish oil; phosphatidylserine; Resperate

HYPERPARATHYROIDISM: ipriflavone; vitamin D

HYPERTENSION: *see* High Blood Pressure

HYPERTENSION, PREGNANCY-INDUCED: calcium

HYPERTHYROIDISM: lachesis

HYPOGLYCEMIA: chromium; fiber; food-sensitivity therapy; glucomannan

HYPOTHYROIDISM: amino acids; iron; glandulars; rhodiola; selenium; sepia; thyroid glandulars

I

IMMUNE ENHANCEMENT: astragalus; bee pollen; colloidal silver; echinacea; fermented wheat germ extract; food-sensitivity therapy; glandulars; goldenseal; lomatium; multivitamins; phytonutrients; probiotics; selenium; spirulina; sulforaphane; vitamin A; vitamin C; vitamin D; vitamin E; vitamin K

IMMUNE SYSTEM: *see* Immune Enhancement

IMPOTENCE: amino acids; arginine; DHEA; ginkgo biloba; glandulars; lycopodium; maca

INCONTINENCE: lycopodium; progesterone; sepia

INDIGESTION: *see* Digestion

INFECTION PREVENTION: *see* Immune Enhancement

INFECTIONS: *see* Immune Enhancement

INFERTILITY, FEMALE: B-complex vitamins; glandulars; maca; progesterone; sepia; vitex

INFERTILITY, MALE: coenzyme Q1O; ginseng; L-carnitine; maca; testicular glandular; vitamin C; zinc

INFLAMMATION: boswellia; bromelain; echinacea; evening primrose oil; fish oil; ginger root; licorice root; MSM; multivitamins; quercetin; turmeric; vitamin D; vitamin E

INFLAMMATORY BOWEL DISEASE (IBD): aloe; amino acids; boswellia; DHEA; fish oil; food-sensitivity therapy; licorice root; phytonutrients; prebiotics; probiotics; quercetin; turmeric

INJECTION PAIN: apis; ledum

INJURIES: arnica; boswellia; bromelain; enzymes; glucosamine; hyaluronic acid; MSM; vitamin C

INSOMNIA: amino acids; ashwagandha; chamomile; kava; melatonin; nux vomica; passionflower; sitz bath; sulphur; tryptophan and 5-HTP; valerian

INSULIN RESISTANCE: chromium; cinnamon; fish oil; glucomannan; gymnema sylvestre; magnesium; vanadium; resveratrol

IRRITABILITY: lachesis; lycopodium; nux vomica; passionflower; Resperate; sepia; valerian; water

IRRITABLE BOWEL SYNDROME (IBS): chamomile; enzymes; fiber; food-sensitivity therapy; gentian root; hydrotherapy; nux vomica; peppermint; prebiotics; probiotics

J

JAUNDICE, NEWBORN: cell salts

JET LAG: gelsemium; melatonin

JOINT PAIN: boswellia; bromelain; cayenne; fish oil; glucosamine; hyaluronic acid; turmeric; vitamin D

JOINTS, WEAK: *see* Joint Pain

K

KIDNEY DISEASE: apis; *Cordyceps sinensis*; hydrotherapy; L-carnitine; N-acetylcysteine; phytonutrients; soy

KIDNEY FAILURE: *see* Kidney Disease

KIDNEY PAIN: apis; water

KIDNEY STONES: magnesium; pyridoxine; uva ursi; vitamin B6

KIDNEY TRANSPLANTS: fish oil

KIDNEYS, DETOXIFYING: *see* Kidney Disease

L

LACTOSE INTOLERANCE: enzymes; probiotics

LEAKY GUT SYNDROME: *see* Digestion

LIBIDO, REDUCED: *Cordyceps sinensis*; ginseng; maca; sepia; testicular glandulars

LICE: tea tree oil

LIGAMENTS, WEAK: cell salts; hyaluronic acid; vitamin C

LIVER DETOXIFICATION: *see* Detoxification

LIVER DISEASE: *see* Detoxification

LIVER HEALTH: *see* Detoxification

LIVER PROTECTION: *see* Detoxification

LOW APPETITE: gentian root

LOW BACK PAIN: cell salts; fish oil; glucosamine; MSM; rhus toxicodendron; sulphur; turmeric

LOW SPERM COUNT: amino acids; coenzyme Q10; ginseng; maca

LUPUS: DHEA; fish oil

LYME DISEASE: cat's claw; colloidal silver; probiotics

M

MACULAR DEGENERATION: B-complex vitamins; bilberry; carotenoids; ginkgo biloba; vitamin C; vitamin E; zinc

MALARIA: wormwood

MALNOURISHMENT: enzymes; spirulina

MANIC DEPRESSION: fish oil; lachesis

MEMORY PROBLEMS: acetyl-L-carnitine; ashwagandha; B-complex vitamins; cell salts; essential oils; flaxseed; ginkgo biloba; ginseng; L-carnitine; phosphatidylserine; phytonutrients; rhodiola; vitamin B12

MENINGITIS: apis

MENOPAUSE: adrenal glandulars; pine bark extract; black cohosh; burdock; dandelion; DHEA; exercise; flaxseed; lachesis; maca; passionflower; phytonutrients; pine bark extract; progesterone; pulsatilla; sepia; soy; sulforaphane; sulphur; vitamin E; vitex

MENSTRUAL CRAMPS: black cohosh; cell salts; chamomile; cinnamon; fish oil; pine bark extract; pulsatilla; valerian

MENSTRUAL DISORDERS: glandulars; progesterone; vitex

MENSTRUATION, HEAVY: cell salts; cinnamon; iron; lachesis; vitex

MENSTRUATION, IRON-DEFICIENCY ANEMIA FROM: ferrum phosphoricum; iron

MENSTRUATION, IRREGULAR CYCLES: pulsatilla; sepia; vitex

MIGRAINE PREVENTION: *see* Migraines

MIGRAINES: amino acids; butterbur; coenzyme Q10; feverfew; ipecacuanha; lachesis; magnesium; progesterone; pulsatilla; riboflavin; sepia

MISCARRIAGE PREVENTION: progesterone; vitex

MITRAL VALVE PROLAPSE: coenzyme Q1O; L-carnitine; magnesium

MONONUCLEOSIS: colloidal silver; echinacea; gelsemium; glandulars; lomatium; selenium; vitamin C

MORNING SICKNESS: ginger root; ipecacuanha; pulsatilla; sepia

MOSQUITO BITES: ledum

MOTION SICKNESS: ginger root

MOUTH CANCER: beta-carotene; spirulina

MOUTH INFECTIONS: tea tree oil

MOUTH SORES: aloe; licorice root

MULTIPLE SCLEROSIS: evening primrose oil; fish oil; flaxseed; gelsemium; vitamin B12; vitamin D; vitamin E

MUSCLE CRAMPS/SPASMS: black cohosh; calcium; cell salts; ignatia; kava; magnesium; potassium; sitz bath; valerian

MUSCLE PAIN: acupressure; arnica; boswellia; cayenne; cell salts; MSM; peppermint; vitamin D

MUSCLE PROBLEMS: *see* Muscle Pain

MUSCLE TENSION: calcium; kava; magnesium

MUSCLE WEAKNESS: vitamin D; vitamin E

N

NAIL HEALTH: biotin; enzymes; MSM; silicon

NAIL PROBLEMS: *see* Nail Health

NASAL CONGESTION: goldenseal; N-acetylcysteine; nettle; quercetin

NAUSEA: acupressure; ginger root; ipecacuanha; nux vomica

NECK PAIN: acupressure; boswellia; MSM; turmeric

NERVE CELLS, PROTECTING: evening primrose oil; fish oil; ginkgo biloba; vitamin B12

NERVOUSNESS: B-complex vitamins; cell salts; passionflower; valerian

NEURAL TUBE DEFECTS: folic acid; vitamin B12

NEUROPATHY: acetyl-L-carnitine; alpha lipoic acid; evening primrose oil; vitamin B1; vitamin B12

NIGHT BLINDNESS: bilberry; vitamin A

NIGHT VISION: bilberry

O

ORCHITIS: pulsatilla

OSTEOARTHRITIS: B-complex vitamins; boswellia; cat's claw; fish oil; flaxseed; glucosamine sulfate; guggul; MSM; SAMe; turmeric

OSTEOPOROSIS: amino acids; calcium; cell salts; DHEA; evening primrose oils; exercise; fish oil; ipriflavone; lysine; maca; magnesium; progesterone; silicon; soy; vitamin C; vitamin D; vitamin K

OSTEOPOROSIS PREVENTION: *see* Osteoporosis

OTOSCLEROSIS: ipriflavone

OVARIAN CYSTS: apis; glandulars; lachesis; progesterone; pulsatilla; sepia; vitex

OVARIAN PAIN: *see* Ovarian Cysts

OVULATION: vitex

P

PAGET'S DISEASE: ipriflavone

PAIN: acupressure; aloe; amino acids; arnica; boswellia; feverfew; kava; MSM; rhus toxicodendron; turmeric

PANCREAS: enzymes; glandulars

PANIC ATTACKS: *Aconitum napellus*; carbo vegetabilis; kava; Resperate

PARASITES: colloidal silver; goldenseal; MSM; oregano; probiotics; wormwood

PARKINSON'S DISEASE: coenzyme Q10; vitamin E

PELVIC CONGESTION/ INFLAMMATION: sitz bath

PEPTIC ULCERS: licorice root; propolis

PERIODONTAL DISEASE: coenzyme Q1O; tea tree oil; vitamin C

PERIPHERAL VASCULAR DISEASE: arginine; enzymes; ginkgo biloba; hawthorn; vitamin E

PEYRONIE'S DISEASE: acetyl-L-carnitine

PHYSICAL TRAUMA: arnica; MSM; rhus toxicodendron

PNEUMONIA: carbo vegetabilis; colloidal silver; echinacea; goldenseal; hydrotherapy; lomatium

POLYCYSTIC OVARIAN SYNDROME: chromium; progesterone; saw palmetto; vitex

POSTPARTUM RECOVERY: arnica; sitz bath

POST-SURGICAL PAIN: boswellia; bromelain; cayenne; MSM; turmeric

PREDNISONE TAPERING: ashwagandha; DHEA; glandulars; rhodiola

PREECLAMPSIA: calcium; magnesium; vitamin C; vitamin E

PREGNANCY: calcium; iron; nettle; pine bark extract; prenatal vitamins

PREGNANCY COMPLICATIONS: *see* Preeclampsia

PREGNANCY EDEMA: dandelion; vitamin B6

PREMATURE EJACULATION: lycopodium; maca

PREMATURE INFANTS: fish oils; L-carnitine

PREMENSTRUAL SYNDROME (PMS): amino acids; black cohosh; burdock; calcium; dandelion; evening primrose oil; exercise; ginkgo biloba; ignatia; lachesis; magnesium; passionflower; phytonutrients; progesterone; pulsatilla; sepia; St. John's wort; vitamin B6; vitamin E; vitex

PROSTATE CANCER: D-glucarate; maitake; pomegranate; vitamin D

PROSTATE CANCER PREVENTION: carotenoids; flaxseed; phytonutrients; vitamin D

PROSTATE ENLARGEMENT: nettle; saw palmetto; sepia; sitz bath; zinc

PROSTATE INFECTIONS: colloidal silver; cranberry; echinacea; goldenseal; quercetin; sitz bath

PROSTATITIS: *see* Prostate Infections

PSORIASIS: aloe; cayenne; cell salts; fish oil; food-sensitivity therapy; licorice root; pulsatilla; sepia

PUNCTURE WOUNDS: ledum

R

RADIATION EXPOSURE: antioxidants; ginkgo biloba; ginseng; melatonin; spirulina

RADIATION POISONING: *see* Radiation Exposure

RASHES: calendula; cell salts; enzymes; fish oil; food-sensitivity therapy; sulphur; water

RAYNAUD'S SYNDROME: ginkgo biloba; sepia

RECTAL PAIN OR ITCH: calendula; sitz bath; sulfur

RESPIRATORY TRACT INFECTIONS: astragalus; bromelain; echinacea; garlic; goldenseal; hydrotherapy; lomatium; lycopodium; oregano; probiotics; N-acetylcysteine; vitamin A

RESTLESS LEG SYNDROME: calcium; iron; magnesium; tryptophan and 5-HTP

RHEUMATOID ARTHRITIS: apis; boswellia; cat's claw; cayenne; echinacea; evening primrose oil; fermented wheat germ extract; fish oil; flaxseed; selenium; turmeric

RETINOPATHY: bilberry; fish oil; zinc

S

SCARS: calendula; vitamin E

SCHIZOPHRENIA: DHEA; fish oil; food-sensitivity therapy; niacin

SEASONAL AFFECTIVE DISORDER (SAD): melatonin; St. John's wort; tryptophan and 5-HTP

SEBORRHEIC DERMATITIS: biotin; fish oil

SEIZURES: cell salts

SHINGLES: apis; cayenne; lachesis; rhus toxicodendron; vitamin B12

SINUSITIS: acupressure; bromelain; cell salts; food-sensitivity therapy; goldenseal; hydrotherapy; MSM; N-acetylcysteine; pulsatilla; quercetin; sepia

SKIN CANCER PREVENTION: carotenoids; selenium

SKIN CONDITIONS: aloe gel; burdock; cell salts; chamomile; echinacea; evening primrose oil; fish oil; hydrotherapy; licorice root; milk thistle; sulphur; tea tree oil

SKIN PROTECTION: calendula; carotenoids; coenzyme Q1O; DHEA; fish oil; pine bark extract

SLOW GROWTH: ashwagandha; fish oil; vitamin D

SMELL, LOSS OF: alpha lipic acid

SMOKING CESSATION: antioxidants; melatonin; nux vomica; tryptophan and 5-HTP; valerian

SORE THROAT: apis; cell salts; colloidal silver; echinacea; ferrum phosphoricum; goldenseal; lomatium; propolis; sulphur

SPINAL PROBLEMS: cell salts

SPRAINS/STRAINS: bromelain; cell salts; ledum; MSM; rhus toxicodendron; turmeric

STIFF NECK: *see* Neck Pain

STOMACH CRAMPS: *see* Digestion

STOMACH UPSET: *see* Digestion

STRESS: ashwagandha; B-complex vitamins; chamomile; DHEA; exercise; ginseng; kava; pantothenic acid; passionflower; phosphatidylserine; Resperate; rhodiola; valerian; vitamin B12; vitamin C

STROKE: alpha GPC; ginkgo biloba

STROKE PREVENTION: enzymes; fish oil; potassium; vitamin D; vitamin E

SUDDEN INFANT DEATH SYNDROME (SIDS): selenium

SUNBURN: aloe gel; cantharis; carotenoids; vitamin C

SURGERY RECOVERY: amino acids; arnica; bromelain; cayenne; multivitamins; vitamin C

SWELLING: arnica; bromelain; cell salts; MSM; turmeric

SYNDROME X: chromium; exercise; glucomannan; gymnema sylvestre; vanadium

SYSTEMIC TOXICITY: chlorella; dandelion; fiber; garlic; hydrotherapy; milk thistle; probiotics; spirulina

T

TEETH, BRITTLE: calcium; cell salts; vitamin D

TEETHING: cell salts; chamomile

TENDONS, WEAK: cell salts; silicon

TENSION HEADACHES: acupressure; black cohosh; ignatia; kava; magnesium; MSM; passionflower; peppermint; valerian

TESTOSTERONE DEFICIENCY: acetyl-L-carnitine; glandulars

THROMBOPHLEBITIS: bromelain; enzymes; horse chestnut

THROMBOPHLEBITIS PREVENTION: bromelain; enzymes; fish oil; ginkgo biloba

TINNITUS: ginkgo biloba; ipriflavone

TMJ SYNDROME: ignatia; magnesium; MSM

TOE FUNGUS: tea tree oil

TONSILLITIS: ardrographis; colloidal silver; echinacea; ferrum phosphoricum; goldenseal; lomatium

TOOTH ABSCESS: cell salts; tea tree oil

TOOTHACHE: cell salts; chamomile

TOOTH DECAY PREVENTION: green tea; probiotics

TOOTH LOSS: calcium; vitamin D

TOXICITY, SYSTEMIC: *see* Systemic Toxicity

TOXINS: *see* Systemic Toxicity

TRAUMA, EMOTIONAL: Bach flower remedies

TRAVELER'S DIARRHEA: *Arsenicum album*; ginger; probiotics

TRIGLYCERIDES: cayenne; chromium; fish oil; garlic; glucomannan; guggul

U

ULCERATIVE COLITIS: boswellia; bromelain; chamomile; chlorella; fish oil; food-sensitivity therapy; hydrotherapy; lycopodium; nux vomica; peppermint; prebiotics; probiotics; propolis; wheatgrass; wormwood

ULCERS: aloe; *Arsenicum album*; calendula; chamomile; hydrotherapy; licorice root; nux vomica; pine bark extract; probiotics; propolis; quercetin

UPPER RESPIRATORY TRACT INFECTIONS: astragalus; colloidal silver; echinacea; lomatium; vitamin C; vitamin D

URINARY TRACT INFECTIONS: apis; burdock; cantharis; colloidal silver; cranberry; goldenseal; lomatium; saw palmetto; sitz bath; uva ursi; water

URTICARIA: quercetin; rhus toxicodendron

UTERINE FIBROIDS: progesterone; vitex

UTERINE, PROLAPSE: progesterone; sepia

V

VAGINAL INFECTIONS: *see* Vaginitis

VAGINITIS: cell salts; echinacea; food-sensitivity therapy; phytonutrients; probiotics; progesterone; pulsatilla; sepia; tea tree oil

VARICOSE VEINS: bilberry; bromelain; butcher's broom; calendula; cell salts; horse chestnut; lachesis; phytonutrients; pine bark extract; pulsatilla; sepia

VEIN CLOTS: bromelain; enzymes; fish oil

VERTIGO: gelsemium; ginkgo biloba

VIRAL INFECTIONS: aloe; astragalus; colloidal silver; echinacea; enzymes; lomatium; phytonutrients; St. John's wort

VISION: bilberry; carotenoids; ginkgo biloba; zinc

VITAMIN A DEFICIENCY: spirulina; vitamin A

VOMITING: *Arsenicum album*; ginger root; nux vomica; probiotics

W

WARTS: garlic; tea tree oil

WATER RETENTION: dandelion; vitamin B6

WEIGHT LOSS: amino acids; arginine; calcium; *Caralluma fimbriata*; chromium; conjugated linoleic acid; dandelion; DHEA; glucomannan; green tea; L-carnitine; lo han; nutritional supplements; stevia; tryptophan and 5-HTP; vitamin D; water; xylitol

WILSON'S DISEASE: zinc

WOUNDS: aloe; amino acids; calendula; cell salts; phytonutrients; propolis; St. John's wort; vitamin C; vitamin E; zinc

WRINKLES: antioxidants; coenzyme Q10; green tea; vitamin C

INDEX

Page numbers in *italic* represent charts.

AAMI. *See* Age-associated memory impairment
Abdominal pain, 425
Acetaminophen poisoning, 334–35
Acetyl-L-carnitine (ALC), 1–3
Acidophilus, 370–71
Acne
   burdock for, 71
   flaxseed for, 190
   goldenseal for, 239
   guggul for, 246
   saw palmetto for, 410
   tea tree oil for, 446
   vitamin A for, 461
   vitamin E for, 477
   vitex for, 485
   zinc for, 498
Aconite. *See Aconitum napellus*
Aconitum napellus (aconite), 3–5
Acupressure, 5–11
   administering, treatment, 7
   chemical reaction, 6–7
   point location chart, 8, 9
   points, 5–6
   Qi and, 6
   recommendations for use, 10–11
   side effects, 7
Acupuncture, 6
Adaptogen, 310
ADD. *See* Attention deficit disorder
ADHD. *See* Attention deficit/hyperactivity disorder
Adrenal glands, 128, 229
Adriamycin, 112
Agaricus blazei, 11–12
Age-associated memory impairment (AAMI), 352.
     See also Memory impairment
Age-related macular degeneration (AMD), 465
Aging
   ashwagandha for, 40
   B-complex vitamins and, 48
   ginseng for, 224

   hyaluronic acid for, 258
   melatonin for, 318
Agitation, 148
AIDS
   aloe for, 15
   arginine for, 32
   selenium for, 416
   vitamin A for, 461
   vitamin E for, 477
   weight loss related to, 32
   zinc for, 498
ALA. *See* Alpha lipoic acid
ALC. *See* Acetyl-L-carnitine
Alcoholism
   lachesis for, 290
   milk thistle for, 323
   nux vomica for, 341
Allergies
   acupressure for, 10
   apis for, 29
   Arsenicum album for, 36
   bee pollen for, 54, 55
   butterbur for, 73, 74
   DHEA for, 129
   eyebright for, 157
   food-sensitivity therapy for, 196
   gentian root for, 208
   milk thistle for, 323
   MSM for, 329
   nux vomica for, 341
   quercetin for, 389
   vitamin C for, 465
Aloe vera, 13–15
Alpha GPC, 16
Alpha lipoic acid (ALA), 16–18
Altitude sickness, 393
Alzheimer's disease
   ALC for, 2
   alpha GPC for, 16
   ginkgo biloba for, 215–16

Alzheimer's disease (cont.)
  huperzine for, 256
  phosphatidylserine for, 352–53
  turmeric for preventing, 452
  vitamin E for, 477
  zinc for, 498
AMD. *See* Age-related macular degeneration
Amenorrhea, 2, 485. *See also* Menstrual pain
Amino acids, 18–21, *21*
Andrographis, 21, 22
Anemia
  ashwagandha for, 40
  ferrum phosphoricum for, 168–70
  gentian root for, 207
  iron deficiency and, 276
  iron for, 279
  nettle for, 337
  spirulina for, 431
Angina
  arginine for, 32
  CoQ10 for, 111
  hawthorn for, 251
  L-carnitine for, 294
  magnesium for, 313
  vitamin E for, 477
Anorexia, 294
Antibiotics, 67, 372
Anti-inflammatory properties, 209
Antioxidants, 22–27, *28*
  arthritis patients and, 25
  athletes and, 26
  bilberry, 57–58
  cancer patients and, 26
  cardiovascular disease and, 26–27
  cayenne as, 94
  chemotherapy and, 26
  cholesterol, high and, 26–27
  detoxification patients and, 26
  diabetes and, 26
  dosage, 25
  free radicals and, 22–23
  pollution and, 23
  recommendations for specific people taking,
    25–26
  side effects, 25
  smokers and, 27
  sources, 28
Anxiety
  Aconitum napellus for, 3
  acupressure for, 10
  Arsenicum album for, 36
  black cohosh for, 62

  carbo vegetabilis for, 87
  exercise for, 155
  gelsemium for, 204
  ignatia for, 267
  kava for, 286
  passionflower for, 348
  pulsatilla for, 384
  Resperate for, 395
  rhodiola for, 398
  St. John's wort for, 436
  tryptophan and 5-HTP for, 449
  valerian for, 458
Aorta elasticity problems, 201
Apis, 29–31
Appetite, loss of, 124, 208
Appetite suppression, 85, 86
Arginine, 31–32
Arnica, 33–34
Aromatherapy, 147–48
Arrhythmia
  CoQ10 for, 111
  hawthorn for, 251
  L-carnitine for, 294
  magnesium for, 313
Arsenic toxicity, 36
Arsenicum album, 34–37
Artery health, 38. *See also* Coronary artery disease
Arthritis
  antioxidants for, 25
  apis for, 29
  ashwagandha for, 40
  bee pollen for, 55–56
  black cohosh for, 63
  boswellia for, 65
  bromelain for, 68
  cayenne for, 95
  enzymes for, 145
  evening primrose oil for, 151
  exercise for, 155
  feverfew for, 172
  fish oil for, 182–83
  flaxseed for, 190–91
  food-sensitivity therapy for, 196
  ginger root for, 210
  hyaluronic acid for, 258
  hydrotherapy for, 262
  ledum for, 297
  lycopodium for, 306
  MSM for, 327–29
  nettle for, 337–38
  pine bark extract for, 358
  pulsatilla for, 384–85

rhus toxicodendron for, 400
turmeric for, 452
vitamin C for, 465
vitamin E for, 477–78
Artichoke, 37–38
Ashwagandha, 38–41
Asthma
   aloe for, 14
   Arsenicum album for, 36
   astragalus for, 42
   boswellia for, 66
   butterbur for, 74
   carbo vegetabilis for, 87
   fish oil for, 183
   food-sensitivity therapy for, 196
   ginseng for, 224–25
   ipecac for, 270
   lachesis for, 290
   magnesium for, 313
   MSM for, 329
   onion for, 344
   pine bark extract for, 358–59
   pulsatilla for, 385
   vitamin C for, 465
Astragalus, 41–44
Atherosclerosis
   CoQ10 for, 111
   guggul for, 246
   pomegranate for, 363
   tocotrienols for, 448
   vitamin C for, 465
   vitamin K for, 482
   zinc for, 498
Athletes
   antioxidants for, 26
   echinacea for, 135
   free radicals and, 109
   ginseng for, 219
   ribose for, 401
Athlete's foot, 346, 446
Attention deficit disorder (ADD)
   evening primrose oil for, 151
   fish oil for, 182
   food-sensitivity therapy for, 196
   ginkgo biloba for, 216
   iron for, 279
   sulphur for, 441
Attention deficit/hyperactivity disorder (ADHD)
   evening primrose oil for, 151
   fish oil for, 182
   food-sensitivity therapy for, 196
   iron for, 279

pine bark extract for, 359
phosphatidylserine for, 353
zinc for, 498
Autism, 196, 471
Autoimmune conditions
   echinacea for, 136–37
   enzymes for, 145
   food-sensitivity therapy for, 196
   MSM for, 329–30
   progesterone for, 377–78
   vitamin D for, 471

Bach flower remedies, 45–47, 46
Back pain, 254
Bacteria, 134–35, 370–71
Bad breath, 491
B-complex vitamins, 47–54
   biotin, 53–54
   dosage, 48
   folic acid, 51–52
   side effects, 49
   vitamin B1, 49
   vitamin B2, 49
   vitamin B3, 49–50
   vitamin B5, 50–51
   vitamin B6, 51
   vitamin B12, 52–53
Bee pollen, 54–56
Bee stings, 29–30
Benin prostatic hypertrophy (BPH), 408, 411
Benzodiazepine withdrawal, 318
Berberine, 237–38
Beta blockers, 112–13
Bifidobacterium, 370
Bilberry, 56–59
Biotin, 53–54
Birth complications, 498
Birth-control pill side effects, 420
Black cohosh, 60–65
Bladder infection
   nux vomica for, 341
   pulsatilla for, 385
   saw palmetto for, 411–12
   sepia for, 420
   sitz bath for, 425
Bleeding, 170, 276
Bloating, 196
Blood clotting, 201. *See also* Circulation
Blood-sugar levels, 103–4
Bone loss, 473
Bone pain, 350
Boswellia, 64–66

BPH. *See* Benin prostatic hypertrophy
Brain injury, 353
Breast cancer, 372–73
Breast pain, 485–86
Breast tenderness, cyclical, 152
Bromelain, 66–69
Bronchitis
    butterbur for, 74
    carbo vegetabilis for, 87
    food-sensitivity therapy for, 196
    hydrotherapy for, 262
    ipecac for, 270
    pulsatilla for, 385
    reishi for chronic, 394
Bruising
    bromelain for, 66
    hyaluronic acid for, 258
    ledum for, 297
    St. John's wort for, 436
Burdock, 70–71
Burnout, 127
Burns
    aloe for, 14
    bromelain for, 68
    calendula for, 82
    cantharis for, 83, 84–85
    St. John's wort for, 436
    vitamin E for, 478
    zinc for, 498
Butcher's broom, 72–73
Butterbur, 73–75

CAD. *See* Coronary artery disease
Caffeine, 166
Calcarea fluorica, 413
Calcarea phosphorica, 413–14
Calcarea sulphurica, 414
Calcidiol, 469
Calcitriol, 469
Calcium, 76, 76–81
Calendula, 81–83
Calorie counting, 161
Cancer. *See also specific types of cancer*
    Agaricus blazei for, 12
    antioxidants for, 26
    Arsenicum album for, 36
    astragalus for, 43–44
    black cohosh and, 62
    bromelain for, 68
    burdock for, 71
    calcium for, 80
    carotenoids for, 89–90

cat's claw for, 93
chlorella for, 102
CoQ10 for, 111
coriolus versicolor as complementary treatment
    for, 119
D-glucarate and, 125
enzymes for, 145–46
fiber for, 177–78
fish oil for, 183–84
flaxseed for, 191
FWGE for, 167–68
garlic for, 201
ginseng for, 225
green tea for, 242–43
hydrotherapy for, 262
maitake as complementary treatment for, 316
melatonin for, 318–19
NAC for, 335
onion for, 344
prebiotics for, 369
quercetin for, 389
red yeast rice for, 392
reishi for, 393–94
selenium for, 416–17
soy for, 427–28
spirulina for, 431
sulforaphane for, 439
tocotrienols for, 448
turmeric for, 452–53
vitamin C for, 465
vitamin D for, 471–72
vitamin E for, 478
wormwood for, 493
Candida
    food-sensitivity therapy for, 196–97
    gentian root for, 207
    oregano for, 346
Canker sores, 14
Cantharis, 83–85
Caralluma fimbriata, 85–86
Carbohydrates, 161
Carbo vegetabilis, 86–87
Cardiac autonomic neuropathy, 17
Cardiomyopathy
    CoQ10 for, 112
    L-carnitine for, 294
    magnesium for, 313
Cardiovascular disease, 466–67, 478–79
    ALA for, 17
    antioxidants and, 26–27
    arginine for, 31
    bromelain for, 68–69

calcium for, 80
carotenoids for, 90
cayenne for, 95–96
DHEA for, 129
enzymes for, 146
exercise for, 155
fish oil for, 179–80, 184
flaxseed for, 191
garlic for, 201–2
ginger root for, 211
green tea for, 243
hawthorn for preventing, 253
red yeast rice for, 392
resveratrol for, 397
selenium for, 417
soy for, 428
vitamin D for, 472–73
Cardiovascular health
    Cordyceps sinensis for, 117
    ginger root and, 209–10
    hawthorn for, 250
    quercetin for, 389
    reishi for, 394
Carotenoids, 87–90
Carotid stenosis, 478
Cartilage rebuilding, 234
Cascara sagrada, 90–91
Cataracts
    bilberry for, 56, 58
    selenium for, 417
    vitamin C for, 466
    vitamin E for, 478
Cat's claw, 91–93
Cavities, 433, 494. *See also* Dental conditions
Cayenne, 93–96
Cellulitis, 82
Chamomile, 96–101
Chemotherapy
    antioxidants and, 26
    astragalus and, 44
    astragalus for, 41
    CoQ10 and, 112
    coriolus versicolor for, 119
    diarrhea induced by, 372
    FWGE for, 167
    infections induced by, 167
    nux vomica for, 341
    pine bark extract for, 359
    probiotics and, 372
Children
    aconite for, 5
    aloe latex and, 14

cascara sagrada and, 91
    multivitamins for, 331–32
Chinese medicine, 42
Chlorella, 101–3
Chlorophyll, 355
Cholecalciferol, 468–69
Cholesterol
    Agaricus blazei for, 12
    aloe for, 15
    antioxidants and, 26–27
    artichoke for, 38
    chromium for, 105
    cinnamon for, 108
    fiber for, 178
    flaxseed for, 191
    garlic for, 202
    ginger root for, 211
    glucomannan for, 232
    guggul for, 244–46
    onion for, 344–45
    pine bark extract for, 359
    pomegranate for, 364
    red yeast rice for, 391, 392–93
    soy for, 428
    spirulina for, 431
    tocotrienols for, 448
    turmeric for, 453
    vitamin D for, 473
    vitamin E for, 479
Chromium, 103–6
Chronic fatigue syndrome. *See also* Fatigue
    CoQ10 for, 112
    DHEA for, 129
    L-carnitine for, 294–95
    ribose for, 401
Chronic obstructive pulmonary disease (COPD), 184
Cinnamon, 106–8
Circulation
    lachesis and, 289
    milk thistle for, 323
    pine bark extract for, 360
Circulatory health
    DHEA for, 129
    ginger root and, 209–10
    ginkgo biloba and, 214
Circulatory problems
    calcium for, 80
    cayenne for, 94
    cinnamon for, 108
    CoQ10 for, 109
    ginkgo biloba for, 216
Cirrhosis, 323–24

CLA. *See* Conjugated linoleic acid
Cluster headache, 319
Coenzyme Q10 (CoQ10), 109–15
Cognitive health
   fish oil for, 184–85
   huperzine for, 256
   vitamin D for, 472
   water for, 490
Cold
   acupressure for, 10
   andrographis for, 22
   astragalus for, 44
   cinnamon for, 108
   echinacea for, 137
   garlic for, 202
   goldenseal for, 239
   lomatium for, 304
   peppermint for, 350
   vitamin C for, 466
   zinc for, 498–99
Cold sores, 14, 446
Colic
   chamomile for, 98
   enzymes for, 146
   garlic and, 200
   nux vomica for, 341
Colitis, 306, 341
Colloidal silver, 115–16
Colon cancer, 80, 372–73
Colorectal cancer, 167, 335
Computer eye irritation, 157
Concentration, 398–99
Concussion, 33
Congestion, 236–37
Congestive heart failure. *See also* Cardiovascular
    disease
   arginine for, 32
   carbo vegetabilis for, 87
   CoQ10 for, 112
   hawthorn for, 251–52
   L-carnitine for, 295
   magnesium for, 313
   ribose for, 401
Conjugated linoleic acid (CLA), 165
Conjunctivitis
   calendula for, 82
   eyebright for, 157
   pulsatilla for, 385–86
Constipation
   acupressure for, 10
   aloe for, 13
   burdock for, 71

   cascara sagrada for, 90–91
   dandelion for, 123–24
   fiber for, 178–79
   food-sensitivity therapy for, 197
   gentian root for, 207
   glucomannan for, 232
   milk thistle for, 324
   nux vomica for, 341
   prebiotics for, 369
   probiotics for, 373
   sitz bath for, 425
Contrast dye-induced kidney damage, 336
COPD. *See* Chronic obstructive pulmonary disease
CoQ10. *See* Coenzyme Q10
Cordyceps sinensis, 116–18
Coriolus versicolor, 118–19
Corns, 203
Coronary artery bypass surgery recovery, 401
Coronary artery disease (CAD), 363–64, 402
Cough
   acupressure for, 10
   elderberry for, 139
   licorice root for, 300
   peppermint for, 350
Coumadin, 110, 113
Cranberry, 120–21
Crohn's disease
   boswellia for, 66
   fish oil for, 185
   wormwood for, 493
Curcumin, 355, 451
Cuts, 498
Cystitis, interstitial, 32

Dandelion, 122–25
Dementia
   ALA for, 17
   DHEA for, 129
   huperzine for, 256
   phosphatidylserine for, 353
Dental conditions, 381
Dental pain, 264
Depression
   ALC for, 2
   black cohosh for, 62
   chromium for, 105
   essential oils for, 148
   exercise for, 155
   fish oil for, 185
   food-sensitivity therapy for, 197
   ginkgo biloba for, 216
   ignatia for, 267

kava for, 286–87
milk thistle for, 324
phosphatidylserine for, 353
pulsatilla for, 386
SAMe for, 406
sepia for, 420
St. John's wort for, 436–37
tryptophan and 5-HTP for, 449
valerian for, 458
vitamin D for, 472
Dermatitis, radiation, 83
Detoxification
  antioxidants and, 26
  burdock for, 70
  dandelion for, 122–23
  exercise for, 155
  green drinks and, 283
  green tea for, 243
  hydrotherapy for, 262
  juicing, recipes for, 282–83
  licorice root for, 299–300
  milk thistle for, 324
  phytonutrients for, 354–55
  spirulina for, 431
  sulforaphane for, 439
  weight loss and, 164
  wheatgrass, 491–92
D-glucarate, 125–27
DHA. *See* Docosahexanoic acid
DHEA, 127–31
Diabetes
  Agaricus blazei for, 12
  ALA for, 17–18
  aloe for, 14–15
  antioxidants and, 26
  burdock for, 71
  calcium for, 80
  chromium for, 104, 105–6
  cinnamon for, 108
  CoQ10 for, 112
  dandelion for, 124
  DHEA for, 129
  evening primrose oil for, 151–52
  exercise for, 155
  fiber for, 179
  ginseng for, 225–26
  glucomannan for, 232
  gymnema sylvestre and, 246–48
  L-carnitine for, 295
  magnesium for, 313–14
  maitake for, 316
  milk thistle for, 324

onion for, 345
pine bark extract for, 360
pomegranate for, 364
quercetin for, 389–90
reishi for, 394
resveratrol for, 397
soy for, 428
stevia for, 433
ulcers, 360
vanadium for, 459
vitamin C for, 466
vitamin D for, 472
vitamin E for, 478
Diabetic foot ulcer, 32. *See also* Ulcer(s)
Diabetic neuropathy, 2, 95
Diabetic retinopathy, 106
Diarrhea
  antibiotic-induced, 372
  Arsenicum album for, 36–37
  bilberry for, 58
  chemotherapy-induced, 372
  food-sensitivity therapy for, 197
  gelsemium for, 204
  ginger root for, 211
  goldenseal for, 239
  infectious, 373
  probiotics for, 372, 373
Diet
  calorie counting and, 161
  carbohydrate, protein, fat ratio and, 161
  consistency and, 162–63
  fat intake and, 160–61
  fiber in, 173, 175
  food sensitivities and, 162, 193–94
  plant food and, 162
  portions and, 161
  potassium in, 365
  prebiotics in, 369
  skipping meals and, 161
  sugar intake and, 159–60
  water intake and, 162
  weight problems and, 159–63
Digestion
  astragalus for, 44
  cinnamon for, 108
  enzymes and, 141–45
  essential oils for, 148
  ginger root and, 209
  green tea for, 243–44
  nux vomica and, 340
  peppermint and, 349

Digestive problems
  bromelain for, 69
  carbo vegetabilis for, 87
  enzymes for, 146
  fiber and, 174
  flaxseed for, 191–92
  gentian root and, 205–6
  goldenseal for, 239
  hydrotherapy for, 262–63
  propolis for, 381
  quercetin for, 390
  sulphur for, 441
  turmeric for, 453
  valerian for, 458
Dizziness, 490
DNA, 24
Docosahexanoic acid (DHA), 180, 181
Down's syndrome, 295
D-ribose, 165
Drug addiction recovery, 323
Drug damage, 112–13
Drug interactions, deficiencies from, 295
Dry eye syndrome, 185, 461.
      See also Eye health
Dry skin, 192. See also Skin conditions

Earache, 98, 170
Ear infections
  food-sensitivity therapy for, 197
  lachesis for, 290
  xylitol for, 494–95
Ear ringing, 218
Eating disorders, 499. See also Anorexia
Echinacea, 132–38
Eczema
  calendula for, 82
  evening primrose oil for, 152
  fish oil for, 185
  flaxseed for, 192
  food-sensitivity therapy for, 197
  licorice root for, 300
  probiotics for, 373
  vitamin E for, 478
ED. See Erectile dysfunction
Edema
  dandelion for, 124
  nettle for, 338
  water for, 491
EFAs. See Essential fatty acids
Eicosapentanoic acid (EPA), 180, 181
Elderberry, 138–39
Ellagic acid, 355

Endometriosis
  lachesis for, 290
  pine bark extract for, 360
  progesterone for, 378
  pulsatilla for, 386
Energy boost, 56, 116
Energy channels, 6
Energy levels
  B-complex vitamins for, 47
  flaxseed for, 192
  rhodiola for, 398
Enzymes, 140–47
  commercial, 143
  deficiency, 141
  dosage, 144
  recommendations for use, 145–47
  side effects, 144–45
  sources of, 140–41
  supplemental, types, 141–42
EPA. See Eicosapentanoic acid
Epilepsy, 336
EPO. See Evening primrose oil
Epstein-Barr, 304
Erectile dysfunction (ED), 32. See also Impotence
Essential fatty acids (EFAs), 187–88
  omega-3, 180, 187
  omega-6, 149–50, 187
Essential oils, 147–49
Evening primrose oil (EPO), 149–52
Exercise, 152–56
Eyebright, 156–57
Eye health, 360–61
Eyelid inflammation, 157
Eye problems, 157, 239, 443
Eyestrain, 10, 58

Fall prevention, 472
Fatigue. See also Chronic fatigue syndrome
  ashwagandha for, 40
  chlorella for, 102
  Cordyceps sinensis for, 117
  exercise for, 155
  eye, 157
  food-sensitivity therapy for, 197
  gelsemium for, 204
  ginseng for, 226
  iron for, 279
  licorice root for, 301
  magnesium for, 314
  phosphatidylserine for, 353
  sulphur for, 441
  water for, 490

Fat intake, 160–61
Fat reduction, 158–66
 natural stimulants, 166
 nutritional supplements, 165–66
 weight loss and, 158
Fermented wheat germ extract (FWGE), 166–68
Ferrum phosphoricum, 168–70, 414
Fertility
 maca for, 310
 pine bark extract for, 361
 sepia for, 420
 vitamin E for, 478
Fever
 burdock for, 71
 cinnamon for, 108
 ferrum phosphoricum for, 170
 hydrotherapy for, 263
Feverfew, 170–72
Fiber, 172–79
 diet and, 173, 175
 dosage, 175
 glucomannan, 231
 insoluble, 174, 176
 juicing and, 281
 recommendations for use, 177–79
 side effects, 175
 soluble, 174, 176
Fibrocystic breasts
 progesterone for, 378
 sepia for, 420
 vitamin E for, 478
 vitex for, 485–86
Fibromyalgia
 black cohosh for, 63
 chlorella for, 102
 magnesium for, 314
 MSM for, 330
 ribose for, 402
 SAMe for, 406–7
 tryptophan and 5-HTP for, 450
 vitamin D for, 472
Fish oil, 179–86
5-HTP. *See* Tryptophan and 5-HTP
Flatulence
 chamomile for, 98
 dandelion for, 123–24
 ginger root for, 210–11
Flavoglycosides, 355
Flavonoids, 388
Flaxseed, 187–93
Flu
 Aconitum napellus for, 4

acupressure for, 10
andrographis for, 22
Arsenicum album for, 37
artichoke for, 37
echinacea for, 137–38
elderberry for, 138, 139
gelsemium for, 204
lomatium for, 304
NAC for prevention of, 336
nux vomica for, 341
rhus toxicodendron for, 400
Folic acid, 51–52
Food sensitivities
 enzymes for, 146–47
 gentian root for, 208
 situations, 193–94
 testing for, 194–95
 weight loss and, 162
Food-sensitivity therapy, 193–98
 avoidance mechanisms and, 195
 recommendations for use, 196–98
 sensitivity situations, 193–94
 testing and, 194–95
FOS. *See* Fructooligosaccharides
Fractures, 443
Free radicals, 22–24, 109
Fructooligosaccharides (FOS), 355
Fungus
 echinacea and, 135
 prebiotics for, 369
 tea tree oil for, 446
FWGE. *See* Fermented wheat germ extract

Gallbladder problems, 197
Gallic acid, 355–56
Gallstones
 milk thistle for, 324–25
 peppermint for, 350
 vitamin C for, 466
Gamma linolenic acid (GLA), 149–50
Garlic, 199–203
Gelsemium, 203–5
Gene expression, 102–3
Genital warts, 304, 421
Gentian root, 205–8
Ginger root, 208–12
Gingivitis, 466
Ginkgo biloba, 212–18
 dosage, 215
 recommendations for use,
  215–18
 side effects, 215

Ginseng, 219–27
  American, 219, 222–24
  Chinese, 219–21, 223
  dosage, 223
  recommendations for use, 224–27
  Siberian, 219, 221–24
  side effects, 223–24
GLA. *See* Gamma linolenic acid
Glandulars, 227–31
Glaucoma
  ALA for, 18
  bilberry for, 58–59
  magnesium for, 314
  vitamin C for, 466
Glucomannan, 231–32
Glucosamine, 233–36
Glucosinolates, 356
Goldenseal, 236–39
Gout, 124, 338
Green tea, 240–44
Grief, 267–68
Growing pains, 80
Guarana, 166
Guggul, 244–46
Gum infections, 446
Gymnema sylvestre, 246–48

HA. *See* Hyaluronic acid
Hair health
  MSM for, 330
  nettle for, 338
  silicon for, 423
Hair loss, 148–49, 410
Hangover, 270, 341–42
Hawthorn, 250–53
Hay fever, 338–39
HCA. *See* Hydroxycitric acid
Headaches. *See also specific types of headache*
  acupressure for, 10
  butterbur for, 73
  food-sensitivity therapy for, 197
  gelsemium for, 204
  gentian root for, 208
  hydrotherapy for, 263
  ignatia for, 268
  kava for, 287
  lycopodium for, 306
  MSM for, 330
  peppermint for, 350
  pulsatilla for, 386
  sitz bath for, 425
  sulphur for, 441

Health protection, 102–3, 321
Hearing loss, 314
Heart attack recovery, 252, 295
Heartburn
  calcium for, 80
  food-sensitivity therapy for, 198
  MSM for, 330
Heart disease. *See* Cardiovascular disease
Heart failure, 226
Heart palpitations, 348, 490
Hemorrhage, 270, 290
Hemorrhagic disease of newborn, 482
Hemorrhoids
  bilberry for, 59
  butcher's broom for, 72, 73
  food-sensitivity therapy for, 198
  horse chestnut for, 254
  sitz bath for, 425
Hepatitis
  dandelion for, 124
  lycopodium for, 306
  milk thistle for, 325
  vitamin C for, 467
Hepatitis B, 117
Hepatitis C, 417
Herpes
  apis for, 30
  lomatium for, 304
  lysine for, 308
  propolis for, 381–82
  rhus toxicodendron for, 400
  sepia for, 421
High blood pressure
  Agaricus blazei for, 12
  arginine for, 32
  calcium for, 80
  chlorella for, 103
  CoQ10 for, 113
  dandelion for, 124
  fish oil for, 185
  garlic for, 202
  ginkgo biloba for, 216
  glucomannan for, 232
  hawthorn for, 252
  magnesium for, 314
  melatonin for, 319
  onion for, 344–45
  passionflower for, 348
  pine bark extract for, 361
  pomegranate for, 364
  potassium for, 366
  Resperate for, 395–96

stevia for, 433
vitamin D for, 473
water for, 490
HIV, 130, 295
Homeopathy. *See also specific homeopathic remedies*
herbs vs., 4
popularity of, 34
resistance to, 35
Homocysteine, 336
Hormone balancing
dandelion for, 124
D-glucarate, 126–27
licorice root for, 301
milk thistle for, 325
pulsatilla for, 383–84
sepia for, 418–19
weight loss and, 163–64
Hormone replacement therapy, 63
Horse chestnut, 253–55
Hot flashes, 155, 486. *See also* Menopause
Huang Qi, 42
HupA. *See* Huperzine A
Huperzine, 255–56
Huperzine A (HupA), 255–56
Hyaluronic acid (HA), 256–58
Hydrotherapy, 258–63, 424
cold, 259, 261
dosage, 261
hot, 259, 261
recommendations for use, 262–63
side effects, 261
Hydroxycitric acid (HCA), 165
Hypericin, 356
Hypericum, 263–64
Hyperparathyroidism
bone loss related to, 473
ipriflavone for, 273
vitamin D for, 473
Hypertension, 291, 458
Hyperthyroid, 291
Hypoglycemia
chromium for, 105–6
fiber for, 179
food-sensitivity therapy for, 198
Hypothyroidism, 398, 421

IBD. *See* Inflammatory bowel disease
IBS. *See* Irritable bowel syndrome
Ignatia, 265–68
Immune system/immunity
astragalus and, 41–43
bee pollen for, 56

coriolus versicolor for, 118
echinacea and, 134
exercise for, 155–56
food-sensitivity therapy for, 198
ginseng for, 226
licorice root and, 299
onion for, 345
probiotics for, 373
selenium for, 417
spirulina for, 431
Impotence
DHEA for, 130
ginkgo biloba for, 216–17
lycopodium for, 306
Indigestion
acupressure for, 10
artichoke for, 38
burdock for, 71
dandelion for, 123–24
gentian root for, 208
milk thistle for, 325
Indoles, 356
Infants, 296
Infections. *See also specific infections*
burdock for, 71
chemotherapy-induced, 167
colloidal silver for, 116
ear, 197, 290
echinacea for, 132–33
eye, 239
FWGE for, 167
hydrotherapy for, 263
licorice root for, 301
propolis for, 382
turmeric for, 453
vitamin C for, 467
vitamin E for, 479
Infectious diarrhea, 373
Infertility, 486
Infertility, male
ALC for, 2
CoQ10 for, 113–14
L-carnitine for, 296
vitamin C for, 467
zinc for, 499
Inflammation, 301
Inflammatory bowel disease (IBD)
aloe for, 15
DHEA for, 130
fiber for, 179
fish oil for, 185–86
food-sensitivity therapy for, 198

Inflammatory bowel disease (cont.)
  licorice root for, 301
  prebiotics for, 369–70
Injection pain, 30
Injuries
  boswellia for, 66
  bromelain for, 69
  enzymes for, 147
  hypericum for, 264
Insomnia
  ashwagandha for, 40
  chamomile for, 98
  kava for, 287
  melatonin for, 319
  nux vomica for, 342
  passionflower for, 348
  sitz bath for, 425
  sulphur for, 441
  tryptophan and 5-HTP for, 450
  valerian for, 458
Insulin resistance
  fish oil for, 186
  glucomannan for, 232
  gymnema sylvestre for, 248
Ipecac. *See* Ipecacuanha
Ipecacuanha (ipecac), 268–70
Ipriflavone, 270–75
  dosage, 272
  recommendations for use, 273–75
  side effects, 272–73
Iron, 275–80
  deficiency, 78, 275–78
  dosage, 278
  heme, 275
  nonheme, 275
  pregnancy and deficiency in,
    277, 279
  recommendations for use, 279–80
Irritability, 490
Irritable bowel syndrome (IBS)
  chamomile for, 98
  fiber for, 179
  food-sensitivity therapy for, 198
  gentian root for, 208
  peppermint for, 350
  prebiotics for, 370
  probiotics for, 373
Isoflavones, 356, 426
Isothiocyanates, 356

Jet lag, 319
Juicing, 281–83

Kali muriaticum, 414
Kali phosphoricum, 414
Kali sulphuricum, 414
Kava, 284–87
Kidney disease
  apis for, 30
  contrast dye-induced, 336
  L-carnitine for, 295
  NAC for chronic, 335
  soy for, 428
Kidney failure
  Cordyceps sinensis for, 117
  ipriflavone for, 273
Kidney pain, 491
Kidney protection, 186
Kidney stones
  magnesium for, 314
  uva ursi for, 455
Kidney toxicity, 117
Krestin, 118

Lachesis, 288–91
Lactose intolerance, 373
L-carnitine, 292–96
  deficiency, 292–93
  dosage, 293
  recommendations for use, 294–96
  side effects, 293
Ledum, 296–98
Libido
  Cordyceps sinensis for, 118
  DHEA for, 127
  ginseng for, 226–27
  maca for, 310
  sepia for, 421
Lice, 446
Licorice root, 298–302
Lignans, 356
"Like cures like," 4
Limonoids, 356
Liver
  D-glucarate for, 126
  glandulars and, 229
  milk thistle for, 325–26
  reishi for, 394
Liver disease
  black cohosh and, 61–62
  dandelion for, 122
  L-carnitine for, 296
  SAMe for, 407
  turmeric for, 453
Lo han, 302

Lomatium, 303–4
Longevity, 397. *See also* Aging
Low back pain. *See also* Back pain
  sitz bath for, 425
  sulphur for, 441
Lung conditions, 117
Lupus
  DHEA for, 130
  fish oil for, 186
Lycopene, 356
Lycopodium, 305–6
Lyme disease, 93
Lysine, 306–8

Maca, 309–11
Macular degeneration
  bilberry for, 59
  carotenoids for, 90
  vitamin E for, 479
  zinc for, 499
Magnesia phosphorica, 414
Magnesium, 311–15
  calcium and, 79
Maitake, 315–16
Malaria, 493
Malnourishment, 432
Manic depression, 291.
     See also Depression
Melanoma, 167–68
Melatonin, 316–20
Memory impairment
  ALC for, 1, 2
  ashwagandha for, 40–41
  B-complex vitamins for, 47
  essential oils for, 149
  flaxseed for, 192
  ginkgo biloba for, 217
  ginseng for, 226
  rhodiola for, 398–99
Meningitis, 30
Menopause
  black cohosh for, 60, 63–64
  burdock for, 71
  calcium deficiency and, 77
  dandelion for, 124
  DHEA for, 130
  flaxseed for, 192
  ginseng for, 226
  lachesis for, 291
  maca for, 310–11
  passionflower for, 348
  progesterone for, 378

  pulsatilla for, 386
  sepia for, 421
  soy for, 428
  St. John's wort for, 437
  sulphur for, 441
  vitamin E for, 479
Menstrual bleeding, 108, 276
Menstrual cramps
  black cohosh for, 64
  chamomile for, 99–100
  cinnamon for, 108
  pulsatilla for, 386
  valerian for, 458
Menstrual disorders, 421, 486
Menstrual pain, 186, 361
Mental imagery, 320–22
  health maintenance and, 321
  positive effects of, 321
  practicing, 321–22
  techniques, 321–22
Methylsulfonylmethane (MSM), 326–30
Migraine headache
  butterbur for, 74–75
  CoQ10 for, 114
  feverfew for, 172
  ipecac for, 270
  lachesis for, 291
  magnesium for, 314
  progesterone for, 378
  sepia for, 421
Milk thistle, 323–26
Mitral valve prolapse
  CoQ10 for, 114
  magnesium for, 314–15
Mononucleosis, 204
Morning sickness
  ginger root for, 211
  ipecac for, 269, 270
  sepia for, 421
Mosquito bites, 297–98
Motion sickness, 211–12
Mouth infections, 446
Mouth sores, 301
MS. *See* Multiple sclerosis
MSM. *See* Methylsulfonylmethane
Multiple sclerosis (MS)
  fish oil for, 186
  flaxseed for, 192–93
  gelsemium for, 205
  vitamin D for, 473
  vitamin E for, 480
Multivitamins, 331–33

Muscle cramps/spasms
  calcium for, 80
  ignatia for, 268
  kava for, 287
  potassium for, 366
  sitz bath for, 425
  valerian for, 458
Muscle injuries, 330
Muscle pain, 10, 350
Muscle recuperation, 33–34
Muscle strength, 480
Muscle tension, 5, 287
Muscular dystrophy, 114

NAC. *See* N-acetylcysteine
N-acetylcysteine (NAC), 334–35
Nail health, 330
Natrum muriaticum, 414–15
Natrum phosphoricum, 415
Natrum sulphuricum, 415
Nausea
  acupressure for, 10
  ginger root for, 212
  sepia for, 421
Neck pain, 10
Nettle, 337–39
Neuropathy
  ALA for, 16, 17, 18
  cayenne for, 95
  evening primrose oil for, 151
Niacin, 49–50
Night vision, 59, 462
Nipples, cracked, 82
Nursing. *See* Pregnant/nursing women
Nutritional deficiencies, 164
Nux vomica, 340–42

Omega-3 fatty acids
  deficiency, 187
  fish oil and, 180
  flaxseed as, 187
  omega-6 fatty acids and, 187
Omega-6 fatty acids, 149–50
  evening primrose oil and, 150–51
  fish oil and, 181
  omega-3 fatty acids and, 187
Onion, 343–45
Oral cancers, 167
Orchitis, 386
Oregano, 345–46
Organosulfur compounds, 356

Organ prolapse, 42
Osteoarthritis
  cat's claw for, 93
  glucosamine and, 233–34
  glucosamine for, 235–36
  guggul for, 246
  SAMe for, 403–4, 407–8
Osteoporosis
  calcium for, 77, 80–81
  carotenoids for, 90
  DHEA for, 131
  evening primrose oil for, 152
  exercise for, 156
  ipriflavone for, 270–71, 273–74
  lysine for, 308
  maca for, 310
  magnesium for, 315
  progesterone for, 378–79
  silicon for, 423
  soy for, 428
  vitamin C for, 467
  vitamin D for, 473
  vitamin K for, 482
Otosclerosis, 274
Ovarian cyst
  lachesis for, 291
  progesterone for, 379
  sepia for, 421
  vitex for, 486
Ovarian pain, 30, 306
Ovaries, 229–30

Paget's disease, 274–75
Pain. *See also specific types of pain*
  feverfew for, 172
  kava for, 287
  MSM and control of, 327
  vitamin D for chronic, 472
Pancreas, 230
Panic attacks
  Aconitum napellus for, 3
  carbo vegetabilis for, 87
  kava for, 287
Pantothenic acid, 50–51
Parasites
  goldenseal for, 239
  oregano for, 346
  wormwood for, 493
Parkinson's disease, 114, 480
Passionflower, 347–48
Peppermint, 348–50

Perimenopause, 310–11, 361. *See also* Menopause

Periodontal disease, 114–15

Peripheral arterial disease, 32

Peripheral neuropathy, 18

Peripheral vascular disease, 480

Peyronie's disease, 2

Pharmaceutical medications, 24. *See also* Drug interactions, deficiencies from; *specific medications*

Pharyngotonsillitis, 22

Phenolic acids, 356–57

Phosphatidylserine (PS), 351–53

Physical performance, 115

Phytonutrients, 354–57

Pineal gland, 317

Pine bark extract, 357–62

Pituitary gland, 230

PMDD. *See* Premenstrual dysphoric disorder

PMS. *See* Premenstrual syndrome

Pneumonia, 87, 262

Pollution, 23–24

Polycystic ovarian syndrome, 106, 412

Pomegranate, 362–64

Post-operative surgery, 34

Postpartum recovery, 425

Potassium, 364–66

Prayer, 367–68

Prebiotics, 368–70

Prednisone tapering, 131

Pregnant/nursing women
   calcium for, 81
   Caralluma fimbriata for, 85
   chlorella for, 102
   iron deficiency and, 277
   iron for, 279
   magnesium for, 315
   multivitamins for, 331
   nettle for, 337, 339
   pine bark extract for, 361
   progesterone for complications in, 379
   selenium for, 418
   sepia for, 421
   vitamin C for, 467
   vitex for, 486

Premature infants, 296

Premenstrual dysphoric disorder (PMDD), 450

Premenstrual syndrome (PMS)
   black cohosh for, 64
   burdock for, 71
   calcium for, 81
   dandelion for, 124

   evening primrose oil for, 152
   exercise for, 156
   ginkgo biloba for, 217
   ignatia for, 268
   lachesis for, 291
   magnesium for, 315
   passionflower for, 348
   progesterone for, 379
   sepia for, 421
   St. John's wort for, 437
   vitamin E for, 480
   vitex for, 486–87

Prenatal infant growth, 418

Priessnitz, Vincent, 259–60

Probiotics, 368–74
   dosage, 372
   recommendations for use, 372–74
   side effects, 372

Progesterone, 374–79

Propolis, 379–83

Prostate, 408–9
   cranberry for, 120, 121
   infections, 120, 121

Prostate cancer
   carotenoids for, 89
   pomegranate for, 364
   saw palmetto for, 412

Prostate enlargement
   nettle for, 339
   saw palmetto and, 408–9
   sepia for, 421
   sitz bath for, 425
   zinc for, 499

Prostatitis
   quercetin for, 390
   saw palmetto for, 412
   sitz bath for, 425

Protein, 18, 161. *See also* Amino acids

PS. *See* Phosphatidylserine

Psoriasis
   aloe for, 15
   cayenne for, 96
   fish oil for, 186
   food-sensitivity therapy for, 198
   licorice root for, 300
   pulsatilla for, 387
   sepia for, 421

Psyllium husks, 174

Pulsatilla, 384–87

Pyridoxine, 51

Pyruvate, 165–66

Qi, 6
Quercetin, 388–90

Radiation
    coriolus versicolor as complementary treatment
        with, 119
    ginkgo biloba for effects of, 217
    melatonin for, 319
    spirulina for poisoning with, 432
Raynaud's syndrome, 217, 421–22
Rectum, itchy, 425
Rectum prolapse, 425
Red yeast rice, 391–93
Reishi, 393–94
Relaxation, 5
Resperate, 394–96
Respiratory mucus, 69. See also Congestion
Respiratory tract infections. See also specific infections
    astragalus for, 42, 44
    goldenseal for, 239
    lomatium for, 304
    lycopodium for, 306
    NAC for, 336
    oregano for, 346
    probiotics for, 373
    vitamin A for, 462
    vitamin D for upper, 474
Restless leg syndrome, 280, 450
Resveratrol, 396–97
Retinopathy, 59, 106
Rheumatoid arthritis. See also Arthritis
    apis for, 29
    boswellia for, 66
    cat's claw for, 93
    FWGE for, 168
    selenium for, 418
Rhodiola, 397–99
Rhus toxicodendron, 399–400
Riboflavin, 49
Ribose, 400–402

SAD. See Seasonal affective disorder
SAMe, 404–8
Saw palmetto, 408–12
Scars, 478
Schizophrenia
    DHEA for, 131
    fish oil for, 186
    food-sensitivity therapy for, 198
Schlussler cell salts, 412–15
Seasonal affective disorder (SAD), 437, 450
Selenium, 415–18

Sepia, 418–22, 419
Shellfish allergies, 235. See also Allergies
Shingles
    apis for, 30
    cayenne for, 96
    lachesis for, 291
    rhus toxicodendron for, 400
Shock, 3
SIDS. See Sudden infant death syndrome
Silica, 415
Silicon, 422–23
Silymarin, 357
Sinusitis
    acupressure for, 10
    food-sensitivity therapy for, 198
    pulsatilla for, 387
    sepia for, 422
Sitz bath, 424–25
Skin aging. See also Aging
    ALA for, 18
    hyaluronic acid for, 258
    vitamin C for, 468
Skin conditions. See also specific skin conditions
    aloe for, 13
    burdock for, 71
    calendula for, 81, 83
    chamomile for, 100
    DHEA for, 131
    echinacea for, 138
    hydrotherapy for, 263
    milk thistle for, 326
    sulphur for, 441–42
    tea tree oil for, 447
Skin health
    CoQ10 for, 115
    pine bark extract for, 361–62
    selenium for, 418
Skin rashes
    calendula for, 83
    enzymes for, 147
    food-sensitivity therapy for, 198
    water for, 491
Smell (sense of), 18
Smoking
    antioxidants and, 27
    melatonin for cessation of, 320
    tryptophan and 5-HTP for cessation, 450
Snakebites, 132
Sore throat
    apis for, 30
    ferrum phosphoricum for, 170
    sulphur for, 442

Soy, 425–28
Spirituality, 164–65
Spirulina, 429–32
Spleen, 230
Sports injuries, 330
Sports nutrition, 362
Sprains, 298
St. John's Wort, 433–37
Stevia, 432–33
Stimulants, natural, 166
Strains, 400. *See also* Eyestrain
Stress
    ashwagandha for, 41
    B-complex vitamins for, 47
    chamomile for, 100
    DHEA for, 131
    exercise for, 156
    ginseng for, 227
    passionflower for, 348
    phosphatidylserine for, 353
    Resperate for, 395
    valerian for, 458
    vitamin C for, 467
Stroke
    alpha GPC for, 16
    ginkgo biloba for, 218
    potassium for, 366
    prevention, 366
Sudden infant death syndrome (SIDS), 418
Sugar intake, 159–60
Sulforaphane, 357, 437–39
Sulphur, 439–42
Sunburn, 90, 468. *See also* Burns
Sunlight, 469–70
Surgery recovery, 69, 96
Symphytum, 442–43
Syndrome X, 248–49
Systemic toxicity, 202. *See also* Toxicity

Tardive dyskinesia, 320
Tea tree oil, 444–47
Teething, 100
Temporomandibular joint disorder (TJD), 266–68
Testicles, 230
Testosterone deficiency, 2
Theophyllin, 312
Thiamin, 49
Thrombocytopenia, 320
Thrombophlebitis, 69
Thymus gland, 230–31
Thyroid gland, 231, 279
Tinnitus, 218

TJD. *See* Temporomandibular joint disorder
Tocotrienols, 447–48
Tonsillitis, 170
Tooth decay, 244. *See also* Cavities
Tooth loss in elderly, 81, 473–74. *See also* Dental
    conditions
Toxemia in pregnancy, 30. *See also* Pregnant/nursing
    women
Toxicity
    garlic for, 202
    ginseng for, 227
    iron, 279
    weight loss and, 164
Toxic metals, 103
Trauma, 33
Triglycerides
    chromium for, 105
    fish oil for, 185
    glucomannan for, 232
    guggul for, 246
● Tryptophan and 5-HTP, 448–50
● Turmeric, 450–53

Ulcer(s)
    aloe for, 15
    Arsenicum album for, 37
    artichoke for, 37
    calendula for, 83
    chamomile for, 100–101
    diabetic, 360
    licorice root for, 301–2
    nux vomica for, 342
    pine bark extract for, 360
Ulcerative colitis
    boswellia for, 66
    chlorella for, 103
    fish oil for, 185
    probiotics for, 374
    wheatgrass, 492
Urinary incontinence, 422
Urinary tract infections
    apis for, 30
    burdock for, 71
    cantharis for, 85
    cranberry for, 120, 121
    goldenseal for, 239
    lomatium for, 304
    sitz bath for, 425
    uva ursi for, 455
Urticaria, 400
Uterine fibroids, 379, 487
Uterine pain, 425

Uterine prolapse, 422, 425
Uva ursi, 454–55

Vaginal infections, 374, 425
Vaginitis
  echinacea for, 138
  food-sensitivity therapy for, 198
  progesterone for, 379
  sepia for, 422
  tea tree oil for, 447
Valerian, 456–58
Vanadium, 458–59
Varicose veins, 73, 83
  bilberry for, 59
  bromelain for, 69
  horse chestnut for, 253–55
  lachesis for, 291
  pulsatilla for, 387
  sepia for, 422
Vegetarianism, 103, 173
Vertigo, 205, 218
Viral infections
  aloe for, 15
  enzymes for, 147
  St. John's wort for, 437
Vision, 218
Vitamin A, 460–62
Vitamin C, 462–68
Vitamin D, 468–74
Vitamin E, 474–80
Vitamin K, 480–82
Vitex, 483–87
Vomiting, 212

Warfarin, 312
Warts, 203, 447
Water, 488–91
  dehydrators, 489
  dosage, 490
  recommendations for use, 490–91
  side effects, 490
Weight gain, 491
Weight loss
  calcium for, 81
  Caralluma fimbriata for, 86
  chromium for, 106
  consistency and, 162–63
  dandelion for, 124

  detoxification and, 164
  DHEA for, 131
  emotional factors in, 164–65
  exercise and, 163
  fat reduction and, 158
  food sensitivities and, 162
  glucomannan for, 232
  green tea for, 244
  hormone balancing and, 163–64
  L-carnitine for, 296
  lo han for, 302
  nutritional deficiencies and, 164
  plant food and, 162
  spiritual factors in, 164–65
  stevia for, 433
  toxicity and, 164
  tryptophan and 5-HTP for, 450
  vitamin D for upper, 474
  water intake and, 162
  xylitol for, 495
Weight problems
  calorie counting and, 161
  carbohydrate, protein, fat ratio and, 161
  causes of, 158–65
  diet and, 159–63
  fat intake and, 160–61
  genetics and, 159
  portions and, 161
  skipping meals and, 161
  sugar intake and, 159–60
Wheatgrass, 491–92
Whole-food supplements, 281
Wilson's disease, 499
Wormwood, 492–93
Wound healing
  aloe for, 14
  propolis for, 382–83
  vitamin E for, 478
Wounds
  ledum for, 298
  puncture, 298
  St. John's wort for, 436
  vitamin C for, 468
  zinc for, 498

Xylitol, 494–95

Zinc, 496–99